Donald School Textbook of

HUMAN REPRODUCTION AND GYNECOLOGICAL ENDOCRINOLOGY

Donald School Textbook of

HUMAN REPRODUCTION AND GYNECOLOGICAL ENDOCRINOLOGY

Editor

Sonal Panchal MD

Consultant, Dr Nagori's Institute for Infertility and IVF
Ahmedabad, Gujarat, India
Professor, Dubrovnik International University
Croatia
National Academic Director
Ian Donald School, India

Co-Editor

Sanja Kupesic-Plavsic MD PhD

Professor of Obstetrics and Gynecology
Associate Academic Dean for Faculty Development
Director of Center for Advanced Teaching and
Assessment in Clinical Simulation (ATACS)
Paul L Foster School of Medicine
Texas Tech University Health Sciences Center El Paso
El Paso, Texas, USA

Foreword

Asim Kurjak MD PhD

JAYPEE The Health Sciences Publisher

New Delhi | London | Panama

Jaypee Brothers Medical Publishers (P) Ltd

Headquarters
Jaypee Brothers Medical Publishers (P) Ltd.
4838/24, Ansari Road, Daryaganj
New Delhi 110 002, India
Phone: +91-11-43574357
Fax: +91-11-43574314
E-mail: jaypee@jaypeebrothers.com

Overseas Offices
JP Medical Ltd.
83, Victoria Street, London
SW1H 0HW (UK)
Phone: +44-20 3170 8910
Fax: +44(0)20 3008 6180
E-mail: info@jpmedpub.com

Jaypee-Highlights Medical Publishers Inc
City of Knowledge, Bld. 235, 2nd Floor, Clayton
Panama City, Panama
Phone: +1 507-301-0496
Fax: +1 507-301-0499
E-mail: cservice@jphmedical.com

Jaypee Brothers Medical Publishers (P) Ltd.
17/1-B, Babar Road, Block-B, Shyamoli
Mohammadpur, Dhaka-1207
Bangladesh
Mobile: +08801912003485
E-mail: jaypeedhaka@gmail.com

Jaypee Brothers Medical Publishers (P) Ltd.
Bhotahity, Kathmandu, Nepal
Phone: +977-9741283608
E-mail: kathmandu@jaypeebrothers.com

Website: www.jaypeebrothers.com
Website: www.jaypeedigital.com

Inquiries for bulk sales may be solicited at: jaypee@jaypeebrothers.com

Donald School Textbook of Human Reproduction and Gynecological Endocrinology

First Edition: **2019**

ISBN: 978-93-5270-200-8

Printed at: Ajanta Offset & Packagings Ltd., Faridabad, Haryana.

Dedicated to

Prof Asim Kurjak and Prof Frank Chervenak for their dedication and passion to spread knowledge through Ian Donald Inter-University School of Medical Ultrasound.

Contributors

Mala Arora MBBS FRCOG (UK)
Chairperson
Indian College of Obstetrician and Gynecologist 2017
Director
Noble IVF Center
Faridabad, Haryana, India
Consultant Obstetrician and Gynecologist
Fortis La Femme
New Delhi, India

Satish Bharadwaj PhD
Research Officer
Manipal Fertility
Bengaluru, Karnataka, India

Saumya Bulusu MBBS MS DNB
Consultant
KB Bhabha Hospital
Mumbai, Maharashtra, India

Natachandra Chimote PhD
Managing Director and
Consultant Clinical Embryologist
Vaunshdhara Fertility Center
Nagpur, Maharashtra, India

Matan Elami-Suzin MD
Department of Obstetrics and Gynecology
Hebrew University
Hadassah Medical Center
Jerusalem, Israel

Tamara Illescas MD PhD
Consultant
Delta Ultrasound Diagnostic
Center in Obstetrics and Gynecology
Madrid, Spain

Kanna M Jayaprakasan
MD DNB MRCOG PhD
Subspecialist and Hon. Associate Professor in Reproductive Medicine and Surgery
Consultant Gynecologist/Fertility Lead
Royal Derby Hospital, Derby
University of Nottingham
Nottingham, UK

Sunil K Jindal MS DNB MNAMS
Scientific Director and Andrologist
Jindal Hospital and
Dr Madhu Jindal Memorial
Test Tube Baby Center
Meerut, Uttar Pradesh, India

Aditya S Khurd DNB FRM FAMS
Fellowship in Reproductive Medicine (Bengaluru)
Fellowship in Minimal Access Surgery (Kochi)
Consultant Endoscopic Surgeon
Fertility and IVF Specialist
Khurd Endoscopy, Infertility and IVF Center
Pune, Maharashtra, India

Radhika KT MBBS DGO
Gynecologist and Laparoscopic Surgeon
Thalassery Mission Hospital
Kannur, Kerala, India

Sanja Kupesic-Plavsic MD PhD
Professor of Obstetrics and Gynecology
Associate Academic Dean for Faculty Development
Director of Center for Advanced Teaching Assessment in Clinical Simulation (ATACS)
Paul L Foster School of Medicine
Texas Tech University Health Sciences Center El Paso
El Paso, Texas, USA

Asim Kurjak MD PhD
Professor of Obstetrics and Gynecology
Medical School
Universities of Zagreb and Sarajevo
President of International Academy of Perinatal Medicine
Zagreb, Croatia

Neha Lad
Director
Dr Lad's Navjeevan Hospital Pvt. Ltd
Nashik, Maharashtra, India

Nitin Lad
Director
Dr Lad's Navjeevan Hospital Pvt. Ltd
Nashik, Maharashtra, India

Jaideep Malhotra MD FRCOG FRCPI
Managing Director
ART Rainbow IVF
Agra, Uttar Pradesh, India

Keshav Malhotra MBBS MCE
Director
Rainbow IVF
Agra, Uttar Pradesh, India

Narendra Malhotra MD FRCOG
Managing Director
Global Rainbow Healthcare
Agra, Uttar Pradesh, India

Neharika Malhotra MD
Senior Consultant
Rainbow IVF
Agra, Uttar Pradesh, India

Sumina Mannur MBBS MS DNB
Deccan Clinics
Hyderabad, Telangana, India

Jayant G Mehta PhD DipRCPath
Barking, Havering and Redbridge
University Hospital NHS Trust
Queen's Hospital, Romford, Essex, UK

Chaitanya Nagori MD DGO
Director
Dr Nagori's Institute for Infertility and IVF
Ahmedabad, Gujarat, India

Sonal Panchal MD
Consultant
Dr Nagori's Institute for Infertility and IVF
Ahmedabad, Gujarat, India
Professor, Dubrovnik International University
Croatia
National Academic Director
Ian Donald School, India

George Paul MBBS MS
Paul's Hospital
Kochi, Kerala, India

PG Paul MBBS DGO
Paul's Hospital
Kochi, Kerala, India

Mandava V Rao
PhD FRE (Madras) FGSA (Gujarat)
Research Director
Supratech-Micropath Labs
Paldi, Ahmedabad, Gujarat
Former Head
Department of Zoology, HG and BMTC
Former Director
School of Sciences, Gujarat University
Ahmedabad, Gujarat, India

Milan Reljič MD PhD
Associate Professor
Department of Reproductive Medicine and Gynecologic Endocrinology
Clinic for Gynecology and Perinatology
University Medical Center Maribor
Maribor, Slovenia

Joseph G Schenker
MD FACOG FRCOG FIAPM
Professor of Obstetrics and Gynecology
Hebrew University of Jerusalem
Chairman
Department of Obstetrics and Gynecology (Emeritus)
Hadassah-University Hospital
Jerusalem, Israel

Mihir Shah MBBS
Registrar
Hitesh Hospital, Navrangpura
Ahmedabad, Gujarat, India

Parth S Shah MD (Int Med)
Chief, Molecular Genetics Division
Supratech-Genopath Laboratory
Supratech Micropath Labs
Ahmedabad, Gujarat, India

Sandip C Shah MD (Pathol and Bact)
Laboratory Director
Supratech-Micropath Research and Diagnostic
Research Labs Pvt. Ltd.
Ahmedabad, Gujarat, India

Tejanshu P Shah MS MCh (Urology)
Urologist, Andrologist and Infertility Microsurgeon at Hitesh Hospital
Hon Urologist to SAL Hospital
Apollo Hospital and Sterling Hospital
Hitesh Hospital
65B Swastic Society, Navrangpura
Ahmedabad, Gujarat, India

Hemant Shintre MBBS DGO DNB
Consultant
Shintre Hospital
Sangli, Maharashtra, India

Surekha Tayade
MBBS MD DNB (Obstetrics and Gynecology)
MNAMS FICOG
Associate Professor
Mahatma Gandhi Institute of Medical Sciences, Sevagram
Wardha, Maharashtra, India

Francis A Tharakan MD MRCOG
Consultant in Reproductive Medicine and Gynecology
CARE Fertility
Nottingham, UK

SS Vasan
DNB (Uro) Fellowship in Andrology and Incontinence (Singapore)
Uroandrologist
Chairman
Manipal Fertility
Bengaluru, Karnataka, India

Foreword

Human reproduction is one of the fastest growing fields of clinical medicine. There are thousands of papers and chapters describing impressive development of this relatively new field. We in the largest education system in the world—Ian Donald School of Ultrasound—have been following this explosive development virtually from its conception. As a final result, we did introduce a specialist postgraduate course for master degree in human reproduction. Soon it became very popular and much wished type of specialized education. We developed several training centers with top world speakers. The most active in the specialized education is center in Ahmedabad with Professor Sonal Panchal as Head. Sonal proved to be not only very good research worker, but also extremely successful teacher. Her own work with students truly proved known sentence that teaching is transmission of enthusiasm. We have recently asked Sonal and her team to edit Textbook on Human Reproduction, which will be used as an official textbook for Ian Donald specialist course Human Reproduction, Reproductive Endocrinology and Infertility.

After more than one year of hard work, she collected an impressive list of co-authors; among them, one of the pioneers in this field professor Sanja Kupesic-Plavsic, leading person in Ian Donald School settlements. Together with other distinguished authors, Sonal and Dr Chaitanya Nagori described precisely and extensively what are the facts and what are the future challenges in this exciting field.

I am sure, the readers of this most useful book will truly enjoy reading it and will definitely find the book both informative and stimulating. I wish the book very good acceptance by the readers and do congratulate the editors and contributors for an excellent piece of work.

Asim Kurjak MD PhD
Founder and Director of Ian Donald School

Preface

It indeed gives me a pleasure to contribute to the extensive Donald school library in the form of this book "*Donald School Textbook of Human Reproduction and Gynecological Endocrinology*". It is designed to cover the vast subject of human reproduction—its physiology, related pathologies, treatment options and the newest advances in the field—in a most concise manner. The book includes majority of the aspects of infertility—female factor of infertility, male factor of infertility, embryology and laboratory aspects of assisted reproductive technology. Having included the very basics of the subject and also the recent advances, it is a book that will be useful and will be appreciated by students as well as practitioners in the field. The contributions from the experts with rich experience in the field and the practical tips given by them will surely be of great help for the busy practitioners.

I sincerely thank the expert contributors for their sincere efforts and valuable contributions that have brought the worth to this book.

Sonal Panchal

Acknowledgments

I am indebted to Prof Asim Kurjak for his confidence and trust in me for this project. It was his persistent support and encouragement that has resulted in the form of this book finally. My sincere thanks to Prof Kupesic for her valuable guidance, help and support for the project.

I am thankful to Shri Jitendar P Vij (Group Chairman), Mr Ankit Vij (Group President), Ms Chetna Malhotra Vohra (Associate Director—Content Strategy), and Ms Nikita Chauhan (Development Editor) of Jaypee Brothers Medical Publishers, New Delhi, India, for giving a go-ahead at the very beginning and helping me in every way possible to bring out this book.

Contents

CHAPTER

1

Ovulation

Chaitanya Nagori, Sonal Panchal

INTRODUCTION

Ovulation is a very complex phenomenon and its clear understanding is essential to understand the abnormalities of the same. Ovulation will be discussed here under the following heads:

- Physiology of ovulation
- Endocrinal control of ovulation
- Clinicopathology of Ovulation
- Tests to detect ovulation
- Causes of anovulation

PHYSIOLOGY OF OVULATION

Detailed understanding of physiology of ovulation is very essential to manage ovulation dysfunction, which is one of the important causes of fertility problems. Ovulation occurs from the ovaries. Each oocyte is surrounded by a number of follicle cells to create a **follicle**. When the menstrual cycle begins, one, or maybe even a few, primary oocytes begin to grow larger and the follicle cells increase in number and cause the follicle to grow larger too. Usually, some of the developing oocytes will degenerate and only leave one follicle that will mature, but every once in a while two, or even more, follicles will mature. As a follicle reaches maturity, the primary oocyte completes its first meiotic division and becomes a secondary oocyte. Very soon after that, the follicle ruptures, and the secondary oocyte is released into the Fallopian or uterine tube, even though the second meiotic division has not occurred yet. The release of a secondary oocyte from the ovaries is called **ovulation**.[1]

During intrauterine life of a woman, there are 7 million oogonia that reduce to only 1 million at the time of birth.[2]

This number is further reduced to only 300–400 thousands at the menarche. At the time of menopause, only 1,500 ova are available. During reproductive age, only 400 ova reach up to ovulation, i.e. only 0.1% of the total available ova at menarche reach up to ovulation and 99.9% become atretic.[3]

Ovulation occurs once in a month in majority of the normal women. It is the result of the integrated and synchronized succession of hormonal action and morphological changes in hypothalamus, pituitary, and ovary. Autocrine and paracrine factors also take part in ovulation induction. So neuroendocrine complex system regulates ovulation and menstrual cycle.

Figure 1.1 explains the influence of different hormones on ovaries and endometrium. Grossly, the GnRHs released from the hypothalamus control the gonadotropin [luteinizing hormone (LH) or follicle-stimulating hormone (FSH)] secretion from the pituitary and these gonadotropins finally control the estrogen (E2) and progesterone secretion from the ovaries. These steroids are responsible for the cyclical changes in ovaries and uterus. The entire control system is thus called hypothalamopituitary-ovarian axis (HPO). This HPO axis should be intact and synchronized for normal ovulation (Fig. 1.2).

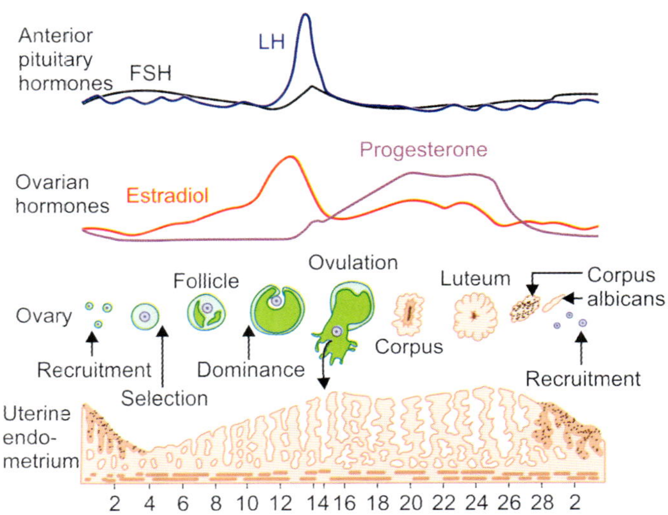

Fig. 1.1: Hormonal and morphological variations during the menstrual cycle—diagrammatic representation.[4]
(FSH, follicle-stimulating hormone; LH, luteinizing hormone).

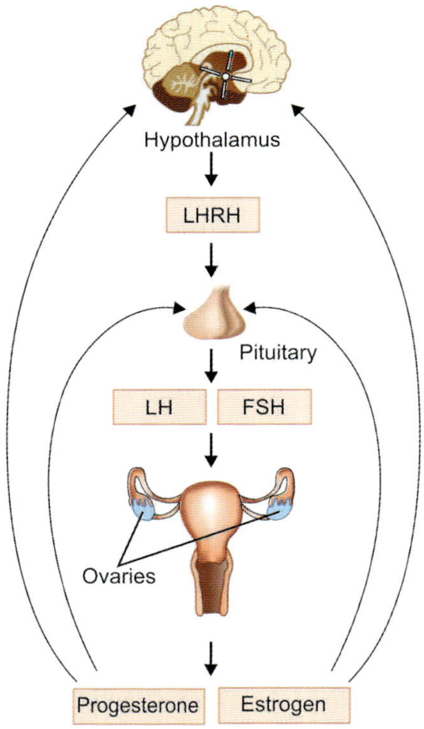

Fig. 1.2: Diagrammatic representation of hypothalamopituitary-ovarian axis.[5]
(FSH, follicle-stimulating hormone; GnRH, gonadotropin-releasing hormone; LH, luteinizing hormone).

ROLE OF INDIVIDUAL HORMONE AND ITS CLINICAL APPLICATION

Gonadotropin-releasing Hormone (GnRH)

A decapeptide is synthesized and secreted from the neuronal endings in anterior and mediobasal part of the hypothalamus. It is released from hypothalamus and acts on the pituitary. Gonadotropin releasing hormone (GnRH) traverses through hypothalamo-hypophyseal portal system. This is a compact blood vessel system and so, it is not detected in circulation. It releases follicle FSH and LH from the pituitary. Its secretion is pulsatile in nature and stimulates pituitary to secrete more LH than FSH. It is always correlated with LH pulse. Each pulse is of 60–90 minutes. It is chiefly influenced by ovarian steroids.

Opiates, catecholamines, and neuropeptides, all have an influence on GnRH secretion. There is enormous release of GnRH before the LH surge and then under the effect of progesterone, the frequency of the GnRH pulse decreases to only one in 8–12 hours.[6] GnRH is suppressed by inhibitory factors till puberty.

Clinical Applications for Ovulation Induction

- It is used for ovulation induction in hypogonadotropic hypogonadism. But unfortunately, it is not yet widely available.
- GnRH agonist (GnRHa) can be used for downregulation in *in vitro* fertilization (IVF).
- GnRHa as short protocol is used for endogenous FSH and LH surge for ovulation induction.
- GnRHa is used for ovulation trigger to elicit endogenous LH surge.
- GnRH antagonist is used for prevention of LH surge in intrauterine insemination (IUI) and IVF cycles.

Follicle-stimulating Hormone

The FSH is secreted from anterior pituitary. FSH secretion is controlled by the feedback system through estradiol and progesterone. When corpus luteum undergoes atresia or regression just before the menstruation, the FSH secretion increases markedly. It acts on the preantral and antral follicles and helps in recruitment and stimulation of the Graafian follicle to make it dominant. It also enhances the conversion of androgens to E2 through the pathway of aromatase enzyme. Secretion of FSH is governed by E2. It frees the oocyte from follicular attachment and converts plasminogen into plasmin. It helps in development of LH receptors for ovulation and for the luteal phase action. It has a definite minimum value, below which it is not sensed by the follicles. This is called FSH threshold. This value is different for every individual. Second peak of FSH is in the midcycle. It has been observed in animals that this second peak of FSH is must for successful ovulation. If this peak is absent, it may cause LUF. But its role in human is not clear. This is so because in humans when surrogate trigger is used in form of LH or human chorionic gonadotropin (hCG), it acts successfully even in absence of FSH. Though the second FSH surge may select the follicles for the next cycle.

Clinical Applications

- It is responsible for LH expression after the follicle size of 10–12 mm. This means FSH rescues the follicle to maturity. So there is no need to increase the dose of FSH for follicular growth after 10–12 mm size. Instead supplementation of LH will grow the follicle.[7]
- FSH secretion decreases during periovulatory period because of progesterone, but bioactivity is highest during this period.

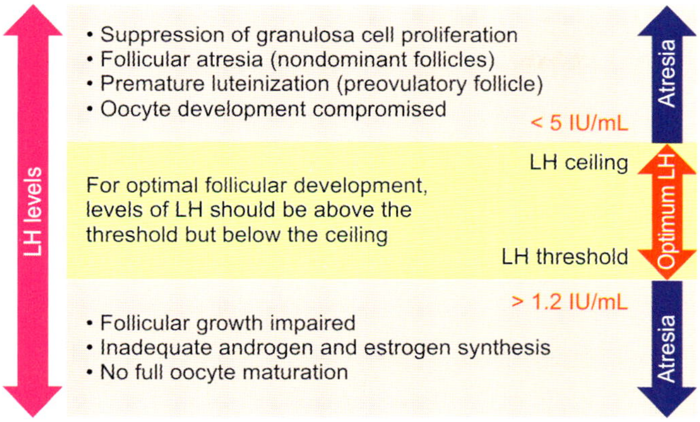

Fig. 1.3: Luteinizing hormone (LH) ceiling and LH threshold—explanation.

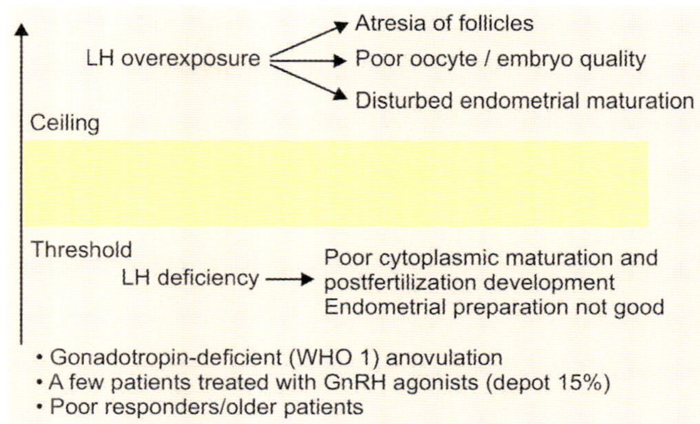

Fig. 1.4: The concept of luteinizing hormone window. (GnRH, gonadotropin-releasing hormone; LH, luteinizing hormone).

- Granulosa cells have androgen receptors. Androgen acts on the immature cells and potentiates action of FSH, e.g. aromatase inhibitor that increases androgen. Dehydroepiandrosterone (DHEA) also potentiates the action of FSH.
- Only 1% of the LH receptors are required for folliculogenesis and so in spite of downregulation with GnRHa in long protocol, the follicle continues to grow.
- FSH can stimulate paracrine signals, which sustains thecal androgen synthesis. So FSH is capable of ovarian androgen synthesis.[7]

Luteinizing Hormone

Luteinizing hormone is another hormone secreted from anterior pituitary. In the first half of the cycle, its level is low and secretion is pulsatile. High levels of LH are detrimental to ova. This can be explained by the LH threshold and LH ceiling concept (Fig. 1.3).[8]

This figure indicates that threshold level, i.e. certain minimum amount is required for growth of follicle. But if the level goes beyond a certain level, it hampers the growth of the follicle. This is known as ceiling effect and that level of LH is called the LH ceiling level. So LH level required for follicle maturation should be between the threshold and the ceiling level. This is known as LH window[9] (Fig. 1.4).

Luteinizing hormone causes luteinization of granulosa cells. LH acts on theca cells to produce androgen. With the rising E2 levels with developing follicle, when the FSH gets a negative feedback, LH gets a positive feedback. LH permits final maturation of follicle forming secondary oocyte and first polar body. It causes disruption of cumulus-oocyte complex and rupture of the follicle. LH surge should start between 14 and 27 hours after estradiol peak for ovum maturation and LH surge lasts for 48–50 hours. The two cell two hormone theory explains the role of LH in ovarian steroidogenesis[10,11] (Fig. 1.5).

Both the gonadotropins, FSH and LH as well as both the cells, i.e. granulosa cells and theca cells are required for maturation of ova. LH stimulates theca cells to produce androgen from cholesterol. Androgen from theca cells go to granulosa cells where under the influence of FSH, androgen is converted into E2 by aromatase activity. So both gonadotropins and both the cells are required for folliculogenesis.

Clinical Applications

- *Luteinizing hormone in clomiphene citrate cycle:* Clomiphene citrate (CC) stimulated FSH and LH from the hypothalamus. This LH may reach the ceiling level especially in polycystic ovary syndrome (PCOS) and is detrimental to ova. The level of LH is therefore checked on day 8–10 of the cycle and if it is more than 10–12 IU/mL, it is less likely that clomiphene can give pregnancy as the follicle quality deteriorates due to high LH.[12]
- *Luteinizing hormone in polycystic ovary:* There is tonically high level of LH that causes abnormal oocyte maturation. There is also premature luteinization that decreases implantation because of progesterone

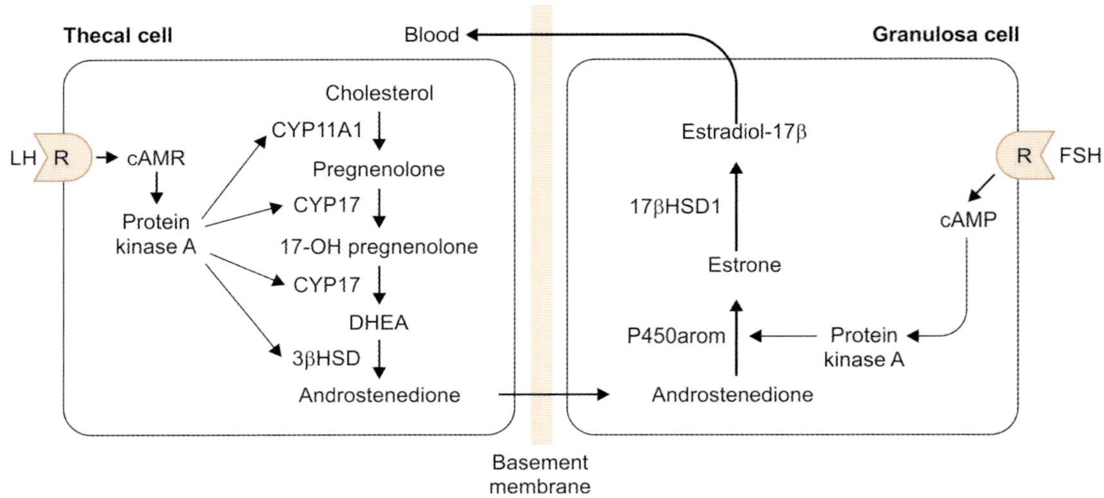

Fig. 1.5: Diagrammatic explanation of two-cell-two-gonadotropin theory.
(cAMP, cyclic adenosine 3',5'-monophosphate; DHEA, dehydroepiandrosterone; FSH, follicle-stimulating hormone; LH, luteinizing hormone).

secretion. So chronic low dose protocol and antagonist protocol in polycystic ovary (PCO) gives very good pregnancy rate. High level of LH causing ceiling effect is clearly seen in PCOS.

- *Luteinizing hormone in downregulated cycle*: In a downregulated cycle, there is low level of LH. When it reaches below the threshold level, the growth of the follicle is hampered. Low level of LH causes poor luteal conversion and so luteal phase defect (LPD) is very common. To compensate this loss, hCG works very well as luteal support but OHSS should be kept in mind in PCOS patients.
- *Luteinizing hormone and ovarian drilling*: By drilling, we are destroying stroma, i.e. theca cells. So androgen production is decreased and this will have negative feedback to hypothalamus and pituitary to decrease in LH secretion. This decrease in LH will revert the LH/FSH ratio and spontaneous ovulation is established.
- *Luteinizing hormone in hypogonadotropic hypogonadism*: LH is must for follicular development as it is discussed in two cell two gonadotropin theory. Without LH, follicular growth is present but it is without E2.
- *Luteinizing hormone in poor responder*: In poor responder rather than increasing dose of FSH, LH or hCG can be added for rescue of the follicle after 10 mm size. Here LH receptors have developed and it can rescue the follicular growth. But dose of more than 150 IU can have an LH ceiling effect.

Estrogen

It is secreted by granulosa cells of the follicles under the influence of FSH as explained in the two cell two hormone theory. It is also produced from androgen by aromatization as discussed earlier. This means for the production of E2, androgen is essential and androgen is produced in theca cells under the effect of LH.

High levels of E2 cause negative feedback mechanism and decrease FSH and LH. But when E2 reaches to certain peak, it causes positive feedback mechanism and causes rise of FSH and LH. This rise causes LH peak and second FSH peak (surge). But LH is more than FSH (Flowchart 1.1).

Estrogen prepares the endometrium and is essential for development of progesterone receptors. Estrogen concentrations are at their lowest at menstruation and rises to maximum at the preovulatory phase. Following ovulation, the E2 level falls and then again rises in the luteal phase with the activity of corpus luteum.

Clinical Applications

- Because of negative feedback mechanism, FSH level decreases after rise of E2 from developing mechanism. This decrease in FSH causes monofollicular development of the follicle. Letrozole does not abolish this negative feedback unlike CC and so letrozole gives monofollicular development.
- Exogenous E2 is given for preparation of endometrium in premature ovarian failure (POF) patients.

Flowchart 1.1: Fine-tuning system of HPO axis—(short-loop and long-loop feedback systems) (Homburg R. The physiology in ovulation. In: Ovulation induction and Controlled ovarian stimulation, A practical guide. Taylor & Francis group. London and New York. 2005. Page 5-18).
(EGF, epithelial growth factor; FSH, follicle-stimulating hormone; GnRH, gonadotropin-releasing hormone; IGF, insulin-like growth factor; IGFBP, insulin-like growth factor binding protein; LH, luteinizing hormone; TGF, transforming growth factor).

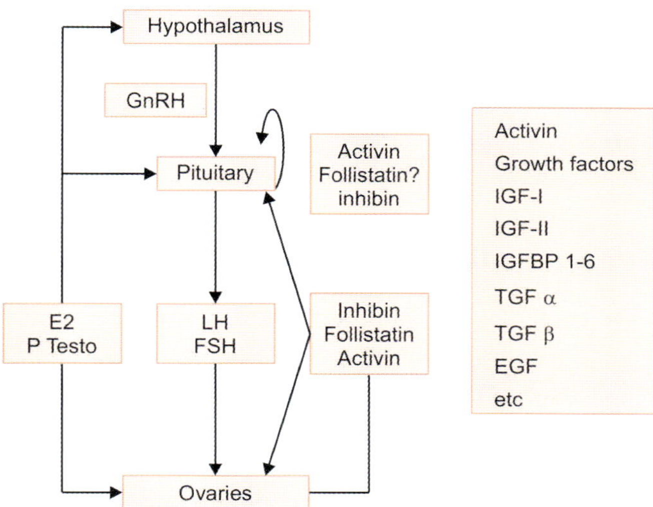

Other Factors

Inhibin

Inhibin is also produced by granulosa cells. It has two dimers, inhibin A and inhibin B, and both differ in their secretion pattern. Inhibin B rises in follicular phase and is inhibitory to FSH (similar to E2). Inhibin A rises in periovulatory period and luteal phase.

Clinical application: Inhibin B is assessed for measuring ovarian reserve, but anti-Müllerian hormone (AMH) and antral follicle count (AFC) are more reliable.

Activin and Follistatin

It increases secretion and promotes action of FSH. This leads to follicular growth and inhibits androgen production. Follistatin being an activin binding protein, neutralizes activin bioactivity.

Growth Factors

Growth factors include insulin like growth factor (IGF), IGF2, IGF-BP 1-6, transforming growth factor α (TGF α), TGF β, epithelial growth factor (EGF), etc. Activity of these

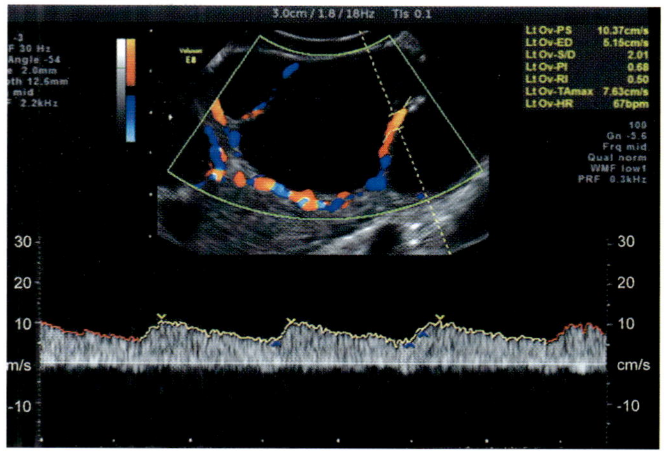

Fig. 1.6: Color and pulse Doppler ultrasound image of a mature follicle.

IGF can be counteracted by IGF binding proteins. Receptors to these are present in ovaries and promote androgen production. All these factors passively help the growth of the follicle.

Ovulation

Ovulation occurs after 34–36 hours of onset of LH surge. Onset of LH surge correlates with perifollicular blood flows. Pre-LH surge, perifollicular resistance index (RI) between 0.4 and 0.48, and peak systolic velocity (PSV) of 10 cm/sec are the indicators of a mature follicle on Doppler ultrasound[13] (Fig. 1.6). Ovulation occurs 10–12 hours after LH peak (Fig. 1.7). E2 peak initiates LH peak and ovulation occurs after 24–26 hours of E2 peak. Inhibitory activities are high before and after ovulation. But it is important to remember that apart from these hormones, normal levels of prolactin, thyroid, and androgen are also essential for normal ovulation.

The hCG plays a major role in inducing influx of blood within follicles. Follicular PSV rises markedly with the rise in the LH levels at the time of preovulatory LH surge.[15] Because of this physiology, when PSV of the follicle is high, it means that the follicle is likely to rupture early and IUI should be done earlier than the conventional protocol of 34–38 hours.

Progesterone

Luteinizing hormone induces the secretion of progesterone from luteinized granulosa cells (Flowchart 1.2). Progesterone rises before ovulation and this rise is because

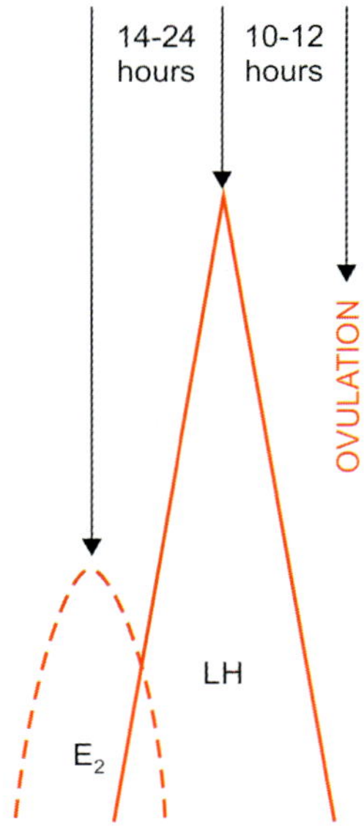

Fig. 1.7: Estradiol (E2) and luteinizing hormone (LH) fluctuations around ovulation.[14]

of rise of FSH. It has a triggering role of high GnRH, which may give LH surge. It helps in increasing proteolytic enzymes for rupture. Progesterone production from corpus luteum keeps on rising till the midluteal period (7–8 days postovulation), when its level is at its peak. Rising progesterone has a negative feedback on the pituitary gonadotropins and decreases the frequency of LH pulse. During this phase, FSH is synthesized but not secreted. It is stored for release when corpus luteum fails and E2 and progesterone levels decrease markedly. Decrease in LH causes demise of corpus luteum and decrease in progesterone secretion toward the end of the cycle, just before menstruation.

Progesterone prepares endometrium for implantation by expressing genes needed for implantation. The hCG of pregnancy rescues corpus luteum and progesterone secretion is maintained till the trophoblastic and placental hormones take over.

Clinical Applications

- Preparation of endometrium occurs with progesterone along with E2 in POF patients.
- The hCG can be used to rescue corpus luteum as a luteal phase support.
- Luteal support with progesterone is given to the patients at high risk of LPD, especially those on agonist cycles and antagonist cycles.

CLINICOPATHOLOGY OF OVULATION

Introduction

For the diagnosis of ovulatory dysfunction, it is extremely important to advice for precise investigations depending

Flowchart 1.2: Diagram of ovarian steroids genesis.[6] (DHEA, dehydroepiandrosterone).

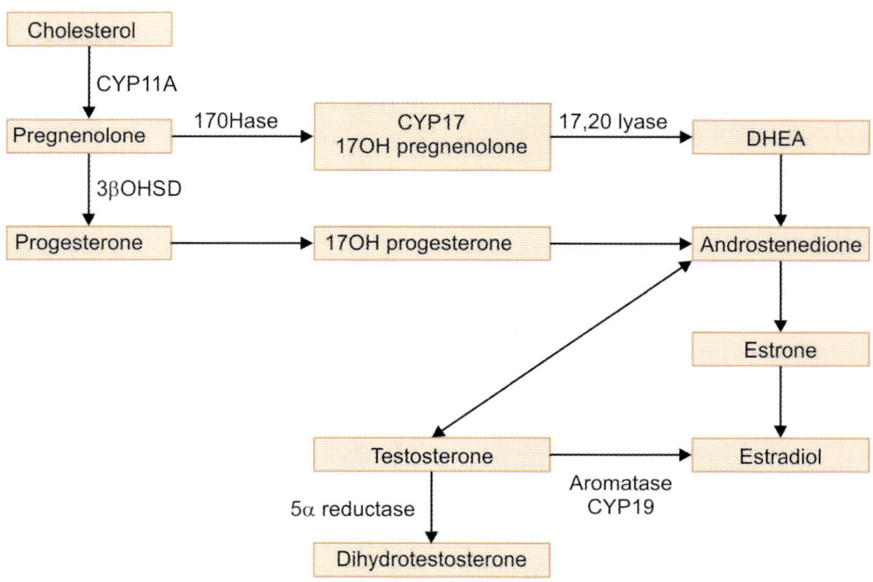

on the history of the patient. It helps the clinician to reach to the correct diagnosis. Reports of unnecessary investigations may create more confusions.

Profiles and packages are useless in infertility and are expensive in clinical practice. In infertility management, specific investigations are required at specific times for correct interpretation. So one has to be very precise when requesting for investigations. The routinely required investigations for infertility and assisted reproductive techniques (ARTs) are discussed here.

Serum Follicle-stimulating Hormone (FSH)

a. Day 2–3 serum FSH (S. FSH) and serum LH (S. LH) are used for diagnosis of polycystic ovarian syndrome (PCOS). High LH indicates anovulation and it is very evident from the history. Therefore, ratio of LH/FSH is not required for diagnosis of PCO. Both high LH and PCO can be diagnosed by an ultrasound scan done on day 2–3 of the menstrual cycle.
b. Serum FSH for diagnosis of menopause: FSH of more than 40 IU/mL indicates ovarian failure. Oral contraceptive (OC) pills can be used to induce withdrawal bleed to confirm menopause. When the patient does not have a withdrawal bleed after giving progesterone for 3–5 days, it indicates she is menopausal. Ultrasound shows hardly any follicles and ovaries are small.
c. FSH for assessment of ovarian reserve: Day 2–3 FSH is done to know the ovarian reserve and also to predict the possibility of pregnancy. Higher the FSH, lesser is the chance for development of good quality follicles/ova, thus resulting in a lesser chance to achieve conception. FSH of less than 8 IU/mL is considered normal. Between 8 and 12 IU/mL FSH, the values are considered high. But when these values are more than 12 IU/mL, there is very little chance of retrieving good quality ova and, therefore, very little chance of achieving pregnancy. Chances of pregnancy beyond FSH level of 15 IU/mL is rare.[16] Though currently age, AFC and AMH are used for assessment of ovarian reserve and thought to be much more accurate and reliable for the purpose than FSH. Utility of FSH as a marker for ovarian reserve has significantly reduced. This is because AFC indicates the number of follicles available in that cycle for recruitment, whereas S. FSH level gives overall impression about the availability of the ova.

   If the patient with low ovarian reserve is given DHEA for 3 months, the AFC may rise, but the FSH still remains high. In these cases, it would be worthwhile to initiate ovulation induction. AFC thus may be a better for patient counseling too. Moreover, repeated FSH assessment is of no significance, because its highest level is decision maker for the possibility of pregnancy. AFC is so far considered the most feasible and reliable parameter for assessment of ovarian reserve.[17,18]
d. Low FSH: Less than 5 IU indicates pituitary or hypothalamic cause for anovulation.

Serum Luteinizing Hormone

a. Serum LH for PCO: Day 2/3 serum level of LH is not required for the diagnosis of PCOS. In PCOS, LH is high and this can be clinically judged by anovulation or oligo-ovulation resulting in delayed menstrual cycles. High LH, leads to high androgen and this can be diagnosed by high stromal volume.[19,20]
b. Serum LH on day 8–10 in clomiphene citrate cycle: CC stimulates hypothalamus to secrete both FSH and LH as it blocks E2 receptors. This high LH is detrimental to ova and gives poor pregnancy rate in spite of good ovulation rate. Therefore, when LH is more than 10–12 IU/mL on day 8–10 of a clomiphene cycle, the subsequent cycles should not be continued with CC, instead the ovulation induction should then be done with gonadotropins. This is more common scenario in PCOS patients.
c. Serum LH in downregulated cycle: In downregulated patients on long protocol, the LH on day 2–3 of the treatment cycle should be between 0.5 and 2 IU to confirm the adequacy of downregulation. Actually, 0.1 IU/mL LH is sufficient for the development of follicle and so assessment of LH levels at this phase of cycle is questionable.
d. Serum LH less than 5 IU/L indicates pituitary or hypothalamic cause for anovulation, especially with low FSH.

Serum Estradiol

a. *Follicular maturity*: When the follicle is mature, serum E2 will be 150 pgm/mL/follicle. If E2 is normal and endometrium is poor, it is a local cause for poor endometrium. But if the E2 level is low, the endometrium is usually poor, and may grow to normal when E2 level rises. Using color Doppler for the assessment of follicular quality can be a useful tool for the same because the flow parameters of the follicle can be correlated with the functional maturity of the follicle, which indirectly indicates estradiol levels.

b. *For poor responder*: In IVF cycles, E2 is assessed on day 2 of the cycle to confirm downregulation. If it is more than 80 pgm/mL, it indicates a possibility of poor response to stimulation. This high E2 is because of high FSH, which is present in poor responders and causes early recruitment of the follicle.
c. *To assess ovarian suppression*: In long agonist protocol IVF cycles, GnRHa is started from day 21 of the previous cycle. This downregulates pituitary, and FSH and LH levels become very low. This also leads to low E2 levels (30–50 pgm/mL). The stimulation is started only thereafter. If E2 level is more than 50 pgm/mL, it is advisable to continue downregulation for 1 or 2 days more before starting the stimulation. In patients on OC pills, E2 should be checked after 12–14 days for starting OC pills.
d. *For suspected risk of hyperstimulation*: In IUI cycles or in non-IVF gonadotropin cycles, hyperstimulation is suspected if E2 is more than 1,600 pgm/mL on the day of trigger. This is common in PCOS patients. In IVF cycles, if E2 is more than 4,000 pgm/mL on the day of trigger, hyperstimulation is suspected. Now with chronic low dose protocol in IUI cycles and ultrasound based scoring systems for deciding the stimulation protocols,[21,22] extremely low OHSS rates are claimed. However, in IVF cycles with antagonist protocol and agonist trigger, OHSS can be almost completely prevented. Therefore, the strategy in PCOS patients should be antagonist protocol with agonist trigger.
   The OHSS can also be predicted by calculating the ovarian volume. If total ovarian volume of both the ovaries together is more than approximately 180 cc, OHSS should be suspected;[23] whereas, if it is less than approximately 110 cc, the risk of OHSS is extremely low. We depend more on ovarian volume than on the E2 levels and withhold hCG trigger when combined ovarian volume of two ovaries is more than 180 cc.

Serum Progesterone

Progesterone is chiefly secreted by corpus luteum in second half of the cycle. Otherwise, it is an intermediate hormone for other steroid hormones during their production and conversion from cholesterol.

Normal Values

- Follicular phase: 1 ng/mL
- LH surge: 1–2 ng/mL
- Ovulation: 3 ng/mL

Midluteal S. progesterone, i.e. a week before menstruation is approximately 10 ng/mL. A level of more than 3 ng/mL indicates ovulation. Therefore, if only ovulation is to be documented, repeated ultrasound scans are not required. In the same way, endometrial biopsy is not required to confirm secretory changes in endometrium and S. progesterone estimation suffices for the same.

Ultrasound with color Doppler is a better modality to assess the secretory phase of the cycle. It can diagnose luteal phase problems viz., LPD or luteinized unruptured follicle. Therefore, it is an inevitable conclusion that random S. progesterone has little value beyond documenting ovulation.

17-OH-Progesterone

This investigation is done in all patients with hirsutism. It is increased due to 21-hydroxylase deficiency. Because of 21-hydroxylase deficiency in patients of heterogeneous carrier, late onset of congenital adrenal hyperplasia is observed. The 17-OH-Progesterone (17-OH-P) is weak androgen and manifests as hirsutism, acne, clitoral enlargement, and menstrual irregularity at puberty.

Normal level of 17-OH-P is less than 200 ng/dL. Whenever the level is between 200 and 800 ng/dL, one should get the adrenocorticotropic hormone (ACTH) levels assessed in serum. Level of more than 800 ng/dL is diagnostic of 21-hydroxylase deficiency. These patients are treated with dexamethasone 0.5 mg daily at bedtime.

Serum Testosterone

Normal value of S. testosterone is 20–80 ng/dL. Its normal production is 0.2–0.3 mg/day. Out of this, 80% binds to sex hormone binding globulin (SHBG) and 19% to albumin. Only 1% is free testosterone. Testosterone may be high in patients with PCOS and tumors. Tumor is suspected, if there is sudden onset of symptoms due to increased testosterone. PCOS patients show gradual rise in testosterone levels. Routine estimation of S. testosterone is not required, as it does not change the line of treatment (Table 1.1).

Dehydroepiandrosterone Sulfate

Dehydroepiandrosterone sulfate is exclusively secreted from adrenal glands. The normal value is 350 ngm/dL. It increases with hyperprolactinemia. In patients with PCOS, prolactin and DHEA-S are a little high and do not require

Table 1.1: Sources of androgen in female.

Hormone	Source
Testosterone	50% Peripheral Conversion
	25% Ovary
	25% Adrenal
Androstenedione	50% Ovary
	50% Adrenal
Dehydroepiandrosterone	90% Adrenal
	10% Ovary
Docosahexaenoic acid	100% Adrenal

any specific treatment except the treatment of PCOS. This rise is secondary to E2 because of anovulation.

Whenever DHEA-S is very high, it is due to adrenal tumor. DHEA-S more than 700 µg/dL is accepted as a marker for adrenal dysfunction. This is rarely found and does not change the management. Ultrasound is better guide to diagnose adrenal tumor. S. testosterone and ultrasound suffices to rule out adrenal tumors. If 17-OH-P is normal, there is no need to search for adrenal enzyme defect. Therefore, routine testing of DHEA-S is not required.

Inhibin A and B

Inhibin B is predominantly secreted by antral follicles. Low day 3 inhibin B level less than 45 pgm/mL indicates poor response to superovulation and patient is less likely to conceive. Same thing can be judged by S. FSH, S. AMH, or AFC and so routine use of inhibin B estimation is not justified.

Inhibin A is secreted from preovulatory follicles. Both inhibin A and B are secreted from granulosa cells and regulate FSH by negative feedback mechanism. Routine estimation of inhibin A does not add any information to change the management of the patient.

Serum Anti-Müllerian Hormone

It is a member of transforming growth factor. It is produced from granulosa cells of small antral follicles. The expression of AMH is localized in granulosa cells of primary preantral and small antral follicles and has important role in human folliculogenesis. AMH expression in follicle decreases in antral follicle more than 8 mm in size. It is now well established that S. AMH concentrations reflect the number of preantral and small antral follicles in the ovary; this would account for raised AMH levels found in both polycystic ovarian morphology (PCOM) and PCOS.[24] In follicles undergoing atresia and in corpus lutea also, the AMH expression is completely lost.[11] AMH levels in women are low until the age of 8 years, rise rapidly until puberty, and decline steadily from the age of 25 until menopause, when AMH production ceases.

Table 1.2: AMH values and implications.

Ovarian fertility potential	pmol/L	ng/mL
Optimal fertility	28.6–48.5	4.0–6.8
Satisfactory fertility	15.7–28.6	2.2–4.0
Low fertility	2.2–15.7	0.3–2.2
Very low/undetectable	0.0–2.2	0.0–0.3
High level	48.5	6.8

Physiology of Anti-Müllerian Hormone

The AMH has an inhibiting role in the ovary, contributing to follicular arrest.[19] It lowers the sensitivity of follicles to FSH, which is required for normal folliculogenesis. *In vitro* studies have shown that the action of FSH in promoting follicular growth is counteracted by AMH.[25] It has a steady level throughout the cycle except for a slight dip just after LH peak.[26]

Some investigators have recorded cyclical fluctuations in AMH with rapid decrease in early luteal phase.[27] This can be correlated with the follicular atresia before recruitment in the late luteal phase.

It can predict ovarian response. It can predict menopause by low levels. High AMH is very high in PCOS, and it predicts OHSS (Table 1.2).

Anti-Müllerian hormone and polycystic ovary: The reported property of AMH to counteract the actions of FSH imply that the high production of AMH by PCO may have an important role in the pathophysiology of the syndrome.[28] In anovulatory PCOS, the failure of follicle development is due to an intrinsic inhibition of FSH action and that this inhibition is due to an intrinsic inhibition of FSH action and due to the high concentration of AMH.[29]

Increased ovarian stromal blood flow in PCOS may be because of overexpression of vascular endothelial growth factor (VEGF), which modulates the permeability of theca cells and increased IGF 1,[30,31] which in turn enhances gonadotropin-stimulated steroid production in granulosa cells and theca cells resulting in increased ovarian androgen production and subsequently increased AMH production.[32]

Anti-Müllerian hormone levels are two to three times higher in PCOS, than in healthy controls.[33] This has been attributed not only to increased number of antral follicles but also to higher production of AMH per follicle in patients with PCOS as compared to size-matched counterparts from normal ovary.[34] In addition, a positive correlation between AMH and both LH and testosterone serum concentrations in PCOS has been reported.[35]

Each individual follicle in women with PCOS produces significantly more AMH than its sized-matched counterpart from a patient with normal ovary.[34] Moreover, it has also been shown that metformin administration in PCOS patients is associated with reduction in AMH concentration in follicle and serum, suggesting that the measurement of AMH can be used to evaluate the treatment efficacy with insulin sensitizers.[36]

Anti-Müllerian hormone and in vitro fertilization: In IVF patients, S. AMH value can predict the response of ovary and so it is useful for counseling the patient. When calculated optimal AMH cut off of less than 1.26 ng/mL was used to predict responses to controlled ovarian stimulation (COS), it was found to have a 97% sensitivity for predicting poor responses (less than four oocytes retrieved) and 98% accuracy in predicting a normal COS response.[37]

Nelson et al. suggested the AMH based strategy for deciding the COS protocol.[38] But we have found AFC as equally effective and more precise for prediction of ovarian response. With extremely low S. AMH levels, moderate, but reasonable pregnancy and live birth rates are still possible. Extremely low AMH levels do not seem to represent an appropriate marker for withholding fertility treatment. Younger women are likely to have better pregnancy rates than their older counterparts with equally low AMH.[39] Constant AMH and inhibin B levels suggest that neither AMH nor inhibin B is an accurate marker of ovarian response after low dose gonadotropins ovulation induction in patients with PCOS.[40] Mashiach et al. have also shown a relationship between follicular fluid AMH concentrations and the quality of embryos in patients with PCOS.[41]

All these references indicate that routine use of AMH does not help in managing non-ART patients. Only one to two mature follicles are required for minimal hyperstimulation with IUI, and AMH will not help to change the line of treatment. Poor responding ovary or low reserve ovary can be very precisely diagnosed by ultrasound.

Serum AMH estimation is indicated in:[42]

- Predicting both over and under response in COS
- Determining the most appropriate treatment regimen
- Pretreatment counseling for couples to make an appropriate and informed choice
- Predicting long-term fertility
- Predicting the age of menopause
- Predicting ovarian aging prior to or following chemotherapy/surgery
- Screening for polycystic ovaries.

Clinical applications of Anti-Müllerian Hormone: Apart from fertility assessment, following are the clinical applications of AMH:

- To confirm presence of testicular tissue in children with low testosterone levels
- Differential diagnosis of intersex disorders
- In patients with bilateral nonpalpable gonads
- Females with granulosa cell tumors
- The inhibitory effect of AMH on folliculogenesis may in future be used for hormonal contraception.

Insulin Resistance

Now it has been proved that in patients of PCOS there is high androgen because of increased insulin level and insulin resistance. It indicates the severity of PCOS. Clinically, waist circumference of 35 inches or 90 cm is predictive of abnormal endocrinology and metabolic function.

There are various methods to diagnose insulin resistance. But 2 hours glucose and insulin response is the one of the most reliable ones.

Two hours glucose tolerance test:

- Normal: <140 mg/dL
- Impaired: 140–190 mg/dL
- Noninsulin dependent diabetes mellitus: ≥200 mg/dL

Two hours insulin response:

- Insulin resistance very likely: 100–150 μU/mL
- Insulin resistance: 151–300 μU/mL
- Severe insulin resistance: >300 μU/mL

In clinical practice, patients with high insulin resistance are the ones who have tonically high LH levels and these patients require ovarian drilling. Alternatively, they may also be benefitted by GnRH antagonist. Antagonist decreases LH levels, prevents premature luteinization, and improves oocyte quality.

Patients who do not want immediate pregnancy are the patients in whom insulin sensitizer alone is the recommended line of treatment. It has been proved beyond doubts that insulin sensitizers do not have any direct effect on ovulation induction, though when given for 3–6 months, the improved insulin sensitivity, improved the hormonal milieu of PCOS patient, thus improving the chance of spontaneous ovulation and conception.

The 3D US is a novel way to diagnose insulin resistance, based on assessment of stromal volume.[43] But when volume ultrasound is unavailable, 2 hours glucose and 2 hours insulin test is the best alternative.

So for chronic anovulation, only three investigations are required:

1. S. prolactin
2. S. TSH
3. Insulin resistance

Serum Prolactin

Prolactin is the hormone secreted by anterior pituitary and is regulated by prolactin inhibitory factor, which is secreted from hypothalamus.

- Normal level of prolactin is 10–25 ng/mL.
- In microadenoma, it is between 100 and 200 ng/mL.
- In macroadenoma, it is more than 200 ng/mL.
- Immunoassay for prolactin does not reflect its bioassay levels always.
- Many a times, patients have no symptoms in spite of high prolactin level because of presence of macromolecules, which are big prolactin molecules (that account for 10–12% of hyperprolactin in symptomatically normal patients).

Galactorrhea with Normal Prolactin Levels

Patients with galactorrhea present with normal S. prolactin levels. This may be mucoid discharge and not actual galactorrhea. Any discharge, therefore, from the breast should be seen under microscope. If it contains fat globules, only then it is galactorrhea.

When ovulation induction is done, in many patients E2 leads to rise in prolactin levels in first half of the menstrual cycle. These patients have night spikes of high prolactin level and are known as spikers. This is transient hyperprolactinemia. The clinical presentation is poor endometrium in spite of good follicles. This condition is difficult to diagnose, but bromocriptine can be given in a dose of 1.25 mg twice a day in these patients in first half of the cycle. It is a therapeutic test. If endometrium improves, it is continued in the subsequent cycle, otherwise it is stopped. Apart from bad oocyte quality, the spikers also have a high chance of LPD.

As discussed earlier, marginally high prolactin levels are also found in PCOS patients due to high E2 and high DHEA-S. In these cases, bromocriptine or cabergoline is not required; PCOS is to be treated.

DIAGNOSIS OF OVULATION

Detection of ovulation is extremely important to decide the further line of treatment in patients for treatment of infertility. There are various tests to detect ovulation and current status of each test is discussed here.

Clinical Presentation

a. Regular menstrual cycle (24–35 days) is in favor of ovulation. Any type of irregularity, beyond the limits (24–35 days), strongly indicate anovulation or dysovulation.
b. '*Mittelschmerz*': This is a midcycle pain in an ovulatory cycle because of contraction of smooth muscles surrounding the follicle about 12–24 hours prior to ovulation. This contraction helps the follicle to rupture and ovulation occurs.
c. Cervical mucus feel: Patient feels watery discharge at the introitus, which becomes thin and copious prior to ovulation. This indicates a mature follicle and not ovulation.
d. Pregnancy is the only surest sign of ovulation.
e. Painful menstruation is also an indicator of the previous cycle being ovulatory.

Basal Body Temperature

The principle of basal body temperature (BBT) measurement is that progesterone secretion after ovulation raises the body temperature. BBT is between 97 and 98°F during the follicular phase. After ovulation, it starts rising and goes high by 0.4–0.8°F, as the progesterone rises. BBT is at its lowest just before ovulation, which is known as nadir. The temperature falls before the period or when progesterone level decreases due to regressing corpus luteum. The rise in temperature persists, in case the patient conceives and patient feels her body temperature as much as low-grade fever. This is because of persistent and high levels of progesterone from the corpus luteum of pregnancy, stimulated by hCG.

Method

Basal body temperature is taken before rising from bed, with glass thermometer placed in oral cavity. The calibration on thermometer is 96–100°F. The change pattern in thermometer is known as biphasic pattern. The next period in normal cycle starts after 12 days of rise in temperature, if pregnancy does not occur. It is a low cost, noninvasive, and simple method and indicates abnormalities of follicular and luteal phase. But the temperature may be altered with smoking and disturbed sleep. It may be stressful for the patient to take temperature daily. There may not be shift in temperature in spite of ovulation and in this case, only after a few days of ovulation, it may be diagnosed. This is not clinically useful. BBT is not commonly used in clinical practice.

Midcycle Luteinizing Hormone Surge Diagnosed by LH Kit

The LH surge occurs for 48–50 hours. LH has short half-life. LH rise can be detected by urinary LH kits. When the threshold level of 40 μ/mL is crossed, test becomes positive on the kit and the color is seen. The intensity of the color increases as LH level increases. LH level normally starts rising early in the morning and may be misinterpreted as negative if urine is tested in the morning as it appears in the urine after 6–8 hours. Therefore, LH assessment in the afternoon is more reliable.

The test is done daily. But doing it twice daily decreases the false negatives. Too much of fluid intake is avoided few hours before the test to prevent dilution of the urine and LH in urine.

Ovulation occurs 20 hours ± 6 hours after detection of urinary LH surge.[44-47] Patient is advised intercourse for 2 days following detection of LH surge as these days are the most fertile ones. If artificial insemination of donor (AID) is planned, it should also be done for 2 days. The specificity and sensitivity for LH surge are 90% and 96% respectively and if test is done twice a day, sensitivity reaches to 99%.[47]

So LH detection kits are noninvasive, self-monitored, and indicates fertile period, so it is useful clinically for planning timed intercourse, IUI and AID. It can diagnose abnormality of follicular phase and luteal phase. But the disadvantage is that it is tedious, may be false negative, and restricts patients from fluid intake. False positive results may occur with OC pills, CC, hCG, human menopausal gonadotropin (HMG), and Danazol. But easy availability of ultrasound has reduced the utility of LH kits.

Endometrial Biopsy

It was used to document secretory changes in the endometrium after ovulation. Endometrial biopsy differentiates follicular phase from secretory phase. An experienced pathologist can date the endometrium after ovulation. The 2 days out of phase endometrium is regarded as LPD.[48] This test is not as preferred as ultrasound or serum progesterone levels as it is inaccurate and highly invasive.

Luteal Serum Progesterone Levels

Progesterone level is below 1 ng/mL during follicular phase. Before ovulation, it rises up to 1–2 ng/mL. The peak reaches after a week of ovulation. Level more than 3 ng/mL indicates ovulation. Normally on 7th postovulatory day, progesterone level is more than 10 ng/mL.[49] Serum progesterone level is only used to document ovulation as it is simple, fairly accurate, noninvasive, and reliable.

Daily assessment of progesterone for diagnosis of LPD is not used as it is inconclusive and multiple levels are required for accuracy.

Estrogen

Clinically, E2 peak will give copious mucous discharge and when dried on a slide will show a 'fern' pattern. Before ovulation, it shows tertiary branches. Normal preovulatory mucous strand can be stretched to 8–10 cm between two ends of artery forceps. Both these tests indicate high E2 level, mostly due to mature follicle but does not indicate ovulation.

Ultrasound

A follicle that is of more than 10 mm in diameter, grows at a rate of 2–3 mm per day, has no internal echogenicity, and has thin (pencil line like) walls is not only more likely to become the leading follicle but will also give mature healthy ovum. The growing follicle can be assessed by transvaginal sonography. A mature follicle is 16–18 mm, has thin walls, regular round shape, and no echogenicity in the lumen. When functionally mature, on color Doppler, the follicle shows blood vessels covering at least three-fourth of the follicular circumference (Fig. 1.3). On pulse Doppler, these blood vessels show an RI of 0.4–0.48[13] and PSV of more than 10 cm/sec. The endometrium starts appearing multilayered on ultrasound as early as midproliferative phase with rising E2. On transvaginal scan, endometrial thickness of 6 mm is considered minimum that is required on the day of ovulation or on the day of hCG trigger for a successful outcome, although 8 mm is generally considered optimum.[50] Segmental uterine artery perfusion demonstrates significant correlation with hormonal and histological markers of uterine receptivity, reaching the highest sensitivity for subendometrial blood flow.[51]

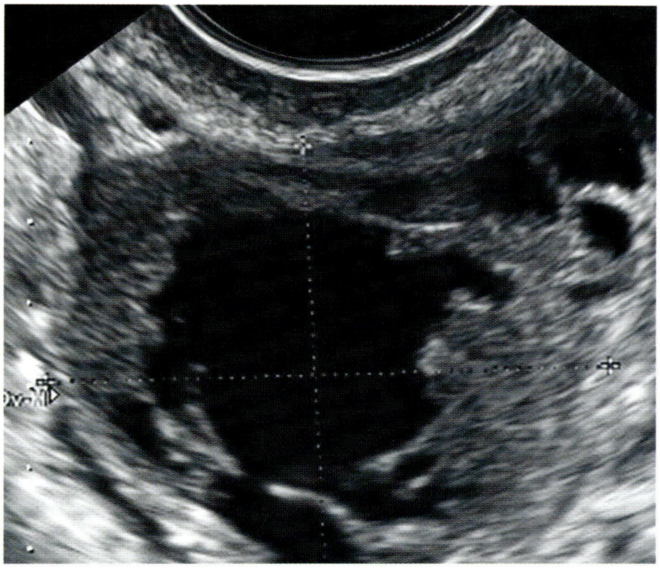

Fig. 1.8: Corpus luteum on B mode ultrasound.

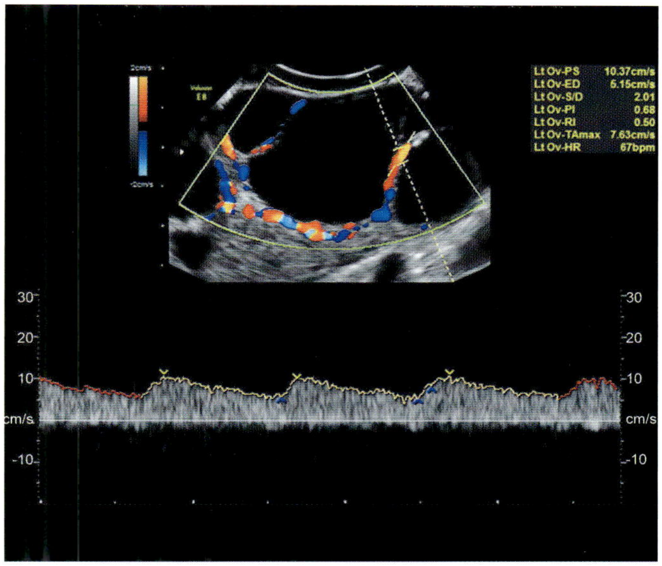

Fig. 1.9: Low resistance pericorpus luteal flow as seen on Doppler.

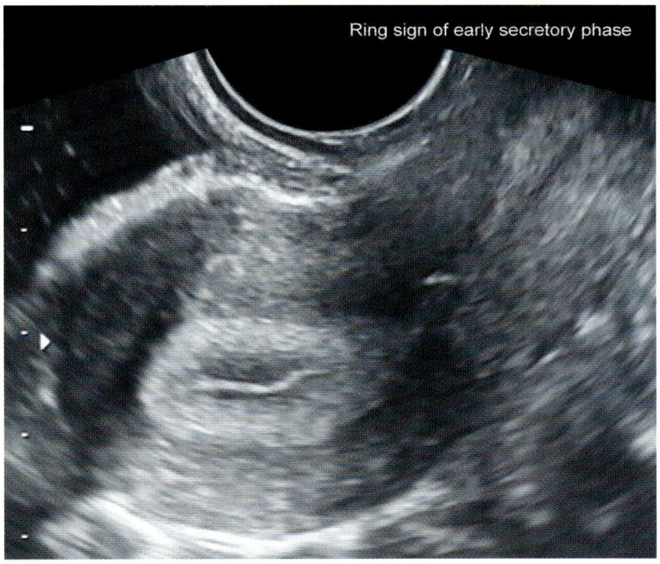

Fig. 1.10: Ring sign of secretory endometrium as seen on B mode ultrasound.

Endometrial vessels on pulse Doppler having RI of between 0.6 and 0.8 have been reported to be a good prognostic factor for implantation.[52] Rupture of the follicle is documented as disappearance of the follicle and it may be replaced by a cystic structure with thick shaggy walls and echogenicity in the lumen. But it is known to have variable appearances (Fig. 1.8) like ground glass echogenicity in lumen or lace like echogenicities.

Corpus luteum can be seen as low resistance vascular structure with internal echogenicities (Fig. 1.9).

Secretory changes are seen in the endometrium in the form of echogenicity of the endometrium which starts from outside, proceeding to the central line making a ring sign of the endometrium.[53] Posterior wall of the uterus also appears more echogenic in this phase due to acoustic enhancement by the endometrium due to fluid accumulation (Fig. 1.10).

Serial ultrasound for documenting ovulation should not be done, if intervention like ovulation trigger or IUI is not planned. Whether ovulation has occurred or not can be known by postovulatory S. progesterone level only.

Summarizing Diagnosis of Ovulation

1. Clinical history suggests ovulation in most cases.
2. Basal body temperature is inconclusive and not used routinely.
3. Urinary LH kit is useful only for patients who cannot visit clinic off and on. It is very rarely used these days.
4. Serum progesterone more than 3 ng/mL postovulatory indicates ovulation and is a most reliable means to document ovulation.
5. Daily ultrasound for just confirming that ovulation has occurred is not required unless some intervention is intended.
6. Endometrial biopsy is not required to assess the secretory phase changes.

7. Fern pattern and Spinnbarkeit indicates high E2 level and not ovulation.

CAUSES OF ANOVULATION

Introduction

The incidence of infertility is 15–17% after 1 year of unprotected intercourse. After 2nd year, only 7–8% of couples remain infertile. After 2.5 years, almost 7% will still remain infertile. Out of these infertile couples, in 20–40%, anovulation or oligo-ovulation is the causative factor.

The classification of causes of anovulation is very well described by World Health Organization (WHO). It is classified as:

I. WHO group I: Hypothalamopituitary failure
II. WHO group II: Hypothalamopituitary dysfunction
III. WHO group III: Ovarian failure
IV. WHO group IV: Hyperprolactinemia
V. WHO group V: Out flow defects (not associated with anovulation)

Hypothalamopituitary Failure (WHO Group I)

It is also known as hypogonadotropic hypogonadism. In this situation, gonadotropin (FSH and LH) concentrations are so low that follicle is not stimulated and, therefore, there is extremely low E2 level. These patients have anovulation and amenorrhea.

Hypothalamic Causes

- Anorexia nervosa: It is weight related. It may be due to crash diet or frank anorexia nervosa.
- Stress: It may be stress related anovulation and amenorrhea. Severe exercises like marathon running can cause amenorrhea.
- Kallmann syndrome: It is associated with anosmia.
- Craniopharyngioma
- Debilitating systemic diseases
- Idiopathic

Pituitary Causes

- Hypophysectomy
- Severe postpartum hemorrhage (PPH) causing Sheehan syndrome
- Radiotherapy for pituitary tumors

In these conditions, GnRH replacement therapy is very useful. But gonadotropins are usually given for ovulation induction.

Hypothalamopituitary Dysfunction (WHO Group II)

As contrast to WHO group I, in patients of this group, FSH is present that stimulates follicle and so E2 is also present. Clinically, this condition presents as oligo-ovulation or anovulation causing amenorrhea. As endogenous E2 is present, 5 days of oral progesterone (10 mg hydroxylprogesterone acetate daily) will give withdrawal bleeding usually within 10 days and this is confirmatory of WHO type II anovulation. PCOS is the most common condition amongst WHO group II. Diagnosis of PCOS is made by Rotterdam criteria (2003). These are as follows:

1. Oligo-/anovulation
2. Clinical and/or biochemical hyperandrogenism
3. Polycystic ovaries on ultrasound

Any two of these three criteria establishes the diagnosis of PCOS.

Oligo-ovulation is ovulation occurring once in 35–180 days. Anovulation is defined as no ovulation in 6 consecutive months.

Hyperandrogenism: Clinical or Biochemical

Clinical signs include hirsutism, acne, alopecia (male type), and female virilization. Biochemical indicators include raised total testosterone, androstenedione, and free androgen index.

Polycystic ovaries on ultrasound: There is presence of 12 or more follicles in either ovary, 2–9 mm in size, and/or ovarian volume more than 10 cc.

The concepts on the number of follicles and ovarian volume for the diagnosis of PCOS are changing. An average value of 26 or more follicles per ovary is a reliable threshold for detecting polycystic ovaries in women with frank manifestation of PCOS. Sensitivity and specificity for diagnosis of PCOS for FNPO (follicle number per ovary) (26) was 85% and 94% and for ovarian volume (OV) (10 cc) was 81% and 84%. But the same study has also quoted that the lower follicle threshold may be required to detect milder variants of the syndrome.[54]

Hyperinsulinemia and high androgen levels are very useful for diagnosis. Postprandial insulin level (2 hours after 75 gm of glucose) is increased in patients with insulin resistance. That is one of the major diagnostic features for PCOS. Along with this, increased stromal volume on 3D ultrasound is diagnostic of PCOS. Management includes life style changes, oral ovulogens, gonadotropins, and ovarian drilling.

Ovarian Failure (WHO Group III)

This group presents with high FSH along with low E2 and amenorrhea. The patient will have symptoms of hypoestrinism. Physiologically, this condition is found with the onset of menopause. But menopause may set in prematurely.

Causes of Ovarian Failure

i. Menopause (>40 years of age)
ii. Premature menopause (<40 years of age)
   a. Familial tendency
   b. Autoimmune disease
   c. Chemotherapy
   d. Radiotherapy
   e. Infections like tuberculosis
   f. Idiopathic
iii. Chromosomal: Turner Syndrome

Diagnosis is confirmed by high FSH more than 25 IU/mL with extremely low AMH. The only available treatment option to achieve a pregnancy in these patients is ovum donation. Hormone replacement therapy is required in these patients to support their physiological needs.

Hyperprolactinemia (WHO Group IV)

Anovulation because of hyperprolactinemia is present when prolactin levels are double the upper normal limits. This leads to anovulation. Marginally high prolactin levels do not require any treatment as it does not lead to anovulation. Mildly high prolactin levels are found in PCOS but in these cases no therapy is required to decrease prolactin levels. Prolactin is regulated by "prolactin inhibiting factor", dopamine. Therefore, any hypothalamic lesion or drugs suppressing hypothalamic activity will increase prolactin level and LH is low.

Outflow Defects

- Primary: imperforate hymen, absent uterus
- Secondary: Asherman syndrome

So chiefly three tests: progesterone withdrawal bleeding, serum prolactin, and serum FSH level assessment can give accurate diagnosis for the management.

CARRY-HOME MESSAGE

1. In all patients of anovulation/amenorrhea (Flowchart 1.3), always assess the prolactin levels as the first investigation to exclude hyperprolactinemia (WHO IV).
2. Progesterone withdrawal bleeding indicates presence of endogenous E2 and diagnosis of hypothalamopituitary dysfunction (WHO II).
3. Low FSH indicates hypogonadotropic hypogonadism (WHO I).
4. High FSH indicates ovarian failure (WHO III).
5. Normal FSH with no withdrawal bleed indicates absent uterus or outflow tract obstruction or Asherman syndrome (WHO V).
6. Clinical examination: Patient's height and weight are assessed for calculation of body mass index (BMI). (BMI = weight in kg/height^2 in meters.) Normal BMI is 20–25; less than 20 is considered underweight; and more than 30 is considered frank obesity. Anovulation is common in patients with abnormal BMI.

With obesity, PCOS must be considered, which is characterized by hirsutism and/or acne, acanthosis nigricans,

Flowchart 1.3: Amenorrhea/anovulation.
(FSH, follicle-stimulating hormone; MRI, magnetic resonance imaging; PCO, polycystic ovary syndrome; TSH, thyroid-stimulating hormone).

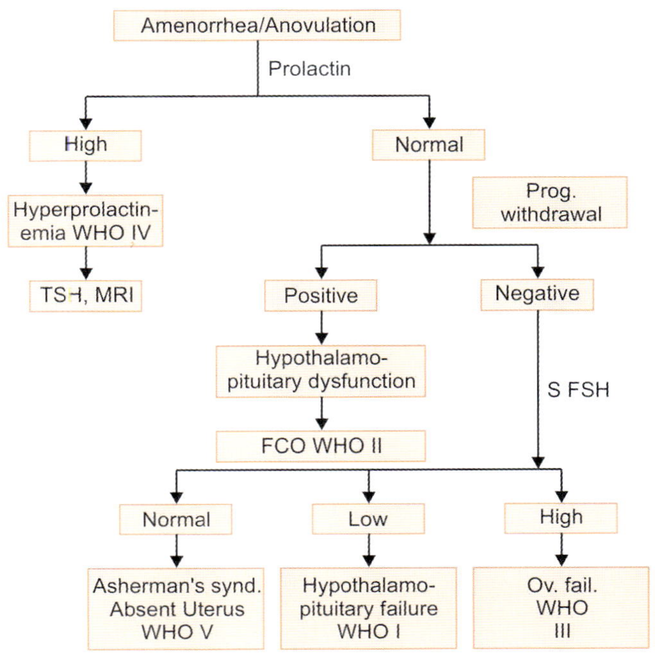

dark discoloration of skin in axilla and neck, and waist circumference more than 35 inches or 90 cm.

The BMI less than 20 may be seen in thin lean PCOS, malnourishment, or anorexia nervosa. Causes of primary amenorrhea and ovarian failures must also be ruled out by excluding the clinical presentation of E2 deficiencies.

REFERENCES

1. Joshua Anderson (Instructor). Oogenesis: How the female reproductive system produces eggs, Chapter 16. CLEP Biology: Study Guide & Test Prep/Science Courses.
2. Lobo RA. Early ovarian ageing: a hypothesis. What is early ovarian ageing? Hum. Reprod. 2003;18(9):1762-4.
3. Gilbert SF, Sunderland MA. The number of ova therefore decides the reserve of the ovary. Developmental biology, 6th edition. Sunderland (MA): Sinauer Associates; 2000.
4. Chaudhary S, Deshpande A. In: Hemant Deshpande (Ed). Physiology of Ovulation in Practical Management of Ovulation Induction. New Delhi: Jaypee, The Health Sciences Publisher; 2016. p. 15.
5. Chaudhary S, Deshpande A. In: Hemant Deshpande (Ed). Physiology of Ovulation in Practical Management of Ovulation Induction. New Delhi: Jaypee, The Health Sciences Publisher; 2016. p. 7.
6. Homburg R. Ovulation Induction and Controlled Ovarian Stimulation. Switzerland: Springer International Publishing; 2014. pp. 7-23.
7. Hiller SG. Current concepts of the roles of follicle stimulating hormone and luteinizing hormone in folliculogenesis. Hum Reprod. 1994;9:188-91.
8. Balasch J, Fabregues. Is luteinizing hormone needed for optimal ovulation induction. Curr Opin Obstet Gynecol. 2002;14(3):265-74
9. Shoham Z. The clinical therapeutic window for luteinizing hormone in controlled ovarian stimulation. Fertil Steril. 2002;14:265-74.
10. Kobayashi M, Nakano R, Ooshima A. Immunohistochemical localization of pituitary gonadotrophins and gonadal steroids confirms the two cells two gonadotrophins hypothesis of steroidogenesis in the human ovary. J Endocrinol. 1990; 126:483.
11. Yamoto M, Shima K, Nakano R. Gonadotrophin receptors in human ovarian follicles and corpora lutea throughout the menstrual cycle. Hor Res. 1992;37(Suppl 1):5.
12. Hughes E, Collins J, Vandekerckhove P. Gonadotrophin releasing hormone analogue as an adjunct to gonadotrophin therapy for clomiphene resistant polycystic ovarian syndrome (Cochrane review). In the Cochrane library. Oxford, Update Software 2001.
13. Kupesic S, Kurjak A. Uterine and ovarian perfusion during the periovulatory period assessed by transvaginal colour Doppler. Fertil Steril. 1993;3:439-43.
14. In: Speroff L, Fritz MA (Eds). Regulation of menstrual cycle in Clinical Gynecologic Endocrinology and Infertility. Lippincott, Williams and Wilkins. p. 213.
15. Bourne T, Jurkovic D, Waterstone J, Campbell S, Collins WP. Intrafollicular blood flow during human ovulation. Ultrasound Obstet Gynecol. 1991;1:53-9.
16. Scott Jr RT, Hofmann GE. Prognostic assessment of ovarian reserve. Fertil Steril. 1995;63:1.
17. Krishnakumar J, Agarwal A, Nambiar D, Radhakrishnan S. Comparison of antral follicle count, anti-Müllerian hormone and day 2 follicle stimulating hormone as predictor of ovarian response and clinical pregnancy rate in patient with an abnormal ovarian reserve test. Int J Reprod Contracept Obstet Gynecol. 2016;5(8):2762-7.
18. Panchal S, Nagori CB. Comparison of anti-Müllerian hormone and antral follicle count for assessment of ovarian reserve. JHRS. 2012;5(3):274-8.
19. Jonard S, Robert Y, Dewailly D. Revisit the ovarian volume as diagnostic criterion for polycystic ovaries. Hum Reprod. 2005;20:2893-8.
20. Balen A, Conway G, Homburg R, Legro R. Polycystic Ovary Syndrome: A Guide to Clinical Management. Taylor & Francis Group. 2005.
21. Panchal S, Nagori CB. Ultrasound based decision making on stimulation protocol for superovulated IUI cycles. IJIFM. 2016;7(1):7-13.
22. Panchal S, Nagori CB. Ultrasound based decision making on stimulation protocol in IVF. DSJUOG. 2016;10(3):330-7.
23. Oyesanya OA, Parsons JH, Collins WP, Campbell S. Total ovarian volume before humanchorionic gonadotrophin administration for ovulation induction may predict the hyperstimulation. Hum Reprod. 1995;10:3211-2.
24. Fanchin R, Maria SL, Righini C, Guibourdenche J, Frydman R, Taieb J. Serum AMH is more strongly related to ovarian follicle status that serum inhibin B, oestradiol, FSH and LH on the day 3. Hum Reprod. 2003;18:323-7.
25. Durlinger AL, Gruijters MJ, Kramer P, Karels B, Kumar TR, Matzik MM. Anti-Müllerian hormone attenuates the effect of FSH on follicle development in the mouse ovary. Endocrinology. 2001;142:4891-9.
26. La MArca A, Stabile G, Artenisio AC, Volpe A. Serum anti-Müllerian hormone throughout the human menstrual cycle. Hum Reprod. 2006;21(12):3103-7.
27. Streuli J, Fraisse T, Chapron C, Bijaoui G, Bischof P, de Ziegler D. Clinical uses of anti-Müllerian hormone assays: pitfalls and promises. Fertil Steril. 2009;91(1):226-30.
28. Pellat L, Rice S, Mason HD. Anti-Müllerian hormone and polycystic ovarian syndrome: a mountain too high? Reproduction. 2010;139:825-33.
29. Pellat L, Rice S, Dilaver N, Heshri A, Galea R, Brincat M, et al. Anti-Müllerian hormone reduces follicle sensitivity to follicle-stimulating hormone in human granulosa cells. Fertil Steril. 2011;96:1246-51.
30. El Behery MM, Diab AE, Mowafy H, Ebrahiem MA, Shehata AE. Effect of laparoscopic ovarian drilling on vascular endothelial growth factor and ovarian stromal blood flow using three dimensional power Doppler. Intern J Gynecol Obstet. 2011;112:119-21.
31. Abd El, Aal DE, Mohamed SA, Amine AF, Meki AR. Vascular endothelial growth factor and insulin like growth factor 1

in polycystic ovary syndrome and their relation to ovarian blood flow. Eur J Obstet Gynecol Reprod Biol. 2005;118: 219-24.
32. Willis D, Mason H, Gilling-Smith C, Franks S. Modulation by insulin of follicle stimulating hormone and luteinizing hormone actions in human granulosa cells of normal and polycystic ovaries. J Clin Endocrinol Metab. 1996;81: 302-9.
33. Pigny P, Merlen E, Robert Y, Cortet-Rudelli C, Decanter C, Jonard S. Elevated serum level of anti-Müllerian hormone in patients with polycystic ovary syndrome: relationship to the ovarian follicle excess and to the follicular arrest. J Clin Endocrinol Metab. 2003;88:5957-62.
34. Pellat L, Hanna L, Brincat M, Galea R, Brain H, Whitehead S, et al. Granulosa cell production of anti-Müllerian hormone is increased in polycystic ovaries. J Clin Endocrinol Metab. 2007;92:240-5.
35. Carlsen SH, Vanky E, Fleming R. Anti-Müllerian hormone concentrations in androgen suppressed women with polycystic ovary syndrome. Hum Reprod. 2009;24: 1732-8.
36. Piltonen T, MorinPapunen L, Koivunen R, Perheentupa A, Ruokonen A, Tapanainen JS. Serum anti-Müllerian hormone levels remain high until late reproductive age and decrease during metformin therapy in women with polycystic ovary syndrome. Hum Reprod. 2005;20(7):1820-6.
37. Gnoth C, Schuring AN, Friol K, Tigges J, Mallmann P, Godehardt E. Relevance of anti-Müllerian hormone measurement in a routine IVF program. Hum Reprod. 2008,23: 1359-65.
38. Nelson SM, Yates RW, Lyall H, Jamieson M, Traynor I, Gaudoin M, et al. Anti-Müllerian hormone based approach to controlled ovarian stimulation for assisted conception. Hum Reprod. 2009;24:867-75.
39. Weghofer A, Dietrich W, Barad DH, Gleicher N. Live birth chances in women with extremely low serum anti-Müllerian hormone levels. Hum Reprod. 2011;26(70):1905-9.
40. Fong SL, Schippe I, de Jong FH, Themmen APN, Visser JA, Laven JSP. Serum anti-Müllerian hormone and inhibin B concentrations are not useful predictors of ovarian response during ovulation induction treatment with rFSH in women with polycystic ovary syndrome. Fertil Steril. 2011;96(2): 459-63.
41. Mashiach R, Amit A, Hasson J, Amzalzg S, Almog B, Ben-Yosef D. Follicular fluid levels of anti-Müllerian hormone as a predictor of oocyte maturation, fertilization rate, and embryonic development in patients with polycystic ovarian syndrome. Fertil Steril. 2010;93(7):2299-302.
42. Loh JS, Maheshwari A. Anti-Müllerian Hormone-is it a crystal ball for predicting ovarian ageing? Human Reprod. 2011;26(11):2925-32.
43. Panchal S, Nagori CB. Correlation of ovarian and stromal volumes to fasting and postprandial insulin levels in polycystic ovarian syndrome patients. Int J Infertil Fetal Med. 2014;5(1):12-4.
44. Filicori M, Butler JP, Crowley WF. Neuroendocrine regulation of the corpus luteum in the human. Evidence for pulsatile progesterone secretion. J Clin Invest. 1984;73:1638-47.
45. Syrop CH, Hammond MG. Diurnal variations in midluteal serum progesterone measurements. Fertil Steril. 1987;47: 67-70.
46. Jordan J, Craig K, Clifton DK, Soules MR. Luteal phase defect: the sensitivity and specificity of diagnostic methods in common clinical use. Fertil Steril. 1994;62:54-62.
47. Miller PB, Soules MR. The usefulness of a urinary LH kit ovulation prediction during menstrual cycles of normal women. Obstet Gynecol. 1996;87:13-7.
48. Duggan MA, Brashert P, Ostor A, Scurry J, Billson V, Kneafsey P, et al. The accuracy and interobserver reproducibility of endometrial dating. Pathology. 2001;33:292-7.
49. Wathen NC, Perry L, Lilford RJ, Chard T. Interpretation of single progesterone measurement in diagnosis of anovulation and defective luteal phase: Observations on analysis of the normal range. Br Med J. 1984;288:7-9.
50. Dickey RP, Olar TT, Taylor SN, Curole DN, Harrigill K. Relationship of biochemical pregnancy to preovulatory endometrial thickness and pattern in patients undergoing ovulation induction. Hum Reprod. 1993;8:327-30.
51. Kupesic S, Kurjak A. Prediction of IVF outcome by three dimensional ultrasound. Hum Reprod. 2002;17:950-5.
52. Kupesic S, Bekavac I, Bjelos D, Kurjak A. Assessment of endometrial receptivity by transvaginal colour Doppler and three dimensional power Doppler ultrasonography in patients undergoing *in vitro* fertilization procedures. J Ultrasound Med. 2001;20(2):125-34.
53. Bald R, Hackeloer BJ.Ultraschall-darstellung verschiendener. Endometriumformen. In: Otto R, Jan FX (Eds). Ultraschall-diagnostik 1982. Stuttgart: Thieme; 1983. p. 187.
54. Lujan ME, Jarrett BY, Brooks ED, Reines JK, Peppin AK, Muhn N. Updated ultrasound criteria for polycystic ovary syndrome: reliable thresholds for elevated follicle population and ovarian volume. Hum Reprod. 2013;28(5):1361-8.

CHAPTER

2 Laboratory Investigations in an Infertile Couple

Chaitanya Nagori

INTRODUCTION

Human reproductive system is based on a very dynamic, intricate and perfectly balanced hormonal orchestra. Each hormone has a specific role at a specific time of the menstrual cycle in female and accordingly at different times of the menstrual cycle, different levels of the same hormones may be considered normal or abnormal. Therefore, different investigations have clinical value, only if done at a particular time. These hormones are produced from pituitary and ovaries and are controlled by hypothalamus. The entire cascade is named as hypothalamo-pituitary-ovarian axis (Fig. 2.1). The pituitary hormones are the follicle-stimulating hormone (FSH) and the luteinizing hormone, whereas those primarily produced from the ovaries are estrogen (estradiol) and progesterone. The others that have a role are 17-hydroxy progesterone, testosterone, anti-Müllerian hormone (AMH), thyroid, prolactin, etc.

INVESTIGATIONS FOR THE INFERTILE WOMEN

Serum Follicle-stimulating Hormone (S. FSH)

- Day 2–3 FSH is done along with luteinizing hormone (LH) for diagnosis of polycystic ovarian syndrome (PCOS). This should not be done as it does not change the line of treatment. PCOS can be diagnosed by history, clinical examination and ultrasound. Ultrasound diagnosis of PCO has been discussed in one of the chapters of this book. We have never used FSH/LH ratio for diagnosis of PCOS. Because abnormal value of this ratio only indicates anovulation, which is otherwise also evident by history.
- Day 2–3 FSH is done before *in vitro* fertilization (IVF). Higher FSH indicates lower chances of pregnancy.[1,2] S. FSH levels up to 10–12 iu/L is considered normal. We do not get day 2–3 S. FSH done as age + antral follicle count (AFC) gives better idea for assessing the ovarian reserve. However, systematic reviews from most studies have failed to define a single threshold or cut off value to describe poor ovarian function.[3]
- Occasionally for the diagnosis of menopause, when progesterone withdrawal bleeding is absent, S. FSH can confirm the diagnosis.
- Earlier, people used to do S. FSH in different cycles, but even raised S. FSH in one cycle can be an indicator of extremely low or no possibility of ongoing pregnancy.[4] Treatment should not be started in selected cycles even when S. FSH is normal.
- Basal FSH provides predictive value for pregnancy which can be judged by baseline scan. High FSH suggests poor ovarian reserve and that can be studied by baseline scan. High FSH is a direct pituitary compensation for the older and less responsive ovary, where reduced oocyte numbers and reduced ovarian hormone production are present and lead to attenuated negative feedback on hypothalamic/pituitary secretion of FSH. High basal FSH levels should be used for counseling women as regards their outcome rather than exclude them from IVF cycles. FSH above 15 U/L in young women still show fair pregnancy rates, indicating that the quality can compensate for quantity of oocytes.[5] Cycling women with high FSH should be offered treatment without further delay.[6] We therefore routinely do not recommend S. FSH assessment, but rely more on baseline scan.

Serum Luteinizing Hormone (S. LH)

- Day 2–3 LH along with S. FSH is done in patients with PCOS. However, high LH indicates only anovulation which can be judged by history. Therefore, routine LH is not done.
- Day 8–9 LH in CC cycles: Clomiphene citrate (CC) stimulated hypothalamus to secrete FSH and LH. High LH is detrimental to ova and gives poor pregnancy

rate with CC in spite of good ovulation rates. Therefore, when LH is more than 10–12 iu/L, CC should not be given for the second cycle and patients should be switched over to gonadotropins.

In IVF/ICSI cycles, OHSS is common for PCOS patients. In these patients, therefore antagonist protocol is preferred to long agonist protocol and agonist is used for ovulation trigger in these patients.[9]

Serum Estradiol Level (E2)

- Follicular maturity: Serum estradiol helps to decide the maturity and quality of the follicle. Especially when the follicle looks mature but the endometrium appears thin, it is E2 level that can decide whether it is the follicular immaturity or local endometrial cause for the same. Normal E2 level is 150 pg/mL/follicle. Lower level than this indicates a bad quality or immature follicle. Normal serum estradiol level with thin endometrium indicates a local cause.
  Though if color Doppler can also be used for assessment of follicular and endometrial quality.
- For poor responder: For IVF cycles, E2 is done on day 2. If E2 more than 80 pg/mL, it indicates poor IVF outcome as it indicates early follicular recruitment due to high FSH and poor ovarian reserve.[7,8] This is not required for IUI cycles and in majority of assisted reproductive technology (ART) cycles.
- To assess ovarian suppression: In IVF cycles with long agonist protocol, gonadotropin-releasing hormone agonist (GnRHa) is started from day 21 of previous cycle. This down regulates pituitary and FSH; LH levels are therefore very low. In turn, it also brings E2 to baseline levels. To assess downregulation, therefore, E2 is done on day 2 of the cycle and stimulation may be started if E2 less than 30 pg/mL, or some may also allow less than 50 pg/mL. In patients who are on downregulation with oral contraceptive pills, E2 levels are checked after 12 days of pills to start stimulation.
- For suspected risk of hyperstimulation: After superovulation in IUI cycles or when gonadotropins are used for ovulation induction, ovaries may develop multiple follicles. Ovarian hyperstimulation syndrome (OHSS) is feared in such patients. E2 level can be measured for these patients. In non-IVF cycles, E2 more than 1,600 pg/mL and in IVF cycles E2 levels more than 4,000 pg/mL on the day of human chorionic gonadotropin (hCG) can cause OHSS. Chronic low-dose gonadotropin ovulation induction protocol is preferred in PCOS patients. In spite of that if 4–5 follicles develop in each ovary, GnRHa can be used for ovulation trigger to avoid OHSS.

Serum Progesterone (S. Progesterone)

Major part of progesterone is secreted by corpus luteum in second half of the cycle. Otherwise, it is an intermediate hormone for other steroid hormones.

Normal values:

Follicular phase	: 1 ng/mL
LH surge	: 1–2 ng/mL
Ovulation	: 3 ng/mL

Midluteal S. progesterone, i.e., a week before menses is approximately 10 ng/mL. A level of more than 3 ng/mL indicates ovulation. Therefore, if only ovulation is to be documented, repeated ultrasound scans are not required. In the same way, endometrial biopsy is not required to confirm secretory changes in endometrium and S. progesterone estimation suffices for the same.

Ultrasound with color Doppler is a better modality to assess the secretory phase of the cycle. It can define all luteal phase problems such as luteal phase defect and luteinized unruptured follicle. Therefore, it is the inevitable conclusion that random S. progesterone has little value beyond documentary ovulation.

Serum Prolactin (S. Prolactin)

Prolactin is the hormone secreted by anterior pituitary and is regulated by prolactin inhibitory factor, which is secreted from hypothalamus.

- Normal level of prolactin is 10–25 ng/mL.
- In microadenoma, it is between 100 and 200 ng/mL.
- In macroadenoma, it is more than 200 ng/mL.
- Immunoassay for prolactin does not reflect the bioassay always.
- Many a times, patients have no symptoms in spite of high prolactin level because of presence of macromolecules, which are big prolactin molecules that account for 10–12% of hyperprolactin in a normal patient.

Galactorrhea with Normal Prolactin Levels

Many a times, patients with galactorrhea present with normal S. prolactin levels. This may be mucoid discharge and not actual galactorrhea. Any discharge therefore from the breast should be checked under microscope. If it contains fat globules, only then it is galactorrhea.

When ovulation induction is done, in many patients estrogen leads to rise in prolactin levels in the first half of the menstrual cycle. These patients are known as spikers. This is transient hyperprolactinemia. The clinical presentation is poor endometrium in spite of good follicles. This condition is difficult to diagnose, but bromocriptine can be given in a dose of 1.25 mg/BD in these patients in first half of the cycle. It is a therapeutic test. If endometrium improves, it is continued in the subsequent cycle; otherwise, it is stopped. If patient is a spiker, she needs treatment; otherwise this condition also deteriorates oocyte quality and causes LPD.

Marginally, high prolactin levels are also found in PCOS patients due to high estrogen and high DHEA-S. In these cases, bromocriptine or cabergolin is not the treatment, PCOS needs to be treated.

17-OH-Progesterone

This investigation is done in all patients with hirsutism. It is increased due to 21-hydroxykase deficiency. Because of 21-hydroxylase deficiency in patients of heterogeneous carrier, late onset of congenital adrenal hyperplasia is observed. 17-OH-P is a weak androgen and manifests as hirsutism, acne, clitoral enlargement and menstrual irregularity at puberty.

Normal level of 17-OH-P is less than 200 ng/dL. Whenever the level is between 200 and 800 ng/dL, it requires ACTH testing. Levels of more than 800 ng/dL is diagnostic of 21-hydroxylase deficiency.[10] These patients are treated with dexamethasone 0.5 mg daily at bedtime.

S. Testosterone

Normal value of S. testosterone is 20–80 ng/dL. Its normal production is 0.2–0.3 mg/day. Out of this, 80% binds to sex hormone binding globulin (SHBG) and 19% to albumin. Only 1% is free testosterone. Testosterone may rise in PCOS and tumors. Tumor is suspected if there is sudden onset of symptoms due to increased testosterone. The PCOS patients show gradual rise in testosterone levels.[11] Routine estimation of S. testosterone is not required as it does not change the line of treatment.

Hormone	*Source*
Testosterone	50% peripheral conversion
	25% ovary
	25% adrenal
Androstenedione	50% ovary
	50% adrenal
DHEA	90% adrenal
	10% ovary
DHA	100% adrenal

S. DHEA-S

DHEA-S is exclusively secreted from adrenal glands. The normal value is 350 ng/dL. It increases with hyperprolactinemia. Therefore, in patients with PCOS, prolactin and DHEA-S are slightly on higher side, which do not require any specific treatment except the treatment of PCOS. This rise is secondary to estrogen because of anovulation.

Whenever DHEA-S is very high, it is due to adrenal tumor. Therefore, ultrasound is better guide to diagnose adrenal tumour. S. testosterone and ultrasound suffices to rule out adrenal tumors.

If there is moderate rise in PCOS and it does not require any treatment. If 17-OH-P is normal, there is no need to search for adrenal enzyme defect. DHEA-S more than 700 μg/dL is accepted as a marker for adrenal dysfunction. This is rarely found and does not change the management. Therefore, routine testing of DHEA-S is not required.

Inhibin A and B

Inhibin B is predominantly secreted by antral follicles. Low day 3 inhibin B level less than 45 pg/mL has poor response to superovulation and patient is less likely to conceive. Same thing can be judged by S. FSH, serum anti-Müllerian hormone (S. AMH) or AFC and so routine use of inhibin B estimation is not justified.

Inhibin A is secreted from preovulatory follicles. Both inhibin A and B are secreted from granulosa cells and regulate FSH by negative feedback mechanism. Routine estimation of inhibin A does not add any information to change the management of the patient.

Serum Anti-Müllerian Hormone (S. AMH)

Introduction

It is a member of transforming growth factor (TGF). It is produced from granulosa cells. The expression of AMH is localized in granulosa cells of primary preantral and small antral follicles and has important role in human folliculogenesis. AMH expression in follicle decreases in antral follicle more than 8 mm in size. In follicles undergoing atresia and in corpus lutea also the AMH expression is completely lost.[12]

AMH levels in women are low until the age of 8, rise rapidly until puberty and decline steadily from the age of 25 until menopause, when AMH production ceases.

It is now well established that serum AMH concentrations reflect the number of preantral and small antral follicles in the ovary, this would account for raised AMH levels found in both PCOM and PCOS.[13]

Physiology

Anti-Müllerian hormone has an inhibiting role in the ovary; contributing to follicular arrest.[14] It lowers the sensitivity of follicles to FSH, which is required for normal foliculogenesis. *In vitro* studies have shown that the action of FSH in promoting follicular growth is counteracted by AMH.[15] It has a steady level throughout the cycle except for a slight dip just after LH peak.[16] Though some investigators have recorded cyclical fluctuations in AMH with rapid decrease in early luteal phase.[17]

AMH and PCO

The reported property of AMH to counteract the actions of FSH implies that the high production of AMH by polycystic ovary may have an important role in the pathophysiology of the syndrome.[14] In anovulatory PCOS, the failure of follicle development is due to an intrinsic inhibition of FSH action and that this inhibition is due to an intrinsic inhibition of FSH action and that this inhibition is due to the high concentration of AMH.[18] Increased ovarian stromal blood flow in PCOS may be because of over expression of vascular endothelial growth factor (VEGF), which modulates the permeability of theca cells and increase insulin like growth factor 1 (IGF 1),[19,20] which in turn enhances gonadotropin-stimulated steroid production in granulosa cells and theca cells resulting in increased ovarian androgen production and subsequently increased AMH production.[21] AMH levels are two to three times higher in PCOS, than in healthy controls.[22] This has been attributed not only to increased number of antral follicles but also to higher production of AMH per follicle in patients with PCOS as compared to size-matched counterparts from normal ovary.[23]

In addition, a positive correlation between AMH and both LH and testosterone serum concentrations in PCOS has been reported.[24]

Each individual follicle in a PCO in women with PCOS produces significantly more AMH than its sized-matched counterpart from a normal ovary.[23] Moreover, it has also been shown that metformin administration in PCOS patients is associated with reduction in AMH concentration in follicle and serum, suggesting that the measurement of AMH can be used to evaluate the treatment efficacy with insulin sensitizers.[25]

It can predict ovarian response. It can predict menopause by low levels. High AMH is very high in PCOS, and it predicts OHSS.

AMH values and implications.[26]

Ovarian fertility potential	*Pmol/L*	*ng/mL*
Optimal fertility	28.6–48.5	4.0–6.8
Satisfactory fertility	15.7–28.6	2.2–4.0
Low fertility	2.2–15.7	0.3–2.2
Very low/undetectable	0.0–2.2	0.0–0.3
High level	>48.5	>6.8

AMH and IVF

In IVF patients, S. AMH value can predict the response of ovary and so it is useful for counseling the patient. When calculated optimal AMH cut off of less than 1.26 ng/mL was used to predict responses to COS, it was found to have a 97% sensitivity for predicting poor responses (<4 oocytes retrieved) and 98% accuracy in predicting a normal COS response.[27] Nelson et al. suggested the following strategy for deciding the COS protocol.[28]

However, we have found AFC as equally effective and more precise for prediction of ovarian response. We never routinely do AMH levels either in IVF or non-IVF cycles. With extremely low-serum AMH levels, moderate, but reasonable pregnancy and live birth rates are still possible. Extremely low-AMH levels do not seem to represent an appropriate marker for withholding fertility treatment. Younger women are likely to have better pregnancy rates than their older counterparts with equally low AMH.[29]

Constant AMH and inhibin B levels suggest that neither AMH nor inhibin B is an accurate marker of ovarian response after low-dose gonadotropins ovulation induction in patients with PCOS.[30] Mashiach et al. have also shown a relationship between follicular fluid AMH concentrations and the quality of embryos in patients with PCOS.[31]

Routine use of AMH does not help in managing non-ART patients. We require 1–2 follicles for superovulation with IUI and AMH will not help us in changing the line of treatment.

Poor responding ovary or low-reserve ovary can be very well judged by ultrasound and very precise.

Serum AMH estimation is indicated in:[32]

- Predicting both over and under response in controlled ovarian hyperstimulation (COH).
- Determining the most appropriate treatment regimen.
- Pretreatment counseling for couples to make an appropriate and informed choice.
- Predicting long-term fertility.
- Predicting the age of menopause.
- Predicting ovarian aging prior to or following chemotherapy/surgery.
- Screening for polycystic ovaries.

The inhibitory effect of AMH on folliculogenesis may in future be used for hormonal contraception.

Clinical applications of AMH, apart from fertility assessment:

- To confirm presence of testicular tissue in children with low testosterone levels.
- Differential diagnosis of intersex disorders.
- In patients with bilateral nonpalpable gonads.
- Females with granulosa cell tumors.

Insulin Resistance

Now it has been proved that in patients of PCOS there is high androgen because of increased insulin level and its sensitivity. It indicates the severity of PCOS. Clinically waist circumference of 35 inches or 90 cm is predictive of abnormal endocrinology and metabolic function.[33]

There are various methods to diagnose insulin resistance. But 2 hours glucose and 2 hours insulin response is the most reliable one.[34]

Two hours glucose tolerance test:

- Normal: <140 mg/dL
- Impaired: 140–190 mg/dL
- Noninsulin dependent DM ≥ 200 mg/dL

Two hours insulin response test:

- Insulin resistance very likely: 100–150 μU/mL
- Insulin Resistance: 151–300 μU/mL
- Severe insulin resistance: >300 μU/mL

In clinical practice, patients with high insulin resistance are the ones who require ovarian drilling. They have tonically high LH levels and therefore drilling helps. Alternatively, they may also be benefitted by GnRHa.

Antagonist decreases LH levels, prevents premature luteinization and improves oocyte quality. Patients who do not want ovulation induction and immediate pregnancy are the patients for Metformin therapy.

3D US is a novel way to diagnose insulin resistance, based on the assessment of stromal volume.[35] However, for all those who do not have volume ultrasound, 2 hours glucose and 2 hours insulin tests are the best alternative.

Therefore, for chronic anovulation, only three investigations are required:

- S. prolactin
- S. TSH
- Insulin resistance

Thyroid Function Tests

- Normal level is 0.5–2.5 miu/mL.
- If TSH is high, measure free T4.
- Any woman after the age of 35 should be assessed for thyroid function.
- Presence of anti-thyroid antibodies indicates future hypothyroidism.
- During pregnancy or in recurrent pregnancy loss, it is done every 2 months.
- Requirement of thyroxine decreases with age.
- For hyperthyroidism, T4 is measured and if it is normal, T3 is measured.

LABORATORY INVESTIGATIONS FOR THE MALE INFERTILITY

In patients of male infertility, there are three important hormonal investigations: S. TSH, S. LH and S. Testosterone used for diagnosis and treatment plan.

There are various permutation combinations of these hormones discussed in this chapter.

High FSH, High LH, Low/Normal Testosterone

This indicates primary testicular failure, due to spermatogenic and Leydig cell damage. Treatment option for these patients will be only donor insemination or adoption. These patients cannot even provide sufficient number of sperms for intracytoplasmic sperm injection (ICSI).

High FSH, Normal LH, Normal Testosterone

Here there is primary spermatogenic failure. As LH is normal, there is no leydig cell damage. This is due to inhibin deficiency. Treatment option to these patients is again donor insemination or adoption.

We have seen that in both the groups FSH is high. Therefore, instead of assessing these three hormones, one can assess only S. FSH and if that is high evaluation of other two hormones is not required. But if S. FSH is normal, LH and testosterone levels need to be assessed.

In patients with high FSH, with normal LH and testosterone, the possible diagnosis is varicocele. In grade 3 varicocele, because of testicular damage, FSH is borderline high. In these patients varicocele ligation + gonadotropins + antioxidants can improve spermatogenesis in many cases.

Normal FSH, High LH, High T (Testosterone)

Normally LH and T are regulated by negative feedback mechanism. But here LH and T both are high as T is not perceived by receptors. This is known as partial androgen resistance. High androgen will be converted into estradiol and so E2/T ratio will be high. This high E2 will cause gynecomastia, that is a diagnostic criterion. This causes oligo-astheno-teratozoospermia, which does not respond to drugs. ART is advised in these patients or adoption if the patient is not affording, after proper counseling.

Normal FSH, Normal LH, Normal T

This is a very common finding in our patients. It may be due to organic cause like obstruction in ductal system, retrograde ejaculation, varicocele or germ cell failure. The treatment is according to the cause.

- Obstruction: surgery or ICSI after PESA/TESA.
- Retrograde ejaculation: α adrenergic blocking drugs + IUI or ART.
- Varicocele: surgery + gonadotropins + antioxidants
- Germ cell failure:
  Spermatogonia arrest: Donor insemination
  Spermatid arrest: FSH + ICSI.

But most commonly patients having azoospermia with normal FSH, LH and T, do not have any pathological cause. These patients have qualitative failure causing azoospermia or severe oligozoospermia.

As discussed in the chapter on medical management of male infertility, these patients can be treated with FSH or human menopausal gonadotropin (HMG) 75–150 units thrice a week and hCG twice a week. It has given excellent results in many cases. In these cases, endogenous bioactivity is poor in spite of normal immunological levels (RIA test). This is why exogenous FSH, LH and hCG are useful.

Low FSH, Low LH, Low T

These are the patients having hypogonadotropic hypogonadism. These patients can be treated by hCG 5,000 iu every fifth day for 5–7 weeks till testosterone becomes normal as it is required for initiation of spermatogenesis. After testosterone becomes normal, FSH is added thrice a week for maturation of sperms. This is given for 3–6 months. But results are excellent and it initiates spermatogenesis.

There may be panhypopituitarism which require replacement of thyroid, corticotrophin and growth hormone (GH). There may be Kallmann syndrome which is congenital. Prolactinoma is normally macro type which requires surgery.

Hyperprolactinemia

Most diagnostic symptom is loss of libido. There is no galactorrhea or gynecomastia. Cause of low testosterone is macroadenoma leading to hyperprolactinemia, and this macroadenoma must be removed. If there is no macroadenoma, oligospermia is because of androgen resistance. Therapy of choice for these patients is long term bromocriptine or cabergolin.

Thyroid Dysfunction

Autoimmune thyroiditis is the most common condition. Hypothyroidism can cause oligospermia. Hypothyroidism

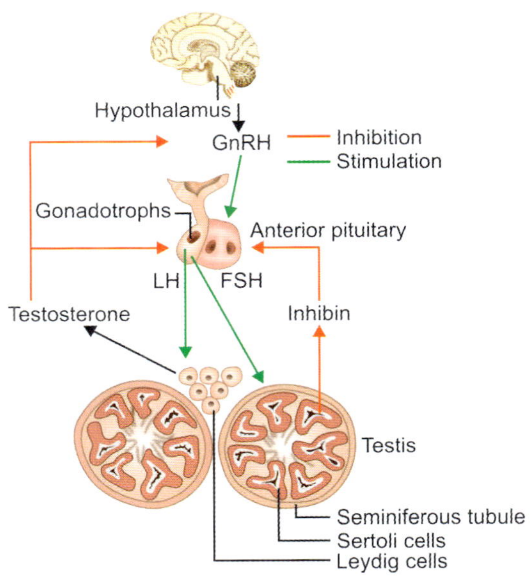

Fig. 2.1: Hypothalamo-pituitary–testicular axis.
(FSH, follicle-stimulating hormone; GnRH, gonadotropin-releasing hormone; LH, luteinizing hormone).

can cause hyperprolactinemia because of high TSH. Hyperthyroidism also causes oligospermia. Therefore, thyroid function assessment is required in patients of oligospermia.

Adrenal Dysfunction

- Infertility may be only manifestation.
- Family history of congenital adrenal hyperplasia.
- Increased DHEA-S causes increased prolactin levels.
- Signs and symptoms of adrenal insufficiency.
- Signs and symptoms of feminization and soft testis.

Endocrine workup:

1.	S. FSH	6.	S. DHEA-S
2.	S. LH	7.	S. Estradiol
3.	S. Testosterone	8.	S. 17-OH-P
4.	S. Prolactin	9.	S. Cortisol
5.	S. TSH & T4	10.	SHBG

REFERENCES

1. Muasher SJ, Oehniger S, Simonetti S, Amtta J, Ellis LM, Liu HC, et al. The value of basal and/or stimulated serum gonadotrophin levels in prediction of stimulation response and *in vitro* fertilization outcome. Fetil Steril. 2003;50:298.
2. Scott RT, Toner JP, Muasher SJ, Oehninger S, Robinson S, Rosenwaks Z. Follicle stimulating hormone levels on cycle day 3 are predictive of *in vitro* fertilization outcome. Fertil Steril. 1989;51:651.
3. Bancsi LF, Broekman FJ, Mol BW, Habbema JD, te Valde ER. Performance of basal follicle stimulating hormone in prediction of poor response and failure to become pregnant after *in vitro* fertilization: a meta-analysis. Fertil Steril. 2003;79:1091-100.
4. Pearlstone AC, Fournet N, Gambone JC, Pang SC, Buyalos RP. Ovulation induction in women age 40 and older: the importance of basal follicle stimulating hormone level and chronological age. Fertil Steril. 1992;58:674.
5. van Rooji IA, de Jong E, Broekmans FJ, Looman CW, Habbema JD, te Velde ER. High follicle stimulating hormone levels should not necessarily lead to the exclusion of subfertile patients from treatment. Fertil Steril. 2004;81:1478-85.
6. Abdalla H, Thum MY. Repeated testing of basal FSH levels has no predictive value for outcome in women with elevated basal FSH. Hum Reprod. 2006;21(1):171-4.
7. Smotrich DB, Widra EA, Gindoff PR, Levy MJ, Hall JL, Stillman RJ. Prognostic value of day 3 estradiol on *in vitro* fertilization outcome. Fertil Steril. 1995;64:1136.
8. Licciardi FL, Lui HC, Rosenwaks Z. Day 3 estradiol serum concentrations as prognosticators of ovarian stimulation response and pregnancy outcome in patients undergoing *in vitro* fertilization. Fertil Steril. 1995;64:991.
9. Homborg R, Hendriks ML, König TE, Anderson RA, Balen AH, Brincat M, et al. Clomifene citrate or low dose FSH for the first-line treatment of infertile women with anovulation associated with polycystic ovary syndrome: a prospective randomised multinational study. Hum Reprod. 2011;27(2):468-73.
10. Kuttenn F, Couillin P, Girard F, Billaud L, Vincens M, Boucekkine C, et al. Late onset adrenal hyperplasia in hirsutism. New Engl J Med. 1985;323:224.
11. Easterling Jr WE, Talbert LM, Potter HD. Serum testosterone levels in the polycystic ovary syndrome. Am J Obstet Gynecol. 1974;120:385.
12. Elvin JA, Clark AT, Wang P, Wolfman NM, Matzuk MM. Paracrine actions of growth differentiation factor-9 in the mammalian ovary. Mol Endocrinol. 1999;13(6):1035-48.
13. Fanchin R, Maria SL, Righini C, Guibourdenche J, Frydman R, Taieb J. Serum AMh is more strongly related to ovarian follicle status that serum inhibin B, oestradiol, FSH and LH on the day 3. Hum Reprod. 2003;18:323-7.
14. Pellat L, Rice S, Mason HD. Anti-Müllerian hormone and polycystic ovarian syndrome: a mountain too high? Reproduction. 2010;139:825-33.
15. Durlinger AL, Gruijters MJ, Kramer P, Karels B, Kumar TR, Matzik MM. Anti-Müllerian hormone attenuates the effect of FSH on follicle development in the mouse ovary. Endocrinology. 2001;142:4891-9.
16. La MArca A, Stabile G, Artenisio AC, Volpe A. Serum anti-Müllerian hormone throughout the human menstrual cycle. Hum Reprod. 2006;21(12):3103-7.
17. Streuli J, Fraisse T, Chapron C, Bijaoui G, Bischof P, de Ziegler D. Clinical uses of anti-Müllerian hormone assays: pitfalls and promises. Fertil Steril. 2009;91(1):226-30.
18. Pellat L, Rice S, Dilaver N, Heshri A, Galea R, Brincat M, et al. Anti-Müllerian hormone reduces follicle sensitivity to follicle-stimulating hormone in human granulosa cells. Fertile Steril. 2011;96:1246-51.
19. El Behery MM, Diab AE, Mowafy H, Ebrahiem MA, Shehata AE. Effect of laparoscopic ovarian drilling on vascular endothelial growth factor and ovarian stromal blood flow using three dimensional power Doppler. Intern J Gynecol Obstet. 2011;112:119-21.
20. Abd El, Aal DE, Mohamed SA, Amine AF, Meki AR. Vascular endothelial growth factor and insulin like growth factor 1 in polycystic ovary syndrome and their relation to ovarian blood flow. Eur J Obstet Gynecol Reprod Biol. 2005;118:219-24.
21. Willis D, Mason H. Gilling-Smith C, Franks S. Modulation by insulin of follicle stimulating hormone and luteinizing hormone actions in human granulosa cells of normal and polycystic ovaries. J Clin Endocrinol Metab. 1996;81:302-9.
22. Pigny P, Merlen E, Robert Y, Cortet-Rudelli C, Decanter C, Jonard S, et al. Elevated serum level of anti-Müllerian hormone in patients with polycystic ovary syndrome: relationship to the ovarian follicle excess and to the follicular arrest. J Clin Endocrinol Metab. 2003;88:5957-62.
23. Pellat L, Hanna L, Brincat M, Galea R, Brain H, Whitehead S, et al. Granulosa cell production of anti-Müllerian hormone

is increased in polycystic ovaries. J Clin Endocrinol Metab. 2007;92:240-5.
24. Carlsen SH, Vanky E, Fleming R. Anti-Müllerian hormone concentrations in androgen suppressed women with polycystic ovary syndrome. Hum Reprod. 2009;24:1732-8.
25. Piltonen T, Morin-Papunen L, Koivunen R, Perheentupa A, Ruokonen A, Tapanainen JS. Serum anti-Müllerian hormone levels remain high until late reproductive age and decrease during metformin therapy in women with polycystic ovary syndrome. Hum Reprod. 2005;20(7):1820-6.
26. Nelson SM, Yates RW, Fleming R. Serum anti-Müllerian hormone and FSH: prediction of live birth and extremes of response in stimulated cycles—implications for individualization of therapy. Hum Reprod. 2007;22:2414-21.
27. Gnoth C, Schuring AN, Friol K, Tigges J, Mallmann P, Godehardt E. Relevance of anti-Müllerian hormone measurement in a routine IVF program. Hum Reprod. 2008,23:1359-65.
28. Nelson SM, Yates RW, Lyall H, Jamieson M, Traynor I, Gaudoin M, et al. Anti-Müllerian hormone based approach to controlled ovarian stimulation for assisted conception. Hum Reprod. 2009;24:867-75.
29. Weghofer A, Dietrich W, Barad DH, Gleicher N. Live birth chances in women with extremely low serum anti-Müllerian hormone levels. Hum Reprod. 2011;26(7):1905-9.
30. Fong SL, Schippe I, de Jong FH, Themmen APN, Visser JA, Laven JSP. Serum anti-Müllerian hormone and inhibin B concentrations are not useful predictors of ovarian response during ovulation induction treatment with rFSH in women with polycystic ovary syndrome. Fertil Steril. 2011;96(2):459-63.
31. Mashiach R, Amit A, Hasson J, Amzalzg S, Almog B, Ben-Yosef D, et al. Follicular fluid levels of anti-Müllerian hormone as a predictor of oocyte maturation, fertilization rate, and embryonic development in patients with polycystic ovarian syndrome. Fertil Steril. 2010;93(7):2299-302.
32. Loh JS, Maheshwari A. Anti-Müllerian Hormone-is it a crystal ball for predicting ovarian ageing? Human Reprod. 2011;26(11):2925-32.
33. Poluit MC, Despres JP, Lemieux S, Moorjani S, Bouchard C, Tremblay A, et al. Waist circumference and abdominal saggital diameter: best simple anthropometric indexes of abdominal visceral adipose tissue accumulation and related cardiovascular risk in men and women. Am J Cardiol. 1994;73:460.
34. Fritz MA. Chronic Anovulation and the polycystic ovary. In: Fritz MA, Speroff L. (Eds). Clinical Gynecologic endocrinology and infertility. Lippincott Williams and Wilkins Publication. p. 495-532.
35. Panchal S, Nagori CB. Correlation of ovarian and stromal volumes to fasting and post-prandial insulin levels in polycystic ovarian syndrome patients. Correlation of ovarian and stromal volumes to fasting and postprandial insulin levels in polycystic ovarian syndrome patients. Int J Infertil Fetal Med. 2014;5(1):12-4.

CHAPTER

3

Assessing Ovarian Reserve

Chaitanya Nagori

INTRODUCTION

Definition

The ovarian reserve (OR) means the capacity of the ovaries to produce fertilizable ova.

Physiology

The number of follicles in the female fetus at 20 weeks of intrauterine age is 6–7 millions and is decreased to approximately 2 million at birth. At puberty, the number decreases to approximately 3–4 lakhs. Fertility decreases after the age of 30 years, when number of follicles are as low as approximately 25,000 only. After the age of 35 years, the prevalence of infertility sharply increases and when the woman reaches the age of 40 years, approximately only 8,000 follicles are available for recruitment. After the age of 45, 99% of women are expected to be infertile.[1] Antral follicle count (AFC) showed the best correlation with women's age and declined linearly at a rate of 3.8% per year.[2]

Another study has also indicated a biphasic pattern of AFC decline. It was documented as 4.8% per year before the age of 37 years compared with 11.7% thereafter.[3]

The number of quantity and quality of the follicles in the ovary thus remaining determine the OR.[4]

When number of ova drops to less than 1,000, menopause occurs. The age of menopause varies between 40 and 60 years with an average age of 51 years. After the age of 42, fertility of the female decreases drastically.[5]

Why Assessment of Ovarian Reserve is Required?

The changing trends and lifestyle has led to late marriages in career oriented women and further delay in planning a family to pursue the career are responsible for decrease in OR in women seeking pregnancy. This social change has increased the incidence of infertility.[6]

Assessing the OR is therefore an essential step before patient counseling to refuse, advance, or postpone fertility treatment and also to decide stimulation protocols. The assessment of OR gives the prognostic information of fertility and allows planning the line of treatment. It helps the couple for choosing the best treatment after counseling. It is therefore essential to assess the OR in the females in whom low reserve is suspected.

According to the literature,[7] the OR needs to be assessed in females who are older than 35 years, have unexplained infertility, and in females who have had a previous cycle of ovulation induction with gonadotropins and had a poor response. In the females, who have a history of ovarian surgery in the past or a smoker also have a risk of low OR and need to be evaluated for the same before recruiting them for fertility therapy. Females who have maternal relations with early menopause also have a higher risk of low OR. In these females, the OR assessment needs to be done at an age much earlier than 35 years as they may be genetically predisposed to low OR and early ovarian failure. These females need special advice for advancement of fertility treatment. But it should be emphasized that decrease in OR does not mean inability to conceive.[7]

Though it is important to mention at this stage here that the pattern of reproductive ageing as assessed by hormonal and ultrasonographic OR tests does not appear to show an abrupt change at a certain age, but follows a continuously increasing rate of decline in the 3rd decade of life. The changes in serum FSH levels and ultrasonographic OR tests follow a quadratic model in regularly menstruating women.[8]

As no test is perfect to comment on fertility potential and plan of treatment, evaluation by combination of tests may be required for the assessment of OR.[8] All the OR tests are considered as screening tests, and abnormal tests should be confirmed by another tests.[7]

OVARIAN RESERVE TESTS

- Clinical markers
- Endocrinal markers
- Ultrasound markers

Clinical Markers

- Age
- Menstrual pattern

Age

It has been already emphasized that advancing age decreases the OR due to apoptosis. This means that age is the single most factor that decides the quantity of the ova in the ovary. Moreover, the quality of the ova available has also been negatively correlated with the increasing age.

But chronological age and ovarian age are not always correlating. A young woman may have low OR and a woman of 40 may also have several antral follicles in her ovaries. Therefore, other tests of OR are required for deciding the line of treatment.

The monthly fecundity rate is about 20% in young couple. With increasing age, fecundity decreases and may take longer time to achieve conception. Society of ART (SART) and disease control and prevention (CDC) have constantly demonstrated that age is the single most factor affecting the probability of success of IVF.

Twenty four percent of oocyte in a woman of less than 35 years will be abnormal, but this number reaches 52% at the age of 35 years. After 40 years, more than 90% of the oocytes are abnormal.[9]

Chronological age is more related to quality of the ova rather than increased follicle-stimulating hormone (FSH). Young women with high FSH may give good ova but old women with low FSH have a high chance of aneuploidy in the ova. This means that the abnormal tests in younger patients have poor prognosis but normal tests do not improve the age related poor prognosis in older patients.

Menstrual Pattern

Length of the menstrual cycle depends on the length of the follicular phase. Length of the normal cycle is 21–35 days (28 days—mean) of which the length of the luteal phase is constant. The quality of the egg deteriorates with increasing age which is responsible for short follicular phase and short cycle length. There will be high FSH and low serum inhibin B level in these patients. This is common as age advances.[10]

Endocrinal Tests

Static Tests

- Day 2/3 serum FSH (S. FSH)
- Day 2/3 serum estradiol (S. E2)
- Day 3 S. FSH and serum liutenizing hormone (S. LH)
- Inhibin B
- Anti-Müllerian hormone (AMH)

Dynamic Tests

- Clomiphene citrate challenge test (CCCT)
- GnRH Analogue stimulation test (GAST)
- Exogenous FSH ORT (EFFORT).

Day 2/3 FSH: FSH level in serum when is assessed, it must be combined and correlated with estrogen. This is because there is a negative feedback system between FSH and estrogen. On day 2–3, all follicles are small (antral), so the estrogen level is low and FSH levels at this stage are the baseline FSH levels. Normal FSH with low E2 indicates normal hypothalamo-pituitary-gonadal axis. The level of FSH increases with increasing age due to falling basal estrogen levels and indicates low OR. Fluctuations in the serum FSH levels in different cycles also indicate diminished OR.[11]

Normal basal FSH is less than 10 μ/mL. Levels between 10 and 15 μ/mL are considered borderline. The OR will be very low when the level of FSH is more than 15 μ/mL. But it has poor predictive value for nonpregnancy. No single cut-off has been established to predict nonpregnancy. Therefore, cycle cancellation should not be advised only on the ground of S. FSH levels. Though a recent study has demonstrated 100% specificity for failure to achieve a live birth at FSH values above 18 μ/mL (Table 3.1).[12]

The FSH is released from anterior pituitary in a pulsatile manner and also has circadian variations. Moreover, isoforms of FSH are also known and there may be fluctuations in these also. This may lead to variable results when serum FSH levels are assessed at different times in the same patient. Single nucleotide polymorphism (SNP) in FSH receptive gene may have normal FSH with poor response. SNPs at 307 and 680 are common.[13]

In this case, it is best to consider the highest value for the decision-making and counseling with the patient for fertility treatment planning. Whatever is the ovarian response, pregnancy rates are poor with high S. FSH levels.

Table 3.1: Correlation of serum FSH levels to ovarian response.

FSH level	*Response*
≤8 μ/mL	Reassure
8–12 μ/mL	Average reserve
12–17 μ/mL	Decreased ovarian reserve
>17 μ/mL	Extremely poor pregnancy rates

Day 2/3 S. Estradiol: Estradiol is secreted from granulosa cells and reflects the follicular activity.

High estradiol level on day 2–3 of the menstrual cycle indicates early follicular recruitment. This is reflected on ultrasound as a follicle of 10 mm or larger on day 2–3 of the cycle. This is because of high basal FSH. Cycle cancellation is much higher when estradiol is 80 pgm/mL or more or 20 pgm/mL or less.[14] High day 2 FSH and estradiol have high predictive value for OR, and when both are high indicates poor OR.[15] High E2 may mask an abnormal FSH concentration in a patient with diminished OR due to negative feedback mechanism.

In patients with polycystic ovarian syndrome (PCOS), estradiol level on day 2 is high because of cumulative estradiol produced from granulosa cells of multiple follicles. E2 level alone is never used as a sole marker for OR.

FSH/LH ratio: High FSH/LH ratio indicates poor OR. FSH rises earlier than LH and frequent measurements may diagnose this rise earlier. FSH/LH ratio is an early indicator of ovarian aging and rising FSH/LH ratio could be the first marker of ovarian aging and decreased OR.[16]

Inhibin B: It is secreted from small antral follicles and selectively inhibits FSH release. As the number of eggs decreases with advancing age, it will lower inhibin B level which in turn gives higher FSH value because of negative feedback mechanism. Decrease in inhibin B occurs earlier than rise in FSH with decreasing OR, but inhibin B assays are variable, requires validation, and there is cycle-to-cycle variability.[17] This is why it is not used as a routine investigation for evaluation of OR.

Though, inhibin B measurement in early stages of the ovarian stimulation provides useful information in making decision to cancel the cycle or to modulate the doses of gonadotropin. The level more than 45 pgm/mL on day 2–3 is indicative of hyper-response to ovulation induction.

Anti-Müllerian hormone: Anti-Müllerian hormone is produced by granulosa cells of primordial, preantral, and small antral follicles.[18] The function of AMH is to modulate primordial follicle recruitment. It inhibits the action of FSH on the follicular growth and selection. Its expression is maintained till the follicle is 6 mm in diameter, beyond which follicles grow under the effect of FSH. The function of AMH is inhibition of initial recruitment of primordial follicles and inhibits the activity of granulosa cells and decreases if follicular growth starts with FSH stimulation.[19-21]

So AMH is a negative regulator of follicular growth and reduces follicular sensitivity to FSH. FSH exerts negative influence on AMH secretion in small follicles.[22]

Therefore, AMH is considered to be reflective of FSH independent follicular growth. AMH reflects quantitative and qualitative assessment of OR. AMH level helps in counseling the woman before chemotherapy as it can predict menopause. Its level becomes negligible, 5 years before actual menopause. It is undetectable before puberty also.

Anti-Müllerian hormone level is constant throughout the menstrual cycle, except that it has lower thresholds in late luteal phase.

In poor response, AMH varies from 0.5 to 1.1 ng/mL, but by this level only exclusion from IVF should not be done. Higher doses of gonadotropins are not much useful in decreased ovarian response, but flare-up protocol and addition of LH can improve the results. Normal AMH has good prognosis and they are normal responders. High AMH indicates exaggerated response after gonadotropin stimulation. So low dose protocol will be useful which avoid ovarian hyperstimulation syndrome (OHSS) as well as improve implantation because of lower steroids.

Anti-Müllerian hormone assays: Formerly two companies having different immunoassays were marketing the kits for AMH assessment. One was DSL, i.e. Diagnostic Systems Laboratory and other one IOT (Immuno tech branded as Beckman Coulter). IOT had four to five times higher values than DSL. This is why there was a confusion and low reliability of the results for AMH assessment numbers and units. Fortunately, now is single new commercially available assay the Gen II enzyme linked immunosorbent assay is available and that has replaced DSL and IOT. Now the new assay is reported as ng/mL like IOT.

Normal values and their interpretation:

- Extremely low levels: Less than 1 pmol/L (DSL) or less than 1.1 pmol/L (gen II assay)
  These patients are poor responders and cycle cancellation rates are very high. These patients may be offered ovum donation.
- Low levels: 1–5 pmol/L (DSL) or between 1.1 and 6.9 pmol/L in gen II assay. These patients are poor responders and have decreased OR and less number of ova can be retrieved when they are stimulated for *in vitro* fertilization. In these cases, 300 IU of FSH should

be used, which is maximum and antagonist protocol should be used.

- Normal levels: 5–15 pmol/L and it is 7–20 pmol/L by gen II assay. These are normal responders. In these cases, agonist protocol is used and maximum dose of FSH required is 225 IU/day for IVF patients.
- High level: When AMH is more than 15 pmol/L (DSL) or more than 20 pmol/L (gen II assay). These patients are hyper-responders. Maximum dose used in these patients is 150 IU daily. But even lower doses and antagonist protocols are preferred.[23,24]

Though AMH assessment done during ovarian stimulation gives erroneous results. With chronic low dose protocol, FSH administration mimics the natural cycle and significant decrease in AMH is observed till the day of follicular dominanace.[25] In IVF cycles with multifollicular development, there is decreased AMH because of decrease in small number of follicles.[26] Assessing AMH during ovarian stimulation is not useful.

Endocrine Dynamic Tests

Clomiphene citrate challenge test: The test is based on the fact that clomiphene citrate (CC), when given for ovulation induction, will stimulate the follicle to produce more inhibin and E2 that will in turn lower FSH on day 10.

Basal level of S. FSH is assessed on day 3 and then is repeated on day 10 after CC stimulation. Higher value of FSH (more than 10 μ/mL) either on day 3 or on day 10 indicates diminished OR. The total of both values more than 26 IU indicates poor reserve.[27,28] Normally LH rises more than FSH after clomiphene stimulation. But in patients with low reserve, FSH rises more than LH. The speculated mechanism is that smaller follicles produce less inhibin B and less estradiol, resulting in less negative feedback to FSH that is released due to clomiphene stimulation.[29,30]

This test does not have a high prognostic value as there is no standardized definition of abnormal test. Because of availability of better tests like AFC and AMH, this test is routinely not used.

GnRH analog stimulation test: In this test, GnRH agonist (leuprolide acetate 1 mg) is given subcutaneously. This causes massive release of FSH and LH from the pituitary which in turn increases the production of estradiol from the follicles within 24 hours time frame. This increase in E2 level (twice the baseline level) or flare-up of E2 level in response to stimulation indicates early development of follicles, indicating good OR.[31,32] But it lacks in standardization in terms of type of the drug, dose, and timing, etc. Therefore, this test is not used routinely in clinical practice.

Exogenous FSH ovarian reserve test: 300 IU of rFSH is given to a patient on day 3 of the cycle. After 24 hours, E2 and inhibin levels are assessed. Increase in E2, more than 30 pgm/mL is predictive of good response.[27,33]

This test like CCCT and GAST is far from uniform and not used in clinical practice.

This means that no dynamic tests can be used at present in routine practice. These are not better than basal tests and these cannot predict nonpregnancy in any patient.

Ultrasound Markers

- Ovarian volume
- Antral follicle count
- Ovarian blood flow

Ovarian Volume

Ovarian volume can be measured by B mode or by 3D ultrasound. To assess it on B mode, the ovary is located first. The probe is rotated to find the long axis of the ovary. The probe is then spanned across the long axis of the ovary to find the longest section of the ovary. Now the probe is rotated 90° to get a true transverse section of the ovary. On the long axis section, measure the largest longitudinal, and AP diameter of the ovary perpendicular to the longitudinal section and measure the transverse diameter on the transverse section. The volume is calculated as D1 × D2 × D3 × 0.523.[34,35] Three-dimensional ultrasound is recommended for more accurate volume calculation. It has low interobserver and intraobserver variability. Volume of 3 cc is taken as a lower cut-off for a normal reserve ovary. Ovarian volume of less than 3 cc was significantly predictive of more than 50% cancellation rates in IVF cycles.[36] (But this has poor predictive value for response to ovulation induction and possibility of pregnancy.)[37]

Ovarian volume of more than 10 cc indicates a possibility of PCOS and may require lower stimulating dose for ovulation induction. But ovarian volume alone is not predictive of OR.

Antral Follicle Count

Antral follicle count is defined as the total number of follicles seen in both ovaries, up to 9 mm in diameter, detected by transvaginal ultrasound (TVS) in early follicular phase (day 2–3 of the menstrual cycle). AFC can predict hyperstimulation as well as poor response after gonadotropin stimulation. Low AFC predicts poor response. AFC is also used to predict hyper-response and thus using in safe and successful stimulation regimes and to prevent OHSS.[38]

Antral follicle count is found to be as effective as AMH in determining ovarian response.[39,40] Smaller follicles (between 2 and 6 mm) decline in number with age and these indicate real OR.[41]

AFC is a better marker than day 3 FSH, estradiol, and inhibin. Another study concludes that AFC and AMH both correlate with each other but have independent significance for estimating follicles larger than 12 mm on the day of hCG. For ova retrieved on ovum pick-up (OPU), in PCO group both AMH and AFC have similar significance.[42] AFC can be correlated to the quality as well as quantity of the oocytes.[43] AFC has low intercycle as well as interobserver variability. Intercycle variability is more significant in young woman when AFC is higher. Low AFC with ovulatory cycle does not indicate poor reserve. The 3D is extremely useful for counting antral follicles. Inversion mode rendering is most convenient when follicles are multiple.

Anti-Müllerian hormone and antral follicle count: Receiver operating characteristic curves showed high accuracy for AMH and AFC for the prediction of poor ovarian response but limited accuracy for nonpregnancy prediction. These data does not show a better predictive ability than AFC.[39,40,44]

For prediction of poor ovarian response, a model including AFC with AMH was found to be almost similar to that of (p value 0.001) using AFC alone.[45]

Ovarian Blood Flow

Ovarian blood flow as a predictor of IVF outcome was assessed by many workers. Though another study shows ovarian stromal PSV after pituitary suppression is predictive of ovarian responsiveness and outcome of IVF treatment.[46] Kupesic et al. have shown correlation in the ovarian stromal flow index (FI) and number of mature oocytes retrieved in an IVF cycle and pregnancy rates. *Stromal FI (<11 low responder, 11–14 good, >15 risk of OHSS).*[47] Measurement of ovarian stromal flow in early follicular phase is related to subsequent ovarian response in IVF treatment.[48]

But it was not found to be accurate and it cannot predict future fertility. It can only predict response to IVF treatment.

The ovarian volume, AFC, vascularization index (VI), flow index (FI), and vascularization flow index (VFI) determined by 3D power Doppler, all have excellent intraobserver and interobserver reproducibility.[49]

The findings of our unpublished study are given (Table 3.2).

Table 3.2: 3D PD parameters in hyper-response, normal-response and poor-response ovaries.

Index	*Hyperresponse*	*Normal*	*Low response*
Vascularization index	5–10	2–5	<2
Vascularization flow index	2–3	1–2	<0.5

It is essential to mention here that AFC, ovarian volume, and ovarian 3D power Doppler flow indices did not significantly change after a short-term treatment of GnRH agonist for pituitary downregulation.[50] It can therefore be reliably used for downregulated as well as non-downregulated cycles for assessment of ovarian response.

Clinical applications: The AMH and AFC are most widely used tests. These can assess the OR quantitatively and qualitatively. No significant difference is observed between the two in terms of accuracy. Both may contribute and act synergistically.[51]

We decide the stimulation protocol based on the parameters like AFC, ovarian volume, ovarian stromal RI, ovarian stromal PSV, stromal FI, age, and body mass index (BMI). The calculation can be simplified by the Table 3.3.[52]

To select the correct stimulation protocol, doses are titrated depending on findings present in a particular patient from high-dose table or low-dose table.

Integrated predictors: La Marca et al. developed an ovarian response predictor index (ORPI). This is based on age,

Table 3.3: Variables that will decide high-dose or low-dose requirement for ovulation induction.

	Increase the dose when..	*Decrease the dose when..*
Age	>35 years	<25 years
BMI	>28 kg/m^2	<20 kg/m^2
AFC	<3 Follicle number per ovary (FNPO)	>12 (FNPO)
Stromal RI	>0.7	<0.5
Stromal PSV	<5 cm/sec	>10 cm/sec
Stromal FI	<11	>15
Ovarian Volume	<3 cc	>10 cc

AMH, and AFC. ORPI less than 0.2 has 86% sensitivity and 89% specificity in predicting poor ovarian response (less than three oocytes), with 88% efficacy. ORPI more than 0.9 has same sensitivity, specificity, and 82% efficacy in prediction of high response (>15 follicles).[53]

Another study has recently been published in which a scoring system has been devised based on the ultrasound parameters: ovarian volume, AFC, ovarian stromal RI, and ovarian stromal PSV with age and BMI.[54] This study has shown zero severe OHSS rate, very low incidence of mild OHSS, and acceptable multiple pregnancy rates.

Bologna criteria:[55] EHRE group has come to the consensus that out of three, two criteria should be present to define poor OR for future research.

a. Maternal age more than 40 or other risk factors for poor OR (genetic or acquired conditions).
b. Previous history of less than three oocytes with a conventional stimulation protocol.
c. Abnormal OR test, i.e. AFC less than 5–7 or AMH less than 0.5–1.1 ng/mL.

Many patients above 40 years of age, may be infertile, though the menstrual cycles are normal. So the patient with good reserve benefit better with IVF and should be offered IVF, if AFC is good.[56]

Genetic predictors: Single nucleotide polymorphism in gonadotropins and its receptors is not associated with change in OR. But some polymorphism in FSH receptors (FSHR) particularly Ser680 genotype are related with resistance to FSH stimulation. These patients require high doses of FSH in spite of other OR markers being normal.[57,58] These observations require further validation by larger studies (Table 3.4).

It has been summarized.[59]

Table 3.4: Ovarian reserve tests and their values suggesting favorable or unfavorable response to ovulation induction.

Ovarian reserve test	*Favorable result*	*Unfavorable result*
Age(in years)	≤35	≥35
FSH (IU/L)	<10	≥10
Day 3 E_2 (pg/mL)	<75	≥75
Day 10 progesterone	≤0.9	≥1.1
AMH (p/mol/L)	15.7–48.5	<15.7
Day 3 Inhibin B (pg/mL)	>45	≤45
AFC	≥5	<5
Ovarian vascularity	Lower PI	Higher PI
Ovarian volume (cc)	≥3	<3
CCCT(FSH only—IU/L)	<12	≥12
GAST	Early E_2 flare	Persistent high E_2/no response

CARRY-HOME MESSAGE

- All ORTs are considered as screening tests, and abnormal test result should be confirmed by another test.
- No test or combined test can predict nonpregnancy.
- Age is the single reliable factor.
- Short follicular phase indicates DOR.
- Day 2–3 FSH more than 12–15 indicates DOR.
- Day 2 E2 more than 80 pgm/mL indicates DOR.
- FSH/LH ratio if high, indicates DOR.
- Inhibin B more than 45 pgm/mL indicates good reserve.
- CCCT, GAST, and EFORT are not used in clinical practice.
- AMH is extremely reliable for counseling (5–15 pmol/L indicates good reserve).
- Ovarian volume is as reliable as AMH, and AFC more than 5 indicates normal reserve.
- Stromal flow decides the doses required and response to stimulation.

REFERENCES

1. Menken J, Trusell J, Larsen U. Age and infertility. Science. 1986;233(4771):1389-94.
2. Ernest Hung Yu Ng, Yeung WSB, Fong DYT, Ho PC. Effects of age on hormonal and ultrasound markers of ovarian reserve in Chinese women with proven fertility. Hum Reprod. 2003;18(10):2169-74.
3. Scheffer GJ, Broekmans FJM, Dorland M, Habbema JDF, Looman CWN, te Velde ER. Antral follicle counts by transvaginal ultrasonography are related to age in women with proven natural fertility. Fertil. Steril. 1999;72:845-51.
4. Broekmans FJ, Kwee J, Hendriks DJ, Mol BW, Lambalk CB. A systematic review of tests predicting ovarian reserve and IVF outcome. Hum Reprod Update. 2006;12:685-718.
5. Van Noord-Zaadstra BM, Looman CW, Alsbach H, Habbema JD, te Velde ER, Karbaat J. Delaying child bearing: effect of age on fecundity and outcome of pregnancy. BMJ. 1991;302:1361-5.
6. Ventura SJ, Mosher WD, Curtin SC, Abma JC, Henshaw S. Trends in pregnancy rates for the United States 1976-97: an update. Natl Vital Stat Rep. 2001;49:1-9.
7. Practice Committee of American Society for Reproductive Medicine. Testing and interpreting measures of ovarian reserve: a committee opinion. Fertil Steril. 2012;98:1407-15.

8. Tufan E, Elter K, Durmusoglu F. Assessment of reproductive ageing patterns by hormonal and ultrasonographic ovarian reserve tests. Hum Reprod. 2004;19(11):2484-9.
9. Alvin ST, Lim BS, Maurine FH, Tsakok MD. Age related decline in fertility: A link to degenerative oocytes? Fertil Steril. 1997;68:265-71.
10. Van Zonneveld P, Scheffer GJ, Broekmans FJ, Blankenstein MA, de Jong FH. Do cycle disturbances explain the age related decline of female fertility? Cycle characteristics of women aged over 40 years compared with a reference population of young women. Hum Reprod. 2003;18(3):495-501.
11. Perloe M, Levy DP, Sills ES. Strategies for ascertaining ovarian reserve among women suspected of subfertility. In J Fertil Women's Med. 2000;45:215-24.
12. Scott RT Jr, Elkind-Hirch KE, Styne Gross A, Miller KA, Frattarelli JL. The predictive value for *in vitro* fertility delivery rates is greatly impacted by the method used to select the threshold between normal and elevated basal FSH. Fertil Steril. 2008;89:868-78.
13. Oschsenkuhn R, von Schonfeldt V, Simoni M. FSH receptor polymorphisms and ovarian function. Gynécologie Endocrinologie. 2009;11(4):265-70
14. Frattarelli JL, Bergh PA, Drews MR, Sharara FI, Scott RT. Evaluation of basal oestradiol levels in assisted reproductive technology cycles. Fertil Steril. 2000;74(3):518-24.
15. de Carvalho BR, Rosa E, Rosa E. Use of ovarian reserve markers and variables of response to gonadotrophic stimulus as predictors of embryo implantation in ICSI cycles. Journal Brasileiro deReproducao Assistida. 2009;13(3):26-9.
16. Mukherjee T, Copperman AB, Lapinski R, Sandler B, Bustillo M. An elevated day three follicle-stimulating hormone: luteinizing hormone ratio (FSH:LH) in the presence of a normal day 3 FSH predicts a poor response to controlled ovarian hyperstimulation. Fertil Steril. 1996;65:588-93.
17. Al-Azemi M, Killick SR, Duffy S, Pye C, Refaat B, Hill N, et al. Multi-marker assessment of ovarian reserve predicts oocyte yield after ovulation induction. Hum Reprod. 2011;26(2):414-22.
18. Visser JA, de Jong FH, Laven JS, Themmen AP. Anti-Müllerian hormone: a new marker for ovarian function. Reproduction. 2006;131:1-9.
19. Durlinger AL, Visser JA, Themmen AP. Regulation of ovarian function: the role of anti-Müllerian hormone. Reproduction. 2002;124:601-9.
20. Di Clemente N, Goxe B, Remy JJ, Cate R, Josso N, Vigier B, et al. Inhibitory effect of AMH upon aromatase activity and LH receptors of granulosa cells of rat and porcine immature ovaries. Endocrine. 1994;2:553-8.
21. Josso N, di Clemente N, Gouedard L. Anti-Müllerian hormone and its receptors. Mol Cell Endocrinol. 2001;179:25-32.
22. Anderson CY, Byskov AG. Estradiol and regulation of anti-Müllerian hormone, inhibin A and inhibin B secretion: analysis of small antral and preovulatory human follicles' fluid. J Clin Endocrinol Metab. 2006;91:4064-9.
23. Faddy MJ, Gosden RG, Gougeon A, Richardson SJ, Nelson JF. Accelerated disappearance of ovarian follicles in mid-life: implications for forecasting menopause. Hum Reprod. 1992;7(10):1342-6.
24. Nelson SM, Yates RW, Fleming R. Serum anti-Müllerian hormone and FSH: prediction of live birth and extremes of response in stimulated cycles-implications for individualization of therapy. Hum Reprod. 2007;22:2414-21.
25. Catteau-Jonard S, Pigny P, Reyss AC, Decanter C, Poncelet E, Dewailly. Changes in serum anti-Müllerian hormone level during low dose recombinant follicle-stimulating hormone therapy for anovulation in polycystic ovary syndrome. J Clin Endocrinol Metab. 2007;92:4138-43.
26. La Marca A, Malmusi S, Giulini S, Tamaro LF, Orvieto R, Levratti P, et al. Anti-Müllerian hormone plasma levels in spontaneous menstrual cycle and during treatment with FSH to induce ovulation. Hum Reprod. 2004;19:2738-41.
27. Maheshwari A, Gibreel A, Bhattacharya S, Johnson NP. Dynamic tests of ovarian reserve: a systematic review of diagnostic accuracy. Reprod BioMed Online. 2009;18(5); 717-34.
28. Kwee J, Schats R, McDonnell J, Schoemaker J, Lambalk CB. The Clomiphene citrate challenge test versus the exogenous follicle stimulating hormone ovarian reserve test as a single test for identification of low responders and hyperresponders to *in vitro* fertilization. Fertil Steril. 2006;85(6):1714-22.
29. Hofmann GE, Danforth DR, Seifer DB. Inhibin B: The physiologic basis of the clomiphene citrate challenge test for ovarian reserve screening. Fertil Steril. 1998;69:474.
30. Yong PY, Baird DT, Thong KJ, McNeilly AS, Anderson RA. Prospective analysis of the relationships between the ovarian follicle cohort and basal FSH concentration, the inhibin response to exogenous FSH and ovarian follicle number at different states of normal menstrual cycle and after pituitary downregulation. Hum Reprod. 2003;18:35.
31. Ravhon A, Lavery S, Micheal S, Donaldson M, Margara R, Trew G. Dynamic assays of inhibin B and oestradiol following buserelin acetate administration as predictors of ovarian response in IVF. Hum Reprod. 2000;15(11):2297-301.
32. Hendriks DJ, Broekmans FJM, Bancsi LFJMM, de Jong FH. Repeated Clomiphene citrate challenge testing in the prediction of outcome in IVF: a comparison with basal markers for ovarian reserve. Hum Reprod. 2005;20(1):163-9.
33. Kwee J, Etling MW, Schats R. Comparison of endocrine tests with respect to their predictive value on the outcome of ovarian hyperstimulation in IVF treatment: results of a prospective randomized study. Hum Reprod. 2003;18(7):1422-7.
34. Gibreel A, Maheshwari A, Bhattacharya S, NP Johnson. Ultrasound tests of ovarian reserve: a systematic review of accuracy in predicting fertility outcomes. Hum Fertil. 2009;12(2):95-106.
35. Syrop CH, Dawson JD, Husman KJ. Ovarian volume may predict assisted reproductive outcomes better than follicle stimulating hormone concentration on day 3. Hum Reprod. 1999;14(7):1752-6.
36. Lass A, Skull J, McVeigh E, Margara R, Winston RM. Measurement of ovarian volume by transvaginal sonography before

ovulation induction with human menopausal gonadotrophin for in-vitro fertilization can predict poor response. Hum Reprod. 1997;12(2):294-97.

37. Hendriks DJ, Kwee J, Mol BW, Lambalk CB. Ultrasonography as a tool for the prediction of outcome in IVF patients: a comparative metaanalysis of ovarian volume and antral follicle count. Fertil Steril. 2007;87:764-75.
38. Broer SL, Dolleman M, Opmeer BC, Fauser BC, Mol BW, Broekmans FJ. AMH and AFC as predictors of excessive response in controlled ovarian hyperstimulation: a meta-analysis. Hum Reprod Update. 2011;17:46-54.
39. Muttukrishna S, McGarrigle H, Wakim R, Khadum I, Ranieri DM, Serhal P. Antral follicle count, anti-Müllerian hormone and inhibin B: predictors of ovarian response in assisted reproductive technology? BJOG. 2005;112: 1384-90.
40. Nardo LG, Christodoulou D, Gould D, Roberts SA, Fitzgerald CT, Laing I. Anti-Müllerian hormone levels and antral follicle count in women enrolled in *in vitro* fertilization cycles: relationship to life-style factors, chronological age and reproductive history. Gynecol Endocrinol. 2007;1-8.
41. Haadsma ML, Bukman A, Greon H et al. The number of small antral follicles(2-6 mm) determines the outcome of endocrine ovarian reserve tests in subfertile population. Hum Reprod 2007; 22:1925-31.
42. Panchal S, Nagori CB. Comparison of anti-Müllerian hormone and antral follicle count for assessment of ovarian reserve. JHRS. 2012;5(3):274-8.
43. Johnstone EB, Rosen MP, Addauan-Andersen C, Sternfeld B, McCulloch C, Cedars MI. Is AFC a marker of oocyte quality? Fertile women have higher AFCs than infertile women. Fertil Steril. 2010;94(4):S-63.
44. Gruijters MJ, Visser JA, Durlinger AL, Themmen AP. Anti-Müllerian hormone and its role in ovarian function. Mol Cell Endocrinol. 2003;211:85-90.
45. Jayakrishnan K, Akansha A, Divya N, Shankar R. Comparison of antral follicle count, anti-Müllerian hormone and day 2 follicle stimulating hormone as predictor of ovarian response and clinical pregnancy rate in patient with an abnormal ovarian reserve test. Int J Reprod Contracept Obstet Gynecol. 2016;5(8):2762-7.
46. Engmann L, Sladkevicius P, Agrawal R, Bekin JS, Campbell S, Tan SL. Value of ovarian stromal blood flow velocity measurement after pituitary suppression in the prediction of ovarian responsiveness and outcome of *in vitro* fertilization treatment. Fertil Steril. 1999;71(1):22-9.
47. Kupesic S, Kurjak A. Predictors of invitro fertilization outcome by three dimensional ultrasound. Hum Reprod. 2002;17(4):950-5.
48. Zaidi J, Barber J, Kyei-Mensah A, Bekir J, Campbell S, Tan SL. Relationship of ovarian stromal blood flow at baseline ultrasound to subsequent follicular response in an *in vitro* fertilization program. Obstet Gynecol. 1996;88:779-84.
49. Merce LT, Gomez B, Engels V, Bau S, Bajo JM. Intraobserver and interobserver reproducibility ov ovarian volume, antral follicle count and vascularity indices obtained with transvaginal 3-dimensional ultrasonography, power Doppler angiography and virtual computer aided analysis imaging program. J Ultrasound Med. 2005;24:1279-87.
50. Ng EHY, Chan CCW, Tang OS, Yeung WSB, Ho PC. Effect of pituitary downregulation on antral follicle count, ovarian volume and stromal blood flow measured by three-dimensional ultrasound with power Doppler prior to ovarian stimulation. Hum Reprod. 2004;19(12):2811-5.
51. Broer SL, Mol BW, Hendriks D, Broekmans FJ. The role of anti-Müllerian hormone in prediction of outcome after IVF: comparison with the antral follicle count. Fertil Steril. 2009;91:705-14.
52. Panchal S, Nagori CB. Baseline scan and ultrasound diagnosis of PCOS. Donald School journal of Ultrasound in Obstetrics and Gynecology. 2012;6(3):290-9.
53. La Marca A, Grisendi V, Guilini S, Argento C, Tirelli A, Dondi G, et al. Individualization of FSH dose in IVF/ICSI cycles using the antral follicle count. J Ovarian Res. 2013;6:11.
54. Panchal S, Nagori CB. Ultrasound based decision making on stimulation protocol for superovulated IUI cycles. IJIFM. 2016;7(1):7-13.
55. Ferraretti AP, Gianaroli L. The Bologna criteria for the definition of poor ovarian responders: is there a need for revision? Hum Reprod. 2014;29(9):1842-5.
56. Klinkert Ellen R, Frank JM, Caspar WN, J Dik FH, Egbert R te Velde. The antral follicle count is a better marker than basal follicle-stimulating hormone for the selection of older patients with acceptable pregnancy prospects after *in vitro* fertilization. Fertil Steril. 2005;83(3):811-4.
57. La Marca A, Siqhinolfi G, Argento C, Grisendi V, Casarini L, Volpe A, et al. Polymorphisms in gonadotrophin and gonadotrophin receptor genes as markers of ovarian reserve and response in *in vitro* fertilization. Fertil Steril. 2013;99: 970-8.
58. Moron FJ, Ruiz A. Pharmacogenetics of controlled ovarian hyperstimulation: time to corroborate the clinical utility of FSH receptor genetic markers. Pharmacogenomics. 2010;11:1613-8.
59. Luciano G, Nardo, Mohiyiddeen L. Ovarian serve as a guide for ovarian stimulation. In: Aboulghar M, Rizk B (Eds). Ovarian Stimulation. Cambridge University Press; 2011. pp. 255-61.

CHAPTER

4

Ovulation Induction

Chaitanya Nagori

INTRODUCTION

Ovulation induction is the most important aspect of any assisted reproductive technology (ART). The success of the ART is dependent on the selection of ovulation induction protocols.

The drugs that are available for the purpose can be used individually or in combination. These chiefly are of two types. These are pharmacological agents, which mimic endogenous gonadotropins to stimulate ovarian function or are agents that manipulate the endogenous gonadotropin secretions through effect on estrogen receptors or estrogen production to stimulate ovaries for producing follicles. The first group are usually injectable gonadotropins and the second group are oral ovulogens. Although researches are being done to produce oral gonadotropin preparations. Amongst the oral ovulogens, those which act on estrogen receptors are called selective estrogen receptor modulators (SERMS) like clomiphene citrate (CC) and those which affect estrogen production are aromatase inhibitors, of which the most commonly used and found to be most effective is letrozole. Gonadotropins commonly used are [follicle-stimulating hormone (FSH)], luteinizing hormone (LH), and human menopausal gonadotropins (HMG). These were earlier produced from menopausal urine but now are produced as recombinant forms.

For the judicious use of these chemicals, it is essential to understand the pharmacology and action of each.

CLOMIPHENE CITRATE

Introduction

Ovarian induction with CC was first published by Green-Blatt et al. in 1961.[1] CC now available commercially is a mixture of two isomers, enclomiphene (trans) 62% and zuclomiphene (cis) 38%. Enclomiphene is more antiestrogenic, and, therefore primarily responsible for ovulation stimulation and has a half-life of few days.[2] Zuclomiphene is more potent, more estrogenic, and responsible for ovulation inducing actions. It is in clinical use since 1967 for dysovulatory infertility. The efficacy of the drug varies in clinical practice, if the proportion of enclomiphene and zuclomiphene are not maintained.[3]

Mechanism of Action

It acts as antiestrogenic agent. It binds with estrogen receptors at hypothalamus signaling lack of estrogen to hypothalamus. This in turn releases gonadotropin-releasing hormone (GnRH) that stimulates pituitary to secret more FSH and LH, which in turn stimulates the ovarian follicular development. As the duration of action is longer, (half-life of 5–21 days, depending on the isomer),[2] it allows more and more FSH and LH and leads to multifollicular development. Clomiphene has direct effect on ovary to stimulate follicular estradiol synthesis also. It increases the GnRH pulse frequency in ovulatory patients and pulse amplitude in anovulatory patients like polycystic ovarian syndrome (PCOS). Clomiphene does not display progestational, corticotropic, androgenic, or antiandrogenic properties.

The disadvantage of CC is that when it binds with the estrogen receptors, it remains there for days or weeks, unlike natural estrogen, which stays there only for hours. This leads to gradual depletion of estrogen receptors.[1]

When to Use Clomiphene Citrate?

It will be effective as ovulation induction in patients in whom reasonable levels of endogenous estrogen are present and hypothalamo-pituitary-ovarian (HPO) axis is intact.

I. WHO group II patients: It is extremely effective in anovulatory patients in whom HPO axis is normal and have normal basal levels of endogenous estradiol (oligo-anovulation, PCOS, etc.). Normal thyroid function tests and prolactin should be confirmed before starting the treatment.[4] It is not effective in hypogonadotropic hypogonadism, i.e. WHO group I as there is no negative feedback mechanism of estrogen.[5]

II. Luteal phase defect (LPD): Short luteal phase is associated with low levels of FSH in follicular phase causing LPD. CC will increase FSH and LH in follicular phase, develops the good follicle, and corrects the abnormality in luteal phase. So CC is the drug of choice in LPD due to short luteal phase.[6]

III. Unexplained infertility: The rationale of using CC in unexplained infertility is that it corrects subtle defects due to deficiency of FSH and LH. It increases the number of follicles available for fertilization and corrects LPD.[7] Cochrane database supports the use of CC in unexplained subfertility.[8] Former belief of cervical dysmucorrhea and decreasing endometrial receptivity in unexplained infertility is not accepted and instead of contraindication, it is the indication for CC in modern era for unexplained infertility.

Clomiphene citrate should not be used in patients with ovarian cyst and abnormal uterine bleeding. It should also not be used in individuals having liver dysfunction, thyroid or adrenal dysfunction, or an organic intracranial pathology. It is a category X drug and is not recommended in pregnancy.

Treatment Regimes

Clomiphene citrate is given as 50 mg dose daily between day 2 and day 5 (both inclusive) for 5 days after spontaneous or induced bleeding. Ovulation, conception, and pregnancy rates are same independent of the day when CC is started. But day 5 is the most accepted day for starting the treatment.

Most women (up to 74%) respond to clomiphene with maximum 100 mg daily dose. Higher doses have very poor pregnancy rate (12% with 150 mg, 7% with 200 mg, and 5% with 250 mg).[9] Prof. Bruno Lunenfeild and Prof. Roy Homburg have recommended only one dose to start with and maximum 100 mg daily. The advantage of using this dose is that it can diagnose clomiphene resistant cases earlier and will cut down superfluous cycles of treatment till ovulation occurs. Highest pregnancy rates with CC has been documented in first three treatment cycles and the chances significantly decrease after six cycles; therefore, it is not recommended to continue CC beyond six treatment cycles.[10]

Monitoring of Clomiphene Citrate Cycles

Serum progesterone in midluteal phase if is more than 3 ng/mL, it is an evidence of ovulation. LH detection kit can help to know the LH surge. Normally LH surge occurs after 7 days of the last dose of CC. Ultrasound is a useful tool to monitor ovulation induction but serial sonography just for documenting ovulation, when no intervention is intended, is not justified.

It is justified to assess S. LH on day 8–9 of the cycle and if it is more than 10 IU/mL, success rate with CC is very low because of poor quality ova and embryo.

Efficacy of the Drug

Clomiphene citrate will induce ovulation in approximately 75–80% of cases. Up to 45–75% of cumulative pregnancy rate can be achieved in 3–9 months.[11] So, if the patient has not conceived within 3–6 months with CC, re-evaluation of the patient and switching over to further management may be required.

Side Effects

Though serious side effects are extremely rare, transient hot flushes (13.6%), mood swings (64–78%), breast tenderness, nausea (2.2%), and pelvic pain (5.5%) may occur.[12] Some may also complain of headache or visual disturbances.[13]

Antiestrogenic effect of CC is one of the major side effects of CC.

Antiestrogenic effect on cervix, endometrium, ovary, ovum, and embryo have been described, but there is no objective evidence that these effects occur or have clinical consequences. Endometrial thickness is within normal range in majority of cases. Very rarely endometrium suppression is observed, which is less than 6 mm in spite of a good mature follicle. It also leads to reduction in glandular density and increase in the number of vacuolated cells.[14] In these cases, patients may be shifted over to other therapy. Decreased uterine blood flow during the early luteal phase has also been found in patients on CC.[15]

Cervical dysmucorrhea can be overcome by intrauterine insemination (IUI). Exogenous estrogen supplementation is of no benefit as the receptors are blocked.[16]

Starting CC early in the cycle or using other SERMs have also been not proved of any benefit.[17,18]

Risks of Clomiphene Citrate

Multiple pregnancy (5–8%) is one of the important unwanted effect of CC due to its long half-life and continued production of FSH and LH.[19] It is because of this effect that the risk of ovarian hyperstimulation is also associated with CC therapy. Though a dreaded complication, it may be seen only in PCOS patients when CC is used as ovulation inducing agent. CC treated patient when conceived had a 23.7% risk of pregnancy loss as compared to 20.4% in spontaneous pregnancies.[20] There is no substantial evidence that CC increases the risk of congenital fetal anomalies or causes any particular birth defects.[21,22] Previous studies suggested that if CC is used for more than 12 months, it can increase the risk of ovarian malignancy. But subsequent studies have proved that fertility drugs are not associated with any invasive cancers. CC does not increase the risk of breast cancer.[23-25] Women on clomiphene therapy must be counseled that no causal relationship has been established between ovulation inducing drugs and breast or ovarian cancer. However, prolonged treatment with CC is futile and should be avoided because it has little success.

Alternative Treatment Regimes with Clomiphene Citrate

Extended Clomiphene Treatment

In patients who did not respond to standard regimes, CC is given for 7–10 days in a dose of 150–250 mg per day or 50 mg/day may be given for 5 days and increment of 50 mg/day is done every 5 days to reach 250 mg/day.[26] No factor has been identified that can predict which patient will respond to extended regime. Such extended regimes have extremely poor pregnancy rates and are not much helpful in clinical practice.

Combination of Clomiphene Citrate with Other Drugs

Clomiphene citrate with glucocorticoids: This combination is very useful in chronic anovulatory patients. It leads to androgen suppression and, therefore, it can be given to those patients who have high dehydroepiandrosterone sulfate (DHEAS). It can be given to all the patients who show increase in adrenal androgen production. It has given good results even with normal DHEAS and unselected population and even PCOS having clomiphene resistance.[27] Those patients who are resistant to 100–150 mg of CC, start ovulating when glucocorticoids are added. Glucocorticoids are given in the form of dexamethasone 0.5 mg daily or prednisolone 5 mg daily continuously for 30 days at bed time.[28] It can be given continuously for 3–6 months. No serious side effects are seen, though water logging and weight gain have been documented. The dose can be reduced to 0.25 mg/day or can be stopped in second phase of the cycle.

Clomiphene citrate with estrogen: Estrogen was tried to improve cervical mucus and endometrial thickness but it has already been discussed earlier that adding estrogen does not help to correct the side effects of CC on cervical mucus or endometrium.[16]

Clomiphene citrate with bromocriptine: Bromocriptine is given to the patients of hyperprolactinemia. But there are two definite indications even with normal prolactin level.

i. Galactorrhea with normal prolactin level. In these cases, galactorrhea must be confirmed by presence of fat globules under the microscope in the secretions expressed from the breast. It must be differentiated from simple mucoid discharge that does have fat globules.
ii. There are patients who are known as spikers. In these patients, there are nocturnal spikes of prolactin in the first half of the cycle when CC is used for ovulation induction. The rise being transient is difficult to confirm even when repeated blood samples are taken. These patients are given bromocriptine in first half of the cycle. It is not to be continued in second half of the cycle as normal level of prolactin is required for maintenance of corpus luteum. Clinically, these patients show poor endometrium even though there is no local cause and follicle is very good and meet all parameters on B mode and color Doppler for optimum maturity. Bromocriptine can be tried in these patients and if endometrium improves, it can be continued for 3–6 months.[29]

Clomiphene citrate with hCG: Routine use of hCG for rupture of the follicle is not justified. If the follicle is mature, it will reflect as serum estradiol (E2) level of more than 150 pgm/mL. This will initiate the LH surge which in turn will cause rupture of the follicle and exogenous hCG is not required. But if the follicle is not mature and if hCG is given as a trigger for ovulation, it will lead to premature luteinization or atresia. Therefore, hCG must not be given just for ovulation.[30,31]

But hCG can be combined with clomiphene when IUI is to be done. hCG in these cases is done to time IUI as follicle ruptures at 34–36 hours after hCG injection. hCG can also be given in patients proved to have absent, inadequate, or delayed LH surge. This is a common occurrence in endometriosis. hCG, therefore, must be used for timed intercourse, to time IUI, and in cases of delayed LH surge.

Clomiphene citrate with gonadotropin: Gonadotropins are often combined with clomiphene with the idea that it would decrease the requirement of gonadotropins. CC by its direct effect on ovary, increases the sensitivity of ovary to gonadotropins. This combination has risks of ovarian hyperstimulation and multiple pregnancies. This combination has been documented to reduce the cost of the treatment.[32] But it does not increase the pregnancy rate to our opinion. The argument is that CC increases FSH and LH both. The poor pregnancy rate with CC is because of high LH which will remain in spite of adding gonadotropins. The effect of high LH will decrease the implantation and pregnancy rate. So even though we get a follicle after adding gonadotropins, in many of these patients, the follicular quality is not good and pregnancy rates are only comparable to CC alone and much less than gonadotropins alone. Instead letrozole is a better drug to be combined with gonadotropins.

Clomiphene citrate with antagonist: This makes a good combination in thin lean PCOS patients where LH is tonically raised. It improves the quality of ovum and also the conception rates. For patients on clomiphene therapy, serum LH levels are checked on day 8–9 of the cycle. If it is more than 10 IU/mL, it is an indicator of poor pregnancy rates. These are the ideal patients to start antagonist. Regular use of antagonist is not justified because it sharply decreases LH and quality of follicle is changed and it causes regression of follicle as well as LPDs.

Clomiphene citrate with metformin: Several workers have shown that metformin is inferior to CC for ovulation induction and metformin alone should not be used for ovulation induction. But in CC resistant cases of PCOS when metformin is combined with CC, it improves ovulation four to nine times more than clomiphene alone. This shall be further discussed in the chapter of PCOS.[33,34]

Prior Treatments

i. Clomiphene after prior treatment with oral contraceptive (OC) pills: The mechanism of action of OC pills is to decrease the LH surge. High LH will cause high androgen, which in turn will cause anovulation. So OC pills when given for 2–3 months will decrease the LH and in turn and androgen and improves sensitivity to clomiphene with the same dose. Therefore, in PCOS patients prior treatment with OC pills was given routinely in CC resistant cases and did show good results.
ii. Micronized progesterone: If it is given for 5 days, it modulates LH pulsatility, reducing LH concentration, and induces more favorable environment for CC.

AROMATASE INHIBITORS: LETROZOLE

Introduction

Letrozole is an aromatase inhibitor used for ovulation induction. It is the third generation of aromatase inhibitor. Another third generation aromatase inhibitor is anastrozole. The main advantage of the drug is that it is a reversible enzyme inhibitor. It was for the first time used by Mitwally et al. in 2001 for ovulation induction.[35]

Mechanism of Induction of Ovulation

Aromatase, a cytochrome P450 dependent enzyme, acts as ultimate step in synthesis of estrogen, catalyzing the conversion of androgen to estrogen. This conversion occurs at peripheral sites such as muscle, fat, and liver. Letrozole inhibits aromatase enzyme by completely binding to the heme of cyto 450 subunits of enzyme, so that androgen is not converted to estrogen.[36,37] The end result is low estrogen causing negative feedback at hypothalamus and pituitary releasing FSH and LH releasing factors resulting in high FSH and LH causing folliculogenesis. As androgen is not converted into estrogen, there is slightly higher level of androgen, which also causes folliculogenesis. Withdrawal of estrogen centrally increases activins also, which are produced by many tissues and pituitary and stimulates FSH synthesis by direct action on gonadotropes.[38] It has no effect on estrogen receptors and acts on hypothalamus. So, it has no deleterious effect on LH surge, cervical mucus, and endometrium. As FSH and LH stimulates folliculogenesis, estrogen will rise and will cause negative feedback on FSH. This is responsible for monofollicular development unlike CC.

It is a potent aromatase inhibitor with a very specific action. After oral administration, it has almost 100% bioavailability, and aromatase inhibitors are cleared from the systemic circulation by liver and have a half life of 30–60 hours.

Indications

Letrozole is widely used in CC resistant cases. Letrozole will reduce estrogen and stimulate hypothalamus to release LHRH to secrete more FSH and induces folliculogenesis, and, therefore, is the drug of choice for patients with PCOS, but this shall be discussed in the chapter dedicated to it. It can also be used in patients with endometriosis. There is an expression of aromatase enzyme in the endometriotic tissue, which leads to progression of endometriosis by highlighting the role of estrogen.[39] Inducing ovulation in these patients with letrozole leads to lower estrogen level and, therefore, protection against progression of the disease. For the same mode of action, it is also a choice of drug for ovulation induction in the survivors of estrogen-dependent malignancies,[40] and in those with high risk of coagulation disorders.[41] It may specifically be more beneficial in patients with implantation failure, especially in women having high levels of aromatase p450 in endometrium.

Characteristics of Letrozole

It causes total suppression of estrogen (up to 97–99%) with doses up to 5 mg/day. Maximum suppression occurs between day 5 and 7. After day 7, estrogen level will rise due to folliculogenesis because of increasing FSH after negative feedback of estrogen due to letrozole. This rise of estrogen will continue for 5–7 days. This E2 peak will cause LH surge for ovulation. So LH surge occurs after 12 days unlike CC when it occurs early. Estrogen rise after 7 days will decrease FSH, which will be responsible for monofollicular development. It has no antiestrogenic effect on cervical mucus or endometrium. Temporary rise of androgen improves the sensitivity of follicle to gonadotropin. It therefore requires lower dose of gonadotropins when it is combined with letrozole.

Advantages of Letrozole

Being almost free from side effects, letrozole is well tolerated and accepted by the patients. It gives monofollicular development,[35,42] so has less chances of multiple pregnancies, has no antiestrogenic effect, and therefore may give higher pregnancy rates. Having no ill effect on the endometrium, the risk of abortion is also decreased. When combined with gonadotropins, lower doses of gonadotropins are required as the androgen is high which sensitizes the follicles to FSH.[43] It has a wide margin of safety and toxicity is rare. Moreover, it is relatively inexpensive.

Regimes

- Recommended dose is 2.5 mg from day 3 to 7.
- Some workers suggest 5 mg dose. The disadvantage of 5 mg dose as a routine is not justified as 2.5 mg can suppress 97–99% of estrogen. A dose of 5 mg may suppress more estrogen causing more FSH to be secreted. So it may not cause monofollicular development. As it is a chemotherapeutic agent, it may be toxic to ovum and embryo.
- Single dose of 20 mg on day 3: It has advantage having short half-life and reduces embryotoxic effect. But symptoms of hypo-estrinism may develop.
- It is superior to anastrozole 1 mg from day 3 to 7.

Side Effects

It may lead to mild gastrointestinal disturbances and rarely asthenia, hot flushes, headache, and back pain. It may give postmenopausal or estrogen withdrawal symptoms. It increases intrafollicular androgen, which may arrest the growth of follicle. But optimum level of androgen is not yet decided.[44-46]

Letrozole with Gonadotropins

Letrozole with recombinant FSH (rFSH) is a good combination for giving equivalent pregnancy rates as gonadotropins with advantage that it decreases the requirement of gonadotropins by sensitizing the follicles to FSH due to high androgen, gives monofollicular development, less multiple pregnancy rates, and less abortion rates.

GONADOTROPINS

Introduction

Since 1958, human pituitary gonadotropin preparations have been used for ovulation induction.[47,48] Lunenfeld et al. first reported the use of HMG, produced from menopausal urine, followed by pregnancy in 1963.[49,50] Now purified preparations and recombinant preparations of gonadotropins are also available.

Physiology of Ovulation and Gonadotropin-induced Ovulation Induction

Ovary has a pool of primordial follicles. Primordial follicles are independent of gonadotropins. Primordial follicles grow into preantral follicles and primary antral follicles. Under the influence of androgen, preantral follicles grow into primary antral and secondary antral follicles. FSH rise in the late luteal phase of previous cycle decides the dominant follicle. Androgen sensitizes the follicles to FSH. For follicular cohort, minimum level of FSH is required and this is called FSH threshold. Large antral follicles can respond to gonadotropin stimulation. As the sensitivity of follicle to FSH increases with development, lower amount of FSH is required. As the amount of FSH decreases, it stops growth of other follicles except the dominant follicle. The process of selection of follicle is completed in 7 days. But when gonadotropins are given from outside, there will be larger number of follicles to grow and ovulate. FSH window means number of days the FSH levels are above threshold. FSH stimulates the follicle to grow. Follicle secretes estrogen which has negative feedback on hypothalamus to secrete less FSH. All oocytes are arrested in prophase stage in meiosis in preantral follicles. When follicle is mature and estrogen secretion is at its peak, pituitary receives a positive feedback for LH surge by the short loop. LH surge causes ovulation to occur. This inhibition is removed by LH surge and first meiotic division will be complete with extrusion of first polar body. Oocytes should be fertilized within 48–72 hours and second meiotic division occurs otherwise oocyte dies. Mature follicle is 16–18 mm and estrogen secretion from such a follicle is 150 pgm/mL/follicle.

Principles of Gonadotropin Therapy

The basic principles were suggested by Insler and Lunenfeld in 1974.[51]

1. Effective dose: Ovarian response is seen when certain dose of FSH is given. Below this dose, the ovaries do not respond.
2. Latent phase: This phase lasts for 3–7 days. It starts with onset of stimulation, but there is no estrogen rise or ultrasound demonstrable follicular growth during this phase.
3. Active phase: This phase starts with ultrasound demonstrable follicle growth to ovulation and it lasts for 4–6 days.

Follicle-stimulating Hormone Preparations Available

1. HMG 75 IU: 75 IU of FSH and 75 IU of LH
2. HMG-HP (highly purified): 75 IU of FSH and 75 IU of LH with less than 5% of urinary proteins
3. Urinary FSH: 75 IU of FSH and 1 IU of LH
4. FSH-HP: 75 IU of FSH with less than 0.1 IU of LH and less than 5% of urinary proteins
5. rFSH: 75 IU of FSH and no LH activity
6. rFSH + rLH combination

The urinary products are prepared from human menopausal urine and are called menotropins. These contain a lot of potentially allergic urinary proteins. These are orally inactive and are to be administered intramuscularly. These menotropins are processed and purified to remove these allergens in highly purified products. These can be given subcutaneously. These products may be called urofollitropins. These have only 1% of LH activity.[52] But these are still contaminated with 95% nongonadotropin related proteins. In 1990s, recombinant gonadotropins were produced by immunochromatography with monoclonal antibodies against gonadotropins. After development of rFSH, rLH was developed in 1994.[53] Where urinary products have the least bioactivity for a particular hormone, it is highest for the recombinant products.

Different Regimes of Gonadotropin Therapy

1. Step up protocol
2. Step down protocol
3. Chronic low dose protocol

Indications of Gonadotropins Therapy

A. Hypogonadotropic hypogonadism (substitutional therapy)
B. Hypothalamo-pituitary dysfunction:
    1. Clomiphene resistant patients
    2. Clomiphene failure patients
    3. Superovulation combined with IUI
    4. Gonadotropin as first line of treatment
    5. Controlled ovarian hyperstimulation (COH) in ART cycles

Step-up Protocol

Baseline scan, done on day 2–3 of the menstrual cycle, before starting stimulation, guides to decide the stimulating dose. Conventionally, in normal reserve, normal responding ovary, 1 amp, i.e. 75 IU of FSH is started from day 5 for 5 days. Ultrasound scan is done on day 5 of stimulation. If this scan shows a follicle of 10–12 mm and/or there is increase in endometrial thickness, the same dose

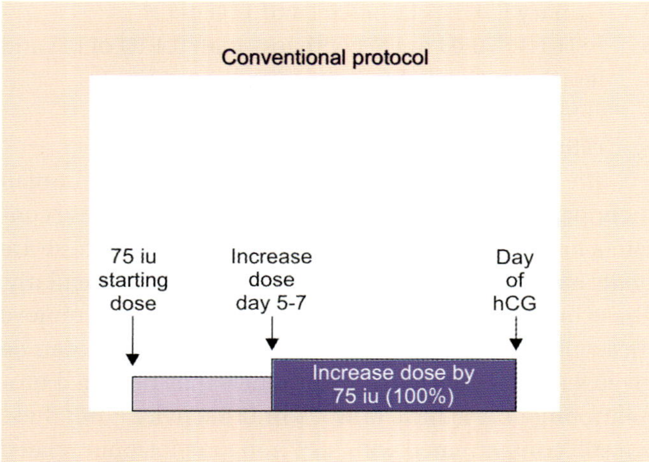

Fig. 4.1: Conventional protocol of gonadotropins in IUI cycles.

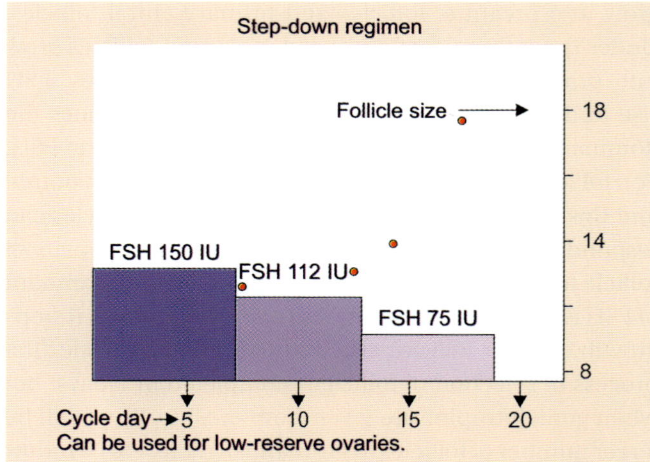

Fig. 4.2: Step-down protocol regimen of gonadotropins for IUI.

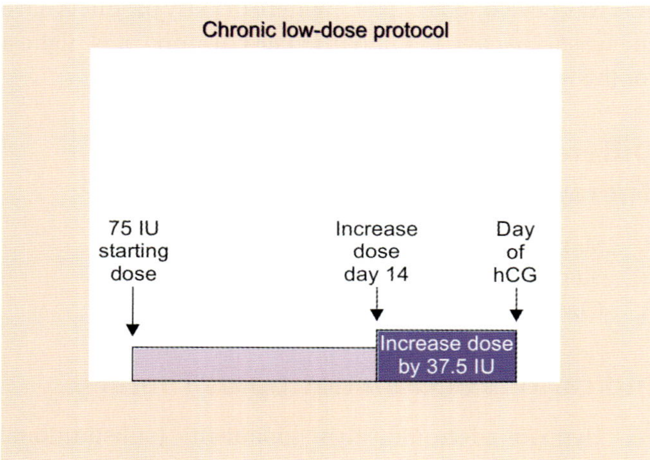

Fig. 4.3: Chronic low-dose protocol of gonadotropins in IUI cycles.

is continued till follicle and endometrium become mature. If there is no increase in the size of the follicle or in the endometrial thickness, the dose is doubled and scan is repeated after 3 days. If the follicle or endometrium grows, the same dose is continued till follicle and endometrium are mature, otherwise dose is further increased by 75 IU/day (Fig. 4.1). But this is rarely the case now as each patient is assessed on day 2–3 of period (baseline scan), and this scan diagnosis poorly responding ovaries, and in these patients stimulation is to be started with higher doses.

This protocol has been blamed for higher rates of multiple pregnancies and ovarian hyperstimulation syndrome (OHSS).[54] Conventional protocol gives excellent pregnancy rates in normal responding ovary. Good ultrasound monitoring can replace hormonal (E_2—estradiol) estimations.

Step-down Protocol

This protocol is very useful for the poor responding ovaries or low reserve ovaries. According to this protocol, stimulation is started with higher dose, i.e. 150–225 IU FSH from day 5 for 5 days. Once the follicle grows to 10–12 mm, the dose is reduced to 75–150 IU FSH; once the follicle size reaches 14 mm, the dose is further reduced, if it was 150 IU, or is continued with 75 IU FSH till follicle and endometrium mature (Fig. 4.2).

Chronic Low-dose Protocol

This protocol is very useful in PCOS patients. PCO contains twice the number of available FSH sensitive antral follicles in cohort as compared to normal ovaries. This protocol gives good pregnancy rates with very little risk of OHSS or multiple pregnancies. But it is essential that PCOS is confirmed on baseline ultrasound scan. In this protocol, stimulation is started with 75 IU of FSH and same dose is continued for 14 days. If follicle or endometrium grows, the same dose is continued till mature follicle and endometrium are achieved otherwise the dose is increased by 37.5 IU for other 7 days. (Fig. 4.3) Almost all the patients develop good follicle and endometrium and incidence of multiple pregnancy and OHSS is extremely low.[55] Majority of the patients develop good follicle within 14 days and we should strongly resist ourselves to increase the dose till then. There may be spotting or some bleeding during this period which should be ignored. With chronic low dose protocol, there is monofollicular development in 70% of cycles, OHSS can be almost totally eliminated and multiple pregnancy rate less than 6% with same pregnancy rate as conventional protocol.[56]

RECOMBINANT FOLLICLE-STIMULATING HORMONE

The invent of rFSH has changed the management of infertile patients. In 1990, 6 lakhs urine donors were required for 120 million liters of urine for urinary gonadotropin production. This was becoming extremely difficult as with developing techniques in ART, the need for gonadotropins were further increasing. Therefore, there was an urgent need for FSH by alternate route. The first rFSH was introduced in 1995. But it was 1992 that Prof Paul Devroey and Germond reported the clinical utility of rFSH.[57] rFSH has highest bioactivity and has no proteins or LH/hCG like activity and best batch-to-batch consistency. As it has no proteins, it is never allergic and also does not produce antibodies against FSH. It has low level of oxidation and/or degradation, i.e.10% compared to 40% with uFSH.

How is Recombinant Follicle-stimulating Hormone Produced?

The objective of recombinant DNA technology is to insert genes in the cell to produce desired proteins. The gene that is coded for desired protein is isolated enzymatically from DNA chain. The isolated gene is put in vector (a large segment of DNA). This is known as rDNA in host cell. This rDNA produces desired proteins-rFSH. Therefore, human DNA genes into a mammalian cell line produces rFSH which is 99.9% pure without LH activity. rFSH has bioactivity of 10,000 IU/mg of protein (Table 4.1).

Preparations

Follitropin α is produced by transfecting Chinese hamster ovary cells with genes for the α and β subunits of human FSH.

The secretory products of these cells undergo six step purification process to get a final preparation which is highly pure biochemically (>99% FSH).

Table 4.1: Specific bioactivity of different gonadotropins.

Product	*Specific bioactivity (IU/mg protein)*
HMG (1950)	8
uFSH (1980)	100–150
uHMG-HP	2,000
uFSH-HP	9,000
rFSH (1995)	10,000

Comparison of Recombinant Follicle-stimulating Hormone with Urinary Follicle-stimulating Hormone

The study conducted by Hedan B clearly indicates superiority of rFSH (Table 4.2).[58]

The meta-analysis conducted by Salim Daya and Gunby of 12 randomized controlled trials has proved that rFSH is 20% more likely to achieve pregnancy than uFSH. The amount of FSH used was 400 IU less.[59]

The meta-analysis data was summarized by the author as "The overall conclusion from this meta-analysis is that rFSH is more effective than uFSH because of the higher rates of clinical pregnancy per cycle started and is more efficient because the total dose of gonadotropin required was lower."[59]

Prospective meta-analysis has proved that clinical pregnancy rate is 5% higher in rFSH and if cryopreserved embryos are taken into account, pregnancy rate is 6.4% higher.[60]

Though a recently published Cochrane review has shown no difference in pregnancy outcomes with fresh embryo transfers when rFSH and urinary FSH were compared. It was concluded that "all available gonadotropins in clinical practice are equally effective and safe" and the choice is based on availability, convenience, and cost.[61]

Comparison of Recombinant Follicle-stimulating Hormone with Urinary Follicle-stimulating Hormone (Highly Purified)

Recombinant FSH is more effective than highly purified FSH in multiple follicular development (Table 4.3).[62]

Frydman and associates also published the data that rFSH gives more number of oocytes, more embryos with lesser number of injections.[63]

Table 4.2: Comparison of recombinant and urinary FSH in terms of doses used and cycle outcome.

	rFSH	*uFSH*
Higher number of oocytes	10.8	8.9
Lower dose of FSH	2,138 IU	2,385 IU
Shorter period	10.7	11.3
High-quality embryos	3.1	2.6
Pregnancy rate with cryopreservation	25.5%	20.4%

Table 4.3: Comparison of recombinant and urinary FSH in ART cycles.

	rFSH	*uFSH*	*P value*
No. of ampoules	21.9 ± 5.1	31.9 ± 13.4	<0.0001
FSH days	11 ± 1.6	13.5 ± 3.7	<0.001
Oocytes retrieved	12.2 ± 5.5	7.6 ± 4.4	<0.0001
Embryos transferred	2 ± 0.19	1.9 ± 0.4	NS
Pregnancy rates	53/119 (45%)	42/114 (37%)	NS
Implantation	32	31	NS

Gearon and Abdalla from Lister hospital, London in an unpublished study have reported for the first time improvement in quality of oocytes in older women treated with rFSH instead of uFSH-HP. Another randomized single blind, multicentric multinational study by Schats et al. also confirmed the same findings.

Recombinant FSH gives more embryos with lesser ampoules. More than four embryos in culture has higher chance of achieving pregnancy.[64] The chances of blastocyst transfer is increased, if more than four oocytes are retrieved.[65]

Recombinant FSH was associated with higher per cycle pregnancy rate than uFSH-HP, when used at the same dose, whereas the pregnancy rates were similar when the dose of r-FSH was 50% lower.[66]

Recombinant Follicle-stimulating Hormone versus Human Menopausal Gonadotropin

Meta-analysis of eight randomized controlled trials comparing rFSH with HMG has shown that rFSH has 50% higher pregnancy rates.[67] The FIVNAT report 1999 showed that the pregnancy rates were higher with rFSH than HMG.

Prospective analysis of 24,000 ART cycles from Germany also showed higher birth rate and lower dosage with rFSH than HMG.[68]

Meta-analysis including 400,000 IVF cycles showed that compared to rFSH, HMG resulted in fewer oocytes and higher doses.[69]

Facts about Highly Purified Human Menopausal Gonadotropin

1. The process is partially successful with specific activity of 2,000 IU/mg of protein.
2. In many cases, LH activity has to be added using hCG which has longer half-life.
3. Presence of variable amount of hCG may further increase variation between different batches of product and result in follicular atresia.[70]
4. HMG-HP contains 30% extraneous proteins including leukocyte elastase inhibitor protein C inhibitor and Zn-α2 glycoprotein apart from hCG.

Different Types of Recombinant Follicle-stimulating Hormone

1. Follitropin α 1995
2. Follitropin β 1996
3. Immunopotency, biopotency, and internal carbohydrate complexity are same for both but follitropin α contains higher proportion of acidic glycoforms.
4. Follitropin α has a specific activity of 13,645 IU/mg whereas that for follitropin β is 9,396 IU/mg.

There is a difference in tolerability between rFSH preparations favoring follitropin α over beta.[71] Though follitropin α has a higher incidence of OHSS as compared to follitropin β (4.1% as compared to 2.7%).[72]

Fill by Mass Concept

Dose of gonadotropin is expressed in international units (IU). But recent fill by mass (FbM) technique reflects a constant relationship between mass and bioactivity and guarantees consistency of dose from batch-to-batch. So drawbacks of vivo bioassay can be avoided. Bioassay of FSH preparation is 50 years old. Steelman-Pohley bioassay which is cumbersome and requires large number of animals and variation can be 10–20%. But FbM is by liquid chromatography supported by glycine mapping isoelectric focusing that demonstrates physicochemical consistency of the product.

Duration of stimulation was significantly shorter in FbM group, and embryo quality and implantation rates were significantly higher—28.6% in FbM versus 18.6% in Filled by International Units (FbIU).[73,74]

Clinical Benefits of Recombinant Follicle-stimulating Hormone[75]

- Improved logistics of pharmaceutical process
- Controlled manufacturing
- Reduced batch-to-batch variability
- Potentially unlimited supply—no shortage
- Not reliant on the urine supply
- No risk of infection

- No risk of contamination with drugs or metabolites
- No seroconversion to antigonadotropin antibodies
- Effective, safe, and less traumatic subcutaneous administration
- Greater purity and specific activity
- Smaller doses required
- More predictable response
- Cost benefit

PROTOCOLS FOR ASSISTED REPRODUCTIVE TECHNIQUE

Gonadotropins in Assisted Reproductive Technique

In ART cycles also, stimulation protocol is decided by baseline scan.

Long Agonist Protocol

Downregulation from 21st day of previous cycle as nasal spray or subcutaneous injections of GnRH agonist (leuprolide acetate 0.5 mg or decapeptyl 0.1 mg) and is continued till periods. The dose is halved from the day of period. Depot preparations of agonist can be used instead of daily agonist injections on day 21 of the previous cycle. The most common starting dose for COS with rFSH is 150–225/day. Increasing the dosage in elderly women does not result in increased oocyte yield.[76] It has been found that 150 IU of rFSH is equivalent to 225 IU of uFSH for follicular growth. The dose of 150 IU is optimum,[74] rather than 100 IU that has been mentioned in a comparative study for IVF patients.

Short Protocol

This protocol exploits the flare-up effect of agonist during the ovarian stimulation. Agonist is started with the beginning of the menstrual cycle and flare-up provides the surge of gonadotropins secretion. A few days later, exogenous gonadotropins is administrated to supplement the flare. Both agonist and gonadotropins are continued till the day of hCG. This protocol is preferred for poor responders.

Ultrashort Protocol

Agonist is given on day 2, 3, 4 of the stimulation cycle in the dose of 500–1,000 µg per day and then gonadotropins are given subsequently till day of hCG.

Antagonist Protocol

High resistance, low velocity stromal flow, fewer antral follicles, smaller ovarian volume, high BMI, and age more than 35 years are the parameters which decide higher doses for stimulation with antagonist protocol; whereas, low resistance, high velocity stromal flow, polycystic ovaries, low BMI, and age less than 24 years are the parameters which would be in favor of lower doses with antagonist protocol. Antagonist is started from day 6 and continued till the day of hCG. In these patients, GnRH agonist can be used for ovulation trigger, instead of hCG. This protocol reduces the incidence of OHSS significantly. This is known as fixed antagonist protocol. Antagonist can also be used as flexible protocol, when antagonist is started when at least one follicle is 14 mm in diameter.[77] Antagonist protocol has high cumulative pregnancy rate in both groups, high AMH (40.1–63.6%), and low AMH (11.1–18.7%).[78] A meta-analysis of 45 randomized controlled trials involving 7,511 women comparing GnRH antagonist protocol and long agonist protocol for COS in ART has found no significant differences in live birth or ongoing pregnancy rates, but marked decrease in OHSS with antagonist protocols.[79] Another meta-analysis comparing agonist and antagonist protocols for poor responders has shown advantage in terms of FSH stimulation, but no statistically significant difference in terms of oocytes retrieved or clinical pregnancy rates.[80,81]

Antagonist–Agonist Protocol

This protocol is especially used for PCOS patients. It is known as OHSS free protocol. Fixed antagonist protocol is used for downregulation and then agonist is used for ovulation trigger.

Antagonist–Agonist Protocol with hCG as Luteal Support

The above mentioned protocol is very likely to lead to LPD. It is therefore recommended to supplement the luteal phase with 1,500 IU of hCG on day 3-7-10 of ovum pick-up.[82]

Predictors of Ovarian Response

These are age, BMI, baseline FSH, AMH, and AFC. A nomogram can be prepared using these predictors. *Howles and colleagues have prepared a manuscript on the same.*[78] The cost effectivity has been mentioned in the results presented here. These are the results of computer modeling study (Tables 4.4 and 4.5).

Table 4.4: Comparison of average cost per cycle with recombinant and urinary FSH in different countries.

	rFSH	uFSH
UK	5,906 pounds	6,060 pounds
US (Social)	40,688 $	47,096 $
(Insurance)	28,481 $	32,967 $
Spain (Public insurance)	12,791 €	13,007 €
Spain (Private)	19,739 €	20,467 €
Germany	21,686 €	22,189 €

LUTEINIZING HORMONE SUPPLEMENTATION: FOR WHOM, WHEN, AND WHY?

Two-cell Two-gonadotropins Theory

Both FSH and LH are required for estradiol synthesis. LH binds to theca cells to induce androgen synthesis. Androgen diffuses into granulosa cells, where FSH-stimulated aromatization leads to estrogen synthesis.[83] LH in follicular phase helps conversion of progesterone to androgen to reduce follicular phase progesterone, which is detrimental to endometrial receptivity.[84] A combination of rFSH and rLH in a ratio of 2:1 is indicated for women with severe gonadotropin deficiency—hypogonadotropic hypogonadism.[85]

Luteinizing Hormone Threshold and Luteinizing Hormone Ceiling Effect

The LH is required for terminal stages of follicular maturation, for meiosis, and ovulation. But high LH causes follicular atresia, premature luteinization, and oocyte quality may be compromised.[86] In patients over-responding to FSH, adding 30 μg rLH leads to monofollicular development.[87] This indicates LH ceiling effect.

CURRENT OPINION

1. Current opinion is that there is no absolute requirement for LH supplementation in unselected patient population.[88]
2. However, LH may have benefit in women aged more than 35 years and those who are poor responders to COS.[89] Though Cochrane review[88] and studies subsequently published have shown that LH supplementation—including for women with advanced age—has no benefit on ongoing pregnancy, with an adjusted OR of 0.99 (CI 0.76—1.29).[88]

Table 4.5: Individualized dose calculation for COS.[83]

AMH level	Predicted response to COS	Treatment strategies
15 pmol/L	High responders (150 IU)	GnRH antagonist protocol Normal oocyte yield, very low excess response, low embryo cryopreservation, high/maintained fresh CPR
5–15 pmol/L	Normal responders (225–300 IU)	GnRH agonist protocol: very low cancellation of oocyte pick-up and OHSS
<5 pmol/L	Poor responders (375 IU)	High-dose FSH: long stimulation, high cancellation Antagonist strategy: short stimulation, moderate cancellation

3. LH supplementation may improve outcomes in patients with suboptimal response to FSH stimulation.[90]
4. No LH cut-off value is known to identify a female requiring LH supplementation and LH assessment is therefore of no use.[91]
5. In antagonist cycle, LH supplementation is controversial. Though some studies have shown that it improves results in selected groups.
6. LH estimation may not be a reliable guide to decide for LH supplementation because of variable bioactivity and polymorphism.

SUMMARY

Adding LH increases the number of developmentally competent oocytes in woman with endogenous LH suppressed below 1 IU/L at the start of stimulation. However, with LH more than 1 IU/L, adding LH is associated with significant lower embryo quality and implantation rate compared with rFSH alone.[92] Recombinant human LH (r-hLH) alone can trigger follicular growth arrest in a significant number of patients supporting the existence of LH ceiling during late follicular maturation.[93] rFSH with r-hLH 150 IU from day 6 might be beneficial in subgroup women in older reproductive age, having LH polymorphism and less sensitivity to LH.

The results of analysis by age showed a trend toward higher implantation rate with rFSH alone in patients aged less than 35 years. In contrast, the group aged more than 35 years had numerically higher implantation rate in the rFSH plus r-hLH group.[94,95] r-hLH supplementation on day 8 in patients having E2 less than 180 pgm/mL and no follicles more than 10 mm, significantly increases the number of oocytes retrieved and requirement of rFSH was also decreased.[96]

CARRY-HOME MESSAGE

1. CC should be used for 3–6 months, 100 mg/day starting from day 5.
2. CC with estrogen has no role.
3. CC with dexamethasone is useful in chronic anovulatory patient and DHEAS is high.
4. CC with bromocriptine is used in patients with normal prolactin levels with galactorrhea and spikers when prolactin is high in first half of the cycle.
5. Routine use of hCG is not justified.
6. CC with GnRHa for downregulation has no role in IUI cycles.
7. CC with gonadotropins do not improve pregnancy rates.
8. CC with metformin can be used in CC resistant PCOS patients.
9. Metformin, OC pills, and progesterone are useful prior to CC.
10. Gonadotropins give better pregnancy rates than CC.
11. Step up protocol is used for normal responding ovaries.
12. Chronic low dose protocol is best for PCO.
13. r-FSH requires lower dosage with better efficacy.
14. rFSH is better than all urinary preparation.
15. rLH is used in poor responders and patients of age more than 35 years.

REFERENCES

1. Greenblatt RB, Barfield WE, Jungck EC, Ray AW. Induction of ovulation with MRL/41. Preliminary report. JAMA. 1961;178:101-4.
2. Practice Committee of American Society for Reproductive Medicine, Birmingham, Alabama, USA. Use of Clomiphene citrate in women. Fertile Sterile. 2004;82(Suppl 1):S90-6.
3. Young SL, Opsahl MS, Fritz MA. Serum concentrations of enclomiphene and zuclomiphene across consecutive cycles of clomiphene citrate therapy in anovulatory infertile women. Fertile Steril. 1999;71:639-44.
4. National Collaborating Centre for Women's and Children's Health. Fertility: Assessment and treatment for people with fertility problems. London, United Kingdom: RCOG press; 2004.
5. Barbeiri RL. Female infertility. In: Strauss JF III, Barbieri RL (Eds). Yen and Jaffe's Reproductive Endocrinology: Physiology, Pathophysiology and Clinical Management, 6th Edition. Philadelphia, Pennsylvania: Elsevier Saunders; 2009. p. 523.
6. Guzick DS, Zeleznik A. Efficacy of clomiphene citrate in treatment of luteal phase deficiency: quantity versus quality of preovulatory follicles. Fertil Steril. 1990;54(2): 206-10.
7. Glazener CM, Coulson C, Lambert PA, Watt EM, Hinton RA, Kelly NG, et al. Clomiphene treatment for women with unexplained infertility: placebo-controlled study of hormonal responses and conception rates. Gynecol Endocrinol. 1990;4(2):75-83.
8. Hughes E, Brown J, Collins JJ, Vanderkerchove P. Clomiphene citrate for unexplained subfertility in women. Cochrane database Syst Rev. 2010;(1):CD000057.
9. Glyser M, March CM, Mishell DR Jr, Bailey EJ. A decades experience with an individualized clomiphene treatment regime including its effect on the post coital test. Fertil Steril. 1982;37:161-7.
10. Garcia J, Jones GS, Wentz AC. The use of clomiphene citrate. Fertil Steril. 1977;28:707-17.
11. Imani B, Eijkemans MJ, te Velde ER, Habbema JD, Fauser BC. A nomogram to predict the probability of live birth after clomiphene citrate induction of ovulation in normogonadotrophic oligoamenorrhic infertility. Fertil Steril. 2003;77(1):91-7.
12. Blenner JL. Clomiphene induced mood swings. J Obstet Gynecol Neonatal Nurs. 1991;20:321-7.
13. Purvin V. Visual disturbances secondary to clomiphene citrate. Arch Opthalmol.1995;113:482-6.
14. Sereepapong W, Suwajanakorn S, Triratanachat S, Sampatanukul P, Pruksananonda K. Effects of clomiphene citrate on the endometrium of regularly cycling women. Fertil Steril. 2000;73:287-91.
15. Hsu CC, Kuo HC, Wang ST, Huang KE. Interference with uterine blood flow by clomiphene citrate in women with unexplained infertility. Obstet Gynecol. 1995;86:917-21.
16. Bateman BG, Nunley WC Jr, Kolp LA. Exogenous oestrogen therapy for treatment of clomiphene citrate-induced cervical mucus abnormalities: is it effective? Fertil Steril. 1990;54:577-9.
17. Wu CH, Winkel CA. The effect of therapy initiation day on clomiphene citrate therapy. Fertil Steril. 1989;52:564-8.
18. Saleh A, Biljan MM, Tan SSSL, Tulandi T. Effects of tamoxifen Tx on endometrial thickness and pregnancy rates in women undergoing superovulation with clomiphene citrate and intrauterine insemination. Fertil Steril. 2000;74:S1-90.
19. Schenker JG, Yarkoni S, Granat M. Multiple pregnancies following induction of ovulation. Fetil Steril. 1981;35:105-23.
20. Dickey RP, Taylor SN, Curole DN, Rye PH, Pyrzak R. Incidence of spontaneous abortion in clomiphene pregnancies. Hum Reprod. 1996;11:2642.
21. Hack M, Lunnenfeld B. Influence of hormone induction of ovulation on the fetus and newborn. Pediatr Adolesc Endocrinol. 1979;5:191.
22. Correy JF, Marsden DE, Schokman FC. The outcome of pregnancy resulting from clomiphene-induced ovulation. Aust N Z J Obstet Gynecol. 1982;22:18-21.
23. Venn A, Watson L, Lumley J, Giles G, King C, Healy D. Breast and ovarian cancer incidence after infertility and *in vitro* fertilization. Lancet. 1995;346:995-1000.

24. Mosgaard BJ, Lidegaard O, Kjaer SK, Schou G, Anderson AN. Infertility, fertility drugs, and invasive ovarian cancer: a case-control study. Fertil Steril. 1997;67:1005-12.
25. Silva I dos S, Wark PA, McCormack VA, Mayer D, Overton C, Little V, et al. Ovulation-stimulation drugs and cancer risks: a long term follow up of a British cohort. Br J Cancer. 2009;100:1824-31. Epub 2009 May 12.
26. Lobo Ra, Granger LR, Davajan V, Mishell DR Jr. An extended regimen of clomiphene citrate in women unresponsive to standard therapy. Fertil Steril. 1982;37(6):762-6.
27. Parsanezhad ME, Alborzi S, Motazedian S, Ormani G. Use of dexamethasone and clomiphene citrate in treatment of clomiphene-citrate resistant patients with polycystic ovarian syndrome and normal dehydroepiandrosterone sulfate levels: a prospective, double blind, placebo-controlled trial. Fertil Steril. 2002;78(5):1001-4.
28. Isaacs JD Jr, Lincoln SR, Cowan BD. Extended clomiphene citrate and prednisone for the treatment of chronic anovulation resistant to CC alone. Feril Steril. 1997;67(4):641-3.
29. Kubota T, Kamada S, Aso T. Combined therapy with bromocriptine and clomiphene citrate for patients with normoprolactinemic amenorrhoea. Int J Fertil. 2004;269: 125-9.
30. Kosmas IP, Tatsioni A, Fatemi HM, Kolibianakis EM, Touraye H, Devroey P. Human chorionic gonadotrophin administration vs luteinizing monitoring for intrauterine insemination timing after administration of clomiphene citrate: a meta-analysis. Fertil Steril. 2007;87:607-12.
31. George K, Nair R, Tharyan P. Ovulation triggers in anovulatory women undergoing ovulation induction. Cochrane Database Syst Rev. 2008;3:CD006900.
32. Lu PY, Chen AL, Atkinson EJ, Lee SH, Erickson LD, Ory SJ. Minimal stimulation achieves pregnancy rates comparable to human menopausal gonadotrophins in the treatment of infertility. Fertil Steril. 1996;65:583-7.
33. Creanga A, Bradley H, McCoemick C, Witkop CT. Use of metformin in polycystic ovary syndrome: a meta-analysis. Obstet Gynecol. 2008;111:959-68.
34. Vandermolen DT, Ratts VS, Evans WS, Stovall DW, Kauma SW, Nestler JE. Metformin increases the ovulatory rate and pregnancy rate from clomiphene citrate-resistant patients with polycystic ovary syndrome who are resistant to clomiphene citrate alone. Fertil Steril. 2001;73:310-5.
35. Mitwally MF, Casper RF. Use of an aromatase inhibitor for induction of ovulation in patients with an inadequate response to clomiphene citrate. Fertil Steril. 2001;75:305-9.
36. Cole PA, Robinson CH. Mechanism and inhibition of cytochrome P-450 aromatase. J Med Chem. 1990;33:2933-42.
37. Santen RJ, Manni A, Harvey H, Redmond C. Endocrine treatment of breast cancer in women. Endocrine Rev. 1990;11:1-45.
38. Roberts V, Meunier H, Vaughan J, Rivier J, Rivier C, Vale W, et al. Production and regulation of inhibin subunits in pituitary gonadotropes. Endocrinology. 1989;124:552-4.
39. Vignali M, Infantino M, Matrone R, Chiodo E. Endometriosis: Novel etiopathogenetic concepts and clinical perspectives. Fertil Steril. 2002;78:665-78.
40. Oktay K, Buyuk E, Libertella N, Akar M, Rosenwaks Z. Fertility preservation in breast cancer patients: a prospective controlled comparison of ovarian stimulation with Tamoxifen and Letrozole for embryo cryopreservation. J Clin Oncol. 2005;23:4347-53.
41. Oktay K. Further evidence on the safety and success of ovarian stimulation with letrozole and tamoxifen in breast cancer patients undergoing *in vitro* fertilization to cryopreserve their embryos for fertility preservation. J Clin Oncol. 2005;23:3858-9.
42. Mitwally MFM, Casper RF. Aromatase inhibition: a novel method of ovulation induction in women with polycystic ovarian syndrome. Reprod Technol. 2000;10:244-7.
43. Reichl H, Balen A, Jansen CA. Prion transmission in blood and urine: what are the implications for recombinant and urinary-derived gonadotrophins? Hum Reprod. 2002;17:2501-8.
44. Winer EP, Hudis C, Burstein HJ, Wolff AC, Pritchard KI, Ingle JN, et al. American Society of Clinical Oncology Technology assessment on the use of aromatase inhibitors as adjuvant therapy for women with hormone receptor-positive breast cancer: status report 2002. J Clin Oncol. 2002;20:3317-27.
45. Buzdar A, Jonat W, Howell A, Jones SE, Blomqvist CP, Vogel CL, et al. Anastrozole, a potent and selective aromatase inhibitor, versus megestrol acetate in postmenopausal women with advanced breast cancer: results of overview analysis of two phase III trials. Arimidex study group. J Clin Oncol. 1996;14:2000-11.
46. Marty M, Gershanovich M, Campos B. Aromatase inhibitors, a new potent, selective aromatase inhibitor superior to aminoglutethimide AG in postmenopausal women with advanced breast cancer previously treated with antioestrogens. Proc Am Soc Clin Oncol. 1997;16:156.
47. Gemzell CA, Diczfalusy E, Tillinger G. Clinical effect of human pituitary follicle-stimulating hormone (FSH). J Clin Endocrinol Metab. 1958;18:1333-48.
48. Bettendorf S. Human hypophyseal gonadotrophin in hypophysectomised women. Jint J Fertil. 1963;45:799-809.
49. Lunnenfeld B, Menzi A, Insler V. Efecti Clinicci della gonadotophina umana della post-menopausa. Rass Clin Terap. 1960;50:213-6.
50. Lunnenfeld B. Treatment of anovulation by human gonadotrophins. J Int Fedn Gynecol Obstet. 1963;1:153.
51. Lunenfield B, Insler V, Rabau E. The principles of gonadotrophin therapy. Acta Endocrinol Suppl (Copenh). 1970;148:52-101.
52. Lunnenfeld B, Eshkol A. Immunology of follicle stimulating hormone and luteinizing hormone. Vitam Horm. 1970;27:131-59.
53. Hull M, Corrigan E, Piazzi A, Loumaye E. Recombinant human Luteinizing hormone: an effective new gonadotrophin preparation. Lancet. 1994;344:334-5.
54. Westergard LG, RRB K, Laursen SB. HMG versus rFSH in normogonadotrophic women down regulated with gonadotrophic releasing hormone agonist who were undergoing IVF and ICSI, a prospective randomised study. Fertil Steril. 2001;76(3):543-9.

55. Homburg R, Levy T, Ben-Rafael Z. A comparative prospective study of conventional regimen with chronic low dos administration of follicle stimulating hormone for anovulation associated with polycystic ovary syndrome. Fertil Steril. 1995;63(4):729-33.
56. Driebergen R, Baer G. Quantification of follicle stimulating hormone (follitropin alpha): is *in vivo* bioassay still relevant in recombinant age? Curr Med Res Opin. 2003;19: 41-6.
57. Germond M, Dessole S, Senn A, Loumaye E, Howles C, Beltrami V, et al. Successful *in vitro* fertilization and embryo transfer after treatment with recombinant human FSH. Lancet. 1992;339(8802):1170-1.
58. Hedon B, Out HJ, Hugues JN, Camier B, Cohen J, Lopes P, et al. Efficacy and safety of recombinant follicle stimulating hormone (Puregon) in infertile women pituitary suppressed with triptorelin undergoing in-vitro fertilization: a prospective randomized, assessor-blind, multicentre trial. Hum Reprod. 1995;10:3102-6.
59. Daya S. Updated meta-analysis of recombinant follicle-stimulating hormone (FSH) versus urinary FSH for ovarian stimulation in assisted reproduction. Fertility and Sterility. 2002;77(4):711-4.
60. Out HJ, Driessen SGAJ, Mannaerts BMJL, Coelingh Bennink HJ. Recombinant follicle-stimulating hormone (follitropin beta, Puregon) yields higher pregnancy rates in *in vitro* fertilization than urinary gonadotropins. Fertil Steril. 1997;68:138-42.
61. van Wely M, Kwan I, Burt AL, Thomas J, Vail A, Van der Veen F, et al. Recombinant versus urinary gonadotrophins for ovarian stimulation in assisted reproductive technology cycles. Cochrane Database Syst Rev. 2011;2:CD005354.
62. Bergh C, Howles CM, Borg K, Hamberger L, Josefsson B, Nilsson L, et al. Recombinant follicle stimulating hormone (r-h-FSH; Gonal-F) versus highly purified urinary FSH (Metrodin HP): results of a randomized comparative study in women undergoing assisted reproductive techniques. Hum Reprod. 1997;12:2133-9.
63. Frydman R, Haverell C, Camier B. A double blind randomized study comparing the efficacy of recombinant human (FSH: Gonal F*) versus highly purified urinary FSH (Metrodin-HP) in inducing superovulation in women undergoing assisted reproductive techniques. Hum Reprod. 1998;13:180-5.
64. Templeton A, Morris JK, Parslow W. Factors that affect outcome of in-vitro fertilisation treatment. Lancet. 1996;348:1402-6.
65. Scholtes MC, Zeilmaker GH. Blastocyst transfer in day-5 embryo transfer depends primarily on the number of oocytes retrieved and not on age. Fertil Steril. 1998;69:78-83.
66. Matorras R, Osuna C, Exposito A, Crisol BS, Pijoan JI. Recombinant FSH versus highly purified FSH in intrauterine insemination: systematic review and meta-analysis. Fertil Steril. 2011;95:1937-42.
67. Daya S, Gunby J, Hughes EG, Collins JA, Sagle MA. Follicle stimulating hormone versus human menopausal gonadotrophins for in-vitro fertilization cycles: a meta-analysis. Fertil Steril. 1995;27:347-54.
68. Ludwig M, Rabe T, Buhler K, Diedrich K, Felberbaum R. Wirksamkeit von recombinanten humane FSH in Vergleich zu urinarem hMG nach Downregulation im langen Protokoll–eine Analyse von 24.764 ART-Zyklen in Deutschland. J Reproduction Med Endocrinol. 1994;4: 284-8.
69. Lehert P, Schertz JC, Ezcurra D. Recombinant human follicle stimulating hormone produces more oocytes with low total dose per cycle in assisted reproductive technologies compared with highly purified HMG: a meta-analysis. Reprod Biol Endocrinol. 2010;8:112.
70. Filicori M, Cognigni GE, Taraborrelli S, Spettoli D, Ciampaglia W, Tabarelli de Fatis C, et al. Luteinizing hormone activity in menotropins optimizes folliculogenesis and treatment in controlled ovarian stimulation. The Journal of Clinical Endocrinology and Metabolism. 2001;86(1).
71. Brinsden P, Akagbosu F, GIbbonset AL. A comparison of the efficacy and tolerability of two recombinant human follicle-stimulating hormone preparations in patients undergoing *in vitro* fertilization-embryo transfer. Fertil Steril. 2003;73: 114-6.
72. Devroey P, Boostanfar R, Koper NP, Mannerts BM, Ijzerma-Boon PC, Fauser BC, et al. A double blind non-inferiority RCT comparing corifollitropin alpha and rFSH during first seven days of ovarian stimulation using GnRH antagonist protocol. Hum Reprod. 2009;24(12):3063-72.
73. Balasch J, Fabergues F, Penarrubia J. Outcome from consecutive assisted reproduction cycles in patients treated with recombinant follitropin alfa filled-by-bioassay and those treated with recombinant follitropin alfa filled-by-mass. Reprod Biomed Online. 2004;8:408-13.
74. Hugues JN, Barlow DH, Rosenwaks Z, Cedrin-Durnerin I, Robson S, Pidoux L, et al. Improvement in consistency of response to ovarian stimulation with recombinant human follicle stimulating hormone resulting from a new method for calibrating the therapeutic preparation. Reprod Biomed Online. 2003;6:185-90.
75. Ludwig M, Diedrich K. Evaluation of luteal phase support protocol in IV. Obstet Gynecol Scand. 2001;80:452-66.
76. Out HJ, Braat DD, Linsten BM. Increasing the daily dose of recombinant follicle stimulating hormone (Puregon) does not compensate for the age-related decline in retrievable oocytes after ovarian stimulation. Hum Reprod. 2000;15:29-35.
77. Ludwig M, Katalinic A, Banz C, Schroder AK, Lonong M, Weiss JM, et al. Tailoring the GnRH antagonist cetrorelix acetate to individual patients' needs in ovarian stimulation for IVF: results of a prospective, randomized study. Hum Reprod. 2002;17(11):2842-5.
78. Nelson SM, Yates RW, Lyall H, Jamieson M, Traynor I, Gaudoin M, et al. Anti-Müllerian hormone based approach to controlled ovarian stimulation for assisted conception. Hum Reprod. 2009;24:867-75.
79. Al-Inany HG, Youssef MA, Aboulghar M, Ayeleke RO, Brown J, Lam WS. Gonadotrophin-releasing hormone antagonists for assisted reproductive technology. Cochrane Database Syst Rev. 2011;5:CD001750.

80. Pu D, Wu J, Liu J. Comparison of GnRH antagonist versus GnRH agonist protocol in poor ovarian responders undergoing IVF. Hum Reprod. 2011;26(10):2742-9.
81. Humadian P, Ejdrup BH, Westergaard LG, Yding AC. 1,500 IU human chorionic gonadotrophins administered at oocyte retrieval rescues the luteal phase when gonadotrophins-releasing hormone agonist is used for ovulation induction: a prospective randomised controlled study. Fertil Steril. 2010;93:847-54.
82. Howles CM. Reproductive Biomed Online Supplement. 2008;16 (2):pS-5.
83. Kobayashi M, Nakano R, Ooshima A. Immunohistochemical localization of pituitary gonadotrophins and gonadal steroids confirms the 'two cell two gonadotrophins hypothesis of steroidogenesis in the human ovary. J Endocrinol. 1990;126(3):483-8.
84. Fanchin R, Righini C, Olivennes F, Taieb J, de Zeigler, Frydman R. Computerised assessment of endometrial echogenicity: clues to the endometrial effects of premature progesterone elevation. Fertil Steril. 1999;71(1): 173-81.
85. Bosch E. Recombinant human FSH and recombinant human LH in a 2:1 ratio combination: a new tool for ovulation induction. Exp Rev Obstet Gynecol. 2009;4(5):491-8.
86. Hillier SG. Current concepts of the roles of follicle stimulating hormone and luteinizing hormone in folliculogenesis. Hum Reprod. 1994;9:188-91.
87. Hughes JN, Soussis J, Calderon I, Balasch J, Anderson RA, Romeu A. Recombinant LH study group 2005. Does the addition of recombinant LH in WHO group II anovulatory women over-responding to FSH treatment reduce the number of developing follicles? A dose-finding study. Hum Reprod. 2005;20:629-35.
88. Mochtar MH, Van der Veen F, Zeich M, van Wely M. Recombinant luteinizing hormone (rLH) for controlled ovarian hyperstimulation in assisted reproductive cycles. Cochrane Database Syst Rev. 2007;2:CD005070.
89. Howles CM. Luteinizing hormone supplementation in ART. In: Kovacs G(Ed). How to improve your ART success rates. Cambridge, UK: Cambridge University Press; 2011. pp. 99-104.
90. Lisi F, Rinaldi L, Fischel S, Lisi R, Pepe G, Picconeri MG, et al. Use of recombinant FSH and recombinant LH in multiple follicular stimulation for IVF: a preliminary study. Reprod Biomed Online. 2001;3(3):190-4.
91. Loumaye E, Engrand P, Howles CM, O'Dea L. Assessment of the role of serum luteinizing hormone an oestradiol response to follicle stimulating hormone on *in vitro* fertilization treatment outcome. Fertil Steril. 1997;67:889-99.
92. Tesarik J, Mendoza. Effects of exogenous LH administration during ovarian stimulation of pituitary down regulated young oocyte donors on oocyte yield and developmental competence. Hum Reprod. 2002;17:3129-37.
93. Loumaye E, Engrand P, Shoham Z, Hillier SG, Baird DT. Clinical evidence for an LH 'ceiling' effect induced by administration of recombinant human LH during the late follicular phase of stimulated cycles in World Health Organization type I and type II anovulation. Hum Reprod. 2003;18:314-22.
94. Marrs RP, Meldrum DR, Muasher SJ. Randomized trial to compare the effect of recombinant human FSH (follitropin alfa) with or without recombinant human LH in women undergoing assisted reproduction treatment. Reprod Biomed Online. 2004;8:175-82.
95. Humadian P, Bungum M, Bungum L, Yding Andersen C. Effects of recombinant LH supplementation in women undergoing assisted reproduction with GnRh agonist downregulation and stimulation with recombinant FSH: an opening study. Reprod Biomed Online. 2004;8:635-43 .
96. De Placido, Alviggi C, Mollo A, Perino A, Strina I, Lisi F, et al. Effects of recombinant LH(rLH) supplementation during controlled ovarian stimulation(COH) in normogonadotrophic women with an initial inadequate response to recombinant FSH (rFSH) after pituitary downregulation. Clin Endocrinol. 2004;60:637-43.

CHAPTER 5

Ovulation Induction in Polycystic Ovarian Syndrome

Chaitanya Nagori, Sonal Panchal

INTRODUCTION

Patients with polycystic ovarian syndrome (PCOS) have high antral follicle count (AFC) and also have high stromal vascularity, both of these make them more prone to ovarian hyperstimulation syndrome (OHSS). This is one of the most dreaded complications of ovulation induction. Therefore, ovulation induction in PCOS requires careful assessment of patient and a careful consideration before deciding on the ovulation induction protocols. Moreover, insulin resistance and high luteinizing hormone (LH), the major components of the PCOS are also challenges for ovulation induction in these patients.

Approximately 20–30% of women in reproductive age group have polycystic ovaries (PCO) and about half of these have signs and symptoms of PCOS. Earliest description of PCO appears to date from 1845 as "sclerocystic ovaries."[1] According to ESHRE/ASRM consensus 2003,[2] the diagnosis of PCOS consists of at least two of the three following criteria:

1. Oligo and/or anovulation
2. Hyperandrogenism: biochemical or clinical
3. PCO on ultrasound: this means an ovary that is 10 cc in volume and/or has more than 12 antral follicles.

PCOS, apart from its endocrinal component, as mentioned in the Rotterdam criteria, also has a metabolic component.

Three major ways to diagnosis of PCOS: (1) clinical findings, (2) laboratory testing, and (3) ultrasound findings. The details of ultrasound diagnosis of PCOS have been discussed in Chapter 13 of this book. The chief components of clinical criteria are irregular menstrual cycles due to oligo-ovulation or anovulation, acne, hirsutism and in severe cases acanthosis nigricans due to hyper androgenemia. Some of these patients may be very obese or absolutely thin lean. Most important among the hormonal criteria are high androgen, high LH and high AMH. The metabolic derangements that are commonly seen in patients with PCOS are hyperinsulinemia and hyperlipidemia. The comprehensive treatment of PCOS may include correction of both metabolic and endocrinal components. In this chapter, the ovulation induction options are discussed for PCOS patients. Ovulation induction in PCOS women is different than ovulation induction in non-PCOS women. In PCOS, women fertility is compromised because of oligo-anovulation, but is also compromised due to poor ovum quality due to high LH and in turn high insulin levels. These patients also have a risk of ovarian hyperstimulation due to high androgen levels and they also have a higher abortion rates both due to bad ovum quality and poor endometrial vascularity. This means improving fertility and ovulation induction in these cases should have a holistic approach to decrease, insulin, androgen and LH and also to decrease the risk of OHSS and abortion rates.

Options for ovulation induction in PCOS patients are:

1. Weight loss
2. Clomiphene
3. Letrozole
4. Insulin-lowering drugs
5. Glucocorticoids
6. Gonadotropins
7. GnRH antagonist
8. GnRH agonist
9. Ovarian drilling
10. *In vitro* fertilization (IVF)/*in vitro* maturation (IVM)

WEIGHT LOSS

It is the first line of treatment in obese PCOS patients. Central obesity is more common to cause metabolic changes. These patients typically have a waist:hip ratio of 0.7–0.8, which is an android type of obesity. Obesity as is known cannot be judged by just the weight. The best parameter to assess obesity is body mass index (BMI). Normal BMI range is 20–24.9 kg/m^2, whereas when it is between 25 and 29 kg/m^2, the individual is called overweight. When BMI is more than 30 kg/m^2, it indicates obesity[3] and BMI of less than 20 kg/m^2 is also considered low and abnormal.

It is the weight loss and decrease in the fat that causes improvement of insulin resistance, decrease in androgen levels and resumption of ovulation. During the initial period of calorie restriction, preferential loss of intra-abdominal fat occurs due to increased lipolysis and its high metabolic activity.[4,5] Only 5% of the total body weight loss is important to induce ovulation.[6] It reduces 30% of visceral fat, this regains reproductive functions in 60–100% of cases. Weight loss reduces hyperinsulinemia, hyperandrogenemia and increases SHBG. It improves the sensitivity for ovulation induction drugs. It also reduces clomiphene resistance. Weight loss decreases the rate of abortions. A retrospective study of 5,019 cycles of IVF revealed that obesity was associated with longer durations and increased amounts of gonadotropin stimulation, increased frequency of cycle cancellation for inadequate response and lower oocyte yields.[7]

Weight loss is an effective way of treating fertility related complications of PCOS and therefore must be emphasized. Weight loss can be achieved by diet control, exercise, group therapy, behavioral counseling, pharmacological treatment and bariatric surgery. Therefore, it is a team work that is required to help the patient to lose weight. But a normal weight PCOS patient may not benefit from weight loss.

CLOMIPHENE CITRATE

Clomiphene citrate (CC) induces ovulation in 70–80% of cases with 30–40% pregnancy rate and gives 30% cumulative live birth rate.[8-10] CC acts on hypothalamus to secrete GnRH, which in turn gives FSH and LH. In PCOS patients, LH is otherwise also high and is a cause of bad oocyte quality. Therefore, if on day 8–9 of the cycle LH <10 iu in the first CC treated cycle, it is not used in the subsequent cycle.[11]

LETROZOLE

This is a very good alternative to CC. It causes borderline hypoestrinism and hyperandrogenism. The mechanism has already been discussed in Chapter 4 of this book. Because of fall in estrogen levels, it leads to rise in FSH and LH levels that stimulate follicular development. The resultant rise in estrogen has negative feedback mechanism and it reduces FSH and LH, thus allowing monofollicular development. Hyperandrogenism caused by letrozole increases the sensitivity of the follicle to FSH. Letrozole with gonadotropins is a synergistic combination.

There are several reports that indicate that letrozole is better than CC for ovulation induction in PCOS[12,13] and some reports have shown that letrozole is at least as effective as CC for ovulation induction.[14,15] Advantages of letrozole in PCOS patients are monofollicular development, lesser incidence of multiple pregnancy, lesser risk of OHSS and lower abortion rates due to fall in LH levels.

INSULIN-LOWERING DRUGS (INSULIN SENSITIZERS)

Insulin resistance in PCOS patients causes hyperinsulinemia, which in turn stimulates theca cells of the ovary to secret more androgen, through LH. Androgen further recruits more follicles and leads to more LH again establishing a vicious cycle. Hypeinsulinemia in women with obesity contributes to anovulation by increased ovarian androgen secretion.[16] More than half of PCOS patients have insulin resistance. Insulin sensitizers like metformin will reduce the insulin levels and thus will break the cycle and thus helps in correcting the hormonal balance. Metformin acts as an insulin-like growth factors and IGF binding proteins. This blocks synergic action of FSH and IGF on granulosa cells, which is the basis of effectiveness of growth hormone.[17]

Earlier metformin was thought to be a useful drug for ovulation induction in PCOS patients. But recent reports indicate that when metformin is used as the only drug for ovulation induction in PCOS patients, the live birth rate is only 7.2% as compared to that with CC which is 22.5%.[18] Findings of two RCTs indicated that metformin does not increase live birth rates above those observed with CC alone.[19]

It has also been proved that metformin does not lower the dose of CC required when it is used in combination with CC.[19] CC, therefore, is the most appropriate first line of treatment for ovulation induction in PCOS patients. It is interesting to know that anthropometrical data and metabolic characteristics do not give grounds for adjustment of dose of metformin as its efficacy is not dose dependent, but side effects are. Therefore, metformin should be preferred in lowest possible doses.[20] ESHRE/ASRM 2007 consensus on the use of metformin as an agent for ovulation induction shows that there is no clear evidence that addition of metformin to CC as a primary therapy for induction of ovulation has a beneficial effect.[21] Therefore, use of metformin in PCOS should be restricted to women with glucose intolerance and frank type II diabetes.[22] Addition of metformin to gonadotropins has no advantage in improving ovulation rates, pregnancy rates, live birth rates, multiple pregnancy rates or incidence of OHSS.[23,24]

Metformin in Patients for IVF

There are several papers that indicate no difference in metformin and nonmetformin group in pregnancy rates in IVF patients.[24,25] Though it is a common practice for gynecologists and endocrinologists to administer or sustain metformin treatment in infertile patients with PCOS scheduled for IVF, irrespective of their basal metabolic status or clinical efficacy of treatment. In patients with PCOS and poor ovarian reserve, metformin worsened the response to gonadotropins and it should be stopped before starting controlled ovarian hyperstimulation for IVF.[26]

In a meta-analysis that evaluated the effectiveness of metformin as a co-treatment during IVF cycles in women with PCOS, metformin reduced the risk of OHSS by approximately 75%.[27] Another study also confirms that in patients with PCOS, who are at a high risk for OHSS and who have been stimulated with gonadotropins for IVF cycles, metformin reduces the risk of OHSS by modulating the ovarian response to stimulation.[28] A study by KjØtrØd et al. concludes that metformin treatment for 12 weeks before and during IVF or ICSI in nonobese women with PCOS significantly increases pregnancy and live birth rates compared with placebo.[29]

Metformin after Conception

Safety of metformin in pregnancy has not been established. A large prospective randomized controlled trial has shown that when metformin is continued in early pregnancy does not decrease the miscarriage rate.[15] Indirect data from a recent meta-analysis has shown no significant benefit of pregestational metformin administration on abortion risk in patients with PCOS, when either used as monotherapy or in combination with other fertility drugs.[30] Metformin crosses the placenta and significant level are found in fetal serum. Therefore, metformin should be stopped after the pregnancy test until more consistent data are available.

Metformin for Young Patients

Metformin for young patients with PCOS have a long timeline to achieve pregnancy. It is a drug of choice in PCOS patients who do not want to conceive immediately. Its action is gradual and within 6 months, it establishes ovulatory cycles by decreasing insulin and androgen level. Other advantage of metformin is that it decreases the incidence of multiple pregnancies with ovulation induction drugs. If the patient does not conceive when on metformin, option of CC remains open for her. A recent meta-analysis revealed that metformin does not result in weight loss among overweight and obese PCOS patients.[12] Addition of Metformin to lifestyle had no significant benefit on ovulation and circulating androgen levels.[31]

Other Insulin Sensitizers

Insulin sensitizers, proglitazone and rosiglitazone and other drugs like acarbose or d-chiroinositol have not been found superior over metformin and so their routine use for infertile patient has not been established.

Clomiphene Citrate and Glucocorticoids

Half of PCOS patients have adrenal component in hyperandrogenism and are evidenced by increased DHEA-S. This is secreted from zona reticularis of adrenal cortex. These patients are resistant to 150 mg of CC and may also require higher doses of gonadotropins. Dexamethosone 0.5 mg daily can be added for 3–6 months in these patients along with CC. Dexamethasone leads to water retention in patients. Water logging can be reduced by adding diuretics once a week or decreasing the dose of Dexamethasone to 0.25 mg or drug may also be discontinued after ovulation. Serious complications are extremely rare and so this drug must be tried in obese CC resistant PCOS.

GONADOTROPINS

Gonadotropins are indicated in patients with CC failure with high LH and having antiestrogenic effect of CC. As LH is already high in PCOS patients, in nondownregulated cycles, it is advisable to use FSH as the ovulation inducing gonadotropin in PCOS patient. Bioactivity of uFSH-HP and rFSH is also higher than other preparations and dose required will be also less of these preparations.

Specific bioactivity of gonadotropins:

HMG (1950)	8 IU/mg of protein
uFSH (1980)	100–150 IU/mg of protein
uHMG-HP	2,000 IU/mg of protein
uFSH-HP (1982)	9,000 IU/mg of protein
rFSH (1995)	10,000 IU/mg of protein

rFSH does not have inhibiting substances like FSH. It has more basic isoforms, higher consistency and has less batch to batch variations. Because of high bioactivity, the dose requirement is less. Though no significant difference is seen in the live birth rate comparing the urinary FSH and rFSH.[32]

rFSH versus HMG

Meta-analysis of eight randomized controlled trials conforming rFSH with HMG has shown that rFSH has 50% higher pregnancy rates.[33] The FINVAT report in 1999 also showed that the pregnancy rates were higher with rFSH than with HMG. The prospective study of 24,000 ART cycles from Germany also showed higher birth rate and lower dosage with rFSH than HMG.[34] But a Cochrane review in 2009 shows a nonsignificant higher live birth rate with HMG as compared to rFSH.[32]

In PCOS patients, gonadotropins are used as chronic low-dose protocol. The incidence of OHSS is reduced from 4.6 to 1% and multiple pregnancy rate is reduced to 5.7% as compared to 22–34% using this protocol. Uniovulatory cycle rate of 70% is achieved with rFSH with chronic low-dose protocol.[35]

In chronic low-dose protocol, 37.5 iu of rFSH is started from day 5 of the cycle. The same dose is continued for 14 days. Increasing the dose before 14 days loses the advantages of chronic low-dose protocol. Though ovulation monitoring is done during this period and in most of the cases a mature follicle develops within these 14 days. If it does not, then the dose of gonadotropin is increased by 37.5 iu for another 7 days. If after that the follicle does not develop again, 37.5 iu rFSH is increased after another 7 days till the mature follicle is achieved.[36] This protocol gives monofollicular development and therefore higher pregnancy rates. Multifollicular development leads to high E2 and progesterone levels, their altered ratios and therefore low implantation rates.

Homburg and Howles published a study on 2005 stating that if low-dose rFSH is used as the first line of treatment for ovulation induction, the pregnancy rates can be doubled to that of CC. This study showed a clear superiority of low-dose FSH over CC for treating anovulatory patients with PCOS. In first cycle pregnancy, rates are 30% with rFSH as compared to 14% with CC, and in second cycle it is 50% with rFSH as compared to 32% with CC.[36] This explains that the time to achieve pregnancy is significantly reduced. If cost is not a prohibiting factor, rFSH in a chronic low-dose protocol is to be preferred over CC.

We have found a combination of letrozole with rFSH very useful. It is cost effective as it reduced the consumption of rFSH and also gives monofollicular development. Letrozole is given from day 3–7 and rFSH is started from day 8. This regime decreases the incidence of OHSS and multiple pregnancies with comparable results as those of rFSH alone.

GnRH ANTAGONIST

In PCOS patients, there is a tonic rise of LH, particularly in thin lean PCOS patients. There is also a possibility of premature LH surge because of high estrogen levels. The advantage of the GnRH antagonist protocol is the growth of fewer follicles, leading to lower peak estradiol levels and lower risk of OHSS.[37,38] Moreover, the risk of OHSS is also reduced as there is an option of using GnRH agonist as a trigger. It has also been proved that the dose of gonadotropins required are also less in GnRH antagonist protocols.[39]

Antagonist is started when at least one follicle has grown to 14 mm, to prevent LH surge and is continued till follicle matures, i.e., the day of hCG. If antagonist is started early and the LH level is not high at that time, the follicle will regress, as certain amount of LH is required for final stages of maturation of the follicle. Gonadotropin dose does not require increment when antagonist is started. Antagonist also helps in correct timing of IUI. But antagonist is not to be added if premature LH surge is not documented in the previous cycle or there is no proof of raised LH on ultrasound. In IVF cycles, GnRH antagonist can be used as a fixed or flexible protocol. In the fixed protocol, GnRH antagonist is started on day 6 of the stimulation where as in flexible protocol it is started when the lead follicle is more than 13 mm or the serum estradiol levels are more than 600 pg/mL. Antagonist used is Ganirelix or Cetrotide 0.25 mg daily. Similar conception rates can be achieved in long agonist and flexible GnRH antagonist protocols.[40]

GnRH AGONIST

GnRH agonist is used for ovulation trigger in PCOS patients. It induces a sustained release of LH from the pituitary gland that lasts for 24 hours.[41] This is effective to induce preovulatory oocyte maturation.[42] The advantage is that the duration of action of GnRH agonist is shorter (24–36 hours) than hCG and is similar to natural surge.[43] It leads to lesser rise in E2 and progesterone levels and therefore gives better implantation rates and chances of OHSS is also reduced. But when agonist is used as a trigger, the chances of luteal phase defect is very high due to lower circulating luteal E2 and progesterone.[44] Some may also have early luteolysis and a short luteal phase.[45] Luteal support is therefore mandatory in these cases.

GnRH agonist for downregulation is an established treatment in IVF cycles, but should not be used in IUI cycles for the same purpose. This is so because, downregulation in IUI cycles, increases gonadotropin consumption, multiple pregnancy rate and incidence of OHSS, without any benefit. For IVF cycles, the recent studies have shown that downregulation with antagonist is a better option in PCOS patients. It significantly reduces the risk of OHSS, and also prevents supraphysiological levels of estrogen, which may be an important cause for implantation failure.

ANTAGONIST AND AGONIST PROTOCOL

In PCOS patients, GnRH antagonist is used for downregulation and agonist is then used for oocyte trigger. Agonist when used as a trigger has 24–36 hours duration of action.

It leads to lower FSH and LH resulting in luteal phase deficiency. Therefore, luteal support with 1,500 iu hCG, every third day can be used[46] along with progesterone. This protocol decreases the risk of OHSS significantly. According to the recent studies, even dual trigger may be given. According to this protocol, agonist trigger is backed by 1500 IU of hCG on the day of oocyte retrieval.[46] This decreases the chance of luteal phase defect but should not be used when the follicles are plenty.

OVARIAN DRILLING

Ovarian drilling is an effective tool for ovulation induction for PCOS patients. The advantage of ovarian drilling is that it induces unifollicular development without the risk of OHSS or high-order multiple pregnancies[47] and its beneficial effects can last for up to 9 years.[48] Cochrane review says that 12-months pregnancy rate after drilling and 6-months gonadotropin stimulation both have similar pregnancy rates.

It has also been quoted by Homburg, that spontaneous pregnancy can occur after several years of drilling. Ovarian drilling gives 70–80% of ovulation rate and 60% of pregnancy rates.[49]

A Cochrane database analysis of four randomized controlled trials comparing laparoscopic ovarian drilling (LOD) with gonadotropin therapy, showed similar cumulative pregnancy rates 6–12 months after LOD and after 3–6 months of gonadotropin therapy.[50]

How Ovarian Drilling Works

Various explanations have been described in literature as to why drilling works. But the most acceptable theory is that drilling decreases androgen level by destroying ovarian stroma. This decrease in androgen will decrease LH and change FSH/LH ratio. Stein-Leventhal had suggested that larger the ovary, larger portion of its stroma needs to be removed to decrease androgen and insulin levels. Therefore, what I have found in my practice, only four punctures does not work in majority of cases. Larger the stromal volume, larger amount of stroma needs to be destroyed and therefore more punctures need to be done to decrease the androgen levels to effective limits. Ovarian drilling leads to destruction of the stromal cells which in turn reduces androgen production, decrease in stromal blood flow, leading to fall in serum levels of VEGF and IGF-1. On drilling along with the stroma, small follicles are also destroyed, which leads to fall in AMH levels and therefore increases the sensitivity of follicles to FSH.[48,51] Failure of ovarian drilling in women with relatively high power Doppler indices along with high levels of AMH may be due to severity of PCOS in these women. It is possible that the extent of follicle destruction by LOD in these women was not enough to reduce intraovarian AMH to a level consistent with resumption of ovulation.[52] Another study has also shown that adjusted diathermy dose based on ovarian volume for LOD of polycystic ovary syndrome has better reproductive outcome compared with fixed thermal dosage.[53] This means that measuring AMH and ovarian stromal 3D power Doppler blood flow for women with anovulatory PCOS undergoing ovarian drilling may provide a useful tool in evaluating the outcome of ovarian drilling.[54]

Method

It may be done with unipolar cautery and has excellent results similar to laser therapy.[55] Various other methods have been described in literature without added advantage. Newer methods for ovarian drilling that are being tried now are transvaginal hydrolaparoscopic drilling, ultrasound guided transvaginal ovarian drilling and laparoscopic ovarian multi-needle intervention. The purpose for trials on these procedures is to ease out the ovarian drilling into a less invasive and a simple procedure.

Advantages of Ovarian Drilling

Ovarian drilling is especially indicated in PCOS patients who are resistant to CC. If ovarian drilling is done before starting gonadotropin therapy, the dose of gonadotropin required can be decreased and risk of OHSS is also reduced. As it destroys stroma and decreases the androgen and in turn LH levels, it improves the ovum quality and decreases the risk of abortions, the incidence of which is higher in PCOS patients as compared to non-PCOS patients. Ovarian drilling is a one-time procedure and therefore is a suitable method to facilitate ovulation induction in PCOS patients who cannot repeated come for monitoring or follow-up.

The mean treatment costs per live birth within 8–12 years after initial treatment are significantly lower per live birth when treatment is started with laparoscopic electrocautery compared with when started with ovulation induction with rFSH, and electrocautery is a rational treatment for clomiphene resistant PCOS.[49] Laparoscopic electrocautery of the ovaries is as effective as ovulation induction with FSH treatment in terms of live births, but reduces the need for ovulation induction or ART in a significantly higher proportion of women and increases the chance for second child.[56]

Disadvantages of Ovarian Drilling

In spite of having significantly advantageous, ovarian drilling has been widely blamed for post procedure ovarian failure, though the risk is probably exaggerated. Ovarian failure after ovarian drilling is possible only when it is done in an ovary that does not have stromal excess or is not a polycystic ovary. Therefore, it is important and essential to do baseline ultrasound scan prior to laparoscopy and diagnosis of PCO is confirmed and preferable stromal volume is also calculated. Api et al. have concluded in their study that there was neither concrete evidence of a decreased ovarian reserve nor premature ovarian failure associated with LOD in women with PCOS.[57]

Variations in the Method of Ovarian Drilling

Unilateral drilling has been suggested by some workers, with an argument that it has an advantage of a short procedure time, minimized adhesions and ovarian tissue damage, but still induces activity in both ovaries.[58] Though according to other authors, this requires further evaluation.[59] In a latest study, Sunj et al. have shown that unilateral ovarian drilling using thermal doses adjusted to the ovarian volume (60 j/cc) was more effective than bilateral drilling done with constant thermal doses for both ovaries.[60] We have not even seen significant adhesions after drilling during caesarean section of the patients in whom we have done ovarian drilling. Ovarian malignancy after drilling has not been proved.

The major concern is that how many punctures should be done per ovary. According to Balen and Armer's technique, four punctures for 4 seconds at 40 W should be done in each ovary.[61] According to Naether et al.,[62] 5–20 punctures for 1 second at 400 W and according to Gjoumas,[63] 5–8 punctures for 5–6 seconds at 300–400 W. If the above data is closely observed and analyzed, puncture duration is decreased when the power of current (Watts) are increased and number of punctures are less if each puncture is continued for longer time.

In our unpublished study that was conducted from 2002 to 2009, the total number of patients with PCOS enrolled was 2,733. Out of these 134 patients did not turn up after initial investigations and 2,699 patients were taken for study. Out of these 2,699 patients, 1,566 patients had come after taking treatment for subfertility for more than a year. In all the patients, a baseline ultrasound scan was done on day 2–3 of the cycle to assess the ovarian volume, stromal volume and the number of antral follicles and in these patients insulin resistance was also confirmed prior to the procedure. Depending on the stromal volume value, 20–40 punctures with 400 W unipolar cautery were done in each ovary and the results are displayed in the table below.

	No drilling	*With drilling*
Conceived	882 (55.68%)	828 (74.26%)
Not conceived	702	287
Total	1,584	1,115

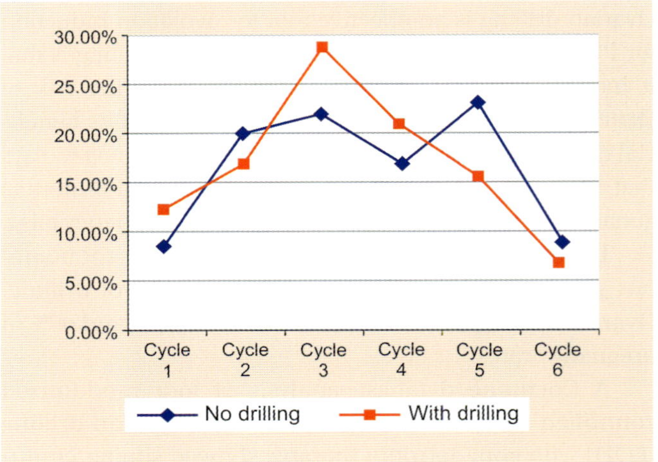

It is seen in the chart above that the number of cycles for conception are fewer when ovarian drilling was done and the author would like to emphasize that there was not a single case of ovarian failure in this series.

IN VITRO MATURATION

In vitro maturation is the future for PCOS patients, as it is 100% OHSS free treatment. The treatment cost is low as consumption of gonadotropins is very low. For this technique, ovulation induction is done with 125 iu/day of FSH (day 3–10 of the menstrual cycle) for 3 days is stopped when the follicle size reaches 10–11 mm. hCG 10,000 iu is given to the patient for final maturation and ovum pick up is done after 33–38 hours. Period for IVM is 24–48 hours. Thereafter, intracytoplasmic sperm injection (ICSI) is done on these mature oocytes. The initial study has documented 8.9 oocytes/retrieval, 64% of maturation rate, 45% of fertilization rate after IVF/ICSI, 15.3% pregnancy rate per transfer and 7.3% live birth rate.[64] The challenges may be adequate laboratory conditions and learning skills for the clinical doing the ovum pick up and also the embryologist.

SUMMARY

1. Weight loss is the first line of treatment.
2. Clomiphene is the time tested drug, but
3. Letrozole is an excellent alternative and may be more preferred.
4. Adding metformin has no advantage on ovulation induction, though corrects the metabolic component, thus supports the pregnancy better.
5. Glucocorticoids may be useful in CC resistant PCOS patients.
6. Chronic low-dose FSH protocol is very effective ovulation induction method for PCOS patients.
7. Agonist may be used as an ovulation trigger.
8. Antagonists to prevent premature LH surge are very useful in thin lean PCOS both in IUI and IVF cycles.
9. Ovarian drilling has excellent results in best hands.
10. IVM is the future.

REFERENCES

1. Thatcher. Defining PCOS—A Perspective. The American Infertility Association News Letter, 2001.
2. Rotterdam ESHRE/ASRM-Sponsored PCOS Consensus Work Group. Revised 2003 consensus on diagnostic criteria and long term health risks related to polycystic ovarian syndrome. Hum Reprod. 2004;19(1):41-7.
3. Erel CT, Senturk LM. The impact of body mass index on assisted reproduction. Curr Opin Obstet Gynecol. 2009;21:228-35.
4. Park HS, Lee K. Greater beneficial effects of visceral fat reduction compared with subcutaneous fat reduction on parameters of the metabolic syndrome: a study of weight reduction programmes in subjects with visceral and subcutaneous obesity. Diabet Med. 2005;22:266-72.
5. Smith SR, Zachwieja JJ. Visceral adipose tissue: a critical review of intervention strategies. Int J Obes Relat Metab Disrd. 1999;23:329-35.
6. Homburg R. Understanding the problems of treating PCOS. In: Homburg R (Ed). Ovulation Induction and Controlled Ovarian Stimulation: A Practical Guide, 2nd edition. Switzerland: Springer International Publishing; 2014. pp. 65-72.
7. Fedorscak P, Dale PO, Stroreng R, Ertzeid G, Bjercke S, Oldereid N, et al. Impact of overweight and underweight on assisted reproduction treatment. Hum Reprod. 2004;19:2523-8.
8. Hammond MG. Monitoring techniques for improved pregnancy rates during clomiphene ovulation induction. Fertil Steril. 1984;42:499-508.
9. Dickey RP, Taylor SN, Curole DN, Rye PH, Pyrzak R. Incidence of spontaneous abortion in clomiphene pregnancies. Hum Reprod. 1996;11:2623-28.
10. Glyser M, March CM, Mishell DR Jr, Bailey EJ. A decade's experience with an individualized clomiphene treatment regimen including its effect on the postcoital test. Fertil Steril. 1982;37:161-67.
11. Panda B, Mohapatra L, Sahu MC, Padhy RN. Success in pregnancy through Intrauterine insemination at first cycle in 300 infertile couples: an analysis. J Obstet Gynecol India. 2014;64(2):134-42.
12. Begum MR, Ferdous J, Begum A, Quadir E. Comparison of efficacy of aromatase inhibitor and clomiphene citrate in induction of ovulation in polycystic ovarian syndrome. Fertil Steril. 2009;92:853-7.
13. Badawy A, Elnashar A, El-Ashry M, Shahat M. Gonadotrophin-releasing hormone agonists for prevention of chemotherapy-induced damage: a prospective randomized study. Fertil Steril. 2009;92:860-3.
14. Badawy A. Clomiphene citrate or letrozole for ovulation induction in women with polycystic ovarian syndrome: a prospective randomized trial, Fertil Steril. 2009;92: 849-52.
15. Casper RF. Letrozole versus clomiphene citrate: which is better for ovulation induction? Fertil Steril. 2009;92:(3):858-59.
16. Bohler H Jr, Mokshagundam S, Winters SJ. Adipose tissue and reproduction in women. Fertil Steril. 2010;94:795-825.
17. Stadtmauer LA, Toma SK, Riehl RM, Talbert LM. Metformin treatment of patients with polycystic ovary syndrome undergoing *in vitro* fertilization improves outcomes and is associated with modulation of the insulin-like growth factors. Fertil Steril. 2001;75:505-9.
18. Creanga AA, Bradley HM, McCormick C, Wiktop CT. Use of metformin in polycystic ovary syndrome: a metaanalysis. Obstet Gynecol. 2008;111(4):959-68.
19. Legro RS, Barnhart HX, Schlaff WD, Carr BR, Diamond MP, Carson SA, et al. Clomiphene, merformin, or both for infertility in polycystic ovary syndrome. N Engl J Med. 2007;356:551-66.
20. Falghesu AM, Romualdi C, Di Florio C, Sanna S, Tagliaferri A, Gambineri A, et al. Is there a dose-response relationship of metformin treatment in patients with polycystic ovary syndrome? Results from a multicentric study. Hum Reprod. 2012;27(10):3057-66.
21. Moll E, Bossuyt PMM, Korevaar JC, Laambalk CB, van der Veen F. Effect of clomiphene citrate plus metformin and clomiphene citrate plus placebo on induction of ovulation in women with newly diagnosed polycystic ovary syndrome: randomized double blind clinical trial. BMJ. 2006;332(7556):1485.
22. Nestler JE. Metformin in the treatment of infertility in polycystic ovarian syndrome: an alternative perspective. Fertil Steril. 2008;90(1):14-6.
23. Palomba S, Orio F Jr, Falbo A, Manguso F, Russo T, Cascella T, et al. Prospective parallel randomised double-blind, double-dummy controlled clinical trial comparing clomiphene citrate to metformin as the first line of treatment for ovulation induction in nonobese anovulatory women with polycystic ovary syndrome. J Clin Endocrinol Metab. 2005;90:4068-74.

24. Costello MF, Chapman M, Conway U. A systematic review and meta-analysis of randomized controlled trials on metformin co-administration during gonadotrophin ovulation induction or IVF in women with polycystic ovary syndrome. Hum Reprod. 2006;21:1387-99.
25. Kjotrod SB, von During V, Carlsen SM. Metformin treatment before IVF/ICSI in women with polycystic ovary syndrome: a prospective, randomized, double blind study. Hum Reprod. 2004;19:1315-22.
26. Palomba S, Falbo A, Cello AD, Cappiello F, Tolino A, Zullo F. Does metformin affect the ovarian response to gonadotrophins for *in vitro* fertilization treatment in patients with polycystic ovary syndrome and reduced ovarian reserve: a randomised controlled trial. Fertil Steril. 2011;96(5):1128-33.
27. Tso LO, Costello MF, Albuquerque LE, Andriolo RB, Freitas V. Metformin treatment before and during IVF or ICSI in women with polycystic ovary syndrome. Cochrane Database Syst Rev. 2009;2:CD006105.
28. Palomba S, Falbo A, Carrillo L, Villani MT, Orio F, Russo T, et al. Metformin reduces the risk of ovarian hypestimulation syndrome in patients with polycystic ovary syndrome during gonadotrophins-stimulated *in vitro* fertilization cycles: a randomized controlled trial. Fertil Steril. 2011;96(6):1384-90.
29. KjØtrØd SB, Carlsen SM, Rasmussen PE, Holst-Larsen T, Mellembakken J, Thurin-Kjellberg K, et al. Use of metformin before and during assisted reproductive technology in non-obese young infertile women with polycystic ovary syndrome: a prospective, randomized, double blind multicentre study. Hum Reprod. 2011;26(8):2045-53.
30. Palomba S, Falbo A, Orio F, Zullo F. Effect of preconceptional metformin on abortion risk in polycystic ovary syndrome: a systematic review and meta-anlysis of randomized controlled trials. Fertil Steril. 2009;92:1646-58.
31. Ladson G, Dodson WC, Sweet SD, Archibong AE, Kunselman AR, Demers LM, et al. The effects of metformin with lifestyle therapy in polycystic ovary syndrome: a randomized double-blind study. Fertil Steril. 2011;95(3):1059-66.
32. Van Wely M, Kwan I, van der Veen F, et al. Recombinant FSH versus urinary gonadotrophins for ovarian hyperstimulation in IVF and ICSI cycles. A systematic review and meta-analysis. Hum Reprod. 2009;24:i134.
33. Daya S, Gunby J, Hughes E.G, Collinns JA, Sagle MA. Follicle stimulating hormone versus human menopausal gonadotrophin for *in vitro* fertilization cycles: a meta-analysis. Fertil Steril. 1995;64:347-54.
34. Ludwig M, Rabe T, Buhler K, Diedrich K, Felberbaum R. Wirksamkeit von recombinantem humane FSH in Vergleigh zu urinarem hMG nach Downregulation im langen Protokoll—eine Analyse von 24,764 ART-Zyklen in Deutschland. J Reproduction Med Endocrinol. 1994;4:284-8.
35. Homburg R, Howles CM. Low-dose FSH therapy for anovulatory infertility associated with polycystic ovarian syndrome: rationale, results, reflections and refinements. Hum Reprod Update. 1999;5(5):493-99.
36. Homborg R, Hendriks ML, Konig TE, Anderson RA, Balen AH, Brincat M, et al. Clomifene citrate or low dose FSH for the first-line treatment of infertile women with anovulation associated with polycystic ovary syndrome: a prospective randomised multinational study. Hum Reprod. 2011;27(2):468-73.
37. Al-Inany HG, Youssef MAFM, Aboulghar M, Broekmans F, Sterrenburg M, Smit J, et al. Gonadotrophin releasing hormone antagonists for assisted conception. Cochrane Database Syst Rev Issue 5 Art No CD001750.
38. Kolbianakis EM, Collins J, Tarlarzis BC, Devroey P, Diedrich K, Griesinger G. Among patients treated for IVF with gonadotrophins and GnRh analogues, is the probability of live birth dependent on the type of analogue used? A systematic review and meta-analysis. Hum Reprod Update. 2006;12:651-71.
39. Navot D, Bergh PA, Laufer N. Ovarian hyperstimulation syndrome in novel reproductive technologies: prevention and treatment. Fertil Steril. 1992;58:249-61.
40. Lainas RG, Sfontouris IA, Zorzovilis IZ, Petsas GK, Lainas GT, Alexapoulou E, et al. Flexible GnRh antagonist protocol versus GnRh long agonist protocol in patients with polycystic ovarian syndrome treated for IVF: a prospective randomized controlled trial (RCT). Hum Reprod. 2010;25(3):683-89.
41. Casper RF, Sheehan KL, Yen SSC. Gonadotrophin-estradiol responses to a superactive luteinizing hormone-releasing hormone agonist in women. J Clin Endocrinol Metab 1980;50:179-80.
42. Itskovitz J, Boldes R, Levron J, Erlik Y, Kahana L, Brandes JM. Induction of preovulatory LH surge and prevention of ovarian hyperstimulation syndrome by gonadotrophin-releasing hormone agonist. Fertil Steril. 1991;56:213-20.
43. Scheele F, van der Meer M, Lambalk CB, Schoute E, Schoemaker J, Hompes PG. Exploring the recovery phase after treatment with gonadotrophin releasing hormone agonist for ovulation induction in polycystic ovarian syndrome: three pilot trials. Eur J Obstet Gynecol Reprod Biol. 1995;62(2):221-4.
44. Itskovitz J, Boldes R, Barlev A, Erlik Y, Kahana L, Brandes JM. The induction of LH surge and oocyte maturation by GnRh analogue (Buserelin) in women undergoing ovarian stimulation for *in vitro* fertilization. Gynecol Endocrinol. 1988;2(suppl):165.
45. Gonen Y, Balkier H, Powell W, Casper RF. Use of gonadotrophin-releasing hormone agonist to trigger follicular maturation for *in vitro* fertilization. J Clin Endocrinol Metab. 1990;71:918-22.
46. Humadian P, Ejdrup Bredkjaer H, Westergard LG, Yding Andersen C. 1500 iu human chorionic gonadotrophin administered at oocyte retrieval recues the luteal phase when gonadotrophin-releasing hormone agonist is used for ovulation induction: a prospective, randomized, controlled study. Fertil Steril. 2010;93:847-54.
47. Balen A. Surgical treatment of polycystic ovarian syndrome. Best Pract Res Clin Endocrinol Metab. 2006;20:271-80.
48. Amer SA, Banu Z, Li TC, Cooke ID. Long term follow up of patients with polycystic ovary syndrome after laparoscopic ovarian drilling: endocrine and ultrasonographic outcomes. Hum Reprod. 2002;17:2851-57.

49. Homburg R. Ovulation Induction and Controlled Ovarian Stimulation. Switzerland: Springer International Publishing; 2014. pp. 109-13.
50. Farquhar C, Vandekerkhove P, Lilford R. Laparoscopiv "drilling" by diathermy or laser for ovulation induction in anovulatory polycystic ovarian syndrome. Cochrane Database Syst Rev. 2001;(4):CD001122.
51. Amer S, Li TC, Leder WL. The value of measuring anti-Müllerian hormone in women with anovulatory polycystic ovary syndrome undergoing laparoscopic ovarian diathermy. Hum Reprod. 2009;24(11):2760-6.
52. Nardo LG, Gelbaya TA, Wilkinson H, Roberts SA, Yates A, Pemberton P, et al. Circulating basal anti-Müllerian hormone levels as predictor of ovarian response in women undergoing ovarian stimulation for *in vitro* fertilization. Fertil Steril. 2009;92:1586-93.
53. Mahmoud S, Kamal MM, Hamed MD. Laparoscopic ovarian drilling in polycystic ovary syndrome:efficacy of adjusted thermal dose based on ovarian volume. Fertil Steril. 2011;95:1115-8.
54. Elmashad AI. Impact of laparoscopic ovarian drilling on anti-Müllerian hormone levels and ovarian stromal blood flow using three-dimensional power Doppler in women with anovulatory polycystic ovarian syndrome. Fertil Steril. 2011;95(7):2342-6.
55. Donesky B, Adashi E. Surgically induced ovulation in the PCO syndrome: ovarian wedge resection revisited. Fertil Steril. 1995;63:439-63.
56. Nahuis MJ, Lohuis EO, Bayram N, Hompes P, Oosterhuis GJE, Kaaijk EM, et al. Long-term follow up of laparoscopic electrocautery of the ovaries versus ovulation induction with recombinant FSH in clomiphene citrate resistant women with polycystic ovary syndrome: an economic evaluation. Hum Reprod. 2012;27(12):3577-82.
57. Api M. Is ovarian reserve diminished after laparoscopic ovarian drilling? Gynecol Endocrinol. 2009;25:159-65.
58. Balen AS, Jacobs HS. A prospective study comparing unilateral and bilateral laparoscopic ovarian diathermy in women with polycystic ovary syndrome. Fertil Steril. 1994;62: 921-5.
59. Fernandez H, Morin-Surruca M, Torre A, Faivre E, Deffieux X, Gervais A. Ovarian drilling for surgical treatment of polycystic ovary syndrome: a comprehensive review. Reprod Biomed Online. 2011;22:556-68.
60. Sunj M, Canic T, Baldani DP, Tandara M, Jeroncic A, Paplada I. Does unilateral laparoscopic diathermy adjusted to ovarian volume increase the chances of ovulation in women with polycystic ovary syndrome? Hum Reprod. 2011;28(9):2417-24.
61. Armar NA, McGarrigle HHG, Honour JW, Holownia P, Jacobs HS, LAchelin GCL. Laparoscopic ovarian diathermy in the management of anovulatory infertility in women with polycystic ovaries.: endocrine changes and clinical outcome. Fertil Steril. 1990;53:45-9.
62. Naether OGJ, Fischer R, Weise HC, Geiger-Kotzler L, Delfs T, Rudolf K. Laparoscopic electrocoagulation of ovarian surface in infertile patients with polycystic ovarian disease. Fertil Steril. 1993;60:88-94.
63. Gjoannaess H. The course and outcome of pregnancy after ovarian electrocautery with PCOS: the influence of body weight. Br J Obstet Gynecol. 1989;96:714-9.
64. Roesner S, Von Wolff M, Eberhardt I, Beuter-Winkler P, Toth B, Strowitzki T. *In vitro* maturation: a five year experience. Acta Obstet Gynecol Scand. 2012;91:22-7.

CHAPTER

Complications of Ovulation Induction

6

Chaitanya Nagori, Sonal Panchal

INTRODUCTION

Rising incidence of infertility and more awareness about its treatment has led to more and more use of ovulation induction drugs. This has in turn also led to more number of patients who have mild, moderate or severe complications of ovulation induction.

The commonest three complications of concern are ovarian hyperstimulation syndrome (OHSS), multiple pregnancies and increasing risk of ovarian cancer.

OVULATION OVARIAN HYPERSTIMULATION SYNDROME (OHSS)

Introduction

Ovarian hyperstimulation syndrome (OHSS) is the most serious and life-threatening complication of ovulation induction. The incidence of mild OHSS is 20–33%, that of moderate OHSS is 3–6% and that of severe OHSS is 0.1–0.2% of the population taken for ovulation induction.[1] Fortunately, with acceptance of antagonist IVF cycles with agonist used as ovulation trigger and freeze all embryos policy in most centers; now the incidence of OHSS has sharply decreased and has reached almost zero in some centers.

Ovarian hyperstimulation syndrome occurs due to excess production of ovarian hormones and vasoactive substances as a result of uncontrolled ovarian hyperstimulation. These together increase the permeability of cell membranes allowing the fluid passage in the third space. It is this accumulation of the fluid in the third space which is responsible for the signs and symptoms of OHSS.

Classification of OHSS

OHSS can be classified as early onset OHSS and late onset OHSS.

Early onset OHSS can be detected from day 3 to 7 after the ovulation trigger with human chorionic gonadotropin (hCG) and is usually due to excessive dosage of drugs given for ovulation induction, especially gonadotropins. Rarely, mutations in FSH receptors may be more susceptible to stimulation by endogenous hCG and spontaneous OHSS may occur.

Whereas the late onset OHSS manifests after 10–12 days after trigger and is usually related to pregnancy. Late onset OHSS is therefore because of endogenous hCG secreted by the products of conception and is more severe. Late onset OHSS cannot be predicted unlike early onset OHSS. Moreover, it is equally common in singleton as well as multiple pregnancies.[2]

This classification is extremely useful for the clinician to decide the severity and consequences of the disease and also to decide as to the patient would require hospitalization and whether she should be taken for medical or surgical line of treatment.

Whether early onset or late onset, OHSS is divided, depending on its severity, into mild, moderate and severe. Mild OHSS as seen earlier is fairly common and does not require any treatment. Therefore, Rizk and Aboulghar et al. ignored this and only considered moderate and severe OHSS as complications of ovulation induction.[3] This classification is useful in defining clinical groups in relation to prognosis and treatment protocols.

Moderate OHSS

This presents as abdominal discomfort, pain, nausea and abdominal distention. Though ultrasound shows ascites and enlarged ovaries, ascites is not evident on clinical assessment. Hematological and biochemical profiles are normal. These patients do not require hospitalization, though regular follow-up is recommended.

Severe OHSS

This stage can be further divided into three grades.

Grade A: Patient presents with dyspnea, nausea, vomiting, diarrhea, abdominal pain with marked distention and oliguria. Acitis in this stage is clinically detected. Hydrothorax may be present. Ultrasound confirms ascites with large ovaries. Biochemical profiles are still maintained within normal range. These patients may require hospitalization but in some centers may also be treated on outpatient basis.

Grade B: The severity of dyspnea, diarrhea, vomiting, oliguria, abdominal distention, pain all increase in severity as compared to grade A. Laboratory investigations show increased hematocrit, abnormal renal function tests (blood urea and serum creatinine levels) and abnormal liver function tests. These patients required hospitalization and vigilant supervision.

Grade C: Apart from all the symptoms and signs of the grade B, the patient then develops acute respiratory distress syndrome. Patients may go into total renal failure. Venous thrombosis is a common complication. These patients are severely ill and require ICU support.

Pathophysiology of OHSS

For prevention and treatment of this severe complication, it is important to understand the pathophysiology of OHSS. OHSS is characterized by ovarian enlargement and shifting of fluid rich in protein specially albumin in third space causing ascites and effusions. Severity of OHSS is directly related to the capillary permeability.

Changes in the Ovary

The ovaries are enlarged due to multiple corpus lutea and stromal edema. There is neovascularization.

Biochemically, there is increased secretion of vascular endothelial growth factor (VEGF), prorenin, active renin, interleukins 1, 2 and 6, prostaglandins, tumor necrosis factor (TNFα), insulin like growth factor (IGF), transforming growth factor (TGF) and N_2O_2. Most of these substances are angiogenic, act through VEGF and are responsible for neovascularization during folliculogenesis and luteinization in the ovary.

Third Space

There is collection of the fluid in the third space presenting as ascites, hydrothorax with massive pleural effusion. This fluid shift is due to increased capillary permeability. This shifting starts after the hCG injection and even before oocyte retrieval. Production of VEGF is depending on hCG, that is given as a trigger or endogenous hCG of pregnancy. VEGF is secreted from granulosa cells. It is responsible for increasing the capillary permeability and fluid shifting.[4] There is rise in the intraperitoneal pressure beyond the intraluminal pressure in inferior vena cava, decreasing the flow in the inferior vena cava. This leads to decreased preload to the heart, decreased cardiac output causing impairment of respiration and renal functions. Antidiuretic hormone (ADH) is also increased because of activation of renin-angiotensin mechanism and this leads to oliguria and hemoconcentration.

Vascular Permeability Factor (VPF)

This is similar to VEGF. It is responsible for vascular leakage. Patients in whom it is present in corpus luteum, follicular fluid, serum and peritoneal fluid are the patients at a high risk of developing OHSS.[5] Being of ovarian origin, its concentration in follicular fluid is high (almost double). When pregnancy occurs, hCG rescues the corpus luteum and VPF secretion increases.

Familial mutations in FSH receptors may increase its sensitivity to trophoblastic hCG and can cause OHSS with spontaneous pregnancy. High E2 is not responsible for OHSS as when hCG is withheld high estradiol alone cannot cause OHSS. This is so because estradiol does not have vasoactivity and cannot cause vascular dysfunction.

Prediction of OHSS can be done before starting stimulation, can be related to stimulation protocols and the stimulation but before hCG. OHSS management is difficult and prognosis is poor so it is important to predict OHSS and prevent it rather than treating it after its occurrence.

Prediction before Stimulation

Risk of OHSS is high in polycystic ovarian syndrome (PCOS) patients, especially the young, thin lean PCOS patients, with antral follicle count of more than 26, with typical peripheral polycystic pattern. Their anti-Müllerian hormone (AMH) levels may be more than 30 pmol/mL or more than 7 ng/mL. In patients with these values of AMH, all cycles were canceled in some centers to prevent OHSS.[6] AMH levels of more than 3.36 ng/mL has 90.5% sensitivity and 81.3% specificity for subsequent development of OHSS.[7] Patients who had OHSS in previous pregnancy are also at a higher risk of developing OHSS.

1. On the baseline (day 2–3) ultrasound scan, if the ovary of a young (<24 years) woman, with body mass index (BMI) of less than 22, is more than 10 cc in volume,

has more than 12–15 follicles in individual ovary, has ovarian stromal resistance index of less than 0.5 and ovarian stromal peak systolic velocity of more than 10 cm/second, ovarian stromal flow index of more than 15, these are the patients who have a very high risk of developing OHSS. In these patients, the doses of gonadotropins should be very low for ovulation induction.[8,9]

2. FSH receptor genotype: FSH receptor mutations and polymorphisms when activated can cause OHSS.[10] To date, 744 single nucleotide polymorphisms have been identified in FSH receptor gene. The N^{680} allele can be associated with hyper-responders and these patients are more prone to develop OHSS. Significant increase in allele N^{680} is observed as severity of OHSS increases. Therefore, it is concluded that genotype in position 680 of FSH receptor cannot predict which patient will develop OHSS but it can predict the severity of OHSS among the patients who develop OHSS.[11]
3. Prediction of OHSS by BMP 15 gene: BMP is bone morphologic protein-15 is related to dose-dependent OHSS. It is a member of TGFβ. It helps to predict the patients likely to develop OHSS.[12]
4. Cystic fibrosis transmembrane conductance regulator (CFTR): Esotradiol upregulates CFTR expression and this phenomenon can cause increase in fluid in peritoneal cavity. This means it may provide a causative link between hyperestrinism and OHSS.[13]

RISK OF OHSS RELATED TO STIMULATION PROTOCOLS

- Long protocol increases the risk of OHSS.
- The number of days of gonadotropin treatment is one of the important factors positively related with the risk of OHSS. In GnRH agonist and antagonist cycles, the number of days of ovulation induction increases and so does the risk of OHSS.
- Using hCG as aluteal support significantly increases the risk of OHSS in patients with multifollicular development.
- On ultrasound monitoring during stimulation, more number of small sized (<9 mm size, >15 in number).[14] Follicles, large volume of the ovary and increased stromal vascularity may be important findings that would suggest increased risk of OHSS.
- The type of gonadotropin did not show any significant difference in development of OHSS. Therefore, the incidence is same with rFSH, urinary FSH and purified HMG.[15] More important is the type of stimulation (chronic low dose, step up, step down) is more important chronic low-dose protocol that has very low rate of OHSS.

Predicting OHSS after the Stimulation and before hCG

1. Estradiol level: Estradiol level of more than 4,000 pg/mL in ART cycle and more than 1,700 pg/mL in ovulation induction is considered high risk for OHSS development.
2. Ultrasound findings: Even when the age of the patient and total number of follicles are similar, the ovarian volume was significantly higher in the patients who developed OHSS (271 ± 87 vs. 157.30 ± 54.20 mL).[16]

PREVENTION OF OHSS

The prevention strategy is divided into primary prevention and secondary prevention.

Primary Prevention

This is by methods and drugs that are selected before stimulation.

- GnRH antagonist protocol: Initial studies showed no difference in severe OHSS in antagonist or long agonist protocols. In antagonist protocols, the pregnancy rate was also found to be lower.[17] But the two recent meta-analysis comparing agonist and antagonist protocol showed significantly lower incidence and severity of OHSS with antagonist protocol.[18,19]
- Laparoscopic ovarian drilling: Both ovarian diathermy and laser vaporization performed prior to stimulation decreases the incidence of OHSS. The transvaginal ovarian diathermy is used in difficult cases. Best results are obtained in thin lean PCOS patients. Ovarian diathermy should be reserved for young patients with severe PCOS who have positive risk factors for hyperstimulation even on prolonged low-dose FSH regimen.
- Metformin: A short-term course of metformin 850 mg twice a day in PCOS patients, given before down-regulation up to the day of oocyte collection decreases the incidence of OHSS and improved the pregnancy rates.[20,21]
- *In vitro* maturation of immature oocyte: This is an alternative management for patients having high risk

of OHSS. It totally avoids OHSS and is the future of assisted reproductive technology (ART).

- Low dose gonadotropins: Low dose FSH with step up protocol should be used to avoid OHSS 150 iu FSH should the starting dose.[22]
- Natural cycle ART completely eliminates the risk of OHSS, though gives significantly low pregnancy rates.
- Avoiding hCG as a luteal support may also decrease the risk of OHSS.

Secondary Prevention of OHSS

- Withholding hCG: Withholding hCG and canceling the cycle when estradiol level is more than 4,000 pg/mL can avoid OHSS. Even when estradiol is less than 4,000 pg/mL, but its values are doubling or more every 2–3 days is also a warning sign against OHSS. This method was commonly used to avoid OHSS, but this increases the financial and emotional burden on the patient. Patients are not happy to drop the cycle. hCG plays a significant role in the development of OHSS as it promotes the secretion of VEGF. Luteinizing hormone (LH) receptors are present on day 8–10 mm size of the follicles. Therefore, more medium sized follicles means, higher risk of OHSS.
- Coasting: It is delaying the administration of hCG. It was one of the most popular methods with long protocol to prevent OHSS. It may help not to cancel the cycle like withholding hCG. Ideally, coasting starts when lead follicle is less than 15–16 mm and E2 level is more than 1,500 pg/mL. No further FSH is given for stimulation. The lead follicle still continues to grow during coasting because it has LH receptors. Normally, follicle continues to grow for 4 more days. Coasting diminishes the functioning of the granulosa cell cohort, causes atresia of small follicles, reduces VEGF secretion and gene expression, thus reducing the risk of OHSS. Coasting should not be done for more than 4 days as it leads to marked fall in estradiol levels and conception rates are low. Human chorionic gonadotropin is given when estradiol (E2) level decreases to less than 3,000 pg/mL. This reduces the risk of OHSS but still allows a reasonable chance of conception.[18]
- Reducing the dose of hCG: Sufficient data is not available on the effects of using lower doses of hCG but there is a general consensus that when E2 is more than 3,000 pg/mL, dose of hCG should be halved. The dose between 3,300 and 5,000 iu of hCG decreases the risk of OHSS.[23]
- GnRH agonist trigger:
  - In patients on antagonist protocol, gonadotropin-releasing hormone agonist (GnRHa) can be used as ovulation trigger. This definitely abolishes the risk of OHSS. It gives the same oocyte quality as hCG trigger with same fertilization rate and cleavage rates. But initial studies showed poor ongoing pregnancy rates due to severe luteal phase defect.
  - This luteal phase defect can be avoided by giving 15,000 iu of hCG on the day of ovum pick up. This rescues the corpus luteum. This may be used of the total number of follicles were less than 24. This regime gives very good pregnancy rates with extremely low risk of OHSS.[24]
  - Grienser et al. proposed to freeze all embryos and do the embryo transfer in the subsequent cycles after GnRHa trigger. Higher cumulative pregnancy rate is claimed by this strategy.[25]
  - One more option is that when the patient was already on agonist downregulation cycle and the risk of OHSS was evident, one may withdraw agonist, replace it with antagonist and then give agonist trigger can reduce the risk of OHSS.[26]
  - Antagonist can be continued in high-risk OHSS patients, who were downregulated by agonist. Coasting with GnRHa has no benefit in preventing OHSS as concluded in a recent Cochrane database.[27] Occasionally, moderate OHSS may occur particularly when pregnancy occurs but severe OHSS is not reported with GnRHa trigger.
- Recombinant LH (rLH) for ovulation: Triggering the ovulation with rLH decreases the risk of OHSS because it does not produce VEGF and so the vascular permeability is not altered. But the pregnancy rates are low. Optimum dose of LH that would maintain the pregnancy rates and still eliminate the risk of OHSS is still not known. Moreover, the ovulating dose of LH is very high and therefore it may prove to be very expensive. The total dose required is 5,000–30,000 iu of rLH. Because rLH has a very short half-life (20 minutes), repeated doses may be required.[28]
- Intravenous (IV) Albumin: There are various reports in favor of and against the use of albumin for prevention of OHSS. Intravenous albumin prevents fluid accumulation the third space and corrects hemodynamic instability by increasing colloidal osmotic pressure. Albumin maintains intravascular volume and prevents hypovolemia, ascites and hemoconcentration.

It counters the vasoactive substances released from corpora lutea. One of the Cochrane reviews has mentioned that albumin is effective in reducing the incidence of OHSS,[29] but the recent reviews do not support this statement. If it is used, it is given 100 mL at the time of oocyte retrieval and 48 hours after oocyte retrieval. In established OHSS, albumin helps to prevent complications of hemoconcentration. But its osmotic pressure lasts for only 36 hours and therefore repeat doses are required.

- Hydroxyethyl starch (HES) solution: HES is a volume expander. It is used as 6% solution in a dose of 1,000 mL at the time of oocyte retrieval and 5,000 mL is given 48 hours after the first one. Hydroxyethyl starch decreases the incidence of moderate and severe OHSS. Recent Cochrane review states the results of HES are better than that of albumin for the purpose.[30]
- Glucocorticoids: It was thought to be useful because of anti-inflammatory action preventing the development of OHSS. It was also tough to have an inhibitory effect on VEGF. But most of the studies could not prove its role in preventing OHSS.[31]
- Ovarian suppression:
  - GnRHa: Continuing GnRHa even after hCG decreases the LH surge and diminishes the occurrence of OHSS. All the embryos are frozen in these cycles and transferred in subsequent cycles. This is useful in ovum donors.
  - E2 and hydroxyl progesterone intramuscular (IM) after embryo transfer also prevents ovarian secretion and prevents OHSS but its role is not yet proved.
  - Aromatase inhibitors in luteal phase have shown promising results. These decrease luteal E2 concentration and thus decrease the incidence of OHSS. This also is useful for ovum donors.
- Dopamine agonist: VEGF increases the vascular permeability. Dopamine agonists acts by VEGF receptor-2 specific inhibition and prevents vascular permeability. The drugs in this group arecabergoline, bromocryptine and quinagolide. There are up to 80 unregulated genes and 7 down regulated genes in those developing OHSS as compared to normal controls.

  Tyrosine hydroxylate is also downregulated in OHSS. Therefore, it is a natural inhibitor for angiogenic process. This suggests dopamine may act as an anti-angiogenic factor and its deficit may lead to OHSS. Dopamine decreases vascular permeability by decreasing VEGF R-2 phosphorylation. Dopamine receptor 2 agonist (cabergoline) inhibits VEGFR-2 dependent vascular permeability without affecting luteal angiogenesis and therefore has no luteolytic effect.[28]

  The recommended dose is 0.5 mg cabergoline from day of hCG up to 8 days. It does not affect fertilization, cleavage or implantation and therefore the reproductive outcome is not changed.[32]

  A study by Alvarez et al. has also shown marked improvement in moderate OHSS but there is no significant benefit in patients with severe OHSS and not in estradiol levels also. Nonergot derived dopamine agonist quinagolide is now promoted instead of cabergoline as the later has a risk of causing vascular disorders in patients with Parkinson's disease. Its recommended dose is 50–100–200 µg/daily for 17–21 days till pregnancy test is done.
- Freeze all policy: Elective cryopreservation is done for all the embryos to avoid late OHSS, which is due to endogenous hCG of pregnancy. The results of fresh embryo transfer and cryopreserved embryo transfer in subsequent cycles are the same.[33] But avoiding late OHSS is a big advantage. Though due to inadequate data, Cochrane database still does not accept this policy for all.[34]
- Follicular aspiration: All the follicles larger or smaller should be aspirated to decrease the incidence of OHSS.[35] Aspiration of all the follicles from one ovary before hCG was recommended earlier but this strategy is no more in practice.
- Intravenous calcium: hCG causes mobilization of calcium from intracellular stores and is related to granulosa cells. Human chorionic gonadotropin and LH receptors are members of protein coupled receptor family whose transducers are represented by calcium dependent kinases and so calcium action in OHSS can be linked to hCG.

  Ten percent, 10 mL of calcium gluconate is given IV at 1.5 mL/minute or in 200 mL saline in 30 minutes on the day of oocyte retrieval and is repeated on day 1, 2 and 3 after oocyte retrieval.[36,37] The relief in clinical symptoms is significant. Ascitic fluid volume is lower from day 3 post oocyte retrieval. Ovarian size decreases from day 10 of oocyte retrieval. It has no detrimental effect on pregnancy rate. Intravenous calcium reduces the fluid transfer to third space. It prevents the damage and repairs the endothelial cell membrane. It is an inexpensive and nontoxic approach to reduce ascites and preserve hematocrit values in OHSS. Intravenous calcium is better than HES in reducing ascites.

TREATMENT OF OHSS

Treatment of OHSS depends on the severity of OHSS the patient presents with.

Moderate OHSS

Though these patients do not require hospitalization, they need a close observation. Patient is asked to report about her signs and symptoms, every day at least on phone and even if she is stable she must be called for clinical assessment at least twice a week. The assessment includes inquiring for abdominal pain, distention, nausea and urine output. Weight, abdominal girth and vital data are assessed and the records are preserved. Ultrasound is done to assess the ovarian size and ascites. And the laboratory investigations include blood count, liver function tests, renal function tests, electrolytes and coagulation profile. Patient must be well educated to report immediately if she develops dyspnea, oliguria or neurological symptoms. Sexual intercourse and any strenuous activities are clearly denied. Patient should take at least 1–2 L if fluid every day and leg exercises are a must to avoid thromboembolism.

Management of Severe OHSS

These patients usually require hospitalization unless they have grade A severe OHSS, whereas hospitalization is advisable for these patients as well.

Hospital Management

Clinical Management

Vigilant records of patient's vital data and general condition is essential. Hypotension and tachycardia may be signs of decreased cardiac preload. Patient's weight and abdominal girth are to be checked daily. Urine output may be affected in these patients. Activation of renin-angiotensin mechanism causes increased ADH secretion leading to oliguria. VPF also plays an important role perfect chart of intake and output must be maintained. Ultrasound must be done to assess ovarian size (Fig. 6.1), free fluid in pelvis (Fig. 6.2), ascites (Fig. 6.3), pleural or pericardial effusion.

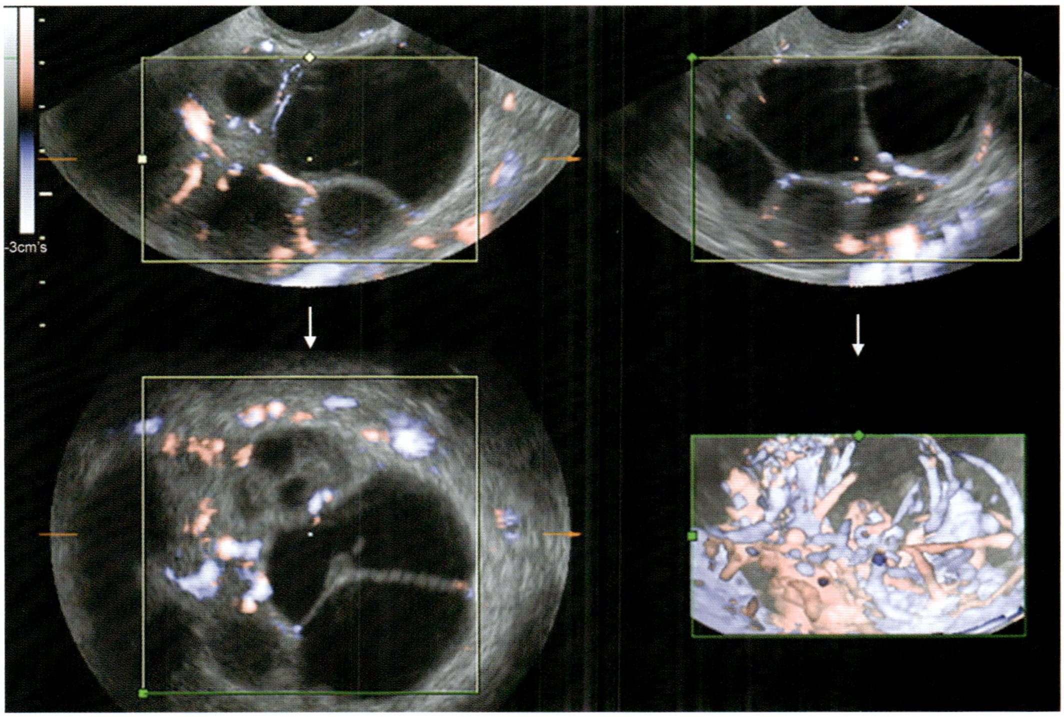

Fig. 6.1: 3D power Doppler (HD flow) ultrasound volume of hyperstimulated ovary.

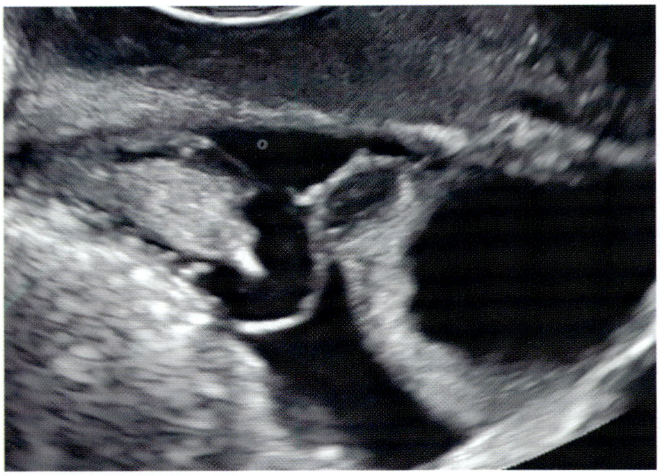

Fig. 6.2: B mode image of free fluid in pelvis.

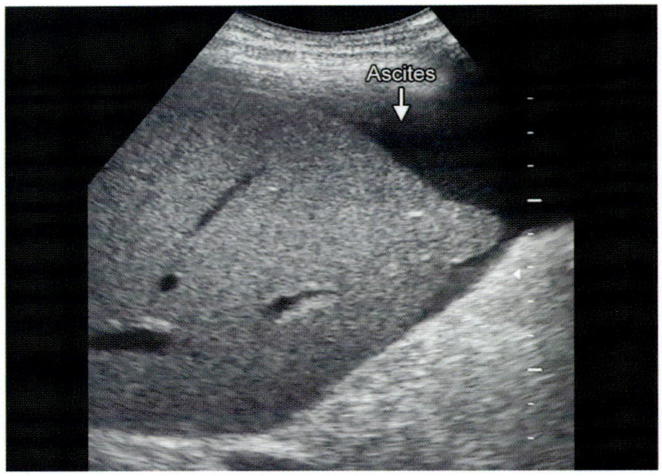

Fig. 6.3: B mode image of ascites.

It is essential to confirm whether the patient has conceived or not because pregnancy can lead to further worsening of the condition. Chest X-ray may be done to confirm pleural effusion. In very critical cases, monitoring of central venous pressure and assessment of pulmonary artery pressure measurement may be required.

Biochemical Monitoring

Blood count and hematocrit values are observed (>55% is considered severe hemoconcentration). Liver function tests and renal function tests are repeated daily. Serum creatinine more than 1.2 mg is alerting. Serum electrolytes must be watched. Sodium less than 135 mEq/L and potassium more than 5 mEq/L should be of concern. Blood gases, coagulation profile and serum beta hCG must be all regularly monitored depending on severity of the condition.

Treatment of OHSS can be divided as medical and surgical.

Medical management consists of:

1. Antibiotic therapy
2. Volume correction
3. Electrolyte replacement
4. Anticoagulants
5. Diuretics
6. Other drugs:
   - Dopamine
   - GnRH antagonist
   - GnRH agonist

1. Antibiotic therapy: Before doping any invasive procedure like ascites or pleural effusion tapping, antibiotic cover is a must. Hypoglobulinemia caused by tapping may lead to severe infections.
2. Volume correction:
   - IV fluids: The main line of treatment is preservation of intravascular volume and electrolyte balance. This is essential to prevent renal damage that may occur due to hemoconcentration. Replacement of fluid in the form of crystalline solutions-normal saline or ringer lactate is preferable. But the volumes replaced must be titrated against urine output to avoid overload complications. Replacement is done at a speed of 125–150 mL/hour to maintain urine output of 20–30 mL/hour.
   - Plasma expanders: These can be used but give only temporary relief but has a disadvantage of increasing fluid in the third space due to increased osmotic pressure. Albumin 0.5–1 g or HES 6% may be used. But both have shown variable results in different reports and may not be of use in established case of OHSS. Though its role in prevention of OHSS is established, repeated hematocrit evaluation is a must when plasma expanders are given. Albumin is given every 2–12 hourly in a dose of 50–100 g at 25% concentration till hematocrit falls below 45% and urine output increases. The risks of using human blood products must be kept in mind. Albumin may be combined with furosemide in patients with oliguria.
3. Electrolyte replacement: Electrolyte imbalance should be corrected. Salt and water restrictions are not required during the treatment.[38] Dextrose 5% with

normal saline is preferred. Avoid hypotonic solutions like ringer lactate which contains potassium.

4. Anticoagulants: Venous thromboembolism is the most serious complication of OHSS. Preventive measures like heparin are extremely beneficial when there is a hypercoagulable state or risk of thromboembolism. Immobilization, pressure from enlarged ovaries and ascites along with hyperestrinism and pregnancy precipitates thromboembolism. Hyperestrinism is a precipitating factor in presence of hypotension and hypovolemia.
   There are diverse views on heparin as prophylaxis in severe OHSS, but should be given to all the patients with congenital thrombophilia or history of familial thrombosis. Prophylaxis is continued for 12–20 weeks according to the condition of the patient. Arterial thrombosis is more common than venous thrombosis which occurs later on.
5. Diuretics: These are contraindicated as they lead to further hemoconcentration, will lead to increased blood viscosity and thromboembolism. The only indication for diuretics in patients with OHSS is pulmonary edema. For oliguria, it should be given only with adequate hemodilution. Abdominal paracentesis instead may be useful.
6. Other drugs:
   - Dopamine: It is extremely useful in patients with oliguria, with OHSS as it improves renal circulation. It is required only for 7 days in nonpregnant patients, but id conception has occurred, it may be required for 10–20 days according to the βhCG levels. Recommended dose is 4.32 mg/kg/24 hours.[39] 750 mg tablet of dopamine 8 hourly will reduce the severity of OHSS.
   - GnRH antagonist on 6th day of pick up and after 4 days of can reduce the intensity of OHSS. But luteal support with both estrogen and progesterone is required.
   - GnRH agonist also can be used for the purpose with estrogen and progesterone as luteal support.
   - Indomethacin: Prostaglandin inhibitors like indomethacin do not cause any clinical improvement and may be instead dangerous because of its renal toxicity.[38]

Surgical Management

Aspiration of the ascetic fluid and tapping of pleural effusion may be required in severe cases. Among the other surgical procedures, required is distortion of the torsed ovary. Torsion ovary is a common complication in patients with OHSS. Rupture of the enlarged ovaries is common and may require emergency surgical intervention. Surgeries are rarely required for thromboembolism and even more rarely a pregnancy termination may be required.

Ascitic tapping: This procedure is especially required for symptomatic relief from abdominal pain and discomfort, dyspnea, respiratory discomfort and oliguria.

Aspiration may be done transvaginally or transabdominally.

1. Transvaginal aspiration is done under ultrasound guidance to avoid ovarian injury. This decreases the pressure in the abdomen and improves renal circulation and improves urine output apart from other ascites related symptoms.
2. Abdominal paracentesis if done blindly without ultrasound guidance has a risk of damaging the ovaries and may lead to hemoperitoneum. Peritoneal pigtail catheter may be placed to avoid multiple punctures if repeated paracentesis may be required in severe cases. Amount of fluid to be tapped on a single sitting may vary from 500 to 4,000 mL depending on the severity of the symptoms. Post tapping albumin replacement is required as proteins are removed in the ascetic fluid.
3. Autotransfusion of ascetic fluid: This is simple and safe and avoids transfusion of exogenous fluids. But the disadvantage is reinjection of cytokines which aggravates OHSS. Peritoneovenous shunting (in antecubital vein) is also recommended.[40]
4. Pleurocentesis: This gives dramatic results. Pulmonary embolism needs to be excluded in patients with severe pulmonary symptoms.
5. Pericardial effusion might also need tapping in severe cases.
6. Acute respiratory distress syndrome (ARDS): It is treated by fluid restriction, dopamine and forced diuresis. It is a result of fluid overload, does not require surgical intervention.

Ovarian torsion: Severe sudden abdominal pain in a patient with OHSS should raise a suspicion of ovarian torsion. Ultrasound may help in diagnosis. Sudden decrease in the ovarian vascularity may be seen. If whirlpool sign is seen, it is diagnostic of torsion, but is not easy to locate in presence of enlarged ovaries (Figs. 6.4A and B).[18] Early diagnosis of torsion may help save the ovary.

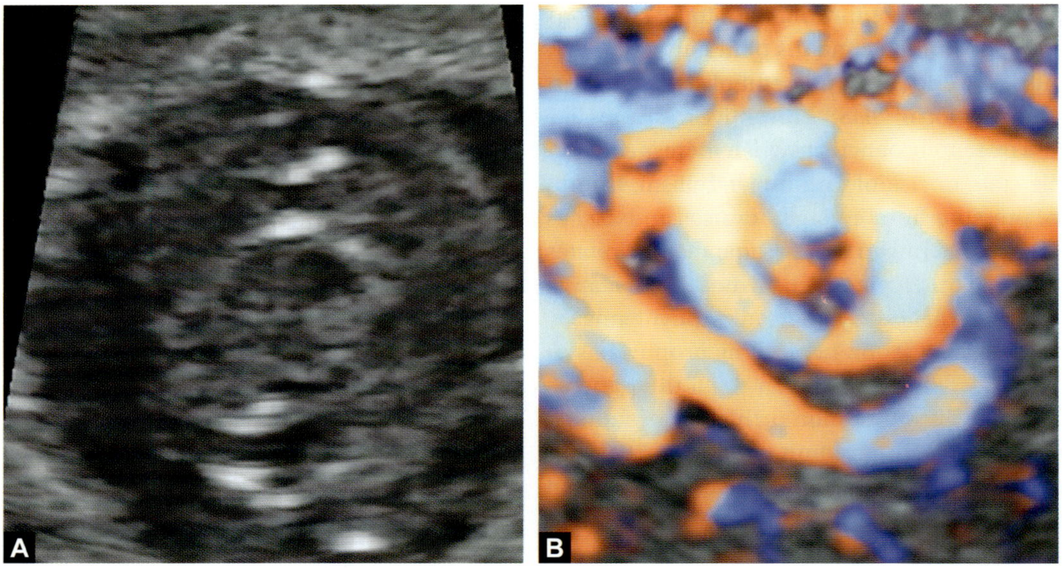

Figs. 6.4A and B: Whirlpool sign as seen on B mode and Doppler.

Laparoscopic unwinding of the ovary and fixing it is the surgical intervention required. This procedure done early during torsion may save a hemorrhagic or ischemic ovary also as this ovary may regain normal circulation in a period of 6–12 weeks.

Ectopic pregnancy: The diagnosis is suspected when transvaginal ultrasound does not show intrauterine gestational sac with βhCG levels higher than 1,500–2,000 iu. However, locating the ectopic gestational sac is a little difficult task in presence of large ovaries. The rupture may lead to severe abdominal pain and fainting attacks, due to hypotension. Clinically, these symptoms are same as that of torsion and differential diagnosis may be difficult.

Ruptured cyst: The clinical scenario is very similar to that of ectopic pregnancy. And in all these cases-suspected, torsion, ectopic or ruptured cyst that present with acute abdomen, surgical exploration with laparoscopy is justified.

Pregnancy termination: Pregnancy termination may be required only in cases with worsening renal, hepatic, neurological and vascular symptoms of severe OHSS in spite of all possible treatment strategies tried.

RECENT ADVANCES

Vascular endothelial growth factor is the critical modulator of the syndrome. The treatment with VEGF receptor antagonist prevents the capillary permeability in OHSS in rat model.[41] Similarly, treatment with chemicals like tyrosine kinase which binds with VEGF and decreases its availability for endothelial effects have similar results in OHSS in rat model.[42]

Second most dreaded complication of ovarian stimulation is cancer. The population based cancer registry identified increased incidence of ovarian cancers in infertile women as compared to general population.[43] The increased risk of ovarian cancer was found in women who were treated with clomiphene citrate for more than a year.[44] But when the same study was extended this increased risk was not confirmed. The women with unexplained infertility are more prone to ovarian cancer and cancer of the body of the uterus, than those with a known cause of infertility.[45] There is no increase in incidence of ovarian or breast cancer with endometriosis. Ovarian stimulation for IVF has shown no increase in the incidence of breast cancer but there is an insignificant increase in the incidence of ovarian cancer.

Ovarian cancer, which is a very common cancer in women, commonly presents at the age of 55–65 years of age. It is usually diagnosed late. Repeated ovulation that causes injury to the ovarian surface and high levels of FSH, LH and E2 have been considered as the root cause of ovarian cancer. Therefore, it may be more feared in the patients undergoing IVF treatment.

MULTIPLE PREGNANCIES

These are common with gonadotropin stimulated cycles that lead to multifollicular development. Multiple pregnancies are thought to be complication of ovulation induction because it leads to lot of pregnancy related complications. The most important is preterm births because this is associated with increased neonatal morbidity and mortality, higher risks of neurological deficits, cerebral palsy, higher susceptibility to severe infections as infancy or child hood complications. These children as they grow also have an increased risk of hypertension, diabetes, cardiac diseases and abnormal lipid profiles. Mothers have higher risk of pregnancy induced hypertension, gestational diabetes mellitus, etc. Multiple pregnancy can prevented or controlled by single embryo transfer policy for IVF cycles, chronic low dose or minimal stimulation protocols.

Though being very commonly used and being safe when judiciously planned, ovulation induction has several risks. If judiciously used ovulation induction is a very important aspect of any ART procedure.

REFERENCES

1. Rizk B, Rizk CB, Nawar MG, Garcia-Velasco JA, Sallam HN. Ultrasonography in the prediction and management of ovarian hyperstimulation syndrome. In: Rizk B (Ed.). Ultrasonography in Reproductive Medicine and Infertility. Cambridge, UK: Cambridge University Press; 2010. pp. 299-312.
2. De Neubourg D, Mangelschots K, Van Roten E, Vercruyssen M, Gerris J. Singleton pregnancies are as affected by ovarian hyperstimulation syndrome as twin pregnancies. Fertil Steril. 2004;82:1961-3.
3. Rizk B, Aboulghar MA. Classification, pathophysiology and management of ovarian hyperstimulation syndrome. In: Brinsden P (Ed.). A Textbook of *In Vitro* Fertilization and Assisted Reproduction, 2nd edition. Cranforth, UK: The Parthenon Publishing Group; 1999. pp. 131-55.
4. Rizk B, Aboulghar MA, Smitz J, Ron-El R. The role of vascular endothelial growth factor and interleukins in the pathogenesis of severe ovarian hyperstimulation syndrome. Hum Reprod Update. 1997;3:255-66.
5. Krasnow JS, Berga SL, Guzick DS, Zelenik AJ, Yeo KT. Vascular permeability factor and vascular endothelial growth factor in ovarian hyperstimulation syndrome: a preliminary report. Fertil Steril. 1996;65(3):552-5.
6. La MArca, Giulini S, Tirelli A, Bertucci E, Marsella T, Xella S, et al. Anti-Müllerian hormone measurement on any day of the menstrual cycle strongly predicts ovarian response in assisted reproductive technology. Hum Reprod. 2007;22:766-71.
7. Lee TH, Liu CH, Huang CC, et al. Serum anti-Müllerian hormone and oestradiol levels as oredictors of ovarian hyperstimulation syndrome in assisted reproductive technology cycles. Hum Reprod. 2008;23:160-7.
8. Kupesic S, Kurjak A. Predictors of IVF outcome by three-dimensional ultrasound. Hum Reprod. 2002;17(4):950-5.
9. Panchal S, Nagori CB. Ultrasound based decision making on stimulation protocol for superovulated IUI cycles. IJIFM. 2016;7(1):7-13.
10. Rizk B. Genetics of ovarian hyperstimulation syndrome. Reprod Biomed Online. 2009;19:14-27.
11. Daelmans C, Smits G, de Maertelaer V, Costagliola S, Englert Y, Vassart G, et al. Prediction of severity of symptoms in iatrogenic ovarian hyperstimulation syndrome by follicle stimulating hormone receptor Ser680Asn polymorphism. J Clin Endocrinol Metab. 2004;89:6310-15.
12. Moron FJ, de Castro F, Royo JL, et al. Bone morphogenetic protein 15 (BMP15) alleles predict over-response to recombinant follicle stimulating hormone and iatrogenic ovarian hyperstimulation syndrome (OHSS). Pharmacogenet Genom. 2006;16:485-95.
13. Ajonuma LC, Tsang LL, Zhang GH, Wong CHY, Lau MC, Ho LK, et al. Estrogen induced abnormally high cystic fibrosis transmembrane conductance regulator expression results in ovarian hyperstimulation syndrome. Mol Endocrinol. 2005;19:3038-44.
14. Blankstein J, Shalev J, Saadon T, Kukia EE, Rabinovici J, Pariente C, et al. Ovarian hyperstimulation syndrome: prediction by number and size of preovulatory ovarian follicles. Fertil Steril. 1987;47:597-602.
15. Bergh C, Howles CM, Borg K, et al. Recombinant follicle stimulating hormone (r-FSH; Gonal F) versus highly purified urinary FSH (Metrodin HP): results of a randomized comparative study in women undergoing assisted reproductive techniques. Hum Reprod. 1997;12:2133-9.
16. Oyesanya OA, Parsons JH, Collins WP, Campbell S. Total ovarian volume before human chorionic gonadotrophin administration for ovulation induction may predict the hyperstimulation syndrome. Hum Reprod. 1995;10:3211-2.
17. Al-Inany H, Aboulghar M. GnRh antagonist in assisted reproduction: a Cochrane review. Hum Reprod. 2002;17: 874-85.
18. Al-Inany HG, Abou-Setta AM, Aboulghar M. Gonadotrophin-releasing hormone antagonists for assisted conception. Cochrane Database Syst Rev. 2006;CD001750.
19. Kolibianakis EM, Collins J, Tarlatzis BC, et al. Among patients treated for IVF with gonadotrophins and GnRh analogues, is probability of live birth dependent on the type of analogue used: a systematic review and meta-analysis. Hum Reprod Update. 2006;12:651-71.
20. Tang T, Glanville J, Orsi N, Barth JH, Balen AH. The use of metformin for women with PCOS undergoing IVF treatment. Hum Reprod. 2006;21:1416-25.
21. Moll E, van der Veen F, van Wely M. The role of metformin in polycystic ovary syndrome: a systematic review. Hum Reprod Update. 2007;13:527-37.
22. Homborg R, Hendriks ML, Konig TE, Anderson RA, Balen AH, Brincat M, et al. Clomifene citrate or low dose FSH for the first-line treatment of infertile women with anovulation associated with polycystic ovary syndrome: a prospective randomised multinational study. Hum Reprod. 2011;27(2):468-73.
23. Chen D, Burmeister L, Goldschlag D, Rosenwaks Z. Ovarian hyperstimulation syndrome: strategies for prevention. Reprod Biomed Online. 2003;7:43-9.
24. Humadian P, Ejdrup Bredkjaer H, Westergard LG, Yding Andersen C. 1500 iu human chorionic gonadotrophin

administered at oocyte retrieval recues the luteal phase when gonadotrophin-releasing hormone agonist is used for ovulation induction: a prospective, randomized, controlled study. Fertil Steril. 2010;93:847-54.

25. Griesinger G, von Otte S, Schroer A, Ludwig AK, Diedrich K, Al-Hasani S, et al. Elective cryopreservation of all pronuclear oocytes after GnRH agonist triggering of final oocyte maturation in patients at risk of developing OHSS: a prospective observational proof-of-concept study. Hum Reprod. 2007;22:1348-52.
26. Martinez F, Rodriguez DB, Buxaderas R, Tur R, Mancini F, Coroleu B. GnRH antagonist rescue of a long protocol IVF cycle and GnRH agonist trigger to avoid ovarian hyperstimulation syndrome: three case reports. Fertil Steril. 2011;95(7):2432.e17-9.
27. Aboulghar M. Agonist and antagonist coast. Fertil Steril. 2012;97(3):523-6.
28. Ludwig M, Katalinic A, Diedrich K. Use of GnRH antagonists in ovarian stimulation for assisted reproductive technologies compared to the long protocol. Meta-analysis. Arch Gynecol Obstet. 2001;265:175-82.
29. Aboulghar M, Evers JH, Al-Inany H. Intravenous albumin for preventing severe ovarian hyperstimulation syndrome. Cochrane Database Syst Rev. 2000;2:CD001302.
30. Youseff MA, Al-Inany HG, Evers JL, Aboulghar M. Intravenous fluids for the prevention of severe ovarian hyperstimulation syndrome. Cochrane Database Syst Rev. 2011;(2):CD001302.
31. Rizk B. Ovarian hyperstimulation syndrome. In: Studd J (Ed.). Progress in Obstetrics and Gynecology. Edinburgh: Churchill Livingstone; 1993. pp. 311-49.
32. Alvarez C. Isabel Alonso-Muriel, Garcia G, Crespo J, Bellver J, Simon C, Pellicer A. Implantation is apparently unaffected by the dopamine agonist Cabergoline when administered to prevent ovarian hyperstimulation syndrome in women undergoing assisted reproduction treatment: a pilot study. Hum Reprod. 2007;22(12):3210-4.
33. Griesinger G, Schultz L, Bauer T, Broessner A, Frambach T, Kissler S. Ovarian hyperstimulation syndrome prevention by gonadotrophin releasing hormone agonist triggering of final oocyte maturation in a gonadotrophin releasing antagonist protocol in combination with 'freeze-all' strategy: a prospective multicentric study. Fertil Steril. 2011;95:2029-33.
34. D'Angelo A, Amso N. Embryo freezing for preventing ovarian hyperstimulation syndrome. Cochrane Database Syst Rev. 2007;(3):CD002806.
35. Zhu WJ, Li XM, Chen XM, Zhang L. Follicular aspiration during the selection phase prevents severe ovarian hyperstimulation in patients with polycystic ovary syndrome who are undergoing *in vitro* fertilization. Eur J Obstet Gynecol Reprod Biol. 2005;122(1):79-84.
36. Yakovenko SA, Sivozhelezov VS, Zorina IU, Dmitrieva NV, Apryshko VP, Voznesenskaya JV. Prevention of OHSS by intravenous calcium. Hum Reprod. 2009;24(suppl 1):i61.
37. Gurgan T, Demirol A, Guven S, Benkhalifa M, Girgin B, Li TC. Intravenous calcium infusion as a novel preventive therapy of ovarian hyperstimulation syndrome for patients with polycystic ovarian syndrome. Fertil Steril. 2011;96:53-7.
38. Rizk B. Ovarian Hyperstimulation Syndrome: Epidemiology, Pathophysiology, Prevention and Management. Cambridge, UK: Cambridge University Press; 2006.
39. Aboulghar M, Mansour RT, Serour GI, Amin Y. Ultrasonically guided vaginal aspiration of ascites in the treatment of severe ovarian hyperstimulation syndrome. Fertil Steril. 1990;53:933-35.
40. Koike T, Araki S, Minakami H, Ogawa S, Sayama M, Shibahara H, et al. Clinical efficacy of peritoneovenous shunting for treatment of severe OHSS. Hum Reprod. 2000;15:113-7.
41. Gomez R, Simon C, Remohi J, Pellicer A. Vascular endothelial growth factor receptor 2 activation induces vascular permeability in hyperstimulated rats, and this effect is prevented by receptor blockade. Endocrinology. 2002;143:4339-48.
42. NcElhinney B, Adrill J, Caldwell C, McClure N. Preventing ovarian hyperstimulation syndrome by inhibiting the effects of vascular endothelial growth factor. J Reprod Med. 2003;48:243-6.
43. Rossing MA, Daling JR, Weiss NS, Moore DE, Self SG. Ovarian tumours in a cohort of infertile women. N Engl J Med. 1994;331:771-6.
44. Venn A, Watson L, Lumley J, Giles G, King C, Healy D. Breast and ovarian cancer incidence after infertility and *in vitro* fertilization. Lancet. 1995;346:995-1000.
45. Venn A, Watson L, Bruisma F, Giles G, Healy D. Risk of cancer after use of fertility drugs with *in vitro* fertilization. Lancet. 1999;354:1586-90.

CHAPTER

7

Tubal Evaluation

Sonal Panchal

INTRODUCTION

Tubal pathology is a cause of subfertility in 25–35% of subfertile couples. Evaluation of fallopian tubes' patency, therefore, forms an essential part of evaluation of a subfertile female.

It has been established that when the follicle grows to maturity in the ovary and luteinizing hormone (LH) surge leads to follicle rupture for release of the ovum, the fimbrial end of the tube proceeds to cover the ovulation site. The fimbrial processes cover the ovary like a ball being held in the palm.

Release of the cumulus oophorus is a slow process, and the cumulus oophorus is not ejected by hydrostatic pressure from within the follicle or by obvious contractions of ovarian smooth muscle cells. Release of the cumulus mass was apparently assisted by fimbrial activity.[1]

The ciliary movement in the tubal lumen leads to development of negative pressure that sucks the ovum from the follicle into the tubal lumen. The ovum then advances in the tubal lumen, where the sperms have reached already after a natural intercourse or intrauterine insemination (IUI). Fertilization occurs in the tube and the embryo advances toward uterine cavity for implantation. fallopian tubes are not just tubular portals, but are motile structures and have peristalsis. This explains that the tubo-ovarian relationship and tubal function in the form of tubal peristalsis and fimbrial function are as important as patency of the fallopian tubes for preservation of fertility.

That is why the best preferred investigation for assessment of the tubes should be the one that not only checks the tubal patency but also assesses the condition of the tubal lumen and the tubo-ovarian relationship.

INVESTIGATIONS FOR ASSESSMENT OF TUBAL STATUS

Various nonsurgical and surgical investigative modalities have been reported to assess fallopian tubes. An ideal test should correctly identify all women with tubal disease with minimal false-negative test results. Further, the tests should be cost-effective, well tolerated by the patient, and should not have any complications. But such an ideal investigation is yet to be found. Therefore, various tests have been tried to assess the tubal status. Nonsurgical techniques such as hysterosalpingogram (HSG) (Carey 1914) and ultrasound-based techniques like saline infusion sonography (SIS) (Corfman and Taylor 1966) and hystero-contrast-sonosalpingography (HyCoSy) (Deichert 1993) are less invasive and associated with less serious risks than surgical technique like laparoscopy and dye test (chromopertubation), though the latter is considered the gold standard for assessment of tubal patency and pathology.

Hysterosalpingography

Hysterosalpingography is widely used for tubal evaluation in subfertile women. This method is fairly accurate in detecting proximal tubal disease, is safe, not much expensive, and may potentially be associated with increased pregnancy rates.[2] HSG provides optimal delineation of the fallopian tubes, allowing detection of tubal patency, tubal occlusion, tubal irregularity, and peritubal disease. HSG is generally done in the proliferative phase of the cycle in order to ensure that woman is not pregnant when the procedure is performed. But HSG should not be done in patients having any comorbidities such as pelvic inflammatory disease.

Method

An analgesic or antispasmodic agent is given to the patient, about 1 hour prior to the procedure to reduce lower abdominal discomfort and to avoid tubal spasm. Testing for chlamydia and/or prophylactic antibiotic is recommended to reduce the risk of pelvic infection. Patient is placed in lithotomy position and aseptic precaution is essential. Speculum is used to expose the cervix. Vagina and cervix are cleaned with antiseptic solution. Anterior cervical lip is grasped with tenaculum, HSG cannula is introduced and stabilized into the cervix. Radio-opaque contrast solution is introduced through the HSG cannula, through cervix into uterus. Solution is warmed to body temperature and very small amount is introduced. Under fluoroscopic guidance, filling of the uterine cavity and passage of the radio-opaque solution into the tubes and its spill from fimbrial end is observed and documented in the form of X-rays (Fig. 7.1).

Hysterosalpingogram allows to study the endometrial cavity and diagnose Müllerian abnormalities and endometrial lesions (Fig. 7.2), in addition to its main use to assess the whole tube, condition of the tubal lumen, and site of block (Fig. 7.3).

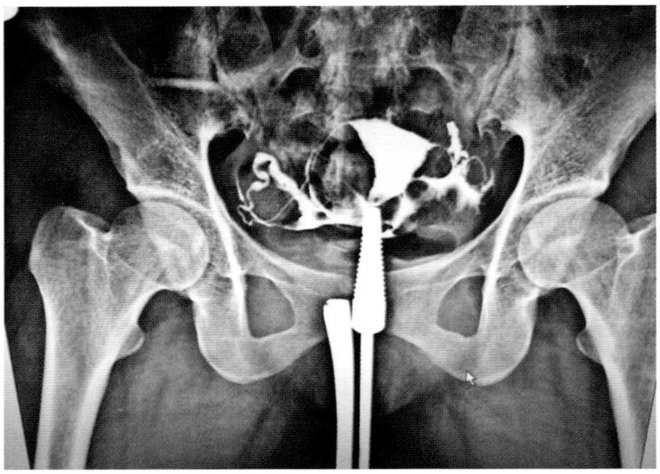

Fig. 7.1: Hysterosalpingogram showing normal endometrial cavity, both tubes, and spill through both tubes.

Moreover, the radio-opaque contrast used for the procedure, contains iodine and, therefore, has a risk of causing a reaction. The procedure is to be done in the radiology set up where both the gynecologist and the patient do not feel very comfortable. However, the main disadvantages are exposure to radiation and its high false negative rates.

Disadvantages

- Extremely painful
- Needs sedation and sometimes rarely anesthesia
- Needs to be done in a radiology set up, which is not comfortable for both patient and clinician
- Moreover it gives a static picture
- Fimbrial condition and tubo-ovarian relation cannot be assessed.

Though HSG has been used for several years for tubal assessment, it has been shown in meta-analysis based on these three studies gave pooled estimates of sensitivity and specificity for HSG as a test for tubal obstruction of 0.65 [95% confidence interval (CI) 0.50–0.78] and 0.83 (95% CI 0.77–0.88), respectively. Tubal block seen on HSG will be confirmed by laparoscopy in only 38% of the women.[3] When HSG suggests that the tubes are patent, this will be confirmed at laparoscopy in 94% of the women and, thus, HSG is a reliable indicator of tubal patency. These findings imply that after abnormal HSG, even in cases of bilateral

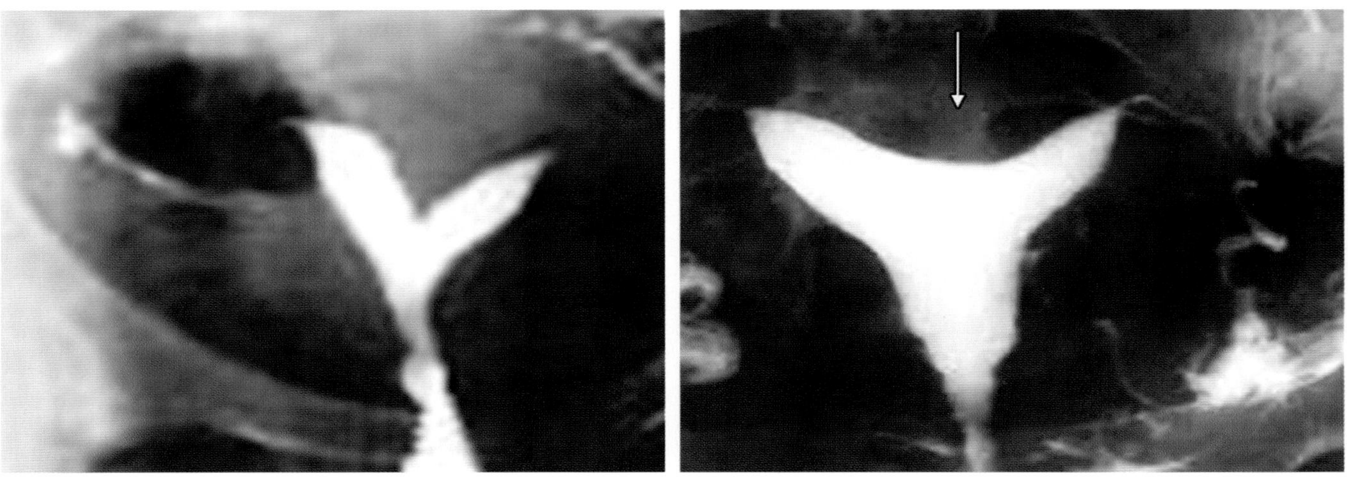

Fig. 7.2: Hysterosalpingogram showing septate uterus and arcuate uterus in figures on left and right, respectively.

pathology such as obstruction, it is still worth performing laparoscopy because, in a considerable number of these patients, the laparoscopic diagnosis allows IUI treatment to remain an option.[4]

Use of ultrasound to test tubal patency may potentially avoid the risk of radiation, while providing the necessary information as provided by HSG. Moreover, ultrasound is an investigation of choice for assessment of uterus and ovaries and was, therefore, tried for the assessment of the fallopian tubes also.

It is because of these reasons that other safer and easier methods for tubal evaluation were sought for.

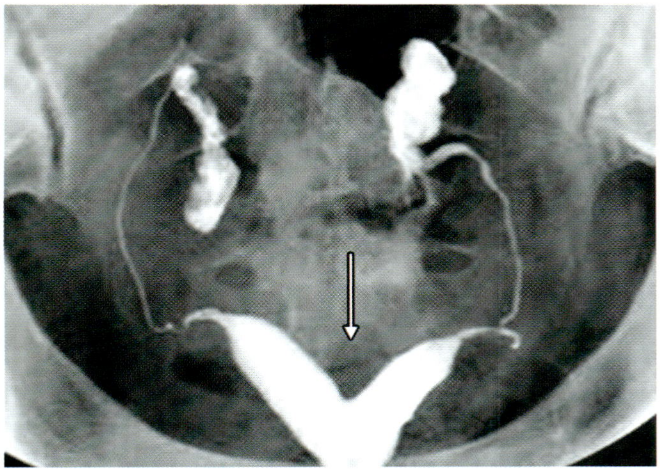

Fig. 7.3: Hysterosalpingogram showing septate uterus (arrow) with normal proximal tubal lumen but bilateral distal hydrosalpinx.

Sonohysterosalpingography (Saline Infusion Sonography)

While transvaginal ultrasound has now proved its place for assessment of uterus and ovaries, normal fallopian tubes are impossible to visualize on ultrasound without any intervention. This is so because there is no tissue-fluid interface when the tubes are normal. fallopian tubes can be identified only when there is fluid in the tubal lumen or outside the tubes. This means that tubes can be identified on ultrasound when either there is hydrosalpinx or free fluid in pelvis (Figs. 7.4A and B) or fluid is introduced in the tubal lumen or in the pelvis. Fluid can be introduced using a catheter through cervix to visualize and assess the fallopian tubes by ultrasound.

Sonographic evaluation of tubes was initially described by various authors, Nanini,[5] Richman,[6] and Randolph,[7] who performed abdominal sonography following intracervical injection of fluid, but was reported first by Richman.

For this procedure, 200 mL of saline was introduced transvaginally, through the cervix into the uterus. Fluid would fill up the uterine cavity and pass through the tubes into the pelvic cavity. Retrouterine fluid seen on abdominal ultrasound was accepted as a criterion for patency. Tufekci also reported use of isotonic saline but with transvaginal ultrasound for tubal patency in 1992.[8] Deichert was the first to report on transvaginal sonographic evaluation of tubal patency, following transcervical injection of echogenic ultrasonic contrast fluid.[9] This investigation was

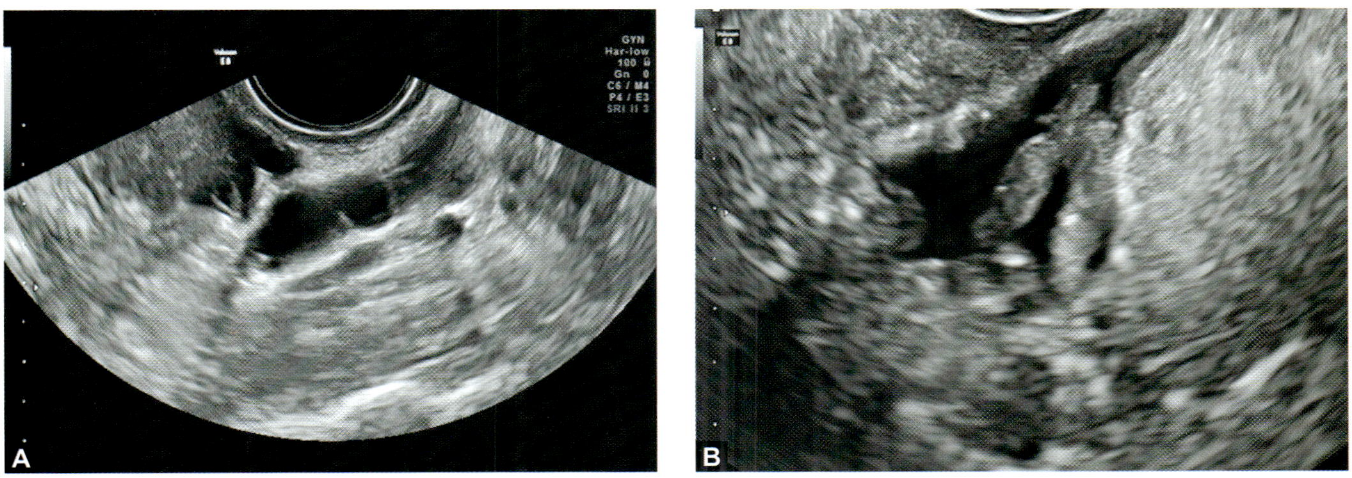

Figs. 7.4A and B: The image (A) shows fluid filled tube—hydrosalpinx, and the image (B) shows the tube floating in free fluid.

given different names by various workers: saline infusion salpingography (SIS), saline sonosalpingography, Saline HyCoSy, etc.

Technique

Sonosalpingography is ideally done in midproliferative phase (day 6–10 of a typical 28 day cycle), after menstruation stops but before ovulation occurs, to reduce the risk of disturbing an early pregnancy. Oral analgesic, ibuprofen 400–600 mg may be given 1–2 hours before the procedure. Preprocedural screening for infections like chlamydia and/or prophylactic oral antibiotics are recommended. Strict asepsis is essential. A detailed transvaginal ultrasound scan is done to assess the position of pelvic organs and to rule out any pathologies, which would come in the way of the procedure. Moreover, any free fluid in pelvis is also checked for.

The probe is removed and speculum is placed in the vagina to visualize the cervix. Vagina and cervix are cleaned with antiseptic solution. If required, cervix is fixed with tenaculum and manipulated to align it with uterus. A 6F–8F balloon catheter or a cannula especially devised for SIS or hysterosalpingography is attached to a 10 mL syringe prefilled with saline. The catheter is introduced through cervix into the uterus. Balloon is distended with 1–2 mL of distilled water or normal saline and is placed just beyond the internal os. Alternatives to this catheter are pediatric feeding tubes or small gauge Foley catheter. Once the catheter is fixed, tenaculum and speculum are removed and transvaginal probe is introduced into the vagina for further assessment.

Saline is injected through the catheter slowly. Scanning is done to assess the uterine cavity that is distended by saline and also passage of saline (fluid) seen through the tubes. When uterine cavity is filled with saline, any endometrial pathology can be demonstrated and diagnosed (Fig. 7.5).

Spill of saline from fimbrial end is seen as fluid flow surrounding the ovary and its collection in pelvis on B-mode scanning (Fig. 7.6).

Absence of spill may indicate blockage. An indirect sign of bilateral tubal block is accumulation of the fluid in endometrial cavity (Fig. 7.7).

It is not always possible to document the spill from the fimbrial end of individual tube. In such cases, fluid accumulation in pouch of Douglas confirms patency of at least one fallopian tube. In patients with bilateral block, distension of the uterine cavity causes severe pain and no spill is observed. Once the procedure is completed, the instruments are removed. Patient is informed that she might get some pelvic cramping or spotting, but the symptoms are short termed and should not worry about it. The accuracy of SIS compared to chromopertubation varies from 81.82%[10] to 100%[11-13]

Complications

The procedure is has no major complication except nausea, vomiting, and mild to moderate pain. The risk of pelvic

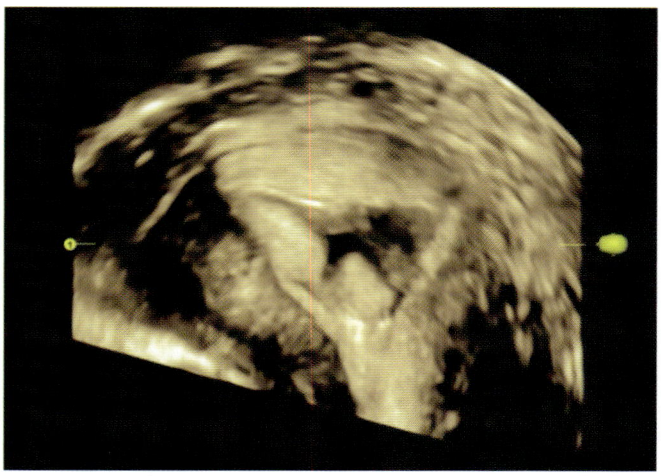

Fig. 7.5: Saline infused in the endometrial cavity shows polyps clearly in endometrial cavity.

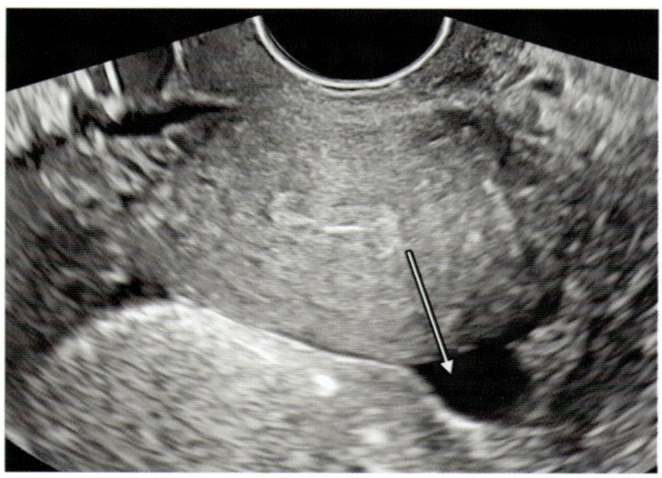

Fig. 7.6: Free fluid collection in the pouch of Douglas (arrow) or around the ovary indicates tubal patency.

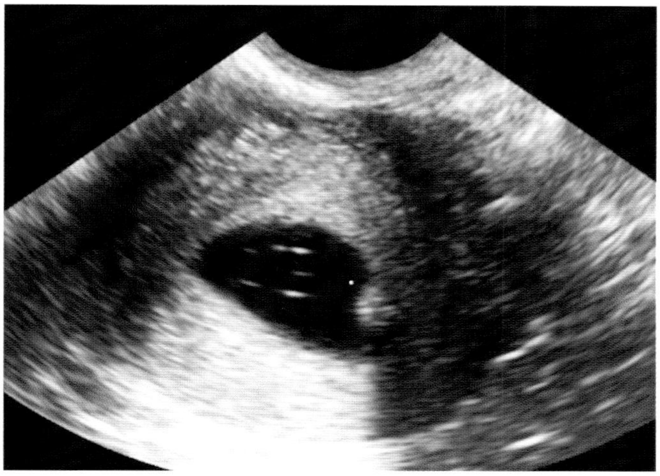

Fig. 7.7: Endometrial cavity distended with fluid.

infection and associated peritonitis is approximately 1%. Vasovagal syncope is rare during or after the procedure. The reported prevalence of complications combined is 8.8%.[14]

Failure to perform or complete the procedure was documented in 7% in a meta-analysis of 24 studies and 2,278 procedures.[15]

Reliability of the Procedure

The agreement of transvaginal salpingosonography compared with X-ray hysterosalpingography was 94%, the sensitivity 50%, the specificity 97%, the positive predictive value (PPV) 50%, and the negative predictive value (NPV) 97%.[16]

Results of SSG correlated positively with laparoscopy in 97% and SSG and HSG showed 93% correlation.[17]

Another study showed sensitivity of SSG as 97.3% for open tubes with specificity of 92%, whereas sensitivity of laparoscopy was 94.6%, and sensitivity of HSG was 94.5% but with a specificity of only 84%.[18]

Saline infusion salpingography in determining fallopian tube patency is as efficient as HSG and can be used instead of HSG for screening infertile patients.[19] HyCoSy showed 97% sensitivity and 82% specificity when HyCoSy was compared to laparoscopy and dye test as a test for tubal patency. HyCoSy is accurate in determining tubal patency and evaluating the uterine cavity and can supplant HSG as the first line diagnostic test in an infertility workup.[20]

The shortcoming of the procedure is that even when patency of individual tube can be confirmed, it does not give any information about the site of the block, condition of the lumen, and tubo-ovarian relationship. Some variations in this technique were tried to overcome this shortcoming.

Modifications

Several modifications have been made to this basic procedure of SIS to improve its diagnostic accuracy as an investigative modality for tubal assessment. The reported modifications are:

- Using pulse Doppler
- Using color Doppler
- Combining air and saline
- Three dimensional (3D) saline sonosalpingography

Using pulse Doppler: If examination during B mode reveals evidence suggesting tubal occlusion or if a small segment of the tube measuring less than 2 cm is not visualized, a pulse Doppler examination can be performed.[21] Doppler gate is placed where the block is expected. This is exactly the point beyond which the tube is not filled with saline or color flow is not seen on injection of saline when examination is done with color Doppler. The gate is reduced to the width of the tube. Brief injections of fluid/saline lasting for 5 seconds are done while Doppler signals are observed.

Patent tube is indicated by a short filling phase with rapid, steep increase in Doppler shift followed by slow uniform fall in Doppler shift. Obstruction presents as short, steep Doppler shift with no subsequent noise signals (Fig. 7.8)[22]

Using color Doppler: Color Doppler can be used with SIS. This is more informative when injection of saline is done selectively toward one of the tubes. Under ultrasound (US) guidance, the tip of the catheter is placed close to either cornu, one by one. First, the color box is placed on the transverse section of the uterus. Color signals following-up the uterine cavity confirm the passage of fluid in the uterus as saline is injected through the cannula in the uterus in short bouts. The field of vision is immediately changed over to ovary and adnexa, by spanning the probe from transverse section of uterus, laterally. While injecting saline, color box is placed to visualize the adnexa and ovary. Filling up of the box with color signals indicates patency of the tube and absence of such signals indicate block[21] (Figs. 7.9A and B). Same procedure is repeated on the opposite side. A detailed evaluation for any pathology is important immediately prior to performing the procedure as hydrosalpinx may create turbulence in the fluid present in the tube and give a false impression of a patent tube.

Adding color Doppler may increase the efficiency and accuracy of SIS for assessment of tubal patency.[23] In a study by Peters and Coloum of 129 infertile patients, Doppler SIS showed complete agreement with X-ray HSG in 81% cases. When compared with the gold standard test of tubal assessment, chromopertubation, Doppler SIS, and SIS showed agreement with chromopertubation findings in 86% of cases, as compared while to 75% for X-ray HSG agreed with chromopertubation only in 75% cases.[21] In a small study by Kupesic et al., in 91.54% of cases, agreement was seen between findings of color Doppler sonosalpingography and that of chromopertubation.[11] Correlation of color Doppler sonosalpingography and X-ray HSG with chromopertubation was 81% versus 60% respectively in one study.[10]

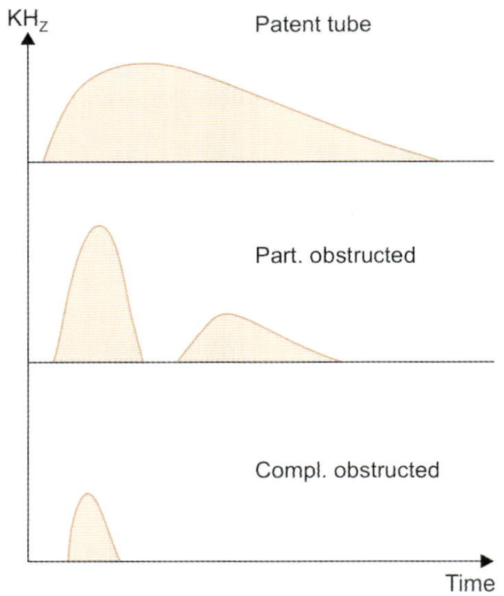

Fig. 7.8: Diagrammatic presentation of fluid flow in patent, partially obstructed, and obstructed tube on pulse Doppler assessment for tubal patency.[22]

Combining saline with air: When air is mixed with saline, bubbles are formed and that makes saline hyperechoic and this helps better outlining of tubal lumen. This can be done either by agitating air and saline or by injecting air after saline has been already pushed in to fill up the uterine cavity and tubes.

This later technique was described by Jeanty et al. and showed 79.4% agreement with results of chromopertubation and showed a sensitivity of 85.7% and specificity of 77.2%.[23]

Transvaginal three-dimensional saline infusion hysterosalpingography: It provides good visualization of the uterine cavity and myometrial walls in three orthogonal planes. However, it does not diagnose tubal occlusion or depict architecture of the fallopian tube as accurately as X-ray HSG. Although the distal fallopian tube and fimbria were seen with real-time imaging, the proximal tube is not satisfactorily imaged with 3D power Doppler (Fig. 7.10). This technique may be reserved as an initial screening test to

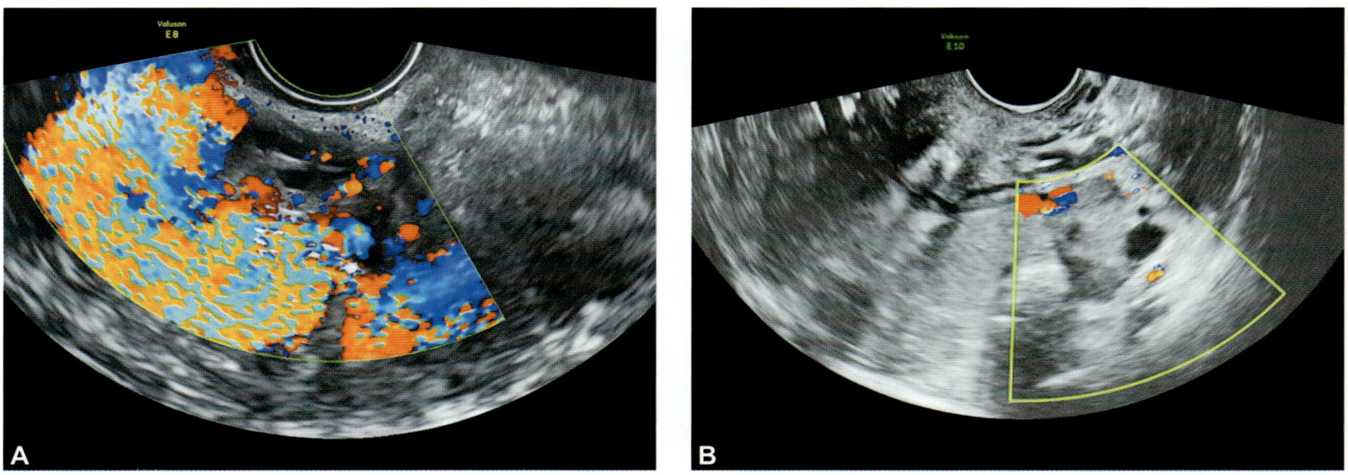

Figs. 7.9A and B: Color Doppler sonosalpingography image of the patent tube on the (A) with entire color box filled with color and blocked tube on the (B) with no filling of the color box.

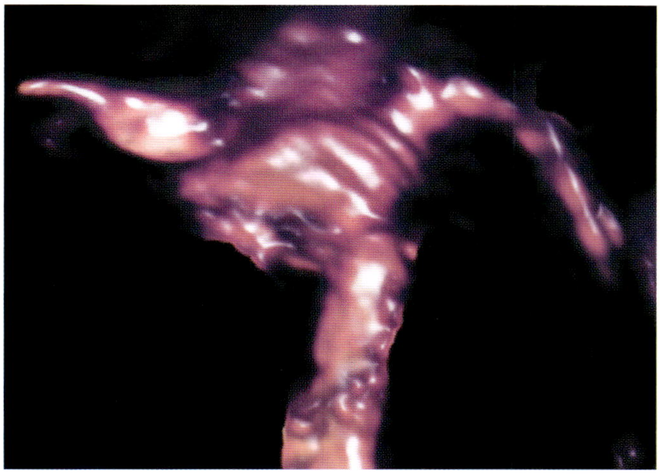

Fig. 7.10: Three-dimensional power Doppler image of saline infusion hysterosalpingography.

evaluate the uterine cavity and test tubal patency. Patients at high risk for tubal disease by history or with suspected tubal occlusion on 3D saline SHSG should be evaluated by either X-ray HSG or laparoscopy with chromopertubation.[24]

Though Kiyokawa et al. have shown that when 3D was added to saline salpingography, the PPV, NPV, sensitivity, and specificity of predicting tubal patency were 100%, 33.3%, 84.4%, and 100%, respectively. Over and above this, this method also has an advantage of assessing the shape of the uterine cavity. The full contour of the uterine cavity was depicted in 96% of cases by 3D-HyCoSy and 64% by X-ray HSG.[25]

Hysterocontrast Salpingography

While intracavitary lesions are clearly delineated by anechoic media, very small hollow cavities, such as normal tubes are not always easily visualized using SIS.[26] Demonstration of the lumen of tubes requires visualization of movement of fluid using highly echogenic medium.[27] Hyperechogenic contrast medium enhances echo signals and allows detection of the flow, both by B mode and Doppler ultrasound.

Experimental and clinical data suggest that insonation of echo-enhancing contrast agents with high acoustic power produces disintegration of microbubbles, resulting in a phenomenon called stimulated acoustic emission (SAE). It is based on this principle that the positive ultrasound contrast media are developed.[28]

Mixing saline with air is a cheap and cost-effective option which produce a high contrast fluid due to the presence of air the bubbles. However, these bubbles stand only for a very short period and, therefore, tubal patency assessment may become practically difficult.

Therefore, commercially available contrast media were introduced with microbubbles that can stand for a longer time.

Echovist and Levovist (Schering AG, Berlin) consists of suspension of microbubbles made of special galactose microparticles. These are suspended either in galactose solution, as in Echovist or in sterile water, as in Levovist. Just before use, these solutions are made by mixing and vigorously shaking the microparticles with the solvent and it can stand for 5–10 minutes. These solutions completely dissolve in the body, within about 30 minutes. These can be used in all patients except those with galactosemia. Non-(embryo-) toxic gel (ExEm-gel® Gynaecologiq BV, Delft, The Netherlands), containing hydroxyethylcellulose and glycerol, has also been used as an intrauterine medium for sonohysterography as an alternative to saline. Gel instillation offers a more stable filling of the uterine cavity. This gel and its compounds have been tested extensively and safely used in medicine. When this gel is pushed rigorously through small openings in syringes or tubes, turbulence causes local pressure drops resulting in air dissolving in the solution, and yielding foam that is stable for several minutes. ExEm-gel® (containing 88.25% purified water), however, is rather viscous for passing into the fallopian tubes. Therefore, 10 mL ExEm-gel® was diluted with 10 mL purified water (to give a mixture containing 94.12% water) and mixed to create foam. The mixture at this ratio creates foam that is sufficiently stable to show echogenicity for at least 5 minutes and sufficiently fluidy to pass through patent tubes. The viscosity of this foam (270 cP) is comparable with that of Echovist (400 cP).[29]

The HyCoSy is a safe outpatient procedure with a relatively low cost and its accuracy has been assessed in a meta-analysis, which compared the results of HyCoSy and laparoscopy and dye tests in 428 infertile women. Sensitivity was 93.3% and specificity was 89.7%.[30]

A meta-analysis of three comparative studies of Echovist-200 (solution of galactose and 1% palmitic acid (Echovist-Schering-AG, Germany), including 1,007 women showed that the results of HyCoSy and chromolaparoscopy were identical in 294 of 428 patients (68.7%) or in 688 of 828 individual tubes (83.1%). HyCoSy showed

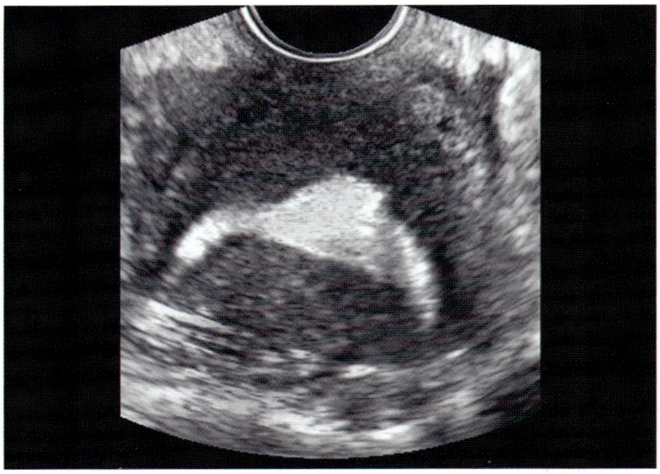

Fig. 7.11: Positive contrast seen in the uterus on B mode ultrasound.

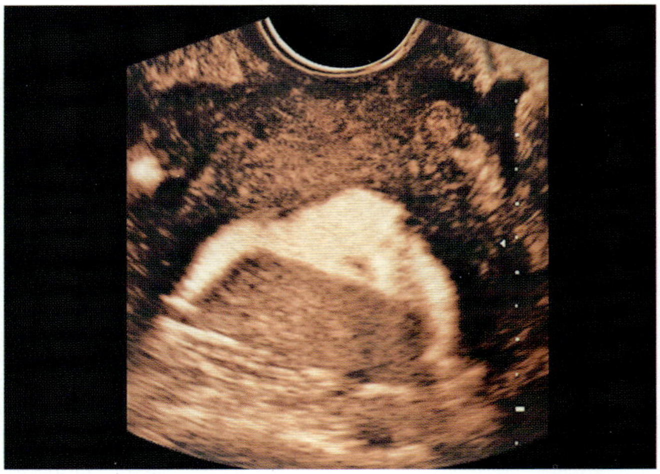

Fig. 7.12: The image shown in Figure 7.11 is shown here on contrast mode.

"false" occlusion in 85 tubes (10.3%) and "false" patency in 55 (6.7%). The results of HyCoSy and HSG were identical in 138 of 202 patients (68.3%) or in 320 of 384 individual tubes (83.3%). HyCoSy showed "false" occlusion in 49 tubes (12.8%) and "false" patency in 15 (3.9%). The findings of chromolaparoscopy and HSG agreed in 49 of 77 patients (63.6%) or in 116 of 152 tubes (76.3%). HSG showed "false" occlusion in 19 (12.5%) tubes and "false" patency in 17 (11.2%).[30]

Contrast agent that is more easily available in most countries including India is Sonovue (Bracco). This contrast agent consists of sodium hexafluoride microparticles in normal saline. For assessment of tubal status, 1 mL of Sonovue is diluted with 4 mL of normal saline and is agitated to create foam for injection into the uterus. This contrast is safe for HyCoSy, as it is for intravascular use also. It is used as an ultrasound contrast agent for vascular studies and for diagnosis of malignancy.

This contrast appears white-echogenic on ultrasound. The scanning technique is the same as that for SIS. Using positive contrast it is possible to delineate the whole tube along with the uterine cavity even on B mode scanning (Fig. 7.11).

There are ultrasound equipment with contrast mode (contrast tuned imaging technology based on harmonics) (Fig. 7.12). The advantage is that it enhances the contrast and makes visualization of tubes even better. Using contrast mode with positive contrast actually makes it easily possible to view the spill from the fimbrial end, if the tube is patent. If the tube is not patent, the contrast column in the tube can identify the site of block.

Technique

The technique for HyCoSy is same as for SIS. As delineation of the tube is better with HyCoSy, total amount of contrast needed is as less as 2–3 mL per tube. For diagnosis of tubal patency, two to three observation phases per tube are needed, with an observation period of continuous flow of about 10 seconds. Visualization of long segments of tube beyond intramural part of the tube usually indicates patency, though whole tube must be observed and spill should be confirmed. Appearance or increase in the fluid in pouch of Douglas may be an indirect sign of tubal patency, same as for SIS. HyCoSy has several advantages over SIS in that it helps clearer visualization of uterine cavity, better assessment of tubal lumen and fimbriae, clearer visualization of spill, and a more exact localization of site of block.

Compared to conventional HSG, HyCoSy provides a simultaneous ultrasound evaluation of pelvis and a more cost-effective evaluation of tubal pathology, and it can be successfully used as a first line noninvasive screening method.[31]

The HyCoSy with contrast is more efficient than with saline solution in determining fallopian tube patency and is as efficient as HSG and can be used instead of HSG for screening infertile patients.[32] In a diagnostic accuracy study of HyCoSy performed with air and saline (hydro-HyCoSy) and with contrast media (SonoVue-HyCoSy) considering hysterosalpingography and/or chromopertubation as reference tests, SonoVue-HyCoSy has been found to be more accurate than Hydro-HyCoSy for the assessment of fallopian tubes.[33] While the sensitivity, specificity, and PPV and NPV of Hydro-HyCoSy were 91%, 71%, 55%, and 95%, respectively, they were 87%, 84%, 69%, and 94%, respectively for SonoVue-HyCoSy. The diagnostic accuracy of Hydro-HyCoSy and of SonoVue-HyCoSy were 77% and 85%, with a Cohen's kappa of 0.52 and 0.66, respectively. In another small study comparing HyCoSy and chromopertubation, there was a high degree of correlation in assessing tubal patency, with sensitivity, specificity, PPV, and NPV of 100%, 55.6%, 80%, and 100%, respectively.[29]

Moreover, the amount contrast agent required for adequate examination was also less with positive contrast. Mean volumes of contrast injections were 35.3 mL of saline, 14.4 mL of infoson, and 13.8 mL of iopamiron 370. Infoson-enhanced HyCoSy provided a significantly larger (P = 0.006) number of correct diagnoses (20/22 fallopian tubes) than did saline HyCoSy (12/24 fallopian tubes), and the same number as that achieved by hysterosalpingography.

HyCoSy is more efficient than any another test of tubal patency that can be compared with it. It has been shown that sensitivity, specificity, and PPV and NPV of Hydro-HyCoSy were 91%, 71%, 55%, and 95%, respectively, while for CnTI-SonoVue-HyCoSy they were 87%, 84%, 69%, and 94%. The diagnostic accuracy of Hydro-HyCoSy and of CnTI-SonoVue-HyCoSy were 77% and 85%, with a Cohen's kappa of 0.52 and 0.66, respectively. CnTI-SonoVue-HyCoSy does not require a learning curve period.[29]

Yet another study has shown that HSG and HyCoSy demonstrated a high concordance with laparoscopy (83% and 80%, respectively). The two methods had a high NPV for tubal disease (HSG, 94%; HyCoSy, 88%), and the PPV were 47% and 75%, respectively.[32]

Study by Exacoustas et al. have also shown that HSG and HyCoSy had the same high concordance as laparoscopy, 86.7% and 86.7%, respectively.

The study concluded that HyCoSy proved to be superior to conventional HSG in evaluating adjacent myometrial structures, adnexa, and degree of follicular maturation, equal to HSG in visualizing the passage of the contrast medium into the peritoneum but inferior to HSG in imaging the fallopian tubes owing to their tortuosity.[34,35]

In spite of all advantages, Balen et al. found that both SIS and HyCoSy are insufficiently accurate and inferior to HSG.[36] They quoted a false positive rate of 9% and false negative rate of 20% for HyCoSy. This is because fallopian tubes are tortuous and usually not confined to a single plane. Moreover, distal parts of the tube may be obscured by bowel gas.

Modifications of Hystero-contrast-sonosalpingography

Additional use of pulsed wave Doppler in HyCoSy can be used as a supplement to gray-scale imaging to improve the diagnostic accuracy in cases of suspected tubal occlusion, and in patients in whom intratubal flow was demonstrated only over a short distance.[12] The 3D power Doppler helps was, therefore, tried to visualize the whole tube and spill.[37] This technique has shown to be superior to conventional HyCoSy with free spill from fallopian tubes was demonstrated in 91% of tubes using 3D-power Doppler as compared to only 46% by conventional HyCoSy and the contrast agent required was almost half for 3D–PD in one this study.[37] There are various advantages with 3D HyCoSy techniques, which allow simultaneous visualization of the uterine cavity and whole tube, short procedure time and reduced patient discomfort, requirement of less amount of contrast, and storage of the 3D volume, which allow offline review and reassessment.

Advantages of 3D Hystero-contrast-sonosalpingography

- Uterine cavity and whole tube can be seen together.
- Condition of lumen and fimbriae can be studied.
- Shortens procedure time and patient discomfort
- Less amount of contrast is required
- Storage of volumes allows reassessment and reviews.
- Spill is better appreciated
- More accurate

Technique of 3D Hystero-contrast-sonosalpingography

Sonovue (Bracco) is used as the contrast agent. Patient preparation, catheter placement, and preparation of contrast media was done according to the method described earlier. Scanning is performed using a 3D ultrasound machine (e.g. Voluson E8 Expert BT 12; GE medical systems). A high frequency transvaginal volume probe (6–9 MHz) is used for pelvic evaluation. Contrast mode is switched on the machine. As the contrast is slowly injected through the balloon catheter into the uterus, transvaginal probe is so oriented that uterine cornu and ovaries are seen on the same plane. Having defined the contrast filling in the tubes, 3D is switched on and volumes are acquired for each side independently (Fig. 7.13).

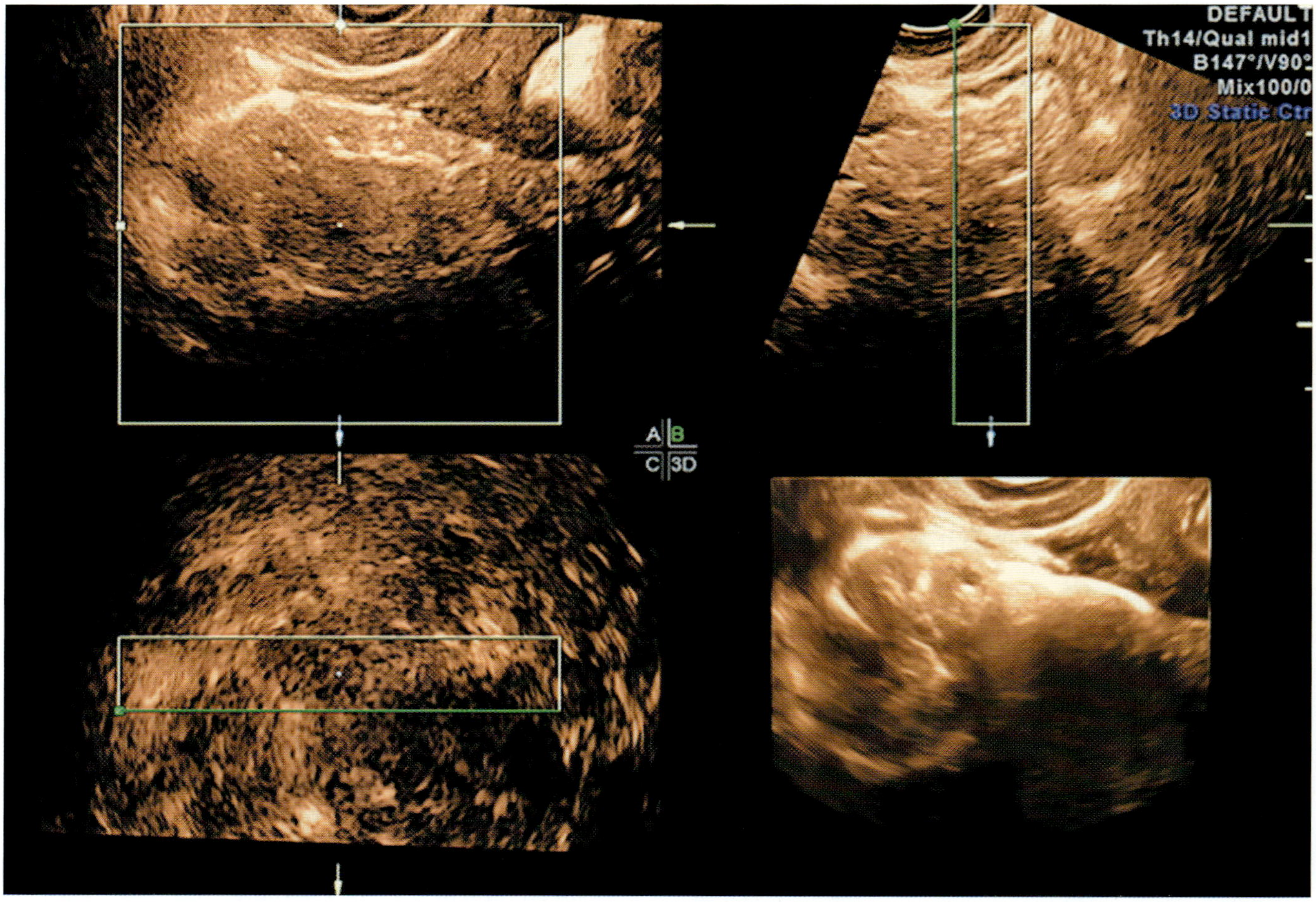

Fig. 7.13: Three-dimensional volume acquired of contrast enhanced tube on HyCoSy.

Rendering is done in front back viewing direction. Surface enhanced mode is used. Threshold is set to make the contrast path more obvious. Magicut (electronic scalpel) is then used to cut all shadows other than the contrast path. Then high definition (HD) live rendering mode is switched on and direction of the light is adjusted to visualize the fimbriae and spill to its best. After the final picture is ready, both the halves are matched and put together to make a complete picture of uterus and both tubes (Figs. 7.14A and B).

We have done a study of 65 infertile females using 3D HyCoSy for tubal assessment and have found to be very reliable.

In a series of 65 subfertile women in whom we performed 3D HyCoSy followed by a laparoscopy and dye test to evaluate tubal patency, the results of 3D HyCoSy were consistent with that of laparoscopy except in two women. One of these two patients had unilateral tubal block on HyCoSy, but the tube was patent at laparoscopy with injection of the methylene blue dye with pressure. In the other patient, the fimbrial end of the tube was not clearly visualized on 3D HyCoSy and was thought to be blocked, but at laparoscopy, the distal tubal portion was buried behind the ovary due to endometriosis and the tube was patent.

This technique is more informative and reliable than 2D HyCoSy. Whole extent of the tubal lumen and fimbrial condition can be visualized. Site of block can be identified. Relation of fimbrial end of tube to ovary can also be defined (Fig. 7.14C).

The HyCoSy with automated 3D-coded contrast imaging (3D-CCI) technology retains the advantages of conventional 2D HyCoSy while overcoming the disadvantages. The 2D HyCoSy is highly observer-dependent and is only accurate in the hands of experienced investigators; by obtaining a volume of the uterus and tubes, automated 3D volume acquisition permits visualization of the tubes in

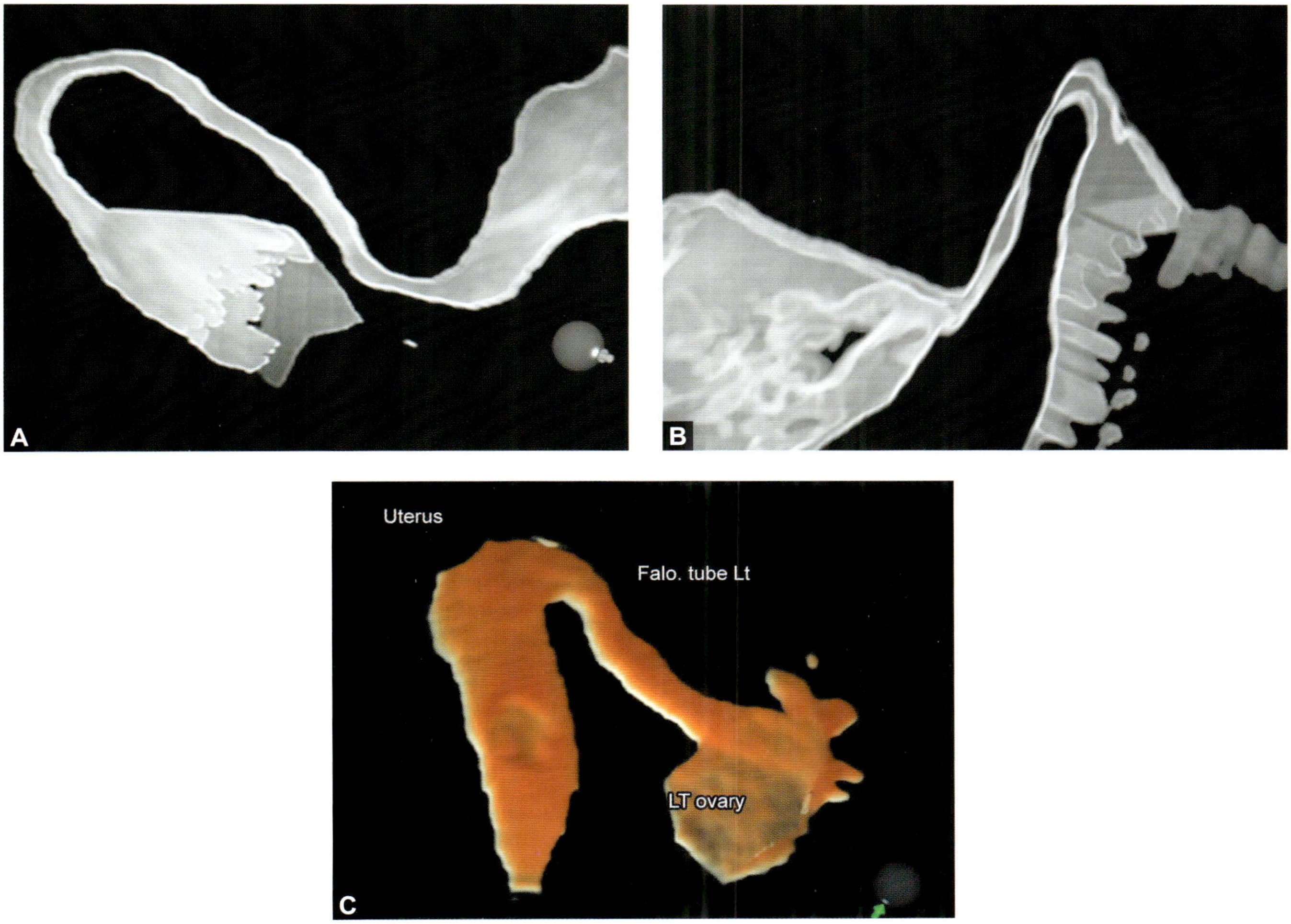

Figs. 7.14A to C: (A and B) Three-dimensional hystero-contrast-sonosalpingography (HyCoSy)-rendered image of half of the uterus and tube of one side individually. (C) High definition live rendered 3D hystero-contrast-sonosalpingography (HyCoSy) showing entire lumen of left fallopian tube with fimbrial end and ovary.

the coronal view and of the tubal course in 3D space, and should allow less experienced operators to evaluate tubal patency status relatively easily.[38]

Large studies have reported that 3D HyCoSy is highly accurate with 100% sensitivity, 67% specificity, 89% PPV, and 100% NPV for tubal patency and concordance rate with laparoscopy of 91%.[39] In a study by Kupesic et al., 3D HyCoSy (sensitivity, specificity, PPV, and NPV of 97.9%, 100%, 97.9%, and 100%, respectively) was found to be marginally superior to 2D HyCoSy (sensitivity, specificity, PPV, and NPV of 93.6%, 97.3%, 98.2%, and 97.3%, respectively) for tubal assessment.[40,41]

It has been shown in another study that for detecting tubal patency among the 150 fallopian tubes assessed, 3D SonoVue-HyCoSy had a sensitivity of 93.5%, specificity of 86.3%, PPV and NPV of 87.8% and 92.6%, respectively, and diagnostic accuracy of 90.0%. The test-positive rates of 3D SonoVue-HyCoSy versus lap and dye were not significantly different (82/150 vs. 77/150, P >0.05).[41] Yet another study by Chan CC et al. have shown that the sensitivity of 3D HyCoSy for detecting tubal patency was 100% with a specificity of 67%. The PPV and NPV were 89% and 100%, respectively; the concordance rate was 91%. The mean duration [+/- standard deviation (SD)] for the 3D HyCoSy was 13.4 +/- 5.5 minutes.[42]

Color coded 3D-power Doppler imaging (3D-PDI) with surface rendering allowed visualization of the flow of contrast through the entire tubal length and free spill of contrast was clearly identified in the majority of cases. The 3D-PDI method appeared to have advantages over the conventional HyCoSy technique, especially in terms of visualization of spill from the distal end of the tube, which was achieved twice as often with the 3D technique. The 3D-PDI technique allowed better storage of the information for reanalysis and archiving than conventional HyCoSy. The mean duration of the imaging procedure was less with 3D-PDI, but the operator time which included postprocedure analysis of the stored information was similar. A significantly lower volume of contrast medium (5.9 +/- 0.6 mL) was used for 3D-PDI in comparison with that (11.2 +/- 1.9 mL) used for conventional 2D HyCoSy.[40]

In spite of all sophisticated imaging technologies, the gold standard is still endoscopy. If any abnormality is found in the tubes on imaging, its confirmation by endoscopy is a must. Endoscopy consists of hysteroscopy to assess the cornual end of the tube and laparoscopy to observe the fimbrial end of the tube.

Hysteroscopy

This allows direct visualization of the entire endometrial cavity, uterocervical canal, and also the cornu. It is usually clubbed with laparoscopy when it is for tubal assessment. The procedure is done under general anesthesia. There are hysteroscopes available with various diameters and various angles. One may use rigid hysteroscope or a flexible hysterofibroscope. After cervical dilatation, the scope attached to the light source and camera is slowly introduced through the cervix under videomonitoring. The cavity is moderately distended with fluid to avoid the contact of the lens of the scope to the mucosa. The selection of the fluid used for distention may depend on whether or not the energy source is used and if it is used it is monopolar or bipolar. Though the energy source is used only for therapeutic purposes. For most diagnostic purposes, normal saline, ringer lactate, or dextrose 5% can be used. To prevent overdistention and also to maintain the clarity of the fluid for easy visualization, the fluid is aspirated or flushed and reinstilled from time to time. Clear visualization of both cornu on hysteroscopy is a sufficient evidence to say that the cornual ends of the tubes are patent (Figs. 7.15A and B).

Laparoscopy

For tubal assessment, hysteroscopy is to be clubbed with hysteroscopy. It is a safe procedure, planned in the proliferative phase of the cycle. Minimum 6 hours of empty stomach is advised. Bowel preparation may also be preferred. The procedure is done under general anesthesia with propofol and atracurium as a muscle relaxant. Endotracheal intubation is required. Intermittent positive pressure ventilation with oxygen, nitrous oxide, and enflurane or isoflurane is used during the surgery. Analgesia is achieved by fentanyl and metoclopramide is used as an antiemetic. Neostigmine is used as a reversal for muscle relaxants.

Patient is placed in modified lithotomy position and is catheterized. Diathermy pads are placed for a possible use of cautery. Veress needle is placed. After that, patient is placed in steep Trendelenburg position. Abdominal cavity is insufflated by CO_2. Once the abdominal cavity is distended, the trocar is put through infraumbilical incision. Through which the laparoscope is introduced. The hysteroscope is still in the uterus. Through this the dye (methylene blue) is slowly injected when the fimbrial end of the fallopian tubes are observed through laparoscope,

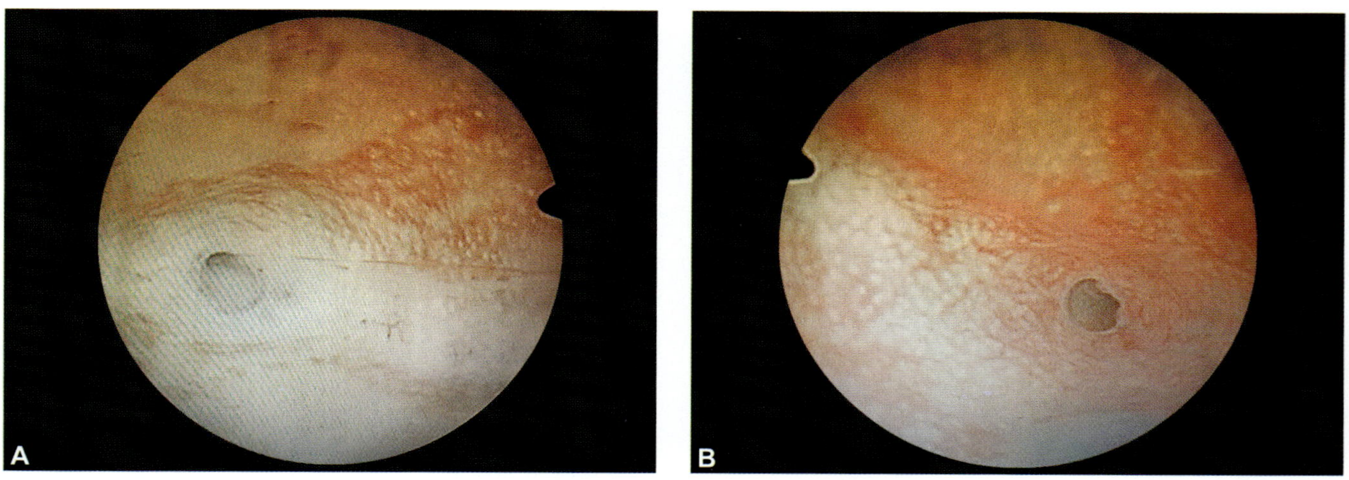

Figs. 7.15A and B: Hysteroscopic image showing bilateral normal cornual ends of the tubes.

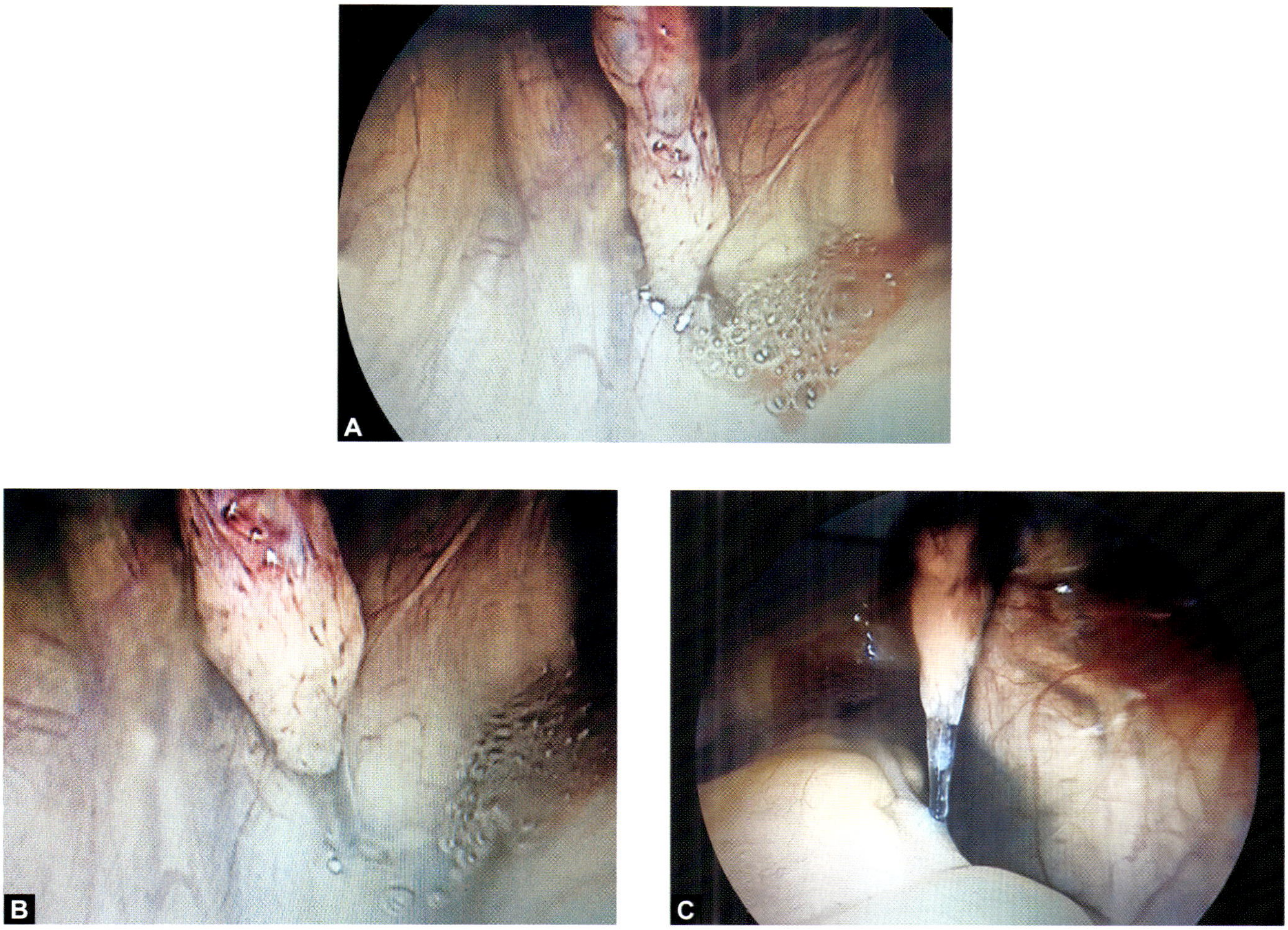

Figs. 7.16A to C: Laparoscopic images of free spill through the fimbrial end of the tube indicating normal patent fallopian tube.

one at a time to see the flow of the dye, which confirms the tubal patency (Figs. 7.16A to C). The block is confirmed by absence of free flow through the tube and distended tube, which is discolored due to methylene blue. Salpingoscopy may be indicated in case of block.

Advantages

- Direct visualization of the tube
- Feel the placidity of the tube
- See the fimbriae floating in the fluid, fimbrial condition and the tubo-ovarian relation.

Complications

- Injury to the blood vessels
- Injury to the bowel
- Both chiefly during insertion of Veress needle or trocar

Contraindications

Absolute contraindications:

- Overdistended bowel due to obstruction or paralytic bowel
- Large abdominal mass
- Generalized peritonitis
- Irreducible external hernia
- Cardiac failure
- Recent myocardial infarction
- Cardiac conduction defects
- Respiratory failure
- Severe obstructive airways disease
- Shock

Relative contraindications:

- Previous surgeries
- Abdominal wall sepsis

- Gross obesity
- Hiatus hernia
- Ischemic heart disease
- Blood dyscrasias and coagulopathies

Salpingoscopy

Salpingoscopy is an extension of laparoscopy using an endoscope of 2.0–2.9 mm. After entry through the abdominal ostium, endoscope enters the tube through the fimbrial end. Tube is distended using normal saline or glycine to evaluate the tubal walls with normal mucosal folds. Abnormalities may be detected in following forms:

- Normal major and minor mucosal folds with slight flattening
- Normal major and minor mucosal folds with focal adhesions or agglutinations
- Extensive adhesions, distorted lumen with formation of pseudospaces
- Dilated lumen, rigid walls, and no mucosal folds

Advantages

It is a gold standard for assessment of the tubes—patency, fimbrial condition, and tubo-ovarian relation.

Identifies the nature of pathology and can treat it simultaneously.

CONCLUSION

Tubal evaluation is essential in subfertile patients. Hysterosalpingography has been used for a long time for assessment of tubal patency. SIS has been proved to be fairly reliable technique for tubal evaluation. This is a transvaginal ultrasound guided procedure. Its diagnostic accuracy dependability can be improved by the use of pulse Doppler and color Doppler. Introduction of ultrasound contrast media and HyCoSy have improved the visibility of the tubal lumen. HyCoSy is accurate in determining tubal patency and evaluating the uterine cavity, suggesting it could supplant HSG not only as the first line diagnostic test in an infertility workup.[29]

Evaluative studies of HyCoSy showed good statistical comparability and concordance with HSG and laparoscopy combined with dye.[38] HyCoSy is well tolerated and can be a suitable alternative outpatient procedure.[43] HyCoSy using contrast agent appears to be more efficient than saline solution in detecting tubal obstruction.[44]

These studies confirm that HyCoSy is as efficient as HSG in assessing tubal patency and have the advantage of simultaneous pelvic evaluation for pelvic pathology and ovarian reserve. HyCoSy can, therefore, be considered as first line investigative tool in low risk women who are not known to have any reproductive comorbidities. HyCoSy combined with 3D ultrasound has the ability to increase the diagnostic accuracy, but this technique is not widely used because of limited availability of 3D ultrasound. It is now considered a first line noninvasive investigation for tubal assessment in a subfertile patient. Though laparoscopic chromopertubation is the gold standard investigative modality for tubal assessment, it use can be restricted to selective group of women as most women could have less invasive ultrasound methods to assess tubal patency.

To quote a few other studies that have concluded similar facts are:

> Saline infusion salpingography can be used as an initial investigation for infertile patients and laparoscopy can be deferred for 6 months. Meanwhile endocrinological and immunological causes are ruled out and then if required laparoscopy may be done.[17] SSG can be used as first ambulatorial evaluation of tubal patency in infertility workup.[45]

The Royal College of Obstetricians and Gynaecologists recommends that where appropriate expertise is available, screening for tubal occlusion using HyCoSy should be considered because it is an effective alternative to HSG for women who are not known to have comorbidities. Women who are thought to have comorbidities should be offered laparoscopy and dye so that tubal and other pelvic pathology can be assessed at the same time.

Because of good degree of statistical comparability and concordance of conventional HyCoSy with HSG and laparoscopy and dye test, the National Institute for Health and Clinical Excellence (NICE) has recommended HyCoSy as a suitable outpatient procedure for tubal patency assessment in women who are not known to have any comorbidity such as pelvic inflammatory disease, previous ectopic pregnancy, or endometriosis.[29,43,46] HyCoSy is well tolerated by women and associated risks are minimal with the risk of pelvic infection is 1%.

Hysterolaparoscopy is the gold standard.

REFERENCES

1. Gordts S, Campo R, Rombauts, Brosens I. Endoscopic visualization of the process of fimbrial ovum retrieval in the human. Human Reprod. 1998;13(6):1425-8.

2. Johnson N, Vandekerckhove P, Watson A, Lilford R, Harada T, Hughes E. Tubal flushing for subfertility (Cochrane Review). The Cochrane Library. 2003;3:CD003718.
3. Belisle S, Collins JA, Burrows EA, Willan AR. The value of laparoscopy among infertile women with tubal patency. J Soc Obstet Gynaecol Can. 1996;18:326-36.
4. Watrelot A, Dreyfus JM, Andine JP. Evaluation of the performance of fertiloscopy in 160 consecutive infertile patients with no obvious pathology. Hum Reprod. 1999;14:707-11
5. Nanini R, Chelo E, Branconi F, Tantini C, Scarselli GF. Dynamic echohysteroscopy: a new diagnostic technique in the study of female infertility. Acta Eur Fertil. 1981;12(2):165-71.
6. Richman TS, Visconi GN, deChurney A, Polan ML, Alcebo LO. Fallopian tubal patency assessed by ultrasound fluid injection. Work in progress. Radiol. 1984;152(2):507-10.
7. Randolph JR, Ying YK, Maier DB, Schmidt CL, Riddick DH. Comparison of real time ultrasonography, hysterosalpingography and laparoscopy/hysteroscopy in the evaluation of uterine abnormalities and tubal patency. Fertil Steril. 1986;46(5):828-32.
8. Tufekci EC, Girit S, Bayirli MD, Durmuþoğlu F, Yalti S. Evaluation of tubal patency by transvaginal sonosalpingography. Fertil Steril. 1992;57:336-40.
9. Deichert U, Schlief R, van de Sandt M, Daume E. Transvaginal hysterosalpingo-contrast sonography(Hy-Co-Sy) compared with conventional tubal diagnostics. Hum Reprod 1989;4(4):418-24.
10. Stern J, Peters AJ, Coulam CB. Colour Doppler ultrasonography assessment of tubal patency: a comparison study with traditional techniques. Fertil Steril. 1992;58(5):897-900.
11. Kupesic S, Kurjak A. Gynecological vaginal sonographic interventional procedures—what does colour add? Gynecol Perinatol. 1994;3:57-60.
12. Deichert U, Schlief R, van de Sandt M, Daume E. Transvaginal hysterosalpingo-contrast sonography for the assessment of tubal patency with gray scale imaging and additional use of pulsed wave Doppler. Fertil Steril. 1992;57(1):62-7.
13. Heikkinen H, Tekay A, Volpi E, Martikainen H, Jouppila P. Transvaginal salpingosonography for the assessment of tubal patency in infertile women: methodological and clinical experiences. Fertil Steril. 1995;64(2):293-8.
14. Dessole S, Farina M, Rubattu G, Cosmi E, Ambrosini G, Battista Nardelli G. Side effects and complications of sonohysterosalpingography. Fertil Steril. 2003;8(3):620-4.
15. de Kroon CD, de Bock GH, Dieben SW, Jansen FW. Saline contrast hysterosonography in abnormal uterine bleeding: a systematic review and meta-analysis. BJOG. 2003;110(10):938-47.
16. Spalding H, Martikainen H, Tekay A, Jouppila P. Transvaginal salpingosonography for assessing tubal patency in women previously treated for pelvic inflammatory disease and benign ovarian tumors. Ultrasound Obstet Gynecol. 1999;14(3):205-9.
17. Kore S, Hegde A, Nair S. Sonography for assessment of tubal patency: our experience. J Obstet and Gynecol India. 2000;50(2):63-6.
18. Seal SL, Ghosh D, Saha D. Comparative evaluation of sonosalpingography, hysterosalpingography and laparoscopy for determination of tubal patency. J Obstet and Gynecol India. 2007;57(2):158-61.
19. Peters AJ, Coulam CB. Hysterosalpingography with colour Doppler sonography. Am J Obstet Gynecol. 1991;164(6 Pt 1):1530-2.
20. Lucaino DE, Exacoustos C, Johns DA, Luciano AA. Transabdominal saline contrast sonohysterography: Can it replace hysterosalpingography in low resource countries? Am J Obstet Gynecol. 2011;204(1):79.
21. Deichert U, van de Sandt M. Transvaginal hystero-salpingo-contrast sonography (Hy-Co-Sy). The assessment of tubal patency and uterine abnormalities by contrast enhanced sonography. Advances in Echo-contrast. 1993;2:55-8.
22. Hüneke B, Lindner Ch, Braendle W. Untersuchung der Tubenpassage mit der vaginalen gepulsten Kontrastmittel-Doppler-Sonographic. Ultraschall Klin.Praax. 4:192-198.
23. Jeanty P, Besnard S, Arnold A, Turner C, Crum P. Air-contrast sonohysterography as a first step assessment of tubal patency. J Ultrasound Med. 2000;19(8):519-27.
24. Sankpal RS, Confino E, Matzel A, Cohen LS. Investigation of the uterine cavity and fallopian tubes using three-dimensional saline sonohysterosalpingography. Int J Gynaecol Obstet. 2001;73(2):125-9.
25. Kiyokawa K, Masuda H, Fuyuki T, Koseki M, Uchida N, Fukuda T, et al. Three-dimensional hystero-salpingo-contrast sonography (3D-HyCoSy) as an outpatient procedure to assess infertile women: a pilot study. Ultrasound Obstet Gynecol. 2000;16(7):648-54.
26. Bonilla-Musoles F, Simon C, Sampaio, Serra V, Sampaio M, Pellicer A. An assessment of hysterosalpingosonography as a diagnostic tool for uterine cavity defects and tubal patency. J Clin Ultrasound. 1992;20(3):175-81.
27. Emanuel MH, Exalto N. Hysterosalpingo-foam sonography (HyFoSy): a new technique to visualize tubal patency. UOG. 2011;37(4):498-99.
28. Prefumo F, Serafini G, Martinoli C, Gandolfo N, Gandolfo NG, Derchi LE. The sonographic evaluation of tubal patency with stimulated acoustic emission imaging. Ultrasound Obstet Gynecol. 2002;20(4):386-9.
29. Boudghene FP, Bazot M, Robert Y, Perrot N, Rocourt N, Antoine JM, et al. Assessment of fallopian tube patency by HyCoSy: comparison of a positive contrast agent with saline solution. Ultrasound Obstet Gynecol. 2001;18(5): 525-30.
30. Holz K, Becker R, Schürmann R. Ultrasound in the investigation of tubal patency: a meta-analysis of three comparative studies of Echovist-200 including 1007 women. Zentralbl Gynakol. 1997;119:366-73.
31. Korell M, Seehaus D, Strowitzki T, Hepp H. Radiologic versus ultrasound fallopian tube imaging. Painfulness of the examination and diagnostic reliability of hysterosalpingography and hysterosalpingo-contrast-ultrasonography with Echovist. Ultraschall Med. 1997;18(1):3-7.
32. Lanzani C,Savasi V, Leone FP, Ratti M, Ferrazzi E. Two-dimensional HyCoSy with contrast tuned imaging technology

and a second generation contrast media for assessment of tubal patency in an infertility program. Fertil Steril. 2009;92(3):1158-61.

33. Tanawattanachaeron S, Suwajanakorn S, Uerpairojkit B, Boonkasemsamti W, Virutamasen P. Transvaginal hystero-contrast sonography (HyCoSy) compared with chromolaparoscopy. The Journal of Obstetrics and Gynecology Research. 2000;26(1):71-5.
34. Strandell A, Bourne T, Bergh C, Granberg S, Asztely M, Thorburn J. The assessment of endometrial pathology and tubal patency: a comparison between the use of ultrasonography and X-ray hysterosalpingography for the investigation of infertility patients. Ultrasound Obstet Gynecol. 1999;14(3):200-4.
35. Exacoustos C, Zupi E, Carusotti C, Lanzi G, Marconi D, Arduini D. Hysterosalpingo-contrast sonography compared with hysterosalpingography and laparoscopic dye perturbation to evaluate tubal patency. J Am Assoc Gynecol Laparosc. 2003;10(3):367-72.
36. Guazzaroni M, Mari A, Politi C, Guazzaroni M, Remedi S, Mallarini G, et al. Ultrasound hysterosalpingography with Levovist in the diagnosis of tubal patency. Radiol Med. 2001;102(1-2):62-6.
37. Balen FG, Allen CM, Gardener JE, Siddle NC, Lees WR. 3-dimensional reconstruction of ultrasound images of the uterine cavity. Br J Radiol. 1993;66:588-91.
38. Sladkevicius P, Ojha K, Campbell S, Nargund G. Three dimensional power Doppler imaging in the assessment of fallopian tube patency. Ultrasound Obstet Gynecol. 2000; 16(7):644-7.
39. Exacoustos C, Di Giovanni A, Szabolcs B, Romeo V, Romanini ME, Luciano D, et al. Automated three-dimensional coded contrast imaging hysterosalpingo-contrast sonography: feasibility in office tubal patency testing. Ultrasound Obstet Gynecol. 2013;41(3):328-35.
40. Chan CC, Ng EH, Tang OS, Ho PC. Comparison of three-dimensional hysteron-contrast-sonography and diagnostic laparoscopy with chromopertubation in the assessment of tubal patency for the investigation of subfertility. Acta Obstet Gynecol Scand. 2005;84(9):909-13.
41. Kupesic S, Plavsic MB. 2D and 3D hysterosalpingocontrast-sonography in the assessment of uterine cavity and tubal patency. Eur J Obstet Gynecol Reprod Biol. 2007;133(1): 64-9.
42. Zhou L, Zhang X, Chen X, Liao L, Pan R, Zhou N, et al. Value of three-dimensional hysterosalpingo-contrast sonography with SonoVue in the assessment of tubal patency. Ultrasound Obstet Gynecol. 2012;40(1):93-8.
43. Tanahatoe S, Hompes PG, Lambalk CB. Accuracy of diagnostic laparoscopy in the infertility work-up before intrauterine insemination. Fertil Steril. 2003;79:361-6.
44. Dijkman AB, Mol BW, van der Veen F, Bossuyt PM, Hogerzeil HV. Can hysterosalpingocontrast-sonography replace hysterosalpingography in the assessment of tubal subfertility? Eur J Radiol. 2000;35:44-8.
45. Ayida G, Kennedy S, Barlow D, Chamberlain P. A comparison of patient tolerance of hysterosalpingo-contrast sonography (HyCoSy) with Echovist-200 and X-ray hysterosalpingography for outpatient investigation of infertile women. Ultrasound Obstet Gynecol. 1996;7:201-4.
46. Volpi E, De Grandis T, Sismondi P, Giacardi M, Rustrichelli S, Patriarca A, Bocci A. Transvaginal salpingo-sonography (TSSG) in the evaluation of tubal patency. Acta Eur Fertil. 1991;22(6):325-8

CHAPTER

Management of Tubal Block (Tubal Infertility)

8

Milan Reljič

INTRODUCTION

Tubal factor infertility accounts for 25–35% of female factor infertility. The most prevalent cause of tubal factor infertility is pelvic inflammatory disease due to *Chlamydia trachomatis* infection. The pathology of tubal disease ranges from intratubal lesion and peritubal adhesion to complete proximal and/or distal tubal blockage. Hysterosalpingography (HSG) and hysterosalpingosonography (HyCoSy) are standard first line tests to assess tubal patency, but laparoscopy remains gold standard to diagnose and evaluate the severity of tubal damage. Reconstructive tubal surgery is the treatment of choice in the young patient with limited tubal pathology. *In vitro* fertilization (IVF) is recommended for women of advance ages, with severe tubal pathology and after unsuccessful tubal surgery. Although we have successful treatment modalities, more effort should be devoted to the prevention of tubal infertility.

PHYSIOLOGY AND PHYSIOPATHOLOGY

The fallopian tubes are fundamental for human reproduction. They are part of the female reproductive system, along with the vulva, the vagina, the uterus, and the ovaries. The fallopian tube is tubal structures that can measure between 7 and 12 cm, formed basically by smooth muscle, covered by a peritoneal layer. In the interior epithelial lining, four types of cells can be seen: secretory cells, ciliated cells, intercalary, and small "indifferent" cells. The fallopian tubes capture the egg when it is released from the ovary and transfer it in their interior where eventually it will meet with the sperm that ascend from the vagina. The tubal ampulla serves as the physiologic site for final gamete maturation and fertilization. The first stage of development of the embryo occurs in the fallopian tubes, during the 4–5 days that it takes for its transfer to the uterine cavity, where finally it is implanted. Tubal epithelium with ciliated and nonciliated cells plays the most important role in transport of gametes and embryo and also enables appropriate conditions for fertilization and early embryonic development. The oviduct serves also as an important reservoir for sperm.

The damage of tubal structure and function can interfere with any step of these processes and may lead to infertility. Due to their structure, the fallopian tubes are easily affected by certain disease. The tubal lumen is narrow and the epithelium is very delicate, which makes it more susceptible to damage than other structures of the female reproductive system. They can suffer various changes related to pathological agents, such as epithelium damage, wall thickening, lumen blockade (distal and proximal), and peritoneal (peritubal) adhesions with disturbance of the tubo-ovarian spatial relationships.

CAUSES OF TUBAL PATHOLOGY

In 9 of every 10 cases, the cause of tubal infertility is an inflammatory pelvic disease (PID) secondary to a sexually transmitted disease (STD). The etiologic relationship between STD, lower genital tract infection, PID, and tubal infertility involves a multifactor multistep process. Acute polymicrobial PID begins with a cervical infection with sexual transmitted pathogens continues with an alteration of the vaginocervical microenvironment and an overgrowth of vaginal facultative and anaerobic flora resulting in lower genital tract infection, to progress with the ascent of pathogens into the endometrium, the fallopian tubes, and the peritoneal cavity. Frequently, the infection is polymicrobial but the primary compromise is usually produced by bacteria that are sexually transmitted. Of the 20 or more microorganisms that are usually transmitted by sexual contact, only 2 or 3 bacteria are capable of producing PID. They are *Neisseria gonorrhea*, *C. trachomatis*, and possibly some species of the Mycoplasma. Infection by *C. trachomatis* accounts for more than 50% of acute PID and it is the most significant cause, not only of because of prevalence but also for its characteristics. It is most frequently (70%) asymptomatic and prolonged, making it more difficult to diagnose. So most women do not know they have damaged tubes until they have problems getting pregnant. In contrast, the gonococcus infection is usually symptomatic and acute, associated with abnormal vaginal discharge, fever, and pelvic pain. Certain kinds of *Mycoplasma* have been cultivated from the endometrium and from the fallopian tubes in cases of PID. Although their pathogenic power is not in doubt, the real role as primary invaders in PID is not completely clear. Infection can also propagate from lower genital tract to the tubes after intrauterine procedures done under inadequate conditions, after spontaneous abortion, and prolonged or traumatic birth. Other infection located in the pelvis can affect the fallopian tubes, due to the proximity, as is the case with appendicitis. A prolonged, misdiagnosed, and untreated infection is more likely to cause permanent endothelial damage, but also after successful antibiotic treatment, the risk for tubal damage is approximately 8–12%.

The tubal ectopic pregnancy is a serious and frequent problem and can damage the fallopian tubes, but more than a cause, is a consequence of a previously established tubal pathology.

Endometriosis is the principal noninfectious cause of definitive damage to the fallopian tubes, due to the peritoneal inflammatory response. Other causes of tubal pathology such as genital tuberculosis, uterine fibromas and tubal agenesia are very rare.

DIAGNOSIS

The most common diagnostic methods that are used for assessing the tubal factor infertility are:

- Hysterosalpingography
- Hysterosalpingosonography
- *C. trachomatis* antibody testing
- Endoscopic techniques [laparoscopy, transvaginal hydrolaparoscopy (THL)]

Hysterosalpingography

Hysterosalpingography consists of the injection of an iodine contrast (liquid opaque to the X-rays) through the neck of the uterus, filling the uterine cavity and the tubes, which allows, in an indirect manner the radiological study of the anatomical characteristics of the lumen of these organs. This technique can reveal several tubal pathologies: obstructions, dilatations, stenosis, polyps, and old tuberculosis infections. It is a method of screening that can be done on an outpatient basis, and it is simple and inexpensive. But generally it does not permit an etiologic diagnosis and it does not reveal the serous plane (external) of the tube, nor the tubal environment. Occasionally, tubal spasms indistinguishable from true obstruction are produced. But this is only one reason that the sensitivity and the specificity of HSG in detecting tubal pathology are not very high (0.65 and 0.83). Complications are rare, but infections (especially in pathological tubes), uterine perforations, anaphylactic shocks, and interruptions of unsuspected pregnancies have been described. Nevertheless, the radiation to which the patient is exposed is minimal and is not considered harmful. Despite these disadvantages, National Institute for Clinical Excellence (NICE) and European Society of Human Reproduction and Embryology (ESHRE) recommend HSG as a first-line approach to assess tubal infertility.

Hysterosalpingosonography

Hysterosalpingosonography may be considered as an alternative to HSG, because it has comparable accuracy, but avoids radiation and allows simultaneous assessment of the uterus and ovaries. It is the ultrasonic exploration of the uterus and of the tubes, while a fluid is injected through the uterine cervix in order to create an acoustic window of differing echogenicity that allows a better observation of the internal wall of these structures. In the normal tubes, the flow of the injected liquid can be seen, especially in the proximal part. On finalizing the exploration, it is observed how the liquid is found in the bottom of the pelvis. If a Doppler velocimetry is available, a continuous signal during the injection of the contrast that confirms the tubal permeability can be detected. Unilateral or bilateral tubal obstructions can be diagnosed. Anyway, the information given is reduced. Only the tubal obstruction can be studied, and even that cannot always be precisely located. Tubal spasm is not rare and could be misdiagnosed as permanent proximal tubal occlusion. Complications are rare. Slight adverse effects like pain, generally light and tolerable, vasovagal reactions, nausea, vomiting, hyperventilation, and sweating have been described.

Chlamydia trachomatis Antibody Test

This is blood test with the objective of determining the Chlamydia immunoglobulin (IgG) antibodies which are thought to persist for years and have, therefore, been used as markers of previous *C. trachomatis* infection. In fact, one positive test alone cannot determine if the infection is current, or an old one. It was showed that between 73 and 79% of infertile women with tubal abnormalities were positive for *C. trachomatis* antibodies. The sensitivity and specificity of this test in detecting tubal infertility vary between 0.20 and 1.00, according to test being considered and cut-off value of antibodies titer being used. There is a marked association between the titer and the likelihood of tubal damage. The higher are the titer, the more likely there would be tubal damage, so the specificity is higher and sensitivity lower and vice versa. And there is also correlation between the severity of disease and antibodies titer. Obviously, it is not an aggressive test and it is inexpensive, but it does not allow for the diagnosis of other possible infectious agents as well as other cases of tubal infertility. We should be aware that it does not offer information about the anatomical state of the tubes and, therefore, should complement other existing methods.

Laparoscopy

Laparoscopy with dye test is generally regarded as being the gold standard for the assessment of tubal pathology. It allows the direct observation of the peritoneal cavity contents, and, therefore, the exterior of the tubes and their surrounding environment. During procedure, a dye such as methylene blue can be injected in a process termed chromopertubation into the uterus and shown to pass through the tubes. Prognostic factors that are identified by laparoscopy are of great importance for management decision between tubal surgery and IVF. If an abnormality is found during laparoscopy, this may be dealt with at the same time thus avoiding another operation. The tubal abnormalities that can be diagnosed correspond to obstructions, stenosis, inflammations, hydrosalpinx, dilatation, diverticula, peritubal adhesions, and agglutinations of phimosis. The salpingoscope may be introduced by laparoscopy and the direct visualization of the internal wall of the ampulla is possible (*salpingoscopy*). The pathological images that can be obtained by salpingoscopy correspond to adhesions, polyps, stenosis, dilatations, obstructions, and atrophy of the mucosa. The laparoscopy requires general anesthesia and hospital admission. Complications are rare but serious, including bowel, vessels, bladder injury, and complications relating to the insufflations of gas and to anesthetic. *Transvaginal hydrolaparoscopy*, which is performed under local anesthesia, is a relatively new culdoscopic technique for exploring the tuboperitoneal infertility. In this procedure, a dilating trocar is inserted through the posterior vaginal wall for endoscopic pelvic examination. Normal saline is used to float the bowel out of the pelvis so that one can evaluate the distal fallopian tubes ovarian surfaces, pelvic sidewalls, and cul de sac. The most common complication of THL is extraperitoneal bowel lesion, which tends to be a minor lesion, managed expectantly. THL is accurate, minimal invasive, and well tolerated diagnostic method which could replace HSG and/or laparoscopy in some cases but its role in infertility evaluation is not yet clearly defined.

THERAPY

There are two options for a couple with tubal infertility to achieve a pregnancy: reconstructive tubal surgery and IVF. In most cases, both techniques may be applied and we should recommend one or the other according to the characteristics of each couple individualizing the strategy to be used in each case. The rationale, potential benefits, complication, advantages, and disadvantages of the proposed treatment should be discussed with the patients. The selection of most appropriate treatment is based on many variables. The age of women, prior fertility, number of children desired, presence of other infertility factor, severity of tubal disease, success and complication rate of surgery and IVF program, patient preference, cost-effectiveness, and reimbursement policy should be taken in consideration. However, IVF and tubal surgery should not be considered as competitive and mutually exclusive, but as complementary procedures which can be applied with appropriate chronological consequences. Anyway, there are clear indications to advise each one of the techniques.

Tubal Surgery

Reconstructive tubal surgery is the treatment of choice in the young patient with limited tubal pathology. The main reason to avoid tubal repair are severe pelvic adhesions with a frozen pelvis, past history of extensive tubal resection for sterilization, thick wall hydrosalpinx, extensive intra-ampullar adhesions and complete destruction of the mucosa, bifocal tube disease, ongoing genital tuberculosis or sequel, the existence of associated, incurable factors for infertility, and the advance age of patient.

Peritubal Adhesiolysis

Peritubal and pelvic adhesions are almost always present in tubal infertility so the first phase of the tubal surgery must always be devoted to adhesiolysis. The salpingo-ovariolysis is essential to restore normal anatomical position of the fallopian tube and the ovary and enables ovum pick-up and gametes transport within fallopian tube. The procedure is done by separating adhesions with laparoscopic scissors, electrocautery, or the laser. It is important to follow microsurgical principles of gentle handling of tissue, constant irrigation, meticulous hemostasis, and precise tissue dissection. Once this adhesiolysis has been carried out, the tubal lesions can be assessed more accurately. The morphology of the tubes is evaluated and their patency checked using methylene blue test. In patients with patent tubes, the intrauterine pregnancy rate after peritubal adhesiolysis vary from 19 to 70%. The success rate is affected by the extent of adhesion, type of adhesion (filmy or dense), degree of tubal damage, and experience of the surgeon. The highest pregnancy rate after adhesiolysis is achieved in women with limited filmy adhesions and otherwise intact tubes. If there is clear benefit of surgery treatment for women with filmy adhesions, this benefit is much less evident in women with dense adhesion and damaged tubes, so these patients are more suited to have IVF treatment.

Distal Tubal Disease

Tubal infertility may be caused by incomplete or complete distal tubal obstruction. In less severe form, fimbrial agglutination and adhesions create incomplete tubal obstruction called *phimosis*. In most patients with distal tubal disease, the fimbriated end of the tube is completely occluded and the distal half of the tube is distended with fluid. This condition is referred as *hydrosalpinx*. In incomplete tubal obstruction, *fimbrioplasty* is performed. The principle of fimbrioplasty is the lysis of fimbrial adhesions, separation of agglutination, or dilatation of fimbrial stricture to restore the original anatomy of the tubal infundibulum. *Neosalpingostomy* consists of creating a new ostium in cases when distal part of the tube is totally occluded. The operation comprises two phases, incision and eversion. In fibroplasty and neosalpingostomy, everted fimbria are secured to the tubal serosa with sutures or electrosurgery.

Pregnancy rates for laparoscopic tubal surgery depend on the severity of the tubal damage and pelvic adhesions. Patients with extensive, dense pelvic adhesions, with dilated tubes (>3 cm), with thick, fibrotic walls and absent luminal mucosa have very low chance for getting pregnant after surgery. There is particularly good correlation between the quality of the mucosa and the intrauterine pregnancy rate, which vary between 0 and 77%. Ectopic pregnancy rate vary between 2 and 17%. According to prognostic factors, decision to repair fallopian tubes or to send patient to IVF should be made intraoperatively. In patients with hydrosalpinx, who are not candidates for reconstructive tubal surgery, salpingectomy or proximal tubal occlusion is indicated. Since it was shown that hydrosalpinx, particularly those visible on ultrasound, have detrimental effect on birth rate after IVF and that salpingectomy and proximal tubal occlusion is effective in restoring IVF outcome.

Proximal Tubal Disease

Proximal tubal blockage accounts for 10–25% of tubal infertility. It may be so called functional or nonstructural obstruction due to tubal spasm or a plug formed mainly of endometrial debris. It was demonstrated by Dessole et al. that nonstructural blockage are very common. In this study, in 60% of patients in whom HSG showed proximal tubal blockage, repeat HSG 1 month later showed tubal patency (Dessole et al., 2000). It was also found that 40% of tubes with proximal occlusion on HSG were occluded by amorphous plug (Kong GWS and Li TC, 2014). Such a nonstructural obstruction can be removed by liquid media flushing into uterus cavity during HSG, dye-test, or hysteroscopy. A true anatomic or structural blockage is caused by sterilization or fibrosis due to salpingitis isthmica nodosa, PID, or endometriosis.

Unless the proximal tubal blockage is a consequence of sterilization or salpingitis isthmica nodosa, tubal cannulation or selective salpingography is first option. Tubal cannulation can be performed under radiographic or hysteroscopic guidance with laparoscopic confirmation. An outer catheter is placed on uterotubal ostium and then flexible inner catheter is gentle advanced through proximal tube. The procedure is successful, if the obstruction is a consequence of a mucosal plug or filmy adhesions (synechiae). It was shown that the obstruction is overcome in 85% of tubes with tubal cannulation and half of them got pregnant. The incidence of tubal perforation was 3–11% and ectopic pregnancy rate 0–6%. If proximal tubal obstruction is due to salpingitis isthmica nodosa or dense intraluminal fibrosis, microsurgical tubocornual anastomosis or IVF is recommended. Tubocornual anastomosis includes the resection of blocked tubal segment, the identification of the intact intramural portion of the tube by careful shaving of the cornua, and then joining healthy isthmus or ampulla directly to the intact intramural portion of the tubes. Published series describe live birth rate ranging from 33 to 56%. The success rate of surgery mainly depends of age of patient, residual length of tubes, distal tubal pathology, surgical techniques, and other factors of infertility.

Sterilization Reversal

These patients differ from other patients who are undergoing fertility treatment. They have better prognosis for pregnancy after surgical procedure and also after IVF. However, appropriate patients selection for tubal anastomosis is crucial since the success rate is depending on patient's age, other infertility factors, the method of sterilization, etc. Microsurgical tubal anastomosis via laparotomy or laparoscopy is technically demanding and should be done by experienced surgeons who have passed special training. In selected group of patient, with good surgical technique, cumulative pregnancy rate up to 80% in 2 years can be achieved. In some countries, extensive electrocoagulation of tube is performed to achieve infertility and there is no data about reversal of sterilization after Essure procedure. The doctors as well as patients should take in mind that in some cases reversal of sterilization is not possible and that IVF procedure is the only option to get pregnant.

In Vitro Fertilization versus Reconstructive Tubal Surgery

Tubal pathology has classically been considered as the major indication for performing IVF. IVF is therapeutic option of choice in cases of severely damaged tubes where the prognosis of tubal surgery is not good, in women older than 35 years, if there are other associated infertility factors, and if the pregnancy has not been achieved 1 year after any type of tubal surgery.

To discover the real efficiency of IVF, we can consult different registers which coincide reasonably well in stating that the live birth rate are influenced by the cause of infertility and above all by the age of the patient. Most statistics publish birth rate between 20.5 and 28.5% per initiated cycles and cumulative probability after three IVF cycles around 50%. From my point of view, it is appropriate to recommend IVF when tubal surgery does not offer a possibility of pregnancy greater than 30–40% after 1 year of follow-up, or a monthly conception rate of less than 2%. Certainly, there are differences between the two techniques since IVF is a palliative technique, which does not cure the tubal pathology while tubal surgery should be considered as a curative treatment. Likewise, there are other aspects to be taken into account such as the reproducibility of IVF, which is greater than that of tubal surgery, as well as the possibility that IVF offers of treating infertility of multifactor origin. One of the mayor advantages of IVF is that the procedure can be performed in an office setting and the pain can be managed with analgesics. In addition, the outcome of the treatment is usually known to the patient within 2 weeks. The medical risk associated with IVF is related to the use of ovarian stimulation. This can lead to the ovarian hyperstimulation syndrome, which occasionally is severe enough to require hospitalization. Multiple pregnancies, preterm labor, and neonatal complications are also more common. Although high older multiple birth can be reduced by limiting the number of embryos transferred, the possibility of twins is still higher than after tubal surgery. There are some data in literature, which shows that children born after IVF have higher risk for congenital malformation and some diseases. The potential risk of cancer resulting from the use of fertility drugs has caused concern, but the evidence for a casual association is still unproven. Complications of follicular aspiration, such as infection and bleeding, can occur but are rather infrequent and are usually easily managed. The overall risk of developing tubal pregnancy after IVF is quite low but is increased in patients with distal tubal disease.

The major advantage of tubal surgery is that it can restore fertility. Consequently, it allows conception without the need for further treatment. Tubal surgery avoids many of the moral ethical and religious dilemmas associated with IVF. The disadvantages of tubal surgery are mainly associated with the performance of a major surgical procedure, the requirement of anesthesia and hospitalization, and risk of ectopic pregnancy. But even in some of the patients where IVF procedure is recommended, laparoscopic surgery cannot be avoided. For example, in patient with hydrosalpinx or dislocated ovaries, tubal surgery is performed to improve success rate or minimize the risk for complications of IVF procedure.

Reconstructive tubal surgery even in the era of assisted reproductive technology remains viable option and should encourage their practice and training.

PREVENTION

The prevention of tubal disease is prevention of STD and its sequel. Prevention can either consist of screening high-risk groups for the presence of disease (post-hoc prevention of tubal infertility by early detection and treatment of pelvic inflammatory disease), or primary prevention of PID (and subsequent tubal infertility) by educational and prevention strategies aimed at adolescent.

Teenagers are at higher risk for STD than any other age group, for a variety of reasons: the presence of cervical ectopy, their relative lack of protecting neutralizing antibodies, the occurrence of anovulatory cycles with easily permeable cervical mucus, the lack of contraceptive usage, their risk-taking behavior, their poor motivation for diagnosis and treatment, and their poor compliance for follow-up. Traditional prevention efforts have frequently been proven ineffective in a teenage population. Peer-led education, training, and skills building backed up by service availability emerges as the most appealing. Adolescents will adopt health behavior more easily from their peers, who are more likely to convince them that they are susceptible to the problem, and that the problem has severe consequences for their future fertility.

The secondary prevention is screening of individual at risk and treating them before PID develops and irreparable tubal damage will have occurred. Among the risk factor for contracting STD are: young at first sexual intercourse, higher life time number of sexual partners, fewer years of education, lower socioeconomic class, lack of contraception, present intrauterine contraceptive device use, and prior history of PID.

Finally, increasing the awareness of doctors and others health care professionals about the (lack of) symptoms of atypical PID and about the need for early treatment will further decrease the risk for tubal infertility developing.

SUGGESTED READING

1. Aristizabal J, Barri PN, Brosens IA. Tubal infertility. IFFS International Consensus. 2001.
2. Briceag I, Costache A, Purcarea VL, Cergan R, Dumitru M, Briceag I, et al. fallopian tubes—literature review of anatomy and etiology in female infertility. J Med Life. 2015;8:129-31.
3. Dessole S, Battista Meloni G, Capobianco G, Manzoni MA, Ambrosini G, Canalis GC. A second hysterosalpingography reduces the use of selective technique for treatment of a proximal tubal obstruction. Fertil Steril. 2000;73:1037-9.
4. European IVF-Monitoring Consortium (EIM), European Society of Human Reproduction and Embryology (ESHRE), Kupka MS, D'Hooghe T, Ferraretti AP. Assisted reproductive technology in Europe, 2011: results generated from European registers by ESHRE. Hum Reprod. 2016;31:233-48.
5. Gomel V. The place of reconstructive tubal surgery in the era of assisted reproductive techniques. Reprod Biomed Online. 2015;31:722-31.
6. Gomel V. Reversal of tubal sterilization versus IVF in the era of assisted reproductive technology: a clinical dilemma. Reprod Biomed Online. 2007;15:403-7.
7. Honoré GM, Holden AE, Schenken RS. Pathophysiology and management of proximal tubal blockage. Fertil Steril. 1999;71:785-95.
8. Hyrapetian M, Loucaides EM, Sutcliffe AG. Health and disease in children born after assistive reproductive therapies (ART). J Reprod Immunol. 2014;106:21-6.
9. Kong GWS, Li TC. Surgical management of tubal disease and infertility. Obstetrics, Gynaecology & Reproductive Medicine. 2014;25:6-11.
10. Moore DE, Spadoni LR, Foy HM, Wang SP, Daling JR, Kuo CC, et al. Increased frequency of serum antibodies to Chlamydia trachomatis in infertility due to distal tubal disease. Lancet. 1982;2:574-7.
11. Pandian Z, Akande VA, Harrild K, Bhattacharya S. Surgery for tubal infertility. Cochrane Database Syst Rev. 2008;16:CD006415.
12. Practice Committee of the American Society for Reproductive Medicine. Role of tubal surgery in the era of assisted reproductive technology: a committee opinion. Fertil Steril. 2015;103:e37-43.
13. Practice Committee of American Society for Reproductive Medicine in collaboration with Society of Reproductive Surgeons. Salpingectomy for hydrosalpinx prior to *in vitro* fertilization. Fertil Steril. 2008;90:S66-8.
14. Schippert C, Garcia-Rocha GJ. Is there still a role for reconstructive microsurgery in tubal infertility? Curr Opin Obstet Gynecol. 2011;23:200-5.
15. Society for Assisted Reproductive Technology. Clinic summary report. [online]. Available from https.//www.sartcorsonline.com/rptCSR_PublicMultYear.aspx?ClinicPKID=0. [Accessed April 22 2015].
16. Thomas K, Coughlin L, Mannion PT, Haddad NG. The value of Chlamydia trachomatis antibody testing as part of routine infertility investigations. Hum Reprod. 2000;15:1079-82.
17. Tulandi T, Akkour K. Role of reproductive surgery in the era of assisted reproductive technology. Best Pract Res Clin Obstet Gynaecol. 2012;26:747-55.

CHAPTER

Etiopathogenesis and Diagnosis of Endometriosis

9

PG Paul, Aditya S Khurd, Radhika KT, Saumya Bulusu

INTRODUCTION

Endometriosis is a common gynecological disorder affecting 6–10% of women in the reproductive age group, rising to 35–50% in women with infertility and or pain.[1] It is classically associated with dysmenorrhea, chronic pelvic pain, and infertility. It is an estrogen-dependent disease and thus usually affects women during the reproductive years. Endometriosis is defined as the presence of endometrial like tissue outside the uterus, which induces a chronic, inflammatory reaction.[2]

ETIOPATHOGENESIS

It is known that endometriosis occurs only in certain women, and there are factors that increase the risk of developing the disease. The risk factors are a family history of endometriosis, early age menarche, short menstrual cycle, heavy and long menstrual flow (>7 days), delayed child bearing, and obstructive type of Müllerian anomalies.

The exact cause and pathogenesis of endometriosis is unclear. Several theories exist that attempt to explain this disease. These theories can be grouped into two, one proposing that endometrial implants originate from the uterine endometrium and the other proposing that the implants arise from tissues other than the uterus.

Retrograde menstruation

Early in the 20th century, Sampson proposed the theory of retrograde menstruation through the Fallopian tube into the peritoneal cavity. Retrograde menstruation is a common physiologic event. Diagnostic laparoscopic studies during perimenstrual periods have shown that it occurs in 90% of women. Conditions that increase the rate of retrograde menstruation, such as congenital obstructive Müllerian anomalies, do increase the risk of endometriosis. But the fact that only 10% of women develop this disease needs more explanation. Genetic, immunologic, and hormonal dysfunction may be modifying factors.

Immunologic Dysfunction

The refluxed endometrial tissue is cleared from the peritoneum by the immune system. Larger tissue fragment has an increased capacity to escape from immune clearance.[3] The eutopic endometrium from women with endometriosis was found to be more resistant to lysis by natural killer (NK) cells than the eutopic endometrium from women without disease.[4] Women with endometriosis have diminished cell-mediated immunity with decreased T cell and NK cell responsiveness.[5] The endometriotic tissue has a higher capacity for biosynthesis of estrogens and increased progesterone resistance compared to eutopic endometrium.[6,7] These effects enhance the survival of the refluxed endometrium.

Metaplasia

The endometrium and peritoneum are derivatives of the same coelomic wall epithelium, and this theory postulates that the peritoneal mesothelium retains its embryologic ability to transform into endometrial tissue. But what causes the transformation of coelomic epithelium into endometrial type glands is not known. Endometriosis in men on a high dose of estrogen therapy can be explained by this theory.

Müllerian Rests or Müllerianosis

Residual cells from embryologic Müllerian duct migration maintain the capacity to develop into endometriotic lesions under the influence of estrogen at the beginning of puberty. Epidemiological studies have shown that there is a twofold increased risk of endometriosis in women exposed to diethylstilbestrol in utero.[8]

Anatomic Spread

Endometriosis is found in the incisional scars after cesarean section and some gynecological procedures due to iatrogenic spread of endometrial tissue. An uncommon site of endometriosis is the thoracic cavity causing cyclical pneumothorax and hemoptysis. A possible mechanism is a hematogenous or a lymphatic spread.

Genetic Factors

Twin and family studies have documented an increased relative risk of endometriosis in families. There is a 7% recurrence risk for all first-degree relatives. Severe endometriosis is more likely when a relative has the disease (61%) than for women without an affected first-degree relative (24%).[9]

Endocrine-disrupting Chemicals (EDCs)

Endocrine-disrupting chemicals (EDCs), such as bisphenol A, phthalates, are structurally similar to endogenous hormones and can mimic or block the effects of the endogenous hormones. A substantial number of environmental pollutants have been shown to disrupt endocrine function.[10]

TYPES AND LOCATION

There are two classic, well-differentiated endometriosis entities:

1. Endometriosis interna or adenomyosis, occurs when ectopic endometrial foci infiltrate the outer myometrium of the uterus. Adenomyoma is an area of encapsulated adenomyosis usually seen on the posterior wall of the uterus.
2. Endometriosis externa, commonly referred to as endometriosis is usually located in the pelvis. Most common sites are ovary, pouch of Douglas, uterosacral ligament, rectosigmoid colon, and vesicouterine pouch. Endometriotic implants can be found in other extragenital locations like gastrointestinal tract (appendix, small bowel), the urinary tract, or the thoracic area. Occasionally it can be seen in episiotomy or laparotomy scars.

There are three clinical forms of endometriosis (endometriosis externa):

1. Peritoneal endometriosis: These are superficial lesions located on pelvic organs or pelvic peritoneum. The classical appearance of the endometriotic implants on peritoneal serosa may present as bluish or blue-black "powder-burn" lesions. Nonclassical or subtle lesions include clear and red "flame-like" lesions or white lesions.
2. Endometrioma or chocolate cyst of the ovary are pseudocysts formed by invagination of endometriosis within the ovarian cortex and contain dense brown chocolate-like fluid. They are usually adherent to the pelvic side wall and the uterus.
3. Deep infiltrating endometriosis: They are lesions that penetrate more than 5 mm below the surface of peritoneum and are found primarily on the uterosacral ligaments or cul de sac, but may also involve the rectovaginal septum. These lesions may present with deep dyspareunia or dyschezia depending on the location.

CLASSIFICATION

Several different classification systems have been developed for staging of endometriosis. The most widely used one is the American Society of Reproductive Medicine (ASRM) classification.[11] However, the stage of endometriosis does not correlate with the severity of clinical symptoms.

Endometriosis is classified in to four stages: minimal, mild, moderate, or severe based on visual observations at laparoscopy. The minimal disease is characterized by isolated implants and no significant adhesions. Mild endometriosis consists of superficial implants without significant adhesions. In the moderate disease, multiple implants with scarring and adhesion around the tubes and ovaries may be present. Severe disease is characterized by multiple implants, ovarian endometriomas along with thick, dense adhesions, and/or complete obliteration of the pouch of Douglas.

DIAGNOSIS

Endometriosis is diagnosed by medical history, clinical examination, ultrasonography, blood tests, and confirmed by laparoscopy.

Clinical Diagnosis

A complete history and physical examination including speculum and bimanual examination help in the diagnosis. The most common symptoms of endometriosis are dysmenorrhea (50–90%), dyspareunia (25–40%), chronic pelvic pain (10–20%), and infertility (30%). The intensity of pain and severity of the disease usually do not correlate. Patients with bowel endometriosis may complain of constipation, diarrhea, dyschezia, or hematochezia. Bladder symptoms include cyclic urinary frequency or urgency. Symptom associated with scar endometriosis is a cyclical pain over the episiotomy or laparotomy scars. Lung endometrial implants can cause respiratory symptoms due to pleural effusion or pneumothorax.

Physical examination may show tenderness or nodularity of uterosacral ligaments or cul de sac during bimanual pelvic examination. Dark blue nodules may be seen in the posterior vaginal fornix in some cases of rectovaginal endometriosis. Enlarged adnexal mass or fixed retroverted uteri with varying mobility restriction are other signs of advanced disease.

Laparoscopy

Laparoscopy with biopsy of lesions is considered as the gold standard for a definitive diagnosis of endometriosis.[12] The classic appearance of the endometriotic implants on laparoscopy may be bluish or blue-black "powder-burn" lesions (Fig. 9.1). Nonclassic or subtle lesions include clear and red "flame-like" lesions or white lesions (Fig. 9.2). These lesions can be associated with local signs of chronic inflammation like fluid-filled vesicles (Figs. 9.3 and 9.4). Ovarian endometriomas may be unilateral or bilateral with varying sizes (Figs. 9.5 and 9.6). Endometriomas contain old blood that has undergone hemolysis. Once the intracystic pressure rises, the cyst contents leak out into the peritoneal cavity causing severe abdominal pain. Endometriomas and deep infiltrating endometriosis are usually associated with adhesions to adjacent structures (Fig. 9.7). Deep infiltrating endometriosis involves the cul de sac, but may also involve

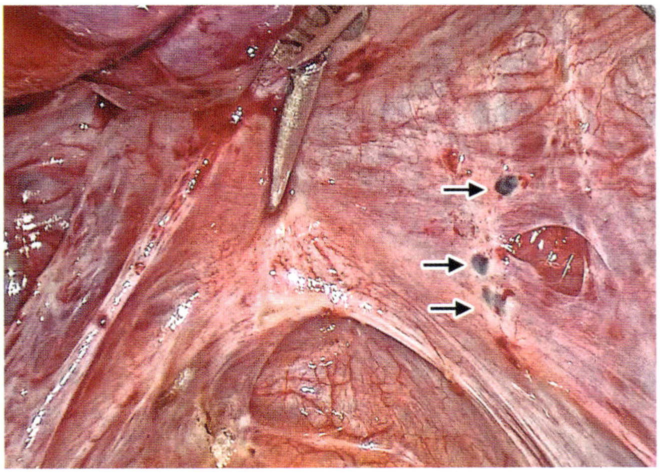

Fig. 9.1: Laparoscopy showing classic bluish or blue-black "powder-burn lesion" above the right uterosacral ligament.

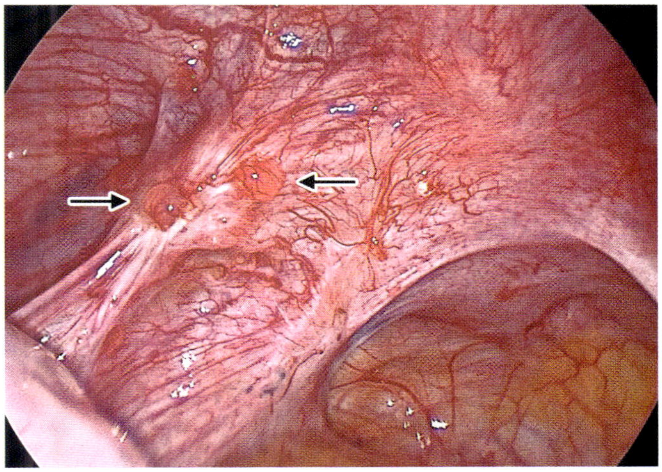

Fig. 9.2: Laparoscopy showing red "flame-like" lesions on left broad ligament.

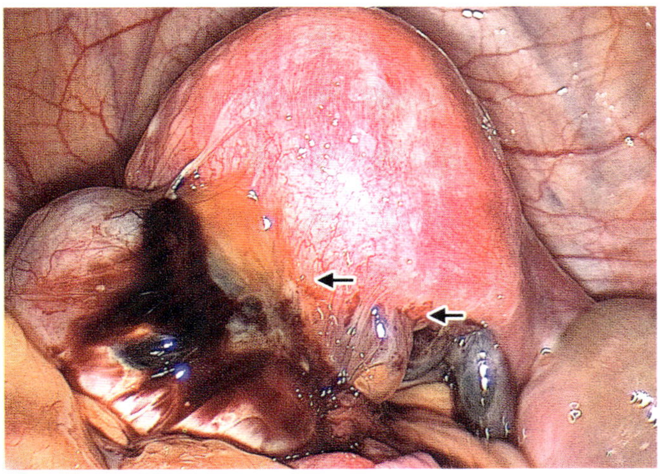

Fig. 9.3: Laparoscopy showing endometriosis with multiple fluid-filled vesicles over the uterus and adnexa.

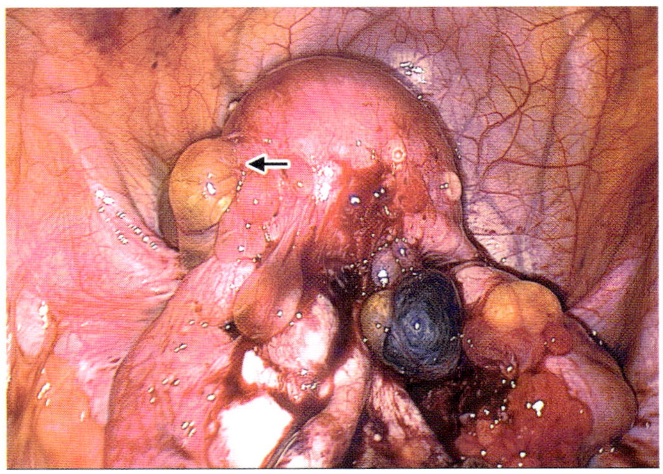

Fig. 9.4: Laparoscopy showing endometriosis with multiple fluid-filled vesicles over the uterus and adnexa.

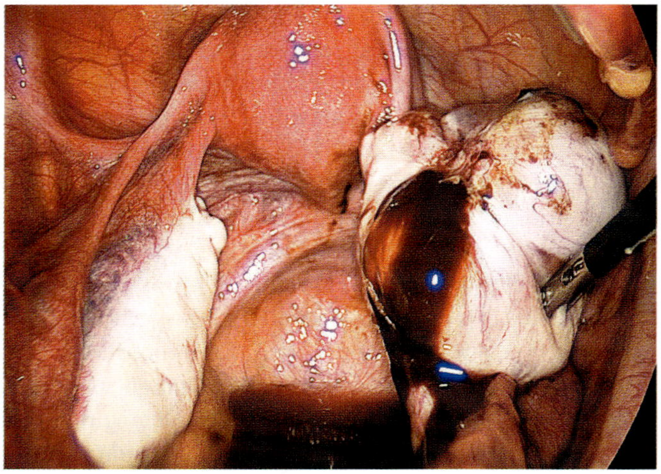

Fig. 9.5: Laparoscopy showing right endometrioma draining chocolate material during dissection.

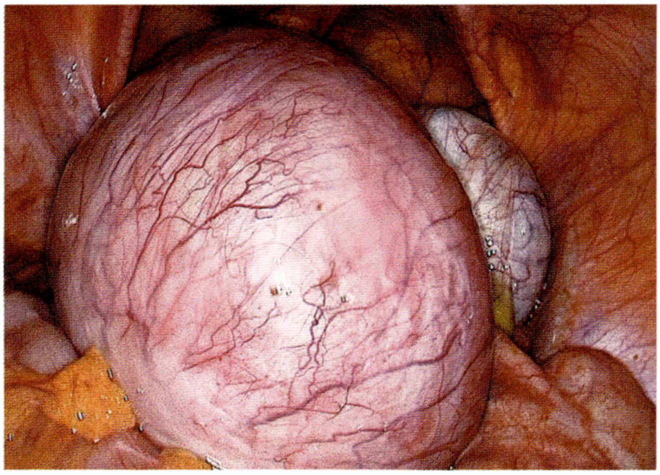

Fig. 9.6: Laparoscopy showing bilateral endometrioma—left endometrioma is larger.

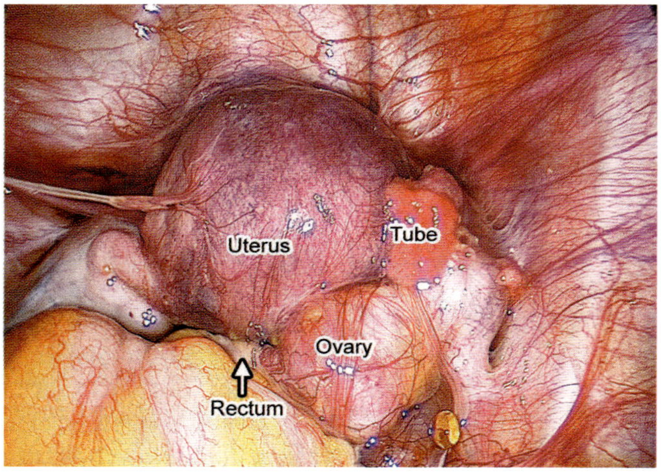

Fig. 9.7: Laparoscopy showing severe endometriosis with pelvic adhesions.

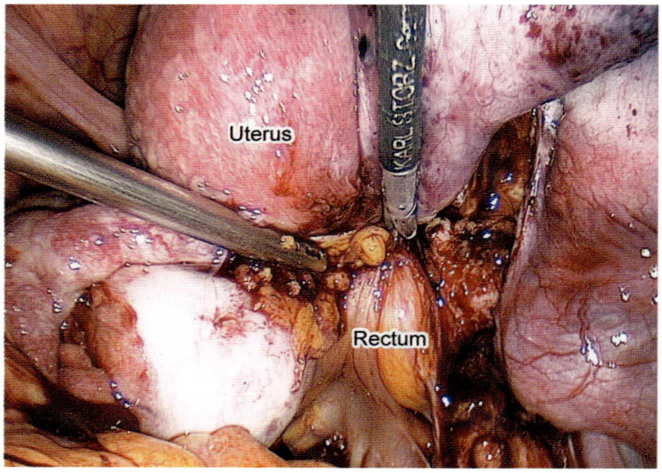

Fig. 9.8: Laparoscopy showing deep infiltrating endometriosis with rectovaginal involvement.

the rectovaginal septum (Fig. 9.8). Deep endometriosis can affect the bladder and laparoscopy may show bladder adhesions to the uterus with endometrial implants (Fig. 9.9A). Cystoscopy can confirm the mucosal involvement (Fig. 9.9B). Endometriotic implants can be found in other extragenital locations like the appendix and diaphragm (Figs. 9.10 and 9.11). Since several studies have demonstrated that visual diagnosis of endometriosis is unreliable, a biopsy is essential to confirm the diagnosis of endometriosis.

Imaging

Several imaging modalities have been proposed to diagnose the presence, location, and extent of endometriosis such as ultrasonography and magnetic resonance imaging (MRI).

Ultrasonography

Transvaginal ultrasonography (TVS) is the first-line diagnostic modality for endometriosis, owing to its relatively high accuracy and easy accessibility. TVS offers a very precise diagnosis of ovarian endometriomas with high sensitivity and specificity.[13] Many studies have described the ultrasound characteristics of endometriomas and defined their typical ultrasound features.[13,14] The "typical" endometrioma is a unilocular cyst in the ovary with homogeneous low-level echogenicity (ground glass echogenicity)

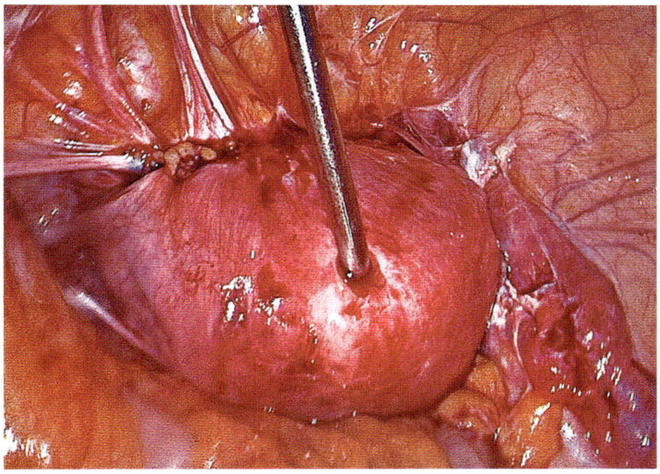

Fig. 9.9A: Laparoscopy showing bladder endometriosis.

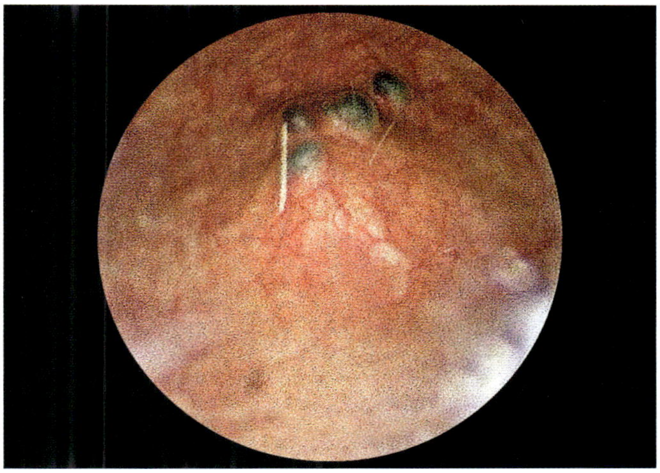

Fig. 9.9B: Cystoscopy of the same patient showing bladder endometriosis.

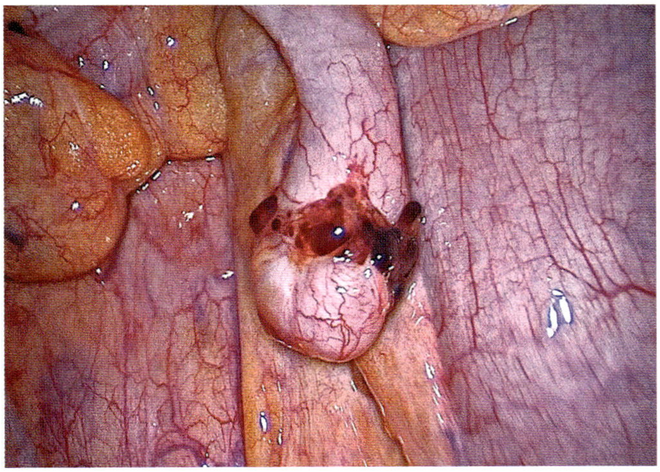

Fig. 9.10: Laparoscopy showing endometriotic implants over the appendix.

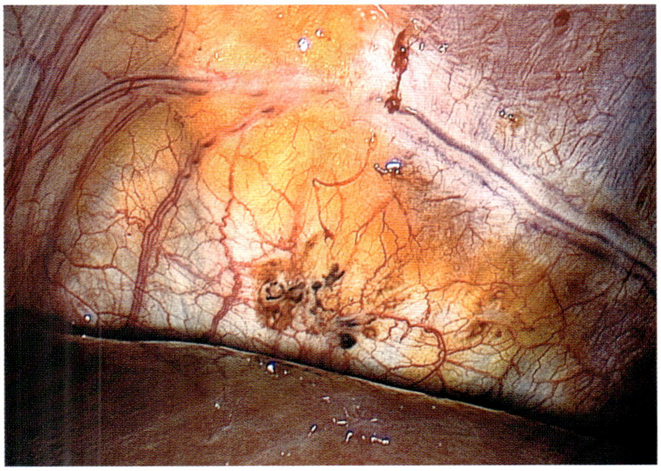

Fig. 9.11: Laparoscopy showing endometriotic implants on the diaphragm.

of the cyst fluid (Fig. 9.12). A large multicentric study identified the following characteristics as the important criteria to diagnose endometrioma:[15]

1. Premenopausal status
2. Ground glass appearance of the cyst fluid
3. Cyst with one to four locules (Fig. 9.13)
4. Absence of papillations with detectable blood flow, i.e. tumors without papillations or tumors with papillations but without flow (Figs. 9.14 and 9.15).

A variety of appearances of endometriomas is possible because of the degradation of internal blood products over time. Many other morphological features have also been described.[16,17] Anechoic cyst or a fluid level may be seen in some of them (Fig. 9.16). When both ovaries are adherent to each other behind the uterus in the cul de sac (kissing ovaries), it is suggestive of severe endometriosis (Figs. 9.17 and 9.18). The other differential diagnoses are dermoid cyst, hemorrhagic cyst, or ovarian abscess (Figs. 9.19 to 9.21).

Conventional ultrasound scans report the presence or absence of pathology such as ovarian endometriomas or hydrosalpinges (hard markers). However, more subtle information is available about the state of the pelvis based on the degree of ovarian and uterine mobility as well as tenderness (soft markers).[18] A combination of hard and soft markers can improve the diagnosis of endometriosis.

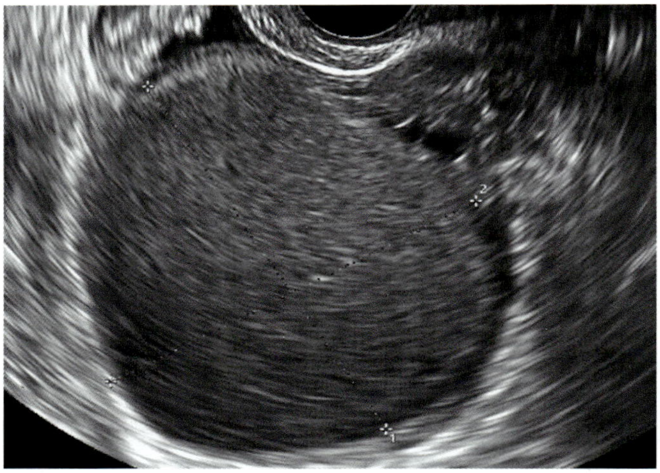

Fig. 9.12: Transvaginal sonography showing a unilocular endometrioma with homogeneous low-level internal echoes (ground glass echogenicity).

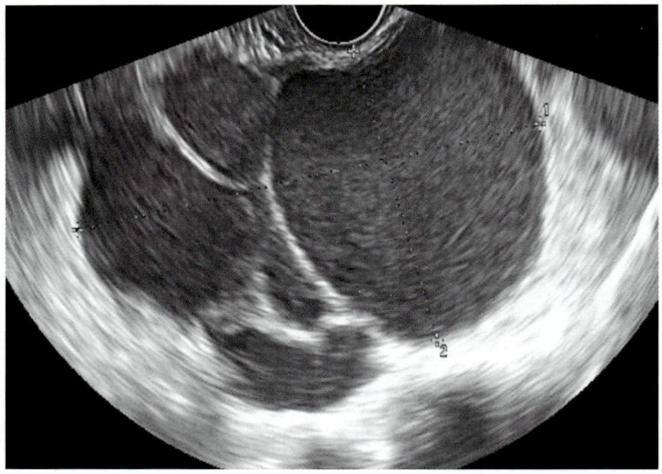

Fig. 9.13: Transvaginal sonography showing a multiloculated endometrioma.

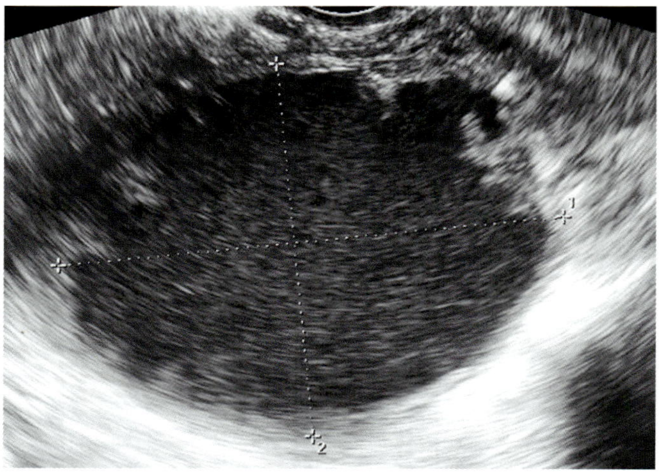

Fig. 9.14: Transvaginal sonography showing an endometrioma with echogenic papillations without color flow.

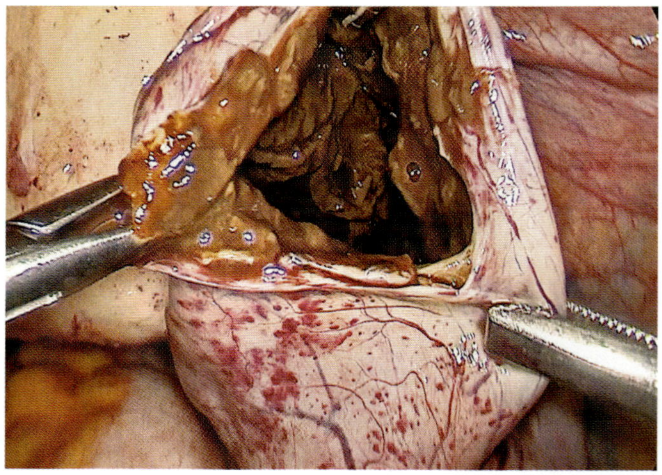

Fig. 9.15: Laparoscopy of the same patient as in Figure 9.14 showing the opened endometrioma with solidified chocolate material causing papillations on transvaginal sonography.

Mobility of ovaries can be assessed by a combination of gentle pressure with the vaginal probe and abdominal pressure with the examiners free hand (Figs. 9.22 and 9.23).

Bladder endometriosis is rare, and presents with dysmenorrhea and associated urinary symptoms. TVS may show a solid nodule within the posterior bladder wall when the bladder is partially filled (Figs. 9.24 and 9.25). Color Doppler may detect low to moderate vascularity. Nevertheless, it has limited value for the diagnosis of smaller endometriotic lesions of the bladder.

Deep infiltrating endometriosis typically involves the uterosacral ligaments, pouch of Douglas or the rectovaginal septum. Since surgery for deep endometriosis requires considerable skill and experience, a preoperative diagnosis is needed to consider the different treatment options. Several imaging techniques, such as TVS, transrectal ultrasonography, rectal endoscopic ultrasonography and MRI have been proposed for the assessment of deep endometriosis. Since transrectal ultrasonography does not allow a good evaluation of other pelvic organs, TVS is preferred in these cases. Endometriotic nodules detected in the uterosacral ligaments, rectovaginal septum, vagina, vesicouterine pouch, bladder, and ureters can be signs of deeply infiltrating endometriosis. Pelvic adhesions can be

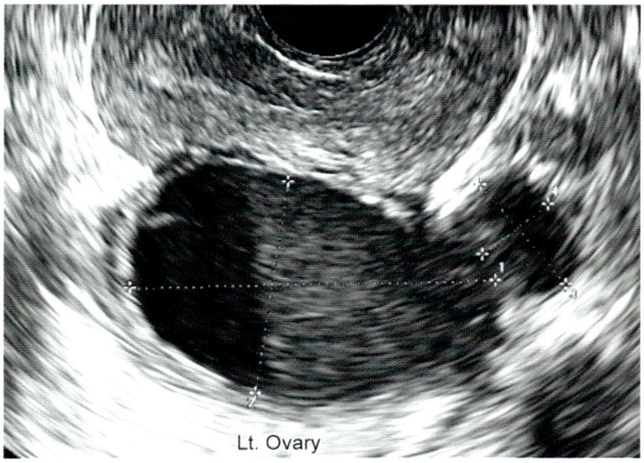

Fig. 9.16: Transvaginal sonography showing an endometrioma with fluid level.

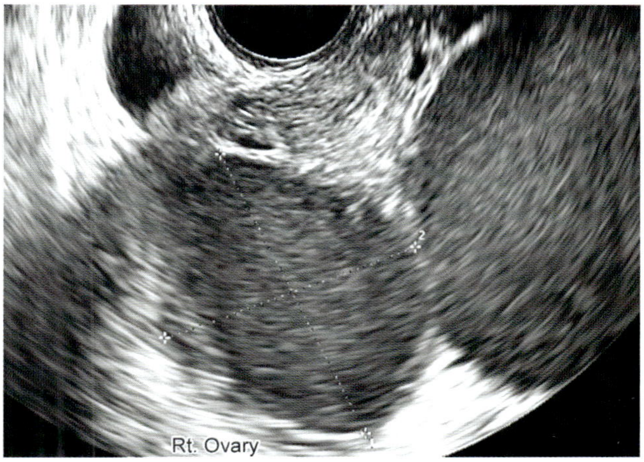

Fig. 9.17: Transvaginal sonography showing kissing ovaries (endometriomas).

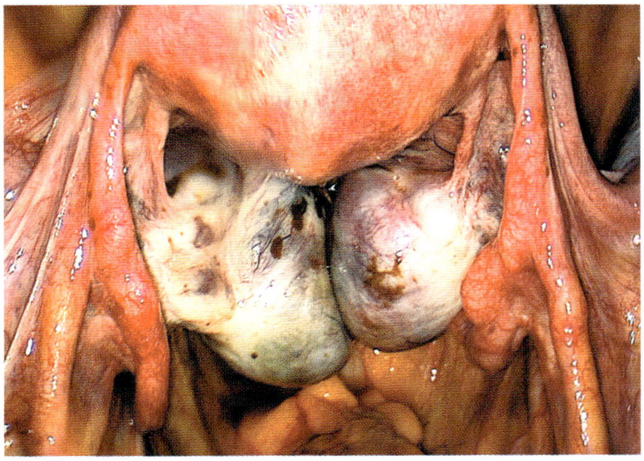

Fig. 9.18: Laparoscopy showing kissing ovaries adherent to uterus and cul de sac.

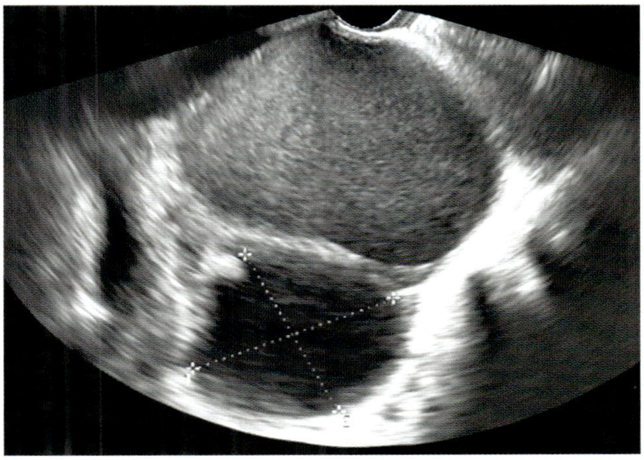

Fig. 9.19: Transvaginal sonography showing an ovarian abscess mimicking an endometrioma.

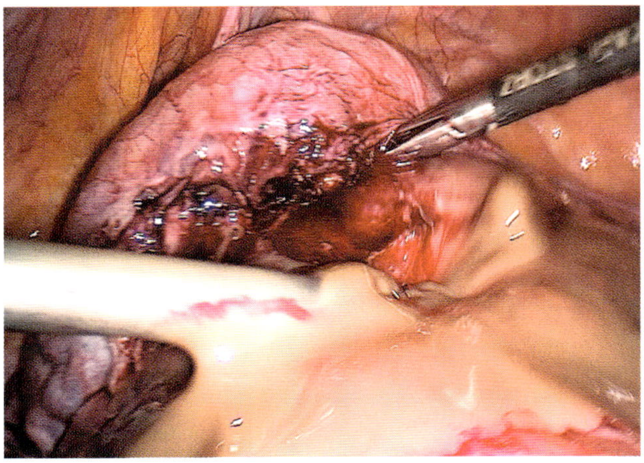

Fig. 9.20: Laparoscopy of the same patient as in Figure 9.19 showing opened ovarian abscess.

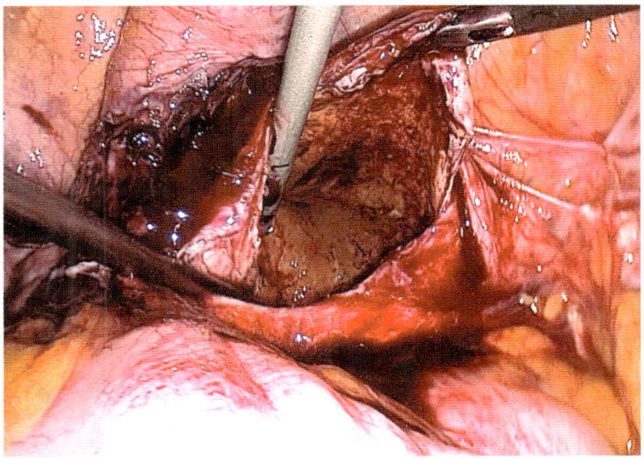

Fig. 9.21: Laparoscopy of the same patient as in Figure 9.19 showing the ovarian abscess cavity after evacuating the pus.

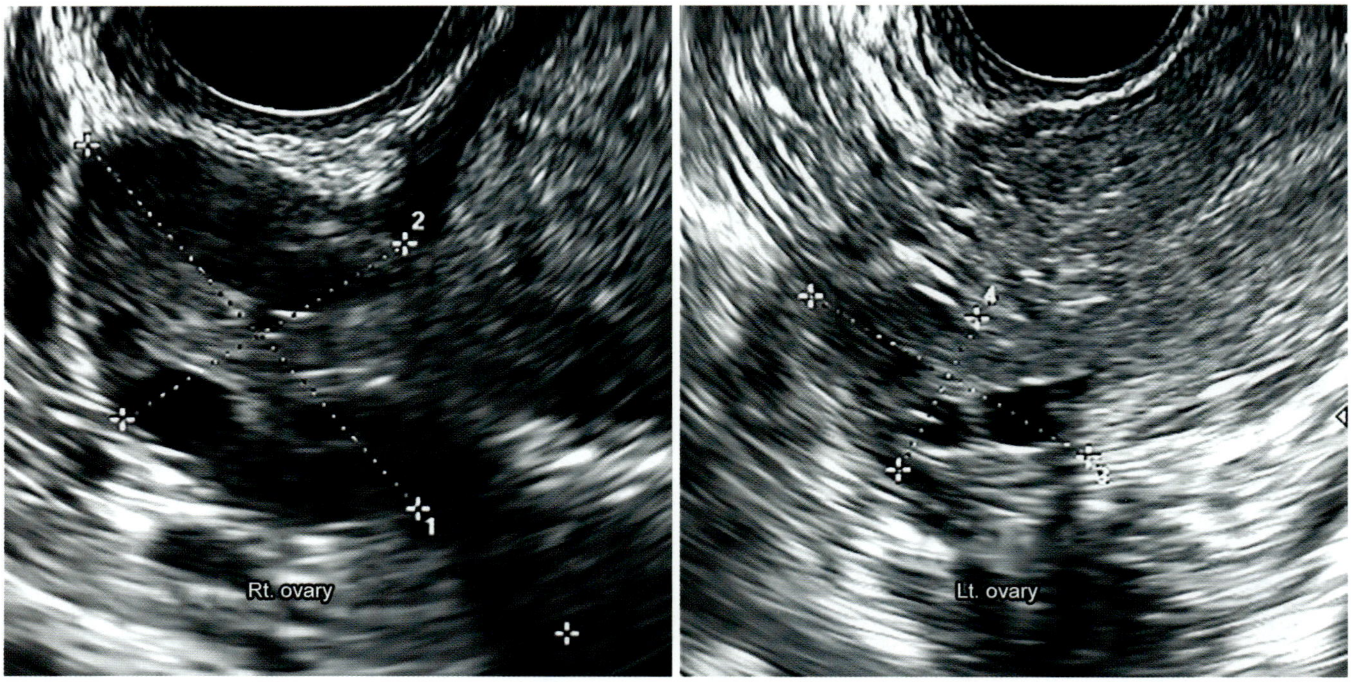

Fig. 9.22: Transvaginal sonography showing a nonmobile left ovary, close to uterus.

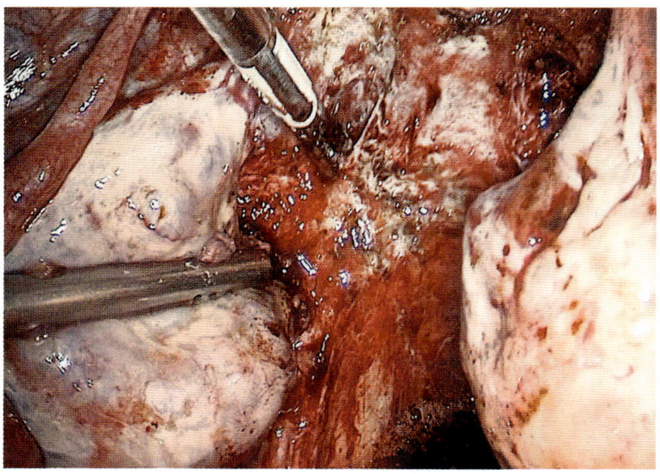

Fig. 9.23: Laparoscopy showing an adherent left ovary behind the uterus.

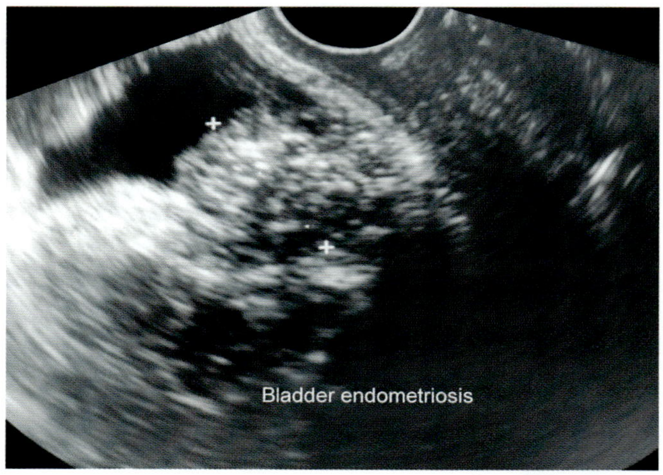

Fig. 9.24: Transvaginal sonography showing bladder endometriosis.

suspected, when pelvic organs appear fixed to each other, when hyperechogenic plaques are found between the serosal surfaces of the different organs, and when the pouch of Douglas is partially or completely obliterated. In women with symptoms and signs of rectal endometriosis, TVS is useful for identifying or ruling out rectal endometriosis.[19] But this is highly operator dependent, and experience is often lacking, hence TVS is not recommended for the diagnosis of rectal endometriosis.[20]

Transabdominal ultrasonography can be used instead of TVS, in young girls and celibate women. However, TVS is more sensitive than transabdominal in detecting adnexal masses and pelvic nodules. Ureteral endometriosis can cause hydronephrosis and thus, transabdominal

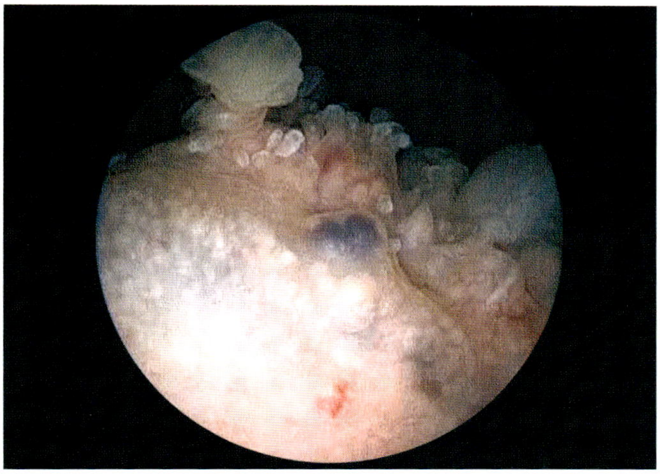

Fig. 9.25: Cystoscopy of the same patient as in Figure 9.24 showing bladder endometriosis.

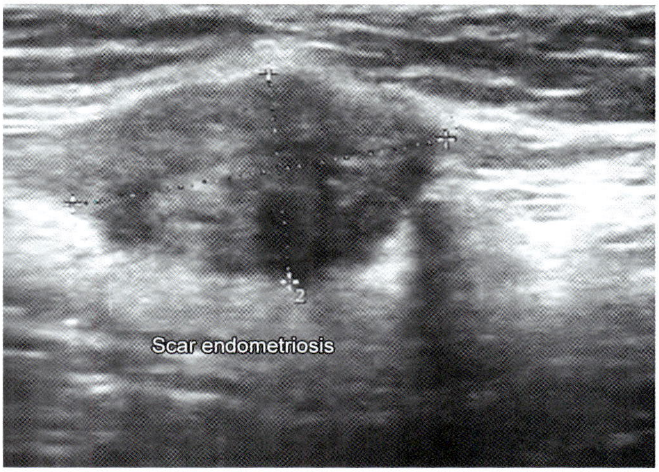

Fig. 9.26: Transabdominal sonography showing scar endometriosis of abdominal wall in a patient with previous cesarean section.

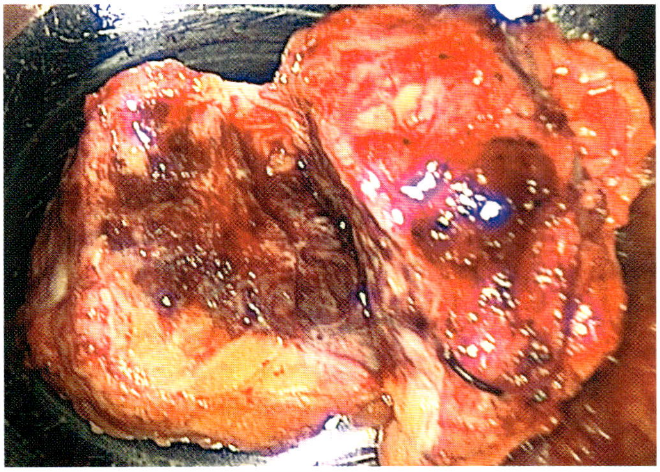

Fig. 9.27: Bisected specimen of an excised scar endometriosis.

ultrasonography of the kidneys is always recommended when deeply infiltrating endometriosis is suspected.

Abdominal scar endometriosis, which usually presents with cyclical pain over the scar, can be diagnosed on transabdominal ultrasound scan (Figs. 9.26 and 9.27).

Magnetic Resonance Imaging

The MRI is less operator dependent than TVS and is more sensitive for detecting the foci of deeply infiltrating endometriosis, because of its ability to completely survey the anterior and posterior compartments of the pelvis. Deep infiltrating endometriosis appear as areas or nodules with regular, irregular, indistinct, or stellate margins on MRI imaging.[21] A distortion of the normal pelvic anatomy or a loculated fluid collection can suggest the presence of adhesions. MRI has a high specificity for the diagnosis of endometriomas as a result of its ability to detect old hemorrhagic content.

Biomarkers

A noninvasive test for endometriosis would be useful for the early detection of endometriosis in symptomatic women who have pelvic pain and/or subfertility with normal ultrasound results. Several noninvasive diagnostic tests are being explored for the diagnosis of endometriosis. These biomarkers of endometriosis can be tested in either plasma or urine or endometrium.

Cancer antigen 125 (CA-125), the most extensively investigated and widely used peripheral biomarker of endometriosis, is produced by endometrial and mesothelial cells. However, CA-125 levels in peripheral blood lack diagnostic power as a single biomarker of endometriosis due to low sensitivity. Although studies have shown that tumor markers, cytokines, and angiogenic and growth factors show altered levels in peripheral blood (plasma or serum) of women with endometriosis when compared with controls, so far none of them, alone or in combination, has been validated as a noninvasive test for endometriosis.[22] Recent studies on circulating microRNAs, a novel class of regulatory molecules with the ability to control gene expression could be used as biomarkers in endometriosis, appear promising. Few studies have shown that endometriosis may be diagnosed by an increased density of nerve fibers in the endometrium of women with endometriosis as compared with controls who lack the disease.[23]

The current recommendation is not to depend on a single or a panel of biomarkers as a noninvasive diagnostic test for endometriosis, as they lack sufficient sensitivity and specificity.[20]

SUMMARY

Endometriosis is a common gynecological disorder affecting women in the reproductive age group. It is more common in women with family history of endometriosis, delayed child bearing, and obstructive Müllerian anomalies. Most common symptoms are dysmenorrhea, chronic pelvic pain, and infertility. Several theories are proposed to explain the cause and pathogenesis of endometriosis. They are retrograde menstruation, immunologic dysfunction, metaplasia, müllerianosis, anatomic spread, genetic factors, and endocrine disrupting chemicals. None of them can explain all the varieties of endometriosis. There are two clinical types of endometriosis—endometriosis interna (adenomyosis) and endometriosis externa. There are three clinical forms of endometriosis externa—peritoneal endometriosis, ovarian endometrioma, and deep infiltrating endometriosis. A good history followed by clinical examination can help the physician to suspect endometriosis. Transvaginal sonography is the main stay of diagnosis. Peritoneal endometriosis cannot be diagnosed by imaging techniques including MRI. Ovarian endometrioma can be diagnosed with TVS with high sensitivity and specificity. Soft markers of endometriosis like ovarian and uterine mobility and tenderness elicited by TVS help to complement the diagnosis of endometriosis. Diagnosis of deep infiltrating endometriosis by TVS is highly operator dependent and MRI may be useful in such situations. At present, biomarkers are not clinically useful, as they lack sensitivity and specificity. Laparoscopy with biopsy is needed for the final confirmation of endometriosis.

REFERENCES

1. Meuleman C, Vandenabeele B, Fieuws S, Spiessens C, Timmerman D, D'Hooghe T. High prevalence of endometriosis in infertile women with normal ovulation and normospermia partners. Fertil Steril. 2009;92:68-74.
2. Kennedy S, Bergqvist A, Chapron C, Dunselman G, Greb R, Hammelshoj L, et al. ESHRE guideline for the diagnosis and treatment of endometriosis. Hum Reprod. 2005;20:2698-704.
3. Nap AW, Groothuis PG, Demir AY, Maas JW, Dunselman GA, de GoeijAF, et al. Tissue integrity is essential for ectopic implantation of human endometrium in the chicken chorioallantoic membrane. Hum Reprod. 2003;18:30-4.
4. Oosterlynck DJ, Cornillie FJ, Waer M, Vandeputte M, Koninckx PR. Women with endometriosis shows a defect in natural killer activity resulting in a decreased cytotoxicity to the autologous endometrium. Fertil Steril. 1991;56:45-51.
5. Mathur S, Peress MR, Williamson HO, Youmans CD, Maney SA, Garvin AJ, et al. Autoimmunity to endometrium and ovary in endometriosis. Clin Exp Immunol. 1982;50(2):259-66.
6. Noble LS, Takayama K, Zeitoun KM, Putman JM, Johns DA, Hinshelwood MM, et al. Prostaglandin E2 stimulates aromatase expression in endometriosis-derived stromal cells. J Clin Endocrinol Metab. 1997;82:600-6.
7. Burney RO, Talbi S, Hamilton AE, Vo KC, Nyegaard M, Nezhat CR, et al. Gene expression analysis of endometrium reveals progesterone resistance and candidate susceptibility genes in women with endometriosis. Endocrinology. 2007;148:3814-26.
8. Missmer SA, Hankinson SE, Spiegelman D, Barbieri RL, Michels KB, Hunter DJ. In utero exposures and the incidence of endometriosis. Fertil Steril. 2004;82:1501-8.
9. Malinak LK, Buttram VC Jr., Elias S, Simpson JL. Heritable aspects of endometriosis. II. Clinical characteristics of familial endometriosis. Am J Obstet Gynecol. 1980;137(3):332-7.
10. Balabanič D, Rupnik M, Klemenčič AK. Negative impact of endocrine-disrupting compounds on human reproductive health. Reprod Fer Develop. 2011;23(3):403-16.
11. American Society of Reproductive Medicine. Revised American Society of Reproductive Medicine classification of Endometriosis: 1996. Fertil Steril. 1997;67:817.
12. Brosens I, Puttemans P, Campo R, Gords S, Kinkel K. Diagnosis of endometriosis:pelvis endoscopy and imaging techniques. Best Practice Res Clin Obstet Gynaecol. 2004;18(2):285-303.
13. Valentin L. Use of morphology to characterize and manage common adnexal masses. Best Pract Res Clin Obstet Gynaecol. 2004;18:71-89.
14. Jermy K, Luise C, Bourne T. The characterization of common ovarian cysts in premenopausal women. Ultrasound Obstet Gynecol. 2001;17:140-4.
15. Van Holsbeke BC, Van Calster S, Guerriero L, Savelli D, Paladini A, Lissoni A, et al. Endometriomas: their ultrasound characteristics. Ultrasound Obstet Gynecol. 2010;35:730-40.
16. Raine-Fenning N, Jayaprakasan K, Deb S. Three-dimensional ultrasonographic characteristics of endometriomata. Ultrasound Obstet Gynecol. 2008;31:718-24.
17. Asch E, Levine D. Variations in the appearance of endometriomas. J Ultrasound Med. 2007;26:993-1002.
18. Okaro E, Condous G, Khalid A, Timmerman D, Ameye L, Huffel S, et al. The use of ultrasound-based 'soft markers' for the prediction of pelvic pathology in women with chronic pelvic pain—can we reduce the need for laparoscopy? BJOG. 2006;113:251-6.
19. Bazot M, Darai E, Hourani R, Thomassin I, Cortez A, Uzan S, et al. Deep pelvic endometriosis: MR imaging for diagnosis and prediction of extension of disease. Radiology. 2004;232(2):379-89.

20. Hudelist G, English J, Thomas AE, Tinelli A, Singer CF, Keckstein J. Diagnostic accuracy of transvaginal ultrasound for non-invasive diagnosis of bowel endometriosis: systematic review and meta-analysis. Ultrasound Obstet Gynecol. 2011;37:257-63.
21. Dunselman GA1, Vermeulen N, Becker C, Calhaz-Jorge C, D'Hooghe T, De Bie B, et al. ESHRE guideline: management of women with endometriosis. Hum Reprod. 2014;29(3):400-12.
22. May KE, Conduit-Hulbert SA, Villar J, Kirtley S, Kennedy SH, Becker CM. Peripheral biomarkers of endometriosis: a systematic review. Hum Reprod Update. 2010;16(6):651-74.
23. Al-Jefout M, Dezarnaulds G, Cooper M, Tokushige N, Luscombe GM, Markham R, et al. Diagnosis of endometriosis by detection of nerve fibres in an endometrial biopsy: a double blind study. Hum Reprod. 2009;24:3019-24.

CHAPTER 10

Management of Endometriosis

PG Paul, Saumya Bulusu, Hemant Shintre, Sumina Mannur, George Paul

INTRODUCTION

Endometriosis is a chronic disease affecting 6–10% of women in their fertile years.[1] The main symptoms of endometriosis are pelvic pain and infertility. Common pain symptoms are dysmenorrhea, chronic cyclical pelvic pain, dyspareunia, and dyschezia. Management of endometriosis depends on the manifestations of disease and patient characteristics. Patients are grouped into two categories for planning treatment strategies—endometriosis with pain and infertility.

ENDOMETRIOSIS AND PAIN

The pain symptoms are very distressing to the patient and need treatment when severe. The cause of pain varies depending on the type of lesions like superficial peritoneal implants, endometrioma, and deep infiltrating lesions, which may involve rectum, vagina, bladder, and ureter. Pain can arise from cyclic bleeding from ectopic endometrial tissue, production of inflammatory mediators like cytokines, and nerve irritation.[2]

Endometriosis-related pain can be managed medically and/or surgically.

MEDICAL TREATMENT

Nonsteroidal anti-inflammatory drugs are helpful in the management of primary dysmenorrhea, and hormonal treatment may be required for chronic pain. Hormonal treatment is based on inducing the stable hormonal environment and suppressing the stimulatory effect of sex steroids on endometriotic lesions leading to its atrophy. All hormonally active drugs are considered equally effective on endometriosis-related pain, and choice of treatment depends on the safety, adverse effect profiles, and cost.

Combined Hormonal Contraceptives

Hormonal contraceptives contain ethinyl estradiol and progestin. They can be used in cyclic or continuous fashion for the treatment of endometriosis, and continuous use appears to result in a better pain control.[3] A low-dose estrogen combination is selected as it can potentiate the antiproliferative action of progestin by inducing progesterone receptors expression *in vitro*.[4] Progestin action results in the decidualization with subsequent atrophy of the ectopic endometrium. Combined oral contraceptive pills (COCs) are usually well tolerated with few severe side effects and can be used for prolonged duration. One randomized controlled trial (RCT) comparing the COCs to placebo in women suffering from endometriosis-related dysmenorrhea found that COCs are more effective at treating dysmenorrhoea compared to placebo.[5]

Progestogens

Synthetic progestins have been widely used for decades for the management of endometriosis-related pain. Progestins act by an antigonadotropic effect causing hypoestrogenism, decidualization of the endometriotic lesion by acting on progesterone receptors, and reducing peritoneal inflammation. A wide variety of oral and injectable progestins have been used as sole therapy or in combination with estrogens. Several studies have shown the efficacy of progestins in treating endometriosis-related pain. However, there is no evidence for an improved efficacy compared to other available hormonal treatment.

Dienogest

Dienogest is a new synthetic oral progestin available for endometriosis-related pain. Although it is a 19-nortestosterone derivative, it lacks the androgenic side effects. Though dienogest inhibits ovulation, studies with the use of dienogest 2 mg daily showed only a moderately reduced estrogen level (normal range of follicular phase) without affecting bone mineral density after treatment for 6 months.[6] Studies comparing dienogest and gonadotropin-releasing hormone agonists (GnRHa) have proven dienogest to be comparable to GnRHa in relieving pain symptoms with advantage of causing less hypoestrogenic side effects." But in the dienogest group, prolonged bleeding and irregular bleeding were more frequent in the first 90 days in 45% of the patients.[7]

Levonorgestrel Intrauterine System

Levonorgestrel intrauterine system (LNG-IUS) is used as a contraceptive and also for the treatment of dysfunctional uterine bleeding. It releases 20 μg/24 h of levonorgestrel for 5 years resulting in a mean plasma concentration of 100–200 pg/mL. Though this is much lower than the concentration achieved with COCs, the endometrial levels achieved with LNG-IUS are much higher. Recently, several studies have shown LNG-IUS as the first line of medical treatment for endometriosis-associated pain symptoms as well as to prevent recurrence in postsurgical patients.[8-10] The exact mechanism of action of LNG-IUS in endometriosis is not known, but suggested mechanisms include atrophy of eutopic endometrium and subsequent reduction in retrograde menstruation and direct inhibitory effect of levonorgestrel on endometrial implants due to the high local concentration in the peritoneal cavity.[11] A recent meta-analysis compared LNG-IUS with GnRHa confirmed this finding and also highlighted the absence of side effects like bone loss and hypoestrogenic symptoms with LNG-IUS.[12] Disadvantages of using LNG-IUS are irregular bleeding usually in first 6 months of use and chances of spontaneous expulsion in 9–10% of patients.[13]

Gonadotropin-releasing Hormone Agonists

Gonadotropin-releasing hormone is a decapeptide secreted by hypothalamic neurons, which act on the pituitary gland to produce a pulsatile secretion of follicle-stimulating hormone (FSH) and luteinizing hormone (LH), which in turn acts on ovaries to produce estrogen and progesterone. GnRH agonists differ from endogenous GnRH by substitution of one or more amino acids. They produce a continuous action on the pituitary receptors producing an initial flare effect followed by deep suppression. So ovarian suppression occurs, and the pseudomenopausal effect is achieved leading to atrophy of the endometrial tissue. GnRHa are available as injectables and nasal spray. Common ones are leuprolide, buserelin, goserelin and nafarelin. A large meta-analysis demonstrated that it improves endometriosis-related pain by 60–100%.[14]

The profound hypoestrogenism due to the use of GnRH agonists leads to frequent adverse effects such as hot flushes and vaginal dryness. Prolonged use has been associated with loss of bone mineral density. Add-back therapy is to minimize the hypoestrogenic side effects and may be started at the initiation of GnRHa therapy. Norethindrone, low dose estrogen, or a combination of low dose estrogen-progestin can be used.[15]

Injectable GnRH antagonists give a quicker onset of action and do not produce the initial flare effect. However, the data are limited, and the cost is prohibitive. New oral GnRH antagonist, elagolix, appears to be a promising drug for treatment of endometriosis-related pain with minimal effect on bone loss.[16,17]

Aromatase Inhibitors

Aromatase inhibitors block the enzyme that catalyzes the conversion of androgens into estrogens in granulosa cells of follicles and other cell types like adipocytes. They are as effective as GnRHa in treating endometriosis and adenomyosis. In premenopausal women, they are used in combination with COCs to prevent ovulation. The combination also takes care of the bone loss associated with the hypoestrogenism. In postmenopausal women, they can suppress gonadotropin-independent local estrogen production by endometriotic implants.

Danazol

Danazol is a synthetic testosterone derivative, which was widely used for the treatment of endometriosis-associated pain in the 1970s and 1980s. It acts by inducing direct atrophy of ectopic endometriotic implants and by antigonadotropic effects. Its use is limited by its androgenic side effects such as acne, hirsutism, weight gain, alopecia, and voice changes.

Nonhormonal Treatments

Several nonhormonal agents, like antiangiogenics, statins, tumor necrosis factor-α (TNF-α) blockers, pentoxifylline, and peroxisome proliferator receptor gamma (PPAR-γ), have been tried in experimental settings. None of the agents is recommended for treatment of endometriosis.

SURGICAL TREATMENT OF ENDOMETRIOSIS

Although surgery is required for definitive diagnosis, it can be used as a therapeutic approach in patients with suspected endometriosis. Surgical treatment is indicated when medical therapy fails or not tolerated, the presence of an endometrioma with the potential to exclude malignancy, management of infertility in selected women, and the presence of bowel or urinary tract obstruction. Laparoscopy is the preferred and standard approach for the surgical management of endometriosis. Laparoscopic view allows visualization of inaccessible areas in pelvis, image magnification, and thereby facilitates precise surgery. The objectives of the surgery are the optimal treatment of all visible and deep disease, restoration of normal anatomy, and adhesion prevention. Options include conservative or definitive management. Conservative surgery involves treatment of endometriosis with preservation of uterus and ovaries. It is offered for infertile patients or as an initial surgical treatment for endometriosis. Definitive surgery consisting of hysterectomy, with or without removal of ovaries, is done for patients in whom conservative surgery has failed. Although hysterectomy with bilateral salpingo-oophorectomy (BSO) is considered as a definitive treatment, it may not cure all patients, and there can be a recurrence of the disease.

Conservative Surgery

Conservative surgery involves adhesiolysis for the restoration of anatomy, destruction of endometrial implants, and surgery for endometriomas.

Endometrial Implants

Endometrial implants can be destroyed by excision, vaporization, and electrosurgical coagulation. Excision can be done using a variety of instruments like scissors, monopolar electrodes, ultrasonic instrument, or rarely laser energy. To excise the implants, the margin of the lesion is identified, and an outline is marked around with the cutting instrument. If vital organs are close by, a relaxing incision is made between the organ and the lesion to avoid inadvertent injury to a vital organ. The implant is now held with a grasper and separated from the underlying tissues with the scissors or energy source (Fig. 10.1). The difficulty of the procedure depends on the location, thickness, and size of the implant. Very small implants can be ablated by sparking with a monopolar electrode (Fig. 10.2). There are many reports of using plasma energy for ablation.[18] Superficial implants can be coagulated with a bipolar forceps (Fig. 10.3). This technique is less precise but easier for the beginners. Advantages of excision are complete removal of the lesion and specimen available for histopathological examination. Disadvantages are risk of injury to adjacent vital organs and requirement for advanced skill. There are two randomized controlled studies that compare ablation with excision.[19,20] These studies did not show any difference in pain scores at 12 months for mild endometriosis. Follow-up of one study at 5 years showed that excision group had lower rates of dyspareunia and were less likely to need medical treatment.[21]

Endometriomas

Surgical management of endometriomas is required when they remain symptomatic or large.[22] Endometriomas of varying size are usually present in moderate to severe endometriosis. There are two types of

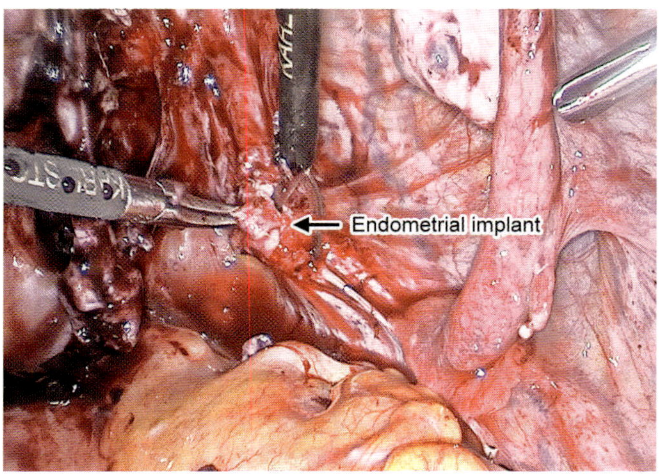

Fig. 10.1: Excision of endometrial implant with scissors.

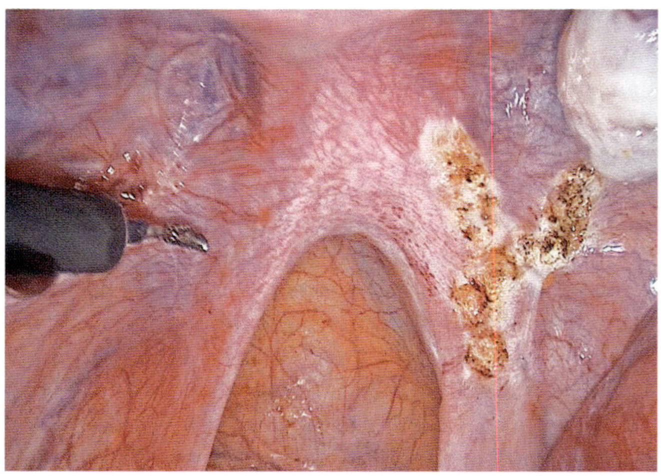

Fig. 10.2: Ablation of endometrial implants using monopolar electrode.

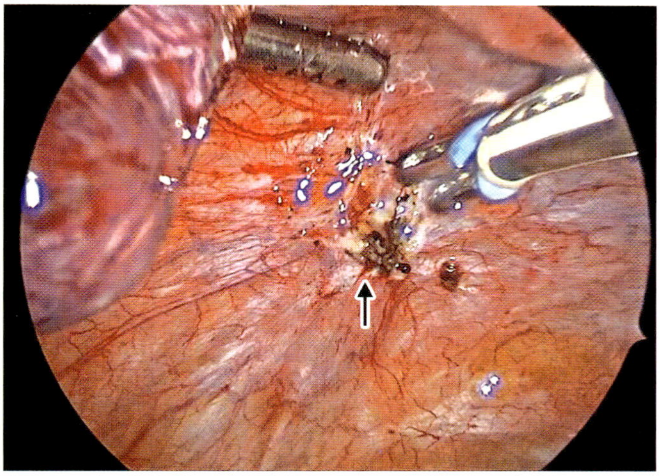

Fig. 10.3: Coagulation of endometrial implants using bipolar electrode.

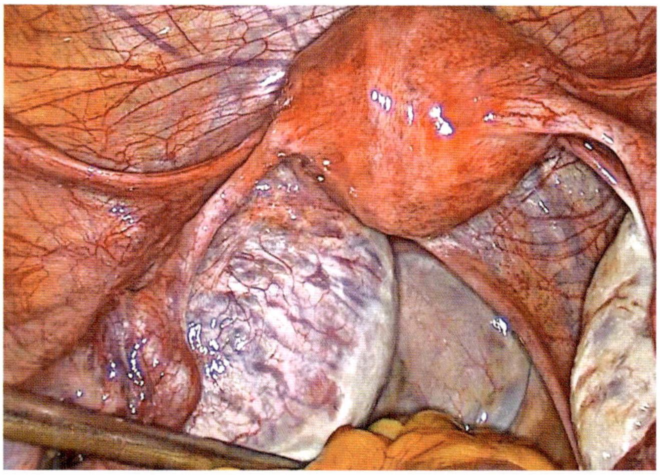

Fig. 10.4: Endometrioma without adhesions on the left side.

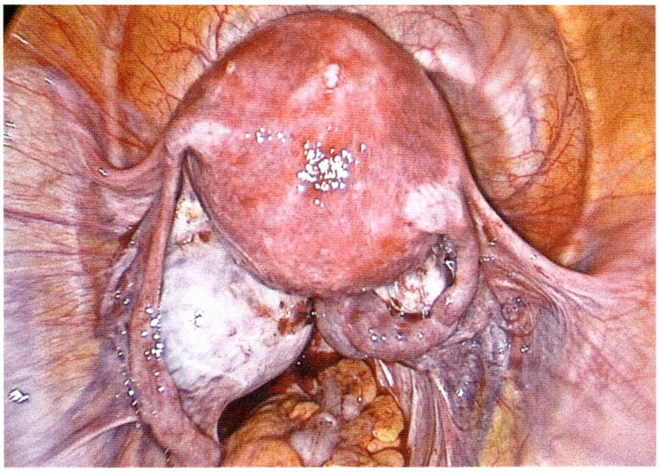

Fig. 10.5: Bilateral endometriomas with adhesions.

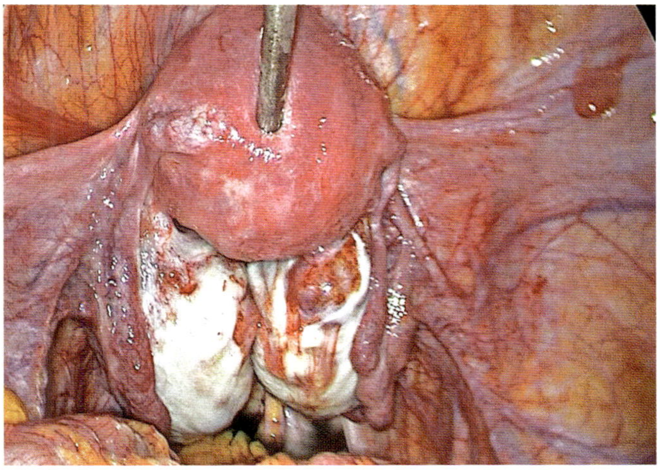

Fig. 10.6A: Injecting dilute vasopressin into the uterus (with bilateral endometriomas).

endometriomas—intraovarian and extraovarion. Intraovarian endometriomas are like any other ovarian cysts without or with minimal adhesions (Fig. 10.4). Most common type is extraovarian, which is formed by the invagination of the endometrial implant on the ovarian cortex with adhesions to the broad ligament or pelvic side wall (Fig. 10.5). The aim of management of endometrioma is the removal of the cyst lining and surface endometriotic implants with minimal damage to the ovarian tissue for preserving the follicles. Extraovarian endometriomas are first released from the pelvic side wall by a combination of blunt and sharp dissection. We use the following technique described earlier.[23] Dilute vasopressin (20 IU in 200 mL of normal saline) is injected into the myometrium till the uterus is blanched, which helps in achieving initial hemostatic dissection of the adnexa and rectosigmoid (Figs. 10.6A and B). After anteverting the uterus with a Spackman cannula, salpingo-ovariolysis is done with sharp dissection. All fleshy adhesions from the uterus and pouch of Douglas are excised. All superficial endometriosis implants are coagulated, and deep ones are excised. The ovary with small endometrioma is mobilized from the pelvic ovarian fossa, and when the chocolate material invariably leaks out, the leaked out contents are aspirated, followed by complete irrigation and aspiration of the cyst. For large endometriomas, we puncture the cyst with a trocar and aspirate the chocolate material (Fig. 10.7). Cyst wall opening is now enlarged to allow complete inspection

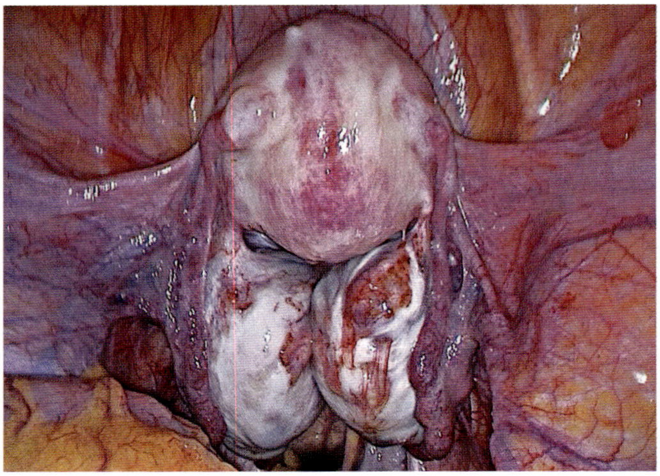

Fig. 10.6B: Blanching of the uterus and adnexae after vasopressin injection.

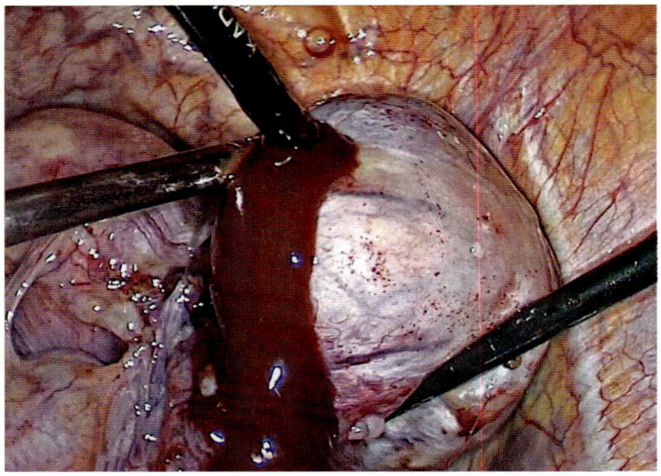

Fig. 10.7: Aspiration of chocolate material from endometrioma.

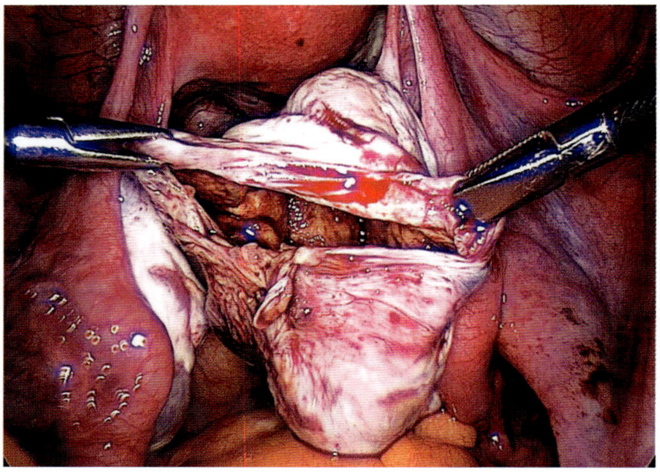

Fig. 10.8: Traction on the cyst wall with two graspers.

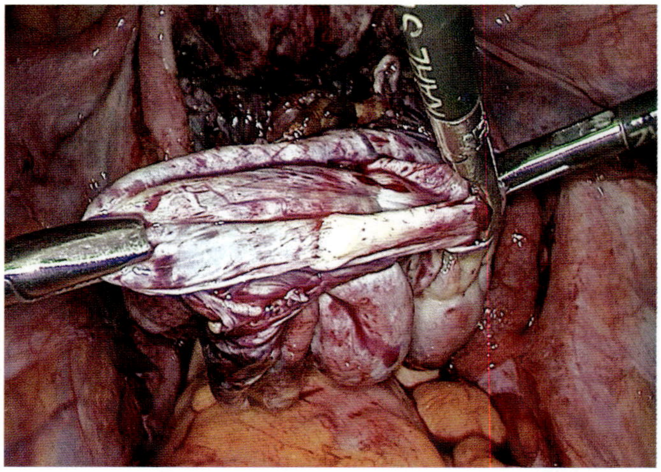

Fig. 10.9: Enucleation of cyst wall.

of the inside of the cyst. Any solid excrescence and number of loculi are now inspected. A controlled tear of 1 cm is made on the edge of the cyst by traction with two graspers, rather than using sharp cutting. This step separates the cyst wall from the ovarian tissue. After identification of the cleavage plane, the cyst wall is enucleated through traction exerted in opposite directions with two grasping forceps (Fig. 10.8). The cyst wall is held with a toothed grasper, and ovarian tissue is held with an atraumatic grasper. Traction and counter traction are done to separate the cyst from the ovarian tissue (Fig. 10.9). Complete removal of the cyst wall is done. Enucleation is done gently near the ovarian ligament and hilum to avoid bleeding and injury. For smaller and multiloculated endometriomas, injection of dilute vasopressin below the cyst wall (Figs. 10.10A and B) is useful to reduce the loss of ovarian tissue. Any residual endometriosis on the edges of the ovary is excised. At the end of the procedure, only the active bleeding vessels are controlled with bipolar coagulation. No sutures are used for approximation of the ovarian edges. The ovarian edges are held together to reconstruct the ovary and then held with a bowel grasper for 5 minutes (Figs. 10.11A and B). Trimming of the ovarian edges is rarely needed and done only to excise endometrial implants. Another alternative for cystectomy or excision is drainage of cyst and ablation, with bipolar coagulation, CO_2 laser, or plasma energy, but studies have shown excision is superior because of high recurrence with the latter.[24]

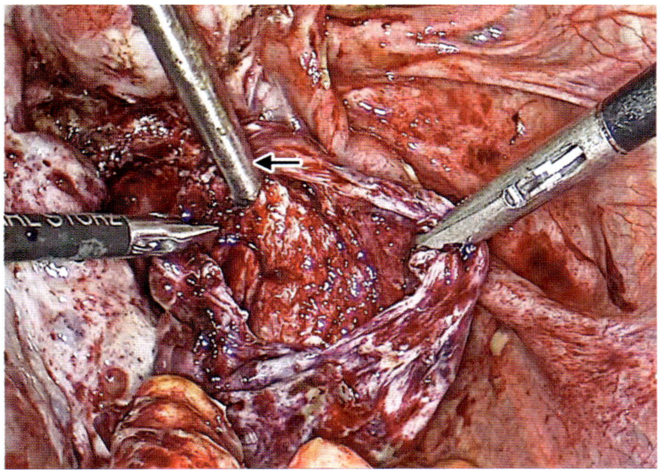

Fig. 10.10A: Injecting dilute vasopressin below the cyst wall.

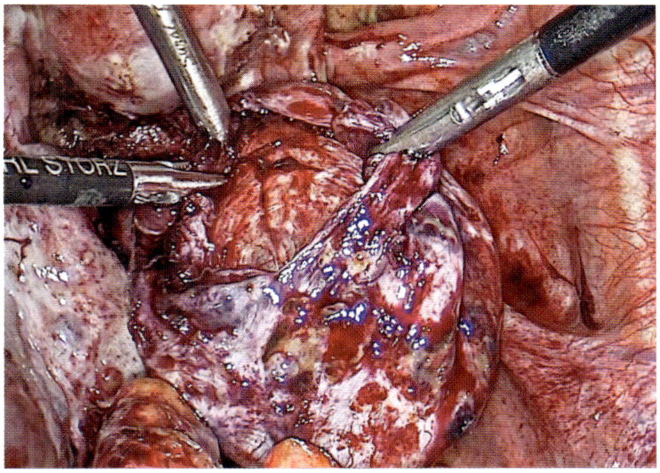

Fig. 10.10B: Bulging of the cyst wall after vasopressin injection.

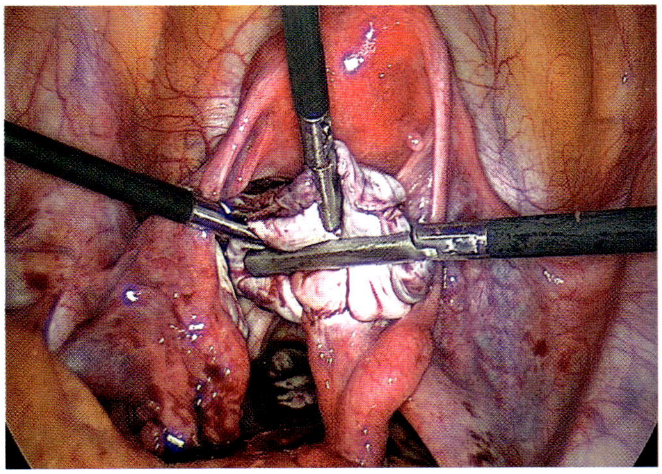

Fig. 10.11A: Reconstruction of right ovary.

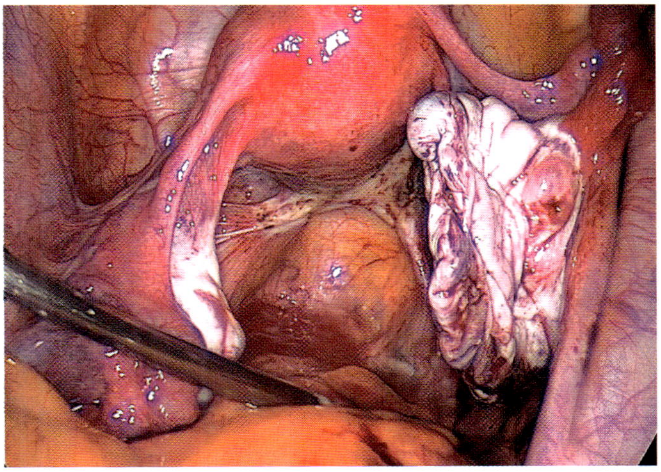

Fig. 10.11B: Right ovary after reconstruction.

Deep Infiltrating Endometriosis

Deep infiltrating endometriosis (DIE) is different from peritoneal and ovarian endometriosis and is characterized by infiltration of more than 5 mm below the peritoneum. Most common locations are uterosacral ligaments, rectovaginal septum, rectum, and vesicouterine pouch. DIE has a strong correlation with severe pelvic pain and dyspareunia but not with infertility. Laparoscopic excision is the preferred approach for DIE.

Posterior Cul-de-sac

Rectovaginal endometriosis typically refers to an infiltrative disease involving the cervix, vagina, rectovaginal septum, and rectum. It can occur in isolation or extend to other pelvic structures causing complete obliteration of the pouch of Douglas (Fig. 10.12). DIE is more common in the posterior compartment with a predisposition for left hemipelvis predominantly affecting uterosacral ligaments. Isolated uterosacral lesions are present in 83%, but in 16.8% of cases involvement of vagina, bowel, and bladder may coexist.[25] Surgical excision of isolated uterosacral ligaments is done after identifying the ureters as they may be more medial due to the fibrotic nature of the disease. If the ureters are not clearly visualized, ureterolysis is done, and any endometriotic nodule on the uterosacral ligaments are excised safely (Fig. 10.13). In cases of bilateral disease with or without vaginal nodule, ureterolysis is

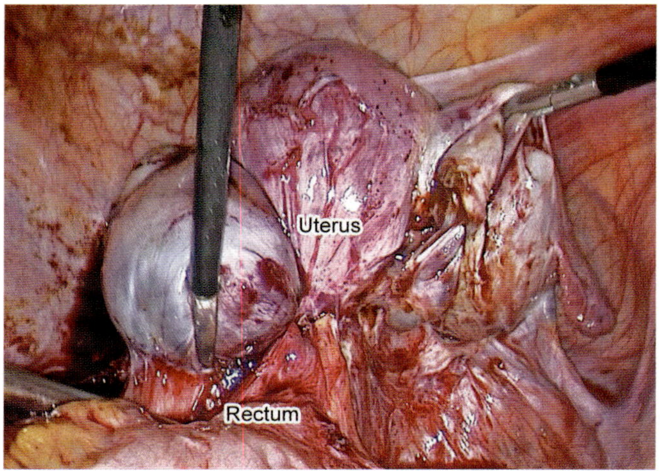

Fig. 10.12: Obliteration of pouch of Douglas due to rectal adhesions to the uterus.

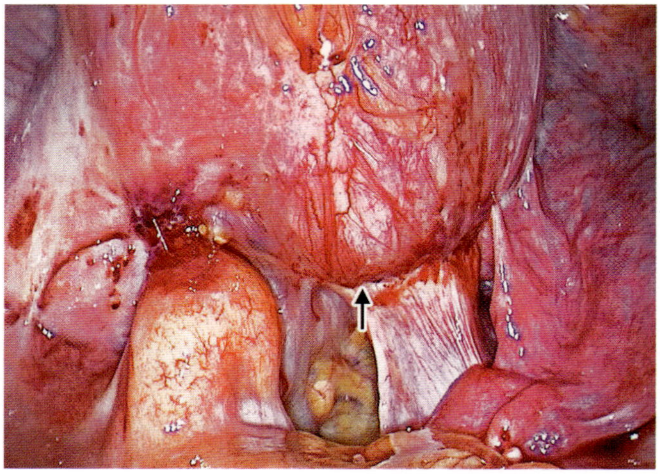

Fig. 10.13: Endometriosis involving uterosacral ligaments.

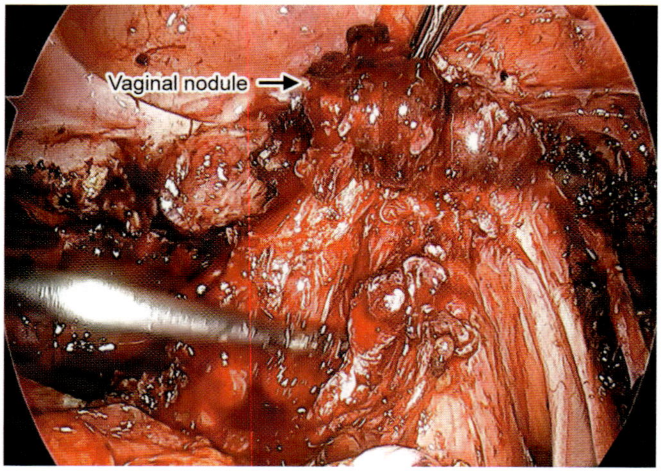

Fig. 10.14: Excision of vaginal nodule.

done bilaterally. When a vaginal nodule is present, it may be adherent to the rectum and need to be released from it before excision (Fig. 10.14). Once released from the rectum, it can be excised along with the cervical and vaginal nodule en masse. Deep dissection of bilateral uterosacral disease can damage the inferior hypogastric plexus resulting in urinary retention and sexual dysfunction. So surgery is aimed at preservation of these nerve plexuses.

Bowel endometriosis occurs in 3–37% of cases and involves the rectum, sigmoid colon, or both in 90% cases.[26]

Rectal endometriosis is challenging surgical situation and can be dealt with three surgical approaches: superficial thickness excision (shaving), full thickness discoid resection, and colorectal segmental resection.[27] Laparoscopic "shaving" involves dissecting the superficial disease from the serosa or muscularis without entering the bowel lumen. The bowel wall is then approximated with interrupted absorbable sutures. Low complication rates have been reported using this technique (1.4% rectal perforation). Discoid resection is described for a lesion of 3 cm or less in diameter and comprises more than 50% of bowel wall infiltration.[28] Initial dissection of the nodule is done by the shaving technique, and anterior resection of a small segment of bowel wall is done using a transanal circular stapler device. This technique offers less operating time and decreased bowel complications. Bowel resection is indicated when lesions are more than 3 cm, infiltration more than 50% of the circumference of the bowel wall, or multifocal disease. It is associated with higher complications like anastomotic leak, bowel obstruction, fistula formation, and long-term complications like incomplete bowel movement and pain. The help of a colorectal surgeon is recommended to perform these advanced procedures.

Urinary Tract Endometriosis

Bladder endometriosis is not rare as considered in the past. It causes urinary symptoms like dysuria, hematuria, and recurrent urinary tract infection in 68.8% of women; 50% of patients show the history of previous pelvic surgery mostly cesarean section.[29] Ultrasonography with full bladder usually shows heterogeneous, hyperechoic, intraluminal lesions protruding from the posterior vesical wall. A cleavage plane can be identified between the uterine wall and bladder lesion. Cystoscopy can confirm the bladder endometriosis, which appears as bluish nodules. Laparoscopy usually shows an anteverted uterus with obliterated anterior cul de sac with the involvement of the round ligaments (Fig. 10.15). The first step is adhesiolysis and restoring the anatomy. The superficial disease can be treated by excision, and deeper lesions may require partial cystectomy for complete removal. The bladder is mobilized from the uterus, and then it is opened after bilateral ureteric stenting, although most of the lesions are above the trigone. After excision of the nodule, the bladder is repaired in two layers, and an indwelling catheter is kept for 10–14 days. Bladder resection is a relatively simple and safe procedure.

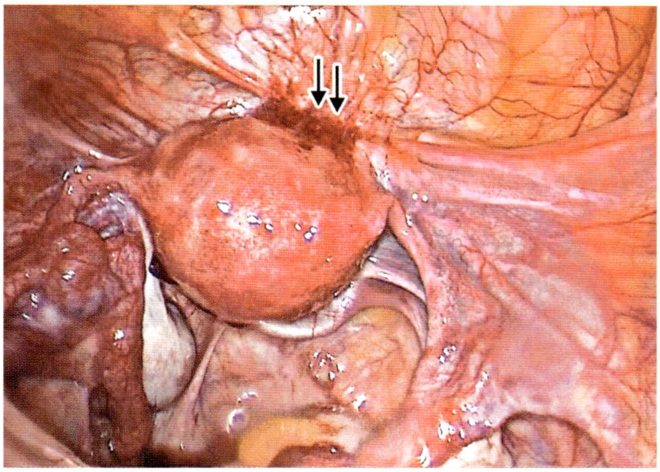

Fig. 10.15: Bladder endometriosis.

Ureteral endometriosis is present in 0.01–1% of women with endometriosis.[30] It often causes nonspecific symptoms like pelvic pain, flank pain or renal colic, and hematuria. Silent kidney loss can also happen in 30% cases.[31] Ureteral endometriosis is usually unilateral and more common on left side involving the lower third of ureter. They are usually involved due to the extension of uterosacral or rectovaginal endometriosis. The initial step is to restore the anatomy by complete adhesiolysis. Congenital sigmoid adhesions to pelvic side wall are released. Ureterolysis is started at the pelvic brim and dissection is done up to the ureteric tunnel (Fig. 10.16A).The endometriotic nodule is completely excised, but care is taken to preserve the vascular network over the adventitia. A double-J ureteric stent may be inserted to reduce the risk of fistula formation (Fig. 10.16B). If there is partial obstruction of the ureter, an end-to-end anastomosis may be required. It is performed after placement of a double-J stent and approximating the ends with three to four fine absorbable sutures. A ureteric implantation is done, if the lesion is less than 2 cm from the bladder. In a series of 91 cases, 85.7% cases required only ureterolysis and only 10% required resection.[32]

Presacral Neurectomy

Presacral neurectomy (PSN) involves the excision of a portion of superior hypogastric plexus, which provides sympathetic innervation to the uterus. This procedure is done

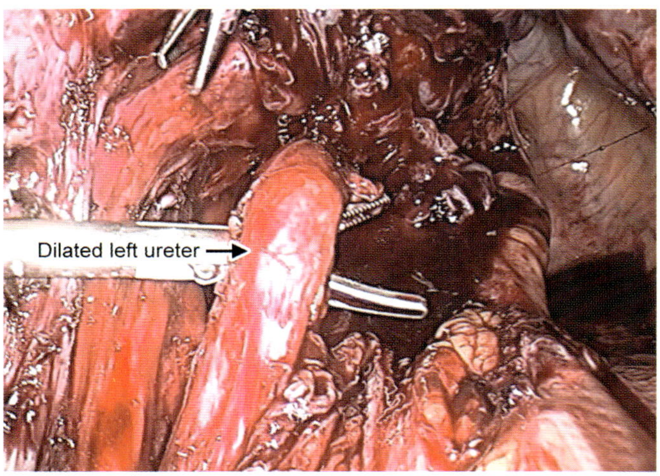

Fig. 10.16A: Ureterolysis of left hydroureter.

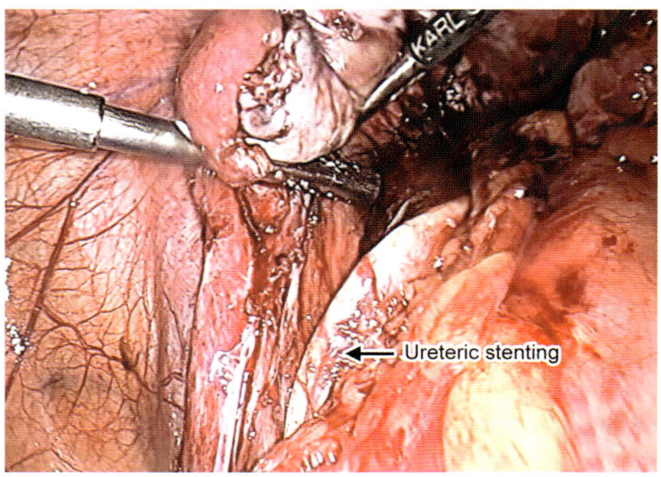

Fig. 10.16B: After ureteric stenting (in the same patient).

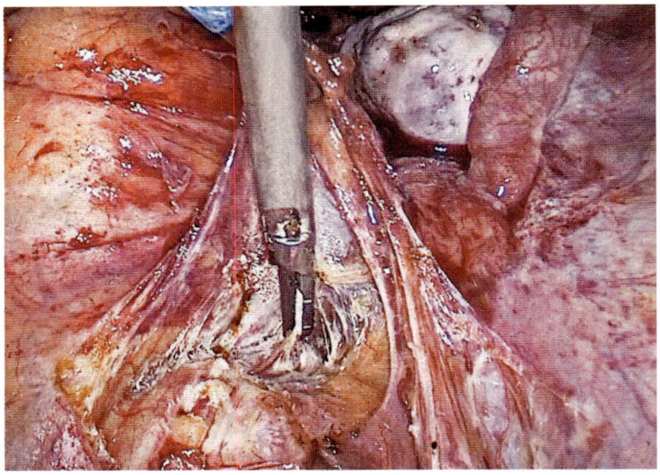

Fig. 10.17: Presacral neurectomy—dividing the nerve plexus with an ultrasonic device.

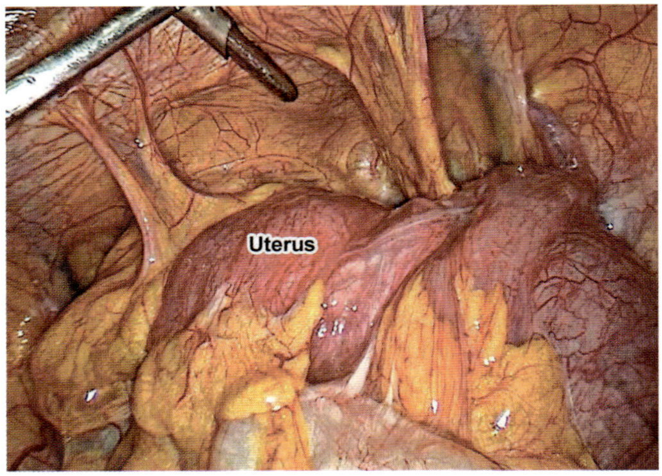

Fig. 10.18: Frozen pelvis.

along with conservative surgery for endometriosis as an additional step to reduce intractable dysmenorrhea. It is more useful when there is associated adenomyosis with central pelvic pain. The peritoneum over the interiliac area at L_5 level is exposed. After careful isolation of right ureter, the superior hypogastric plexus is identified and incised (Fig. 10.17). PSN has a beneficial effect on long-term pain control compared with conservative surgery alone.[33] The possible adverse effects of PSN include constipation, alteration of the sensation of bladder fullness, and occasional vaginal dryness.

Definitive Surgery

Hysterectomy

Hysterectomy with BSO and optimal clearance of endometriosis disease is the definitive management of endometriosis, and it has the lowest risk of recurrence.[34] It is offered to patients who have completed childbearing and those not responding to other conservative measures. It is associated with detrimental effects of surgical menopause and should be considered when deciding this type of surgery. Conservation of at least one ovary during hysterectomy should be attempted in young women although it carries a sixfold risk of recurrence.[35] Dilute vasopressin (20 IU in 200 mL of normal saline) is injected into the myometrium till the uterus is blanched, which helps in achieving initial hemostatic dissection of the adnexa and rectosigmoid. Adhesions between bowel loops, posterior uterine surface, and bilateral adnexae are released with sharp and blunt dissection after identification and isolation of both the ureters. Bilateral round ligaments and infundibulopelvic ligaments are coagulated and divided. The uterovesical fold of peritoneum is opened, and the bladder is pushed down. Both the uterine vessels are coagulated and divided. Anterior culdotomy is done and the incision extended posteriorly to separate the cervix from the vagina. The vaginal vault is then sutured after retrieval of the specimen. In patients with frozen pelvis (Fig. 10.18), we perform a retrograde adhesiolysis technique described earlier.[36] In this technique, we first do the hysterectomy with minimal rectosigmoid adhesiolysis followed by the rectal adhesiolysis and removal of adnexa. Younger women undergoing hysterectomy with BSO will require hormone therapy with progestin-only pills or combined hormone therapy to prevent the proliferative effect of unopposed estrogen on the residual endometriosis.[22]

ENDOMETRIOSIS AND INFERTILITY

Although the relationship between infertility and endometriosis is not well established, the presence of endometriosis in 50% of infertile women compared with 5–10% in women with proven fertility is suggestive of a causal relationship.[37] Various mechanisms suggested to explain infertility in endometriosis are pelvic anatomical distortion due to adhesions, intraperitoneal inflammation, abnormal tubal transport, and implantation defects.[38] Medical treatment has a limited role in the management of endometriosis-associated infertility with the exception of a short course of pretreatment with GnRH analogue before assisted reproductive technique (ART).[39]

Surgery for Peritoneal and Ovarian Endometriosis

Laparoscopic surgery for endometriosis appears to have a beneficial effect on endometriosis-associated infertility. For early stage (stages I and II) disease, laparoscopic excision or ablation of endometriosis has a small but significant improvement in pregnancy rate (26% versus 18%).[40] There are no RCT studies to show that surgical treatment for moderate to severe endometriosis is beneficial, but various uncontrolled studies show an overall pregnancy rate of 50%.[41] Surgical management of endometriomas for improving fertility is a widely debated issue. Cystectomy or opening the cyst and coagulation of implants are the two common approaches as described earlier. A Cochrane review has shown that cystectomy for endometriomas greater than 4 cm improves fertility outcome compared with drainage and coagulation.[42] The disadvantage of cystectomy is a loss of ovarian tissue during the surgery, which can be reduced by employing finer surgical technique and expertise. Although cystectomy can diminish ovarian reserve as measured by anti-Müllerian hormone (AMH), it does not impair the ovarian response to ovulation induction.[43,44]

Rectovaginal Endometriosis

Endometriosis involving retrocervical and anterior rectal wall usually causes severe pain symptoms and surgeries are usually performed for symptom relief. There are not many studies on the outcome of pregnancies in women with rectovaginal endometriosis. One of the RCTs suggests that excision of rectovaginal endometriosis does not improve the pregnancy rate nor reduces the time-to-conception in this group of women.[41] The authors also explain these findings by process of "pseudoperitonealization" of implants leading to a reduction of the biochemical impact of deep lesions on fertilization process.

Recurrent Endometriosis

Recurrent endometriosis is a difficult clinical problem not only because of the inconvenience and increased morbidity for the patient but also the technical difficulties during surgery. Fedele et al. compared the pregnancy outcome after laparoscopic excision in the primary surgery versus recurrent endometrioma in the same ovary and found similar results.[45] American Society for Reproductive Medicine (ASRM) guidelines recommend *in vitro* fertilization embryo transfer (IVF-ET) in women who had previous one or more surgeries for moderate to severe endometriosis.[38]

Ultrasound-guided Aspiration

Ultrasound-guided aspiration was suggested as an alternative treatment for recurrent endometriomas.[46] Difficulties in aspirating thick chocolate material and a high chance of recurrence (60–90%) have been reported.[47] Ultrasound-guided aspiration with sclerotherapy with tetracycline and ethanol has been suggested to reduce the recurrence.[46,48] The recurrence rates were 25% after tetracycline injection, 15% after ethanol, and 31% after methotrexate.[48-50] Pregnancy outcomes in these studies were difficult to interpret. Aspiration of ovarian endometrioma before Intracytoplasmic Sperm Injection (ICSI) was compared with nonaspiration in one RCT and found the number of oocytes retrieved and fertilized, implantation, and pregnancy were similar.[51]

Complications which can arise from this procedure are leakage of chocolate-like material. Also the fluid used for sclerotherapy can cause chemical irritation resulting in pelvic adhesions. A major complication of transvaginal aspiration is the risk of an ovarian abscess, which may necessitate oophorectomy.[52] Occult malignancies also can be missed during these procedures.

A recent report by Zhu et al. performed repeated aspiration of endometrioma and had a recurrence of 5.4% after 3.1 mean aspirations with an overall pregnancy rate of 43.4%.[53] Wang et al. reported a 96% cure rate following ultrasonography-guided aspiration and sclerotherapy with 95% ethanol.[54] Both groups did not report any major complications in their series. Ultrasonography-guided aspiration of endometrioma does not seem to have a role in the current management of endometrioma, because of its poor efficacy and high risk of recurrence and infection. However, it may have a role in facilitating oocyte retrieval in patients who decline or are not fit for surgery to improve access to follicles.[55]

SUMMARY

Endometriosis is a common disease affecting women in their reproductive age group and is grouped into two categories for planning treatment strategies—endometriosis with pain and infertility. Medical management is the first line approach to the treatment of endometriosis-related pain. Common agents used are COCs, progestins, GnRH agonists, LNG, and aromatase inhibitors. All of these have fairly comparable efficacy and varying safety profile. Surgical treatment is indicated when medical therapy fails or not tolerated and in the presence of an endometrioma where malignant potential cannot be excluded. It is also the mainstay of treatment in infertile women. Laparoscopy is the preferred approach for the surgical management of endometriosis. Conservative surgery aims at restoring the pelvic anatomy and excising the endometrial tissues. Larger endometriomas are enucleated rather than draining and coagulating the surface because of the higher chance of recurrence. The management of deep infiltrating endometriosis needs advanced laparoscopic surgical skill. It can involve the urinary tract and bowel, which need good preoperative evaluation for planning an optimal surgery with assistance from other specialists. A definitive surgery like a hysterectomy is needed when other treatments fail. Patients with infertility are primarily treated surgically with good results. But the results not only depend on the stage of the disease but also the age of the patient, duration of infertility, ovarian reserve, and the male factor. Repeated surgeries can reduce the ovarian reserve and should be avoided. Ultrasonography-guided aspiration of endometrioma does not seem to have a role in the current management of recurrent endometrioma. Patients who fail to conceive after surgical treatment should be counseled for ARTs.

REFERENCES

1. Giudice LC, Kao LC. Endometriosis. Lancet. 2004; 364(9447):1789-99.
2. Howard FM. Endometriosis and mechanisms of pelvic pain. J Minim Invasive Gynecol. 2009;16(5):540-50.
3. Vercellini P, Frontino G, De Giorgi O, Pietropaolo G, Pasin R, Crosignani PG. Continuous use of an oral contraceptive for endometriosis-associated recurrent dysmenorrhea that does not respond to a cyclic pill regimen. Fertil Steril. 2003;80(3):560-3.
4. Bono Y, Kyo S, Kiyono T, Mizumoto Y, Nakamura M, Maida Y, et al. Concurrent estrogen action was essential for maximal progestin effect in oral contraceptives. Fertil Steril. 2014;101(5):1337-43
5. Harada T, Momoeda M, Taketani Y, Hoshiai H, Terakawa N. Low-dose oral contraceptive pill for dysmenorrhea associated with endometriosis: a placebo-controlled, double-blind, randomized trial. Fertil Steril. 2008;90:1583-8.
6. Strowitzki T, Marr J, Gerlinger C, Faustmann T, Seitz C. Dienogest is as effective as leuprolide acetate in treating the painful symptoms of endometriosis: a 24-week, randomized, multicentre, open-label trial. Hum Reprod. 2010;25:633-41.
7. Strowitzki T, Marr J, Gerlinger C, Faustmann T, Seitz C. Detailed analysis of a randomized, multicenter, comparative trial of dienogest versus leuprolide acetate in endometriosis. Int J GynaecolObstet. 2012;117:228-33.
8. Abou-Setta AM, Houston B, Al-Inany HG, Farquhar C. Levonorgestrel-releasing intrauterine device (LNG-IUD) for symptomatic endometriosis following surgery. Cochrane Database Syst Rev. 2013;(1):CD005072.
9. Lockhat FB, Emembolu JO, Konje JC. The efficacy, side-effects and continuation rates in women with symptomatic endometriosis undergoing treatment with an intra-uterine administered progestogen (levonorgestrel): a 3 year follow-up. Hum Reprod. 2005;20(3):789-93.
10. Lockhat FB, Emembolu JO, Konje JC. The evaluation of the effectiveness of an intrauterine-administered progestogen (levonorgestrel) in the symptomatic treatment of endometriosis and in the staging of the disease. Hum Reprod. 2004;19(1):179-84.
11. Lockhat FB, Emembolu JE, Konje JC. Serum and peritoneal fluid levels of levonorgestrel in women with endometriosis who were treated with an intrauterine contraceptive device containing levonorgestrel. Fertil Steril. 2005;83(2):398-404.
12. Lan S, Ling L, Jianhong Z, Xijing J, Lihui W. Analysis of the levonorgestrel-releasing intrauterine system in women with endometriosis. J Int Med Res. 2013;41(3):548-58.
13. Youm J, Lee HJ, Kim SK, Kim H, Jee BC. Factors affecting the spontaneous expulsion of the levonorgestrel-releasing intrauterine system. International Journal of Gynecology & Obstetrics. 2014;126(2):165-9.
14. Prentice A, Deary AJ, Goldbeck-Wood S, Farquhar C, Smith SK. Gonadotrophin-releasing hormone analogues for pain associated with endometriosis. Cochrane Database Syst Rev. 2000;(2):CD000346.
15. Barbieri RL. Endometriosis and the estrogen threshold theory. Relation to surgical and medical treatment. J Reprod Med. 1998;43(Suppl 3):287-92.
16. Carr B, Dmowski WP, O'Brien C, Jiang P, Burke J, Jimenez R, et al. Elagolix, an oral GnRh antagonist, versus subcutaneous depot medroxyprogesterone acetate for the treatment of endometriosis: effects on bone mineral density. Reprod Sci. 2014;21(11):1341-51.
17. Diamond MP, Carr B, Dmowski WP, Koltun W, O'Brien C, Jiang P, et al. Elagolix treatment for endometriosis-associated pain: results from a phase 2, randomized, double-blind, placebo-controlled study. Reprod Sci. 2014;21(3):363-71.
18. Roman, H. Deep rectal shaving using plasma energy for endometriosis causing rectal stenosis–a video vignette. Colorectal Dis. 2014;16:834-6.
19. Wright J, Lotfallah H, Jones K, Lovell D. A randomized trial of excision versus ablation for mild endometriosis. Fertil Steril. 2005;83:1830.

20. Healey M, Ang WC, Cheng C. Surgical treatment of endometriosis: a prospective randomized double-blinded trial comparing excision and ablation. Fertil Steril. 2010;94:2536.
21. Healy M, Cheng C, Kaur H. To excise or ablate endometriosis? A prospective randomized double-blinded trial after 5-year follow-up. J Minim Invasive Gynecol. 2014;21:999-1004.
22. Practice Committee of the American Society for Reproductive Medicine. Treatment of pelvic pain associated with endometriosis: a committee opinion. Fertil Steril. 2014;101(4):927-35.
23. Paul PG, Kaur H, Narasimhan D, Chopade G, Kandhari D. Laparoscopic ovarian reconstruction without suturing after cystectomy for endometrioma. Gynecol Surg. 2014;11(3):219-26.
24. Chapron C, Vercellini P, Barakat H, Vieira M, Dubuisson JB. Management of ovarian endometriomas. Hum Reprod Update. 2002;8(6):591-7.
25. Chapron C, Fauconnier A, Dubuisson JB, Barakat H, Vieira M, Bréart G. Deep infiltrating endometriosis: relation between severity of dysmenorrhoea and extent of disease. Hum Reprod. 2003;4:760-6.
26. Campagnacci R, Perretta S, Guerrieri M, Paganini AM, De Sanctis A, Ciavattini A, et al. Laparoscopic colorectal resection for endometriosis. Surg Endosc. 2005;19(5):662-4.
27. Alabiso G, Alio L, Arena S, di Prun AB, Bergamini V, Berlanda N, et al. How to manage bowel endometriosis: the ETIC approach. J Minim Invasive Gynecol. 2015;22:517-29.
28. Remorgida V, Ragni N, Ferrero S, Fulcheri E, Martin DC. How complete is full thickness disc resection of bowel endometriotic lesions? A prospective surgical and histological study. Hum Reprod. 2005;20:2317-20.
29. Knabben L, Imboden S, Fellmann B, Nirgianakis K, Kuhn A. Urinary tract endometriosis in patients with deep infiltrating endometriosis: prevalence, symptoms, management, and proposal for a new clinical classification. Fertil Steril. 2015;103:147-52.
30. Jubanyik KJ, Comite F. Extrapelvic endometriosis. Obstet Gynecol Clin North Am. 1997;24(2):411-40.
31. Yohannes P. Ureteral endometriosis. J Urol. 2003;170(1):20-5.
32. Gabriel B, Nassif J, Trompoukis P, Barata S, Wattiez A. Prevalence and management of urinary tract endometriosis: a clinical case series. Urology. 2011;78(6):1269-74.
33. Zullo F, Palomba S, Zupi E, Russo T, Morelli M. Long-term effectiveness of presacral neurectomy for the treatment of severe dysmenorrhea due to endometriosis. J Am Assoc Gynecol Laparosc. 2004;11(1):23-8.
34. Yeung P Jr. The laparoscopic management of endometriosis in patients with pelvic pain. Obstet Gynecol Clin North Am. 2014;41(3):371-83.
35. Berlanda N, Vercellini P, Fedele L. The outcomes of repeat surgery for recurrent symptomatic endometriosis. Curr Opin Obstet Gynecol. 2010;22(4):320-5.
36. Paul PG, Shabnam K, Bhosale SA, Kaur H, Talwar P, Thomas T. Laparoscopic hysterectomy in frozen pelvis—an alternative technique of retrograde adhesiolysis. Gynecol Surg. 2013;10(4):285-90.
37. D'Hooghe TM, Debrock S, Hill JA, Meuleman C. Endometriosis and subfertility: is the relationship resolved? Semin Reprod Med. 2003;21(2):243-54.
38. Practice Committee of the American Society for Reproductive Medicine. Endometriosis and infertility: a committee opinion. Fertil Steril. 2012;98(3):591-8.
39. Sallam HN, Garcia-Velasco JA, Dias S, Arici A, Abou-Setta AM. Long-term pituitary down-regulation before *in vitro* fertilization (IVF) for women with endometriosis. Cochrane Database Syst Rev. 2006;(1):CD004635.
40. Jacobson TZ, Barlow DH, Koninckx PR, Olive D, Farquhar C. Laparoscopic surgery for subfertility associated with endometriosis. Cochrane Database Syst Rev. 2002;(4):CD001398.
41. Vercellini P, Somigliana E, Viganò P, Abbiati A, Barbara G, Crosignani PG. Surgery for endometriosis-associated infertility: a pragmatic approach. Hum Reprod. 2009;24(2):254-69.
42. Hart RJ, Hickey M, Maouris P, Buckett W. Excisional surgery versus ablative surgery for ovarian endometriomata. Cochrane Database Syst Rev. 2008;(2):CD004992.
43. Raffi F, Metwally M, Amer S. The impact of excision of ovarian endometrioma on ovarian reserve: a systematic review and meta-analysis. J Clin Endocrinol Metab. 2012;97(9):3146-54.
44. Alborzi S, Ravanbakhsh R, Parsanezhad ME, Alborzi M, Alborzi S, Dehbashi S. A comparison of follicular response of ovaries to ovulation induction after laparoscopic ovarian cystectomy or fenestration and coagulation versus normal ovaries in patients with endometrioma. Fertil Steril. 2007;88(2):507-9.
45. Fedele L, Bianchi S, Zanconato G, Berlanda N, Raffaelli R, Fontana E. Laparoscopic excision of recurrent endometriomas: long-term outcome and comparison with primary surgery. Fertil Steril. 2006;85(3):694-9.
46. Aboulghar MA, Mansour RT, Serour GI, Rizk B. Ultrasonic transvaginal aspiration of endometriotic cysts: an optional line of treatment in selected cases of endometriosis. Human Reprod. 1991;6(10):1408-10.
47. Chan LY, So WW, Lao TT. Rapid recurrence of endometrioma after transvaginal ultrasound-guided aspiration. Eur J Obstet Gynecol Reprod Biol. 2003;109(2):196-8.
48. Koike T, Minakami H, Motoyama M, Ogawa S, Fujiwara H, Sato I. Reproductive performance after ultrasound-guided transvaginal ethanol sclerotherapy for ovarian endometriotic cysts. Eur J Obstet Gynecol Reprod Biol. 2002;105(1):39-43.
49. Fisch JD, Sher G. Sclerotherapy with 5% tetracycline is a simple alternative to potentially complex surgical treatment of ovarian endometriomas before *in vitro* fertilization. Fertil Steril. 2004;82(2):437-41.
50. Agostini A, De Lapparent T, Collette E, Capelle M, Cravello L, Blanc B. In situ methotrexate injection for treatment of recurrent endometriotic cysts. Eur J Obstet Gynecol Reprod Biol. 2007;130(1):129-31.
51. Pabuccu R, Onalan G, Goktolga U, Kucuk T, Orhon E, Ceyhan T. Aspiration of ovarian endometriomas before intracytoplasmic sperm injection. Fertil Steril. 2004;82(3):705-11.

52. Mikamo H, Kawazoe K, Sato Y, Itoh M, Tamaya T. Ovarian abscess caused by *Peptostreptococcus magnus* following transvaginal ultrasound-guided aspiration of ovarian endometrioma and fixation with pure ethanol. Infect Dis Obstet Gynecol. 1998;6(2):66-8.
53. Zhu W, Tan Z, Fu Z, Chen X, Zhou Y. Repeat transvaginal ultrasound-guided aspiration of ovarian endometrioma in infertile women with endometriosis. Am J Obstet Gynecol. 2011;204:61.e1-61.e6.
54. Wang L-L, Dong X-Q, Shao X-H, Wang S-M. Ultrasound-guided interventional therapy for recurrent ovarian chocolate cysts. Ultrasound Med Biol. 2011;37:1596-602.
55. Dimitrios Psaroudakis, Martin Hirsch, Colin Davis. Review of the management of ovarian endometriosis: paradigm shift towards conservative approaches. Curr Opin Obstet Gynecol. 2014;26:266-74.

CHAPTER

11

Congenital Uterine Anomalies

Sanja Kupesic-Plavsic, Sonal Panchal

INTRODUCTION

The aim of this chapter is to present the most recent literature on the prevalence and diagnosis of congenital uterine anomalies, and discuss the current dilemmas on their treatment. An interested reader will be guided from the embryological development of the uterus, through most recent classifications of the uterine anomalies, accuracy of invasive and noninvasive diagnostic techniques, to reproductive outcomes of different types of congenital uterine anomalies. Finally, the benefits of hysteroscopic metroplasty and the role of intra- and postoperative imaging will be reviewed in details.

PREVALENCE AND TYPE OF CONGENITAL UTERINE ANOMALIES IN GENERAL AND HIGH-RISK POPULATIONS

The reported prevalence of congenital uterine anomalies in the general population of reproductive age women ranges from 3 to 4%.[1] A recent study using 3D ultrasound (3D US) reported that the rate of congenital uterine anomalies in the subfertile female population is estimated to 13.3%.[2] Congenital uterine anomalies are uncommonly diagnosed because of the different diagnostic procedures used. Müllerian defects are highly prevalent in women seeking assisted reproductive treatment (ART), and apparently the most common types of anomalies diagnosed are arcuate and septate uterus.[2-4]

The 3D US is highly accurate due to its ability to visualize the uterine cavity and external contours of the uterine myometrium and fundus, which establishes its relevance as a gold imaging method to detect congenital uterine anomalies. In a study which was performed to investigate the diagnostic accuracy and precision of 3D US, a 93% positive and 100% negative predictive value was confirmed.[4] Because of multiplanar imaging and surface rendering, the 3D US can detect uterine anomalies that are more inconspicuous, such as arcuate uterus, which can be even overlooked by invasive procedures like hysteroscopy. Recent introduction of 3D saline infusion sonography (SIS) confirmed that this method is highly accurate in the diagnosis of uterine cavity abnormalities (Fig. 11.1). Another advantage is that the 3D US and 3D SIS can group the congenital uterine anomalies into subclassifications.

Maneschi et al. attempted to assess the prevalence of uterine anomalies and relative reproductive function in 322 women with abnormal uterine bleeding (AUB) evaluated by diagnostic hysteroscopy.[5] Uterine contours were classified as septate, bicornuate, arcuate, or normal on the basis of hysteroscopy. A complete medical history was obtained from all the subjects; it included a questionnaire on menstrual characteristics, reproductive history, and pregnancy outcome. Diagnostic hysteroscopy in women with AUB detected a 10% prevalence of uterine anomalies, which were associated with a significantly higher incidence of spontaneous abortion and lower cumulative live birth rates. Overall, women with uterine malformations showed a significantly higher miscarriage rate ($P < 0.05$) and a significantly lower term delivery rate ($P < 0.05$) than women with a normal uterus.

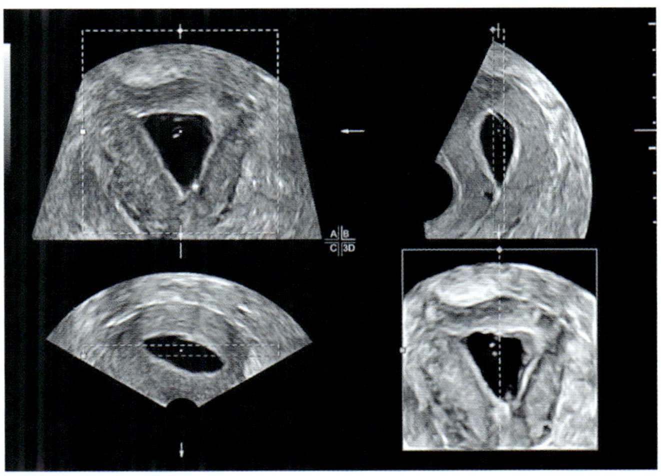

Fig. 11.1: Three-dimensional (3D) saline infusion sonography. Multiplanar and surface rendering of normal uterine cavity.

Jurkovic et al. investigated the prevalence of congenital uterine anomalies in 1,046 women attending gynecological ultrasound clinics for a variety of indications.[6] Using 3D US, anomalies were found in 55 women (5.4%), including 32 (3.1%) with an arcuate uterus and 23 (2.3%) with major anomalies. The prevalence of uterine anomalies was similar to the findings in women undergoing elective sterilization, but lower than in studies of women with recurrent miscarriage.

Saravelos and Cocksedge performed MEDLINE search of the studies from 1950 to 2007 and reviewed all relevant references reporting on the prevalence and diagnosis of congenital uterine anomalies in women with reproductive failure.[7] They found that the most accurate diagnostic procedures are combined hysteroscopy and laparoscopy, SIS, and 3D US. Two-dimensional ultrasound (2D US) and X-ray hysterosalpingography (HSG) are less accurate and are thus inadequate for diagnostic purposes. Magnetic resonance imaging (MRI) is proposed as a relatively sensitive tool, but its practicality remains unclear. A critical analysis of studies suggests that the prevalence of congenital uterine anomalies is approximately 6.7% in the general population, approximately 7.3% in the infertile population, and approximately 16.7% in the population with recurrent miscarriages. The arcuate uterus is the commonest anomaly in the general and recurrent miscarriage populations in this study. In contrast, the septate uterus is the commonest anomaly in the infertile population, suggesting a possible association. The authors recommend that women with recurrent miscarriage, who are likely to have a high prevalence of congenital uterine anomalies should be thoroughly investigated. HSG and/or 2D US are proposed to be used as initial screening tools, while combined hysteroscopy and laparoscopy, SIS, and 3D US should be used for a definitive diagnosis.

Jayaprakasan et al. estimated the prevalence of congenital uterine anomalies in subfertile women and evaluated their influence on early pregnancy following ART.[2] In the study of 1,385 patients, uterine anomalies were demonstrated in 13.3% subjects. Arcuate uterus represented the commonest anomaly (11.8%), followed by septate (0.5%), unicornuate (0.4%), subseptate (0.4%), bicornuate (0.1%), and T-shaped uteri (0.1%). Interestingly, diagnostic hysteroscopy study following a missed or an incomplete abortion consisting of 151 patients revealed congenital uterine anomalies in 20.4% of the patients and acquired uterine pathologies in 18.5%.[8] Among the congenital uterine anomalies, 9.3% were septate uterus, 6.6% were subseptate uterus, 2.6% were arcuate uterus, and 1.9% were uterine hypoplasia. Among acquired abnormalities, 9.3% were uterine synechia, 7.9% were endometrial polyps, and 1.3% were submucous myoma.

A systematic review of MEDLINE, EMBASE, Web of Science, and the Cochrane register analyzed studies utilizing "optimal" and "suboptimal" tests for congenital uterine anomalies.[9] Meta-analyses were performed to establish the prevalence of uterine anomalies and their subtypes within the various populations comprising 89,861 patients from 94 observational studies. The prevalence of uterine anomalies diagnosed by "optimal tests" was 5.5% in the unselected population, 8.0% in infertile women, 13.3% in those with a history of miscarriage, and 24.5% in those with miscarriage and infertility. Arcuate uterus is most commonly detected in the unselected population (3.9%), and its prevalence is not increased in high-risk groups. In contrast, septate uterus is the most common anomaly in high-risk populations. This study clearly indicated that women with a history of miscarriage or miscarriage and infertility have higher prevalence of congenital uterine anomalies compared with the unselected population.

Study by Dreisler and Stampe-Sorensen analyzed the prevalence of congenital uterine anomalies in a general population using SIS.[10] The overall prevalence of Müllerian anomalies in 622 women aged 20–74 years was 9.8%. The majority had arcuate uteri (6.8%), partial septate (2.7%), complete septate (1.6%), and unicornuate uterus (1.6%). Müllerian anomalies were significantly more frequently diagnosed in nulliparous (20%) compared with parous women (7%). Müllerian anomalies were more frequent in women with oligomenorrhea compared with women with normal menstrual periods (19% vs. 10%). One 1st trimester miscarriage or multiple miscarriages were not significantly more frequent in premenopausal women with Müllerian anomalies as compared with women with normal-shaped uteri (24% vs. 22%).

Clearly, differences in prevalence and types of congenital uterine anomalies in general and high risk populations could be explained by diagnostic and selection bias, lack of objective diagnostic criteria for the different anomaly types, and heterogeneity of study designs.[11]

EMBRYOLOGY OF THE UTERUS

The uterus develops from fusion of the paramesonephric ducts, which join in the midline at about the 10th week of gestation to form the unified body of the uterus.[12]

Paramesonephric (Müllerian) ducts are precursors to the uterus, the cervix, the upper two-thirds of the vagina, and the Fallopian tubes. Organogenesis of these structures is the first stage of uterus development. Problems at this stage lead to formation of unicornuate uterus. Then lateral fusion of the paramesonephric ducts occurs in the 7th to 9th weeks of development. Improper lateral fusion leads to bicornuate uterus and didelphic uterus. During this stage, a midline septum forms in the uterine cavity and it gets resorbed within 20 weeks. Failure of the septal resorption causes arcuate uterus and septate uterus. Abnormalities in the resorption of the fused midline tissues occur by the 20th week and can result in the formation of uterine septa of variable length and position. Apoptosis has recently been proposed as a mechanism by which the uterine septum regresses.[13] Bcl-2, a protein involved with regulating apoptosis, was found to be absent from the septa of four uteri using a monoclonal antibody for Bcl-2 and immunohistochemical analysis.[13] The absence of Bcl-2 results in failure of regression of the septum. The partial uterine septum is limited to the uterine fundus, whereas the complete septum extends from the fundus into the cervical canal.[14] On occasion, a longitudinal vaginal septum may be present. In rare cases, cervical duplication may be seen in conjunction with complete uterine and vaginal septa, often confounding attempts at clinical diagnosis.[14,15]

CLASSIFICATION OF UTERINE ANOMALIES

The American Fertility Society (based on the previous work of Buttram and Gibbons) classified the anomalies of the female reproductive tract into groups according to the degree of failure of normal development with similar clinical manifestations, treatment, and possible prognoses for their reproductive performance.[14,16,17] The various Müllerian anomalies are the consequence of four major disturbances in the development of the female genital system during fetal life. These disturbances are as follows:

1. Failure of one or more Müllerian ducts to develop (agenesis, unicornuate uterus without rudimentary horn)
2. Failure of the ducts to canalize (unicornuate uterus with rudimentary horn without proper cavities)
3. Failure to fuse or abnormal fusion of the ducts (uterus didelphys, bicornuate uterus)
4. Failure of resorption of the midline uterine septum (septate uterus, arcuate uterus)

The new European Society of Human Reproduction and Embryology/the European Society for Gynaecological Endoscopy (ESHRE/ESGE) classification system of female genital anomalies aims to provide a more suitable classification system for the accurate, clear, correlated with clinical management, and simple categorization of female genital anomalies.[18] Until now, three systems have been proposed for their categorization, but all of them are associated with serious limitations. ESHRE and ESGE have established a common Working Group, under the name CONUTA (CONgenital UTerine Anomalies), with the goal of developing a new updated classification system. A scientific committee has been appointed to run the project, looking also for consensus within the scientists working in the field. The new system is designed and developed based on: (1) scientific research through critical review of current proposals and preparation of an initial proposal for discussion between the experts; (2) consensus measurement among the experts through the use of the Delphi technique; and (3) consensus development by the scientific committee, taking into account a convergence of opinion and the comments of the experts. In the ESHRE/ESGE classification system, based on anatomy, anomalies are classified into the following main classes, expressing uterine anatomical deviations deriving from the same embryological origin: U0, normal uterus; U1, dysmorphic uterus; U2, septate uterus; U3, bicorporeal uterus; U4, hemiuterus; U5, aplastic uterus; and U6, for still unclassified cases.[18] Main classes have been divided into subclasses expressing anatomical varieties with clinical significance. Cervical and vaginal anomalies are classified independently into subclasses having clinical significance. The ESHRE/ESGE classification of female genital anomalies seems to fulfill the expectations and the needs of the experts in the field, but its clinical value needs to be proved in everyday practice.

Table 11.1 illustrates ESHRE/ESGE classification system using original 3D US images.

The CONUTA (CONgenital UTerine Anomalies) ESHRE/ESGE group conducted a systematic review of the literature to examine if the anomalies that could not be properly classified with the American Fertility Society (AFS) system could be effectively classified with the use of the new ESHRE/ESGE system.[19] An electronic literature search through MEDLINE, EMBASE, and Cochrane library was carried out from January, 1988 to January, 2014. Three participants independently screened selected articles of potential interest and finally extracted data from all the

Table 11.1: Illustration of ESHRE/ESGE classification system using 3D US images.

Normal uterus (U0)	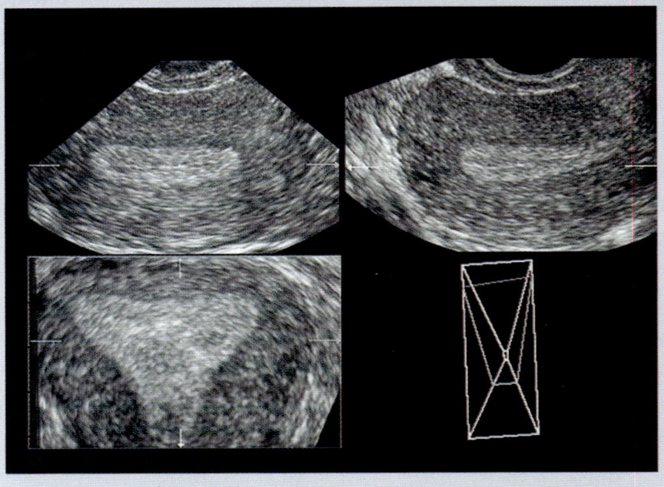
Dysmorphic uterus (U1): • T shaped • Infantile (hypoplastic) • Other	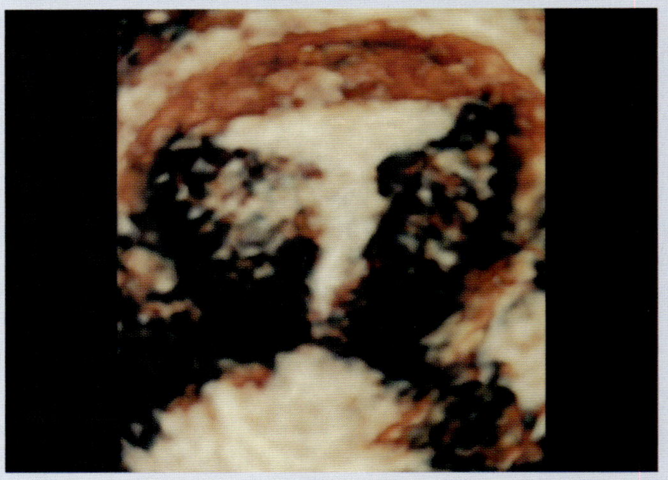
Septate uterus (U2): • Partial • Complete	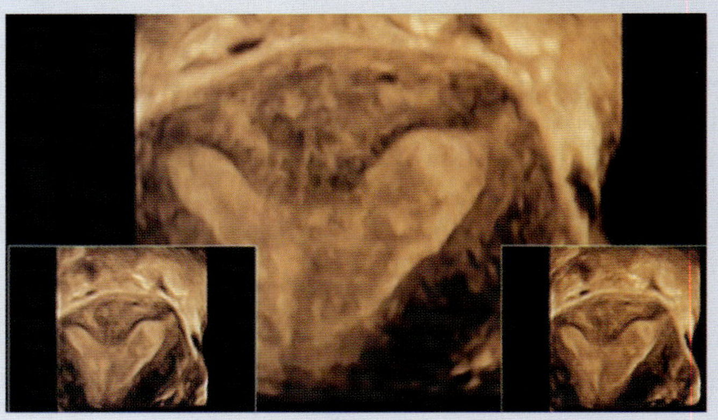

(Contd…)

(Contd...)

Table 11.1: Illustration of ESHRE/ESGE classification system using 3D US images.

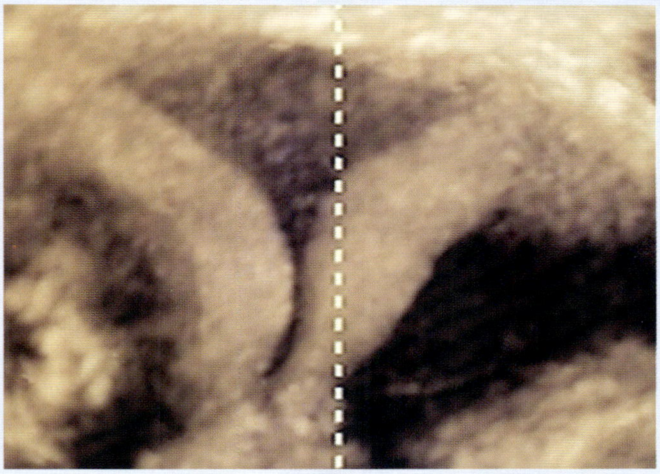

Bicorporeal uterus (U3):
- Partial
- Complete

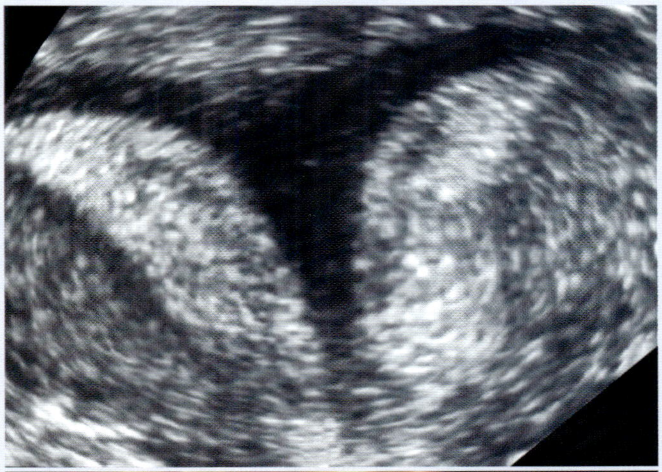

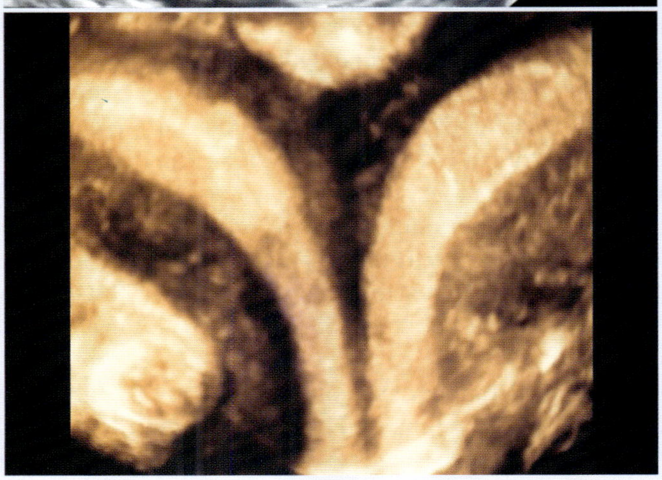

(Contd...)

(*Contd...*)

Table 11.1: Illustration of ESHRE/ESGE classification system using 3D US images.

Hemiuterus (U4): • With rudimentary cavity • Without rudimentary cavity	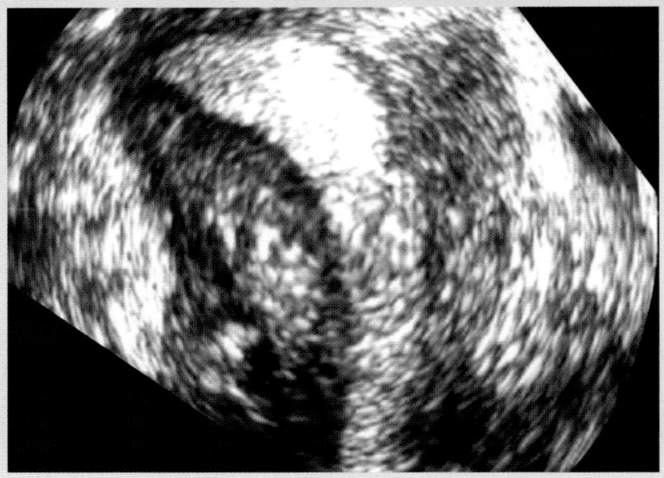
Aplastic uterus (U5) Unclassified cases (U6)	

included studies. Any disagreement was discussed and resolved after consultation with a fourth reviewer and the results were assessed independently and approved by all members of the CONUTA group. Among the 143 articles assessed in detail, 120 were finally selected reporting 140 cases that could not properly fit into a specific class of the AFS system.[19] Those 140 cases were clustered in 39 different types of anomalies. Uterus was the organ most frequently involved (76.9%), followed by cervix (66.7%) and vagina (59%). In all 39 types, the ESHRE/ESGE classification system provided a comprehensive description of each single or complex anomaly. A precise categorization was reached in 38 out of 39 types studied. Only one case of a bizarre uterine anomaly, with no clear embryological defect, could not be categorized and thus was placed in Class 6 (unclassified) of the ESHRE/ESGE system. The conclusion of this review was that comprehensiveness of the ESHRE/ESGE classification adds objective scientific validity to its use.[19] This is likely to further promote its dissemination and acceptance, which may have a positive outcome in clinical care and research related to congenital uterine anomalies.

Most recent study by Graupera et al. aimed to establish the accuracy of 3D US, compared with MRI, for diagnosing uterine anomalies, using the ESHRE/ESGE consensus on the classification of congenital anomalies of the female genital tract.[20] Sixty women with congenital uterine anomalies suspected after examination by conventional 2D US were evaluated with 3D US and MRI. The imaging data were analyzed retrospectively to confirm the presence and type of uterine malformation in accordance with the ESHRE/ESGE consensus. Compared with MRI, for the diagnosis of normal uteri, 3D US had a sensitivity of 83.3%, specificity of 100%, positive predictive value (PPV) of 100%, and negative predictive value (NPV) of 98.2%. For dysmorphic uteri and for hemiuteri, the sensitivity, specificity, PPV, and NPV were all 100. For septate uteri, the sensitivity was 100%, specificity was 88.9%, PPV was 95.5%, and NPV was 100%. For bicorporeal uteri, the sensitivity was 83.3%, specificity was 100%, PPV was 100%, and NPV was 98.2%. In conclusion, 3D US is highly accurate for diagnosing uterine malformations, having a good level of agreement with MRI in the classification of different anomaly types based on the ESHRE/ESGE consensus.[20]

Finally, what is the recommended diagnostic workup of female genital anomalies according to the ESHRE/ESGE system? The consensus was developed based on evaluation of the currently available diagnostic methods and their diagnostic accuracy by performing a systematic review of evidence, and on the definition of where and how to measure the uterine wall thickness.[21] Uterine wall thickness is defined as the distance between the interostial line and external uterine profile at the midcoronal plane of the uterus; alternatively, if a coronal plane is not available, the mean anterior and posterior uterine wall thickness at the longitudinal plane could be used. Gynecological examination and 2D US are recommended for the evaluation of asymptomatic women. 3D US is recommended for the diagnosis of female genital anomalies in "symptomatic" patients belonging to high-risk groups for the presence of a female genital anomaly and in any asymptomatic woman suspected to have an anomaly from routine evaluation. MRI and endoscopic evaluation are recommended for the subgroup of patients with suspected complex anomalies or in diagnostic dilemmas. Adolescents with symptoms suggestive for the presence of a female genital anomaly should be thoroughly evaluated with 2D US, 3D US, MRI, and endoscopically.[21]

ACCURACY OF DIAGNOSTIC (IMAGING AND ENDOSCOPIC) METHODS

Many methods are used to identify Müllerian tract defects from gynecologic examination, HSG, hysteroscopy, laparoscopy, MRI, transvaginal 2D and 3D US, and 2D and 3D SIS.

Gynecologic examination is very important starting point in the diagnostic workup of the patients with congenital uterine anomalies. Direct inspection of the vagina and cervix may detect vaginal aplasia, septum, and cervical malformations.

X-ray HSG provides valuable information about the uterine cavity and tubal patency. However, it does not provide definitive information about the external contour of the uterus, making a distinction between different types of lateral fusion defects often impossible.[12] Hysteroscopy enables direct visualization of the uterine cavity and immediate operative intervention/treatment of the uterine abnormality. Similar to HSG, it cannot be used for evaluation of the external contour of the uterus. Therefore, it should be used in conjunction with laparoscopy. Hysteroscopy carries certain risks such as uterine perforation, infection, and bleeding.[12]

Concurrent laparoscopy is essential for classification of the uterine anomalies and is necessary to confirm normal external uterine configuration before attempts at uterine septum resection. If the anomaly is of a bicornuate variety, a hysteroscopic approach may be contraindicated. Throughout the procedure, laparoscopic visualization is useful for assessing the progress of resection and identifying uterine perforation promptly should it occur. Laparoscopy helps identifying and treating other causes of infertility, such as endometriosis and pelvic adhesions.

By its ability to delineate both internal and external uterine morphology, MRI is an alternative diagnostic method for evaluation of the congenital uterine anomalies. High cost and lack of information on tubal patency are major limitations of this imaging method.

Noninvasive nature of ultrasound, low cost, and ease of performance are major advantages of ultrasound. Transabdominal US is inaccurate for differentiation between different types of Müllerian defects, but it has advantage of concomitant assessment of symmetric and asymmetric renal anomalies.[22] Improved visualization due to the use of high frequency probes and avoidance of subcutaneous fat are main advantages of transvaginal US, leading to better anatomical delineation of pelvic organs in addition to providing images with better contrast and detail resolution.[12] When used as a screening test for congenital uterine anomalies, transvaginal 2D US has a sensitivity around 70%.[23]

A transverse or oblique transverse view of the uterus by 2D US is not optimal in diagnosing congenital uterine defects. Ultrasound is operator dependent and hard copy and/or digital images can be difficult for a third party to interpret. For optimal imaging of the endometrium in certain cases, sonographer needs enhancement with negative contrast medium (e.g. saline) to separate the walls of the uterus, outline the endometrial surface, and detect intracavitary abnormalities and/or endoluminal lesions. Before SIS, detailed transvaginal US is required to assess the appearance of the uterus before saline instillation and determine the orientation of the uterus to facilitate cervical cannulation.[12] If possible, SIS should be performed during the follicular phase of the menstrual cycle, after the cessation of menstrual bleeding. In the study of Keltz et al., the sensitivity and specificity of SIS were 100% when compared with hysteroscopy.[24] The specificity of HSG was significantly lower (20%) than SIS ($p = 0.015$) using surgical confirmation as the gold standard. The accuracy of diagnosis by SIS of congenital uterine anomalies was 100%, whereas HSG accurately diagnosed uterine defects in only 45.5% of cases based on surgical confirmation ($P < 0.01$). SIS is a sensitive and specific screening and diagnostic method for detection of intrauterine defects in patients presenting with recurrent pregnancy loss. Soares et al. evaluated the diagnostic accuracy of SIS in uterine cavity diseases in infertile patients and compared results with HSG and transvaginal 2D US.[25] SIS revealed 100% diagnostic accuracy for detection of polypoid lesions and endometrial hyperplasia, while HSG had a sensitivity of 50% and a

PPV of 28.6% for polypoid lesions and a sensitivity of 0% for endometrial hyperplasia.[25] SIS and HSG had similar sensitivities (75%) in the detection of intrauterine adhesions; both SIS and HSG were of limited use in the diagnosis of minor uterine malformations, although global results of SIS in diagnosing congenital uterine anomalies were superior to HSG.

Transvaginal 3D US is a noninvasive imaging technique with the ability to simultaneously assess multiplanar and surface images of the endometrial cavity and external contour of the uterus.

By obtaining a coronal view of the uterus and through meticulous analysis of three orthogonal planes, Jurkovic et al. reported overall sensitivity and specificity of 98% and 100%, respectively, compared with 88% sensitivity and 94% specificity for transvaginal 2D US.[26] For arcuate uterus, the sensitivity and specificity of transvaginal 3D US were 100%, compared with 67% and 94%, respectively for transvaginal 2D US. For major Müllerian anomalies, the sensitivity and specificity of transvaginal 3D US were 100%, compared with 100% sensitivity and 95% specificity for transvaginal 2D US. The PPV reported for major Müllerian defects was 100% for 3D US, compared with 50% for 2D US.[26] Jurkovic et al. also elaborated on the use of ultrasound screening for congenital uterine anomalies in an unselected population, estimating their prevalence to be between 5 and 6%.[6]

Later studies aimed to establish actual incidence and effect of the different types of uterine malformations on reproductive performance in women willing to conceive in order to define which abnormalities are related to a poor prognosis and which should be surgically corrected prior to an attempt to conceive. The most useful plane obtained by 3D US is the coronal view of the uterus, which is usually not obtainable on 2D US because of anatomical limitations (the vaginal probe has limited mobility within the confines of the vagina). The coronal view enables the assessment of the relationship between the endometrium and the myometrium at the uterine fundus, simultaneously delineating the entire cervical canal, and depicting the cornual angles (Figs. 11.2 to 11.4).[12,27] Recent study on 204 women with fertility problems showed that 3D US has a high level of accuracy for most uterine anomalies.[28] The sensitivity of 3D US was 86.6%, and specificity was 96.9%. The PPV was 99.3%, and the NPV was 54.4%, with an 88.2% accuracy rate. For classification, the PPV of 3D sonography was 82.3%, and accuracy was 76%. In the case of an arcuate uterus and short septa, increased operator's experience improves accuracy and precision. Ghi et al. analyzed 284 patients undergoing office hysteroscopy to assess the accuracy of 3D US in the diagnosis of congenital uterine anomalies.[29]

Women with negative ultrasound findings subsequently underwent office hysteroscopy, whereas a

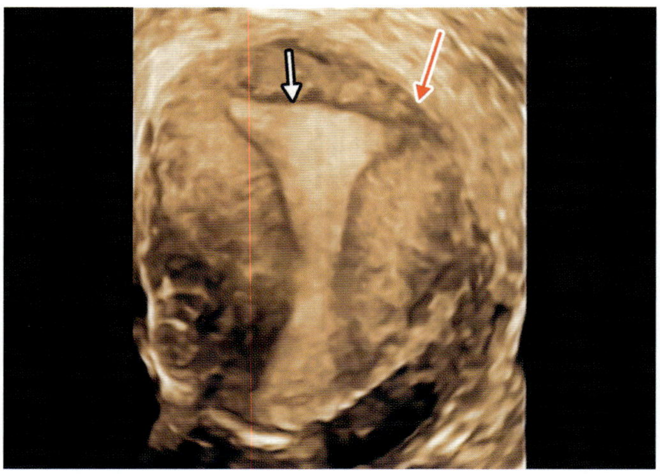

Fig. 11.2: The 3D ultrasound acquired volume of the normal uterus, rendered in surface mode showing coronal image of the uterus. The endometrial cavity is hyperechoic and shows a normal triangular shape. It is surrounded by a thin hypoechoic line, the endometrial-myometrial junction (white arrow), surrounded by a thick myometrial wall. The serosa of the uterus is visualized as outer margin (red arrow).

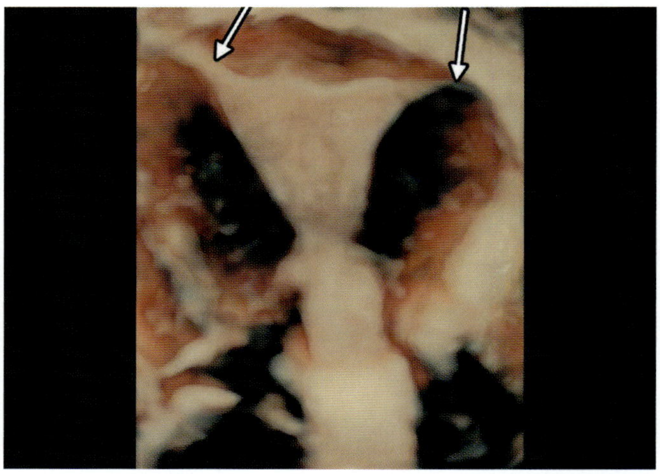

Fig. 11.3: The 3D ultrasound acquired volume of the uterus, rendered in high-definition (HD) live mode shows normal endometrial cavity and cervix. Internal os is seen as a narrowing between the uterine body and cervix. Both cornua (white arrows) are seen as thin sideward extensions from the fundal end of the endometrial cavity.

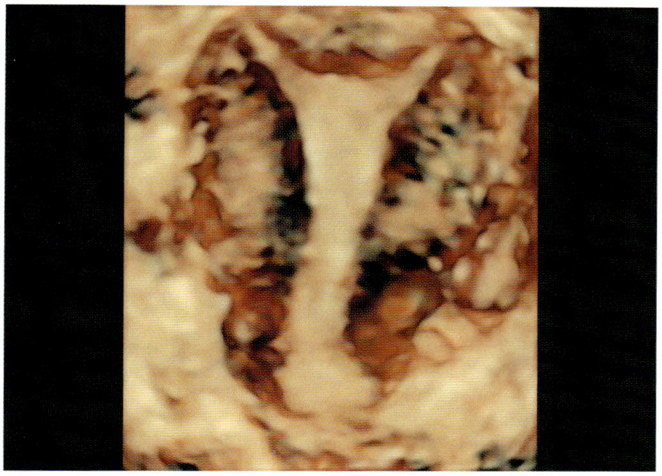

Fig. 11.4: The 3D ultrasound acquired volume of the uterus, rendered in HD live mode shows normal endometrial cavity and cervix. Both cornua are visualized, but in a little different direction than in Figure 11.3.

combined laparoscopic-hysteroscopic assessment was performed in cases of suspected Müllerian anomaly. A specific Müllerian malformation was sonographically diagnosed in 54 women of the 284 included in the study group. All negative ultrasound findings were confirmed at office hysteroscopy. Among the women with abnormal ultrasound findings, the presence of a Müllerian anomaly was endoscopically confirmed in all.[29] Concordance between ultrasound and endoscopy around the type of anomaly was verified in 52 cases, including all those with septate uterus and two out of three with bicornuate uterus. 3D transvaginal ultrasound appears to be extremely accurate for the diagnosis and classification of congenital uterine anomalies, and may conveniently become the only mandatory step in the assessment of the uterine cavity in patients with a history of recurrent miscarriage. A prospective blinded study evaluated the costs, accuracy, risks, and benefits of 3D US compared to HSG.[30] A total of 101 women aged 26–44 years with evidence of uterine anomalies were enrolled. All participants had routine HSG as part of their infertility evaluation as well as 3D transvaginal US as part of the study. Surgical findings were used as the standard for final diagnosis; total of 6 normal uteri and 119 uterine anomalies were classified: 30 congenital uterine anomalies (3 arcuate, 1 unicornuate, 4 bicornuate, 2 didelphys, and 20 septate uteri) and 89 acquired anomalies (38 polyps, 30 fibroids, 17 synechiae, and 4 adenomyosis). The conclusion of this study is that 3D US provides visualization and evaluation of the uterine cavity with similar or better accuracy than standard HSG in the office setting, with lower cost and morbidity.[30]

Turkgeldi et al. confirmed that 3D US's sensitivity and specificity is reported to be close to 100% for diagnosing congenital uterine anomalies, comparable with those of MRI and hysteroscopy with laparoscopy.[31] 3D US may not perform well in thin endometria, but combining it with SIS overcomes this problem. Research shows that 3D US is more sensitive and specific than 2D US in defining and mapping uterine lesions, such as fibroids, adenomyosis, and intrauterine synechia.

Seshadri et al. recently performed a systematic review to assess the diagnostic accuracy of SIS in the evaluation of the uterine cavity in subfertile women.[32] Twenty relevant studies (including 1,645 procedures) were identified and a subsequent meta-analysis was performed comparing SIS with hysteroscopy. Electronic databases were searched for relevant studies and references of relevant studies were cross-checked; validity was assessed and data were extracted independently by two authors. SIS had a high pooled sensitivity and specificity in the detection of congenital uterine anomalies of 85% (95% CI: 0.79–0.90) and 100% (95% CI: 0.99–1.00), respectively.[32] Based on this systematic review and meta-analyses, SIS is a highly sensitive investigative modality, comparable to the gold standard tool, hysteroscopy in the detection of intrauterine abnormalities in subfertile women. SIS is highly sensitive and specific test in the diagnosis of congenital uterine anomalies, uterine polyps, submucous myomas, and intrauterine adhesions, and can be used as a screening tool for subfertile patients prior to IVF treatment.

Table 11.2 reviews benefits and limitations of gynecological examination, HSG, 2D US, 3D US, SIS, MRI, hysteroscopy, and combined hysteroscopy and laparoscopy for detection of congenital uterine anomalies.

COMPARATIVE SONOGRAPHIC STUDIES

Kupesic and Kurjak attempted to evaluate the combined use of transvaginal 2D US, transvaginal color and pulsed Doppler sonography, SIS, and transvaginal 3D US in the preoperative diagnosis of septate uterus.[33,34] A total of 420 infertile patients undergoing operative hysteroscopy were included in this study. The final diagnosis of the uterine disorder was confirmed by hysteroscopy, and 278 patients had an intrauterine septum corrected surgically. Forty three of the patients with a septate uterus had a history of repeated spontaneous miscarriage, 71 had one spontaneous miscarriage (56 in the 1st trimester, and 15 in the 2nd

Table 11.2: Benefits and limitations of gynecological examination, HSG, 2D US, 3D US, SIS, MRI, hysteroscopy, and combined hysteroscopy and laparoscopy for detection of congenital uterine anomalies.

Diagnostic method	*Advantages*	*Disadvantages*
Gynecological examination	• Inspection of the vagina and cervix allow detection of vaginal (aplasia, septum) and cervical malformations	• Lack of precision for diagnosis of congenital uterine anomalies
X-ray HSG	• Provides a good outline of the uterine cavity	• Minimally invasive • Exposure to radiation and iodine contrast media • Lack of visualization of the uterine fundus • Inaccurate for detection of minor anomalies • Impossible distinction between different types of fusion and resorption disorders
2D ultrasound	• Noninvasive • Uterine cavity can be visualized in longitudinal and transverse planes • Detection of the two endometrial echoes in the upper portion of the uterine cavity in transverse plane indicates duplication anomaly of the uterus • Good screening tool	• Does not visualize coronal plane • Morphology of the uterus cannot be objectively analyzed • Operator dependent
3D ultrasound	• Noninvasive • Visualization of the coronal plane and surface rendering of the uterine cavity • Assessment of planar reformatted sections through the uterus • Simultaneous assessment of the uterine wall and fundal shape • Visualization of the ovaries and other pelvic structures with the exception of the tubes	• Operator dependent (requires experience, technical competence, and expertise) • Limitations: shadowing caused by uterine fibroids, thin and/or irregular endometrial lining, and decreased volume of the uterine cavity (in cases of intrauterine adhesions)
Saline infusion sonography	• Simultaneous visualization of the uterine cavity and demonstration of tubal patency	• Minimally invasive • Operator dependent • Avoids radiation exposure • Patients' discomfort (uterine contractions)
MRI	• Noninvasive • Simultaneous visualization of the uterine cavity and fundal shape • High diagnostic precision and accuracy • Visualization of other pelvic structures	• Expensive • Does not visualize tubal patency
Hysteroscopy	• Gold standard for direct inspection of the cervical canal and uterine cavity	• Minimally invasive • Cannot accurately differentiate between the different subtypes of congenital uterine anomalies
Hysteroscopy with laparoscopy	• Gold standard in the investigation of patients with congenital uterine anomalies • Allows concurrent diagnosis and treatment	• Invasive • Expensive

Adopted from Tabi S. and Kupesic-Plavsic S. (2012).[33]

trimester), 82 had primary infertility, and 20 had premature delivery, including 6 with breech and 2 with transverse presentations. A positive history of ectopic pregnancy was found in 76 patients.

Each patient underwent transvaginal ultrasound and transvaginal color Doppler examination during the luteal phase of the menstrual cycle. Color and pulsed Doppler were superimposed to visualize intraseptal and myometrial vascularity in each patient. Eighty-six patients undergoing hysteroscopy were examined by 3D US, while distension of the uterine cavity with saline was performed in 76 patients. The 2D US, SIS, and 3D US reached sensitivity of 95.2%, 98.2%, and 98.4%, respectively; sensitivity of 92.2%, 100%, and 100%, respectively, and PPV of 95.9%, 100%, and 100%, respectively.[34]

Interestingly, no correlation was found between septal height and occurrence of obstetrical complications (P >0.05). Miscarriages and late pregnancy complications occurred with the same rate in patients with small septa dividing less than one third of the uterine cavity (86 of 126), and septa which were dividing more than two thirds of the uterine cavity (108 of 152). The same was true of septal thickness: obstetrical complications were found in the same proportion of the patients with thin (64 of 92) and those with thick (130 of 186) septa (P >0.05). Interestingly, previous obstetrical performance correlated significantly with septal vascularity. Patients with vascularized septa had significantly higher prevalence of early pregnancy failure and late pregnancy complications (169 of 198) than those with avascularized septa (25 of 80) (P <0.05). This difference may be explained by an increased amount of muscle in the septum producing local uncoordinated myometrial contractility. In our study, early miscarriages occurred at a significantly higher rate than did those in a control group (41% vs. 15%). Late miscarriages and premature deliveries occurred in 35 of 278 (12.6%) patients compared to the rate of 7% for normal pregnancies. Intrauterine growth restriction was diagnosed in two patients (8.7%) with septate uterus, compared to 6% in general patient population. Intrauterine fetal death occurred in one patient, and placental abruption and placenta previa were also found in one patient. Breech presentation was found in six (26.1%) pregnancies complicated by an intrauterine septum, whereas transverse presentation occurred in two (8.7%) patients. Since abnormal fetal presentation was significantly more frequent in patients with a septate uterus, a significantly higher rate of Cesarean section (34.8%) was noticed in patients with septate uterus. Cervical incompetence during pregnancy appeared in nine (25.7%) women with an intrauterine septum.

Kupesic et al. confirmed that 3D US allows a precise assessment of the uterine morphology, including the endometrial lining and outer shape of the uterine muscle.[35] Color and power Doppler ultrasound allowed simultaneous visualization of uterine morphology and vascular network giving accurate information on the type of anomaly and the extent of the defect. The visualization of the myometrial portion is further enhanced by detection of the myometrial vessels using color/power Doppler ultrasound.[36] Furthermore, Doppler imaging can detect deficient intraseptal vascularity and/or inadequate endometrial development in patients with a septate uterus. The 3D US (coronal plane and planar reformatted sections through the uterus) enable precise evaluation of the fundal indentation and the length of the septum. Shadowing caused by the uterine leiomyoma, irregular endometrial lining, and decreased volume of the uterine cavity (in cases of intrauterine adhesions) are obvious limitations of 3D US. Results of our study on screening for uterine abnormalities by 3D US indicated that timely detection of congenital uterine anomalies and acquired uterine pathologies may improve the results of ART and perinatal outcome of subfertile patients.[37]

Nazzaro et al. used 2D and 3D power Doppler to differentiate between septate and bicornuate uterus.[38] Seventy-three patients with septate uterus, with or without cervical and vaginal duplication, and 36 patients with bicornuate uterus were selected for inclusion in the study. Irregular vascular networks were detected between the two hemicavities in the patients with septate uterus. All bicornuate uteri showed a peculiar vascular network between the two hemicavities: the main recognizable vessels formed a network depicting the Greek letter γ at the level of the uterine midline. This finding was also confirmed in patients who underwent intravenous contrast medium-enhanced ultrasound examination. This study confirmed that power Doppler assessment and detection of the γ sign can be used to differentiate septate from bicornuate uterus.[38]

According to estimates, 65–85% of patients with bicornuate or septate uteri have a successful pregnancy outcome after metroplasty.[39] However, 59.5% of the patients with such anomalies have a successful subsequent pregnancy without surgery, with a cumulative live birth rate of 78%.[39] There is no case control study to compare live birth rates in women who had surgery compared with those who did not. Noninvasive ultrasound and Doppler criteria to distinguish between the bicornuate and septate uterus, vascularized and non-vascularized septa may contribute to our understanding who are the patients who may benefit from metroplasty.

Ludwin et al. estimated the diagnostic accuracy and compared the diagnostic value of 3D US, 3D SIS, 2D US and 2D SIS (initial and expert diagnosis) in the differential diagnosis of septate, bicornuate, and arcuate uteri.[41] Hysteroscopy performed in conjunction with laparoscopy (HL) detected 23 arcuate, 60 septate, 22 bicornuate, and 12 normal uteri. 3D SIS showed perfect diagnostic accuracy (100.0%) in general detection of uterine abnormalities, compared with initial 2D US (77.8%), expert 2D US (90.6%), 2D SIS (94.0%), and 3D US (97.4%). In the overall diagnosis of uterine anomalies, all of the diagnostic methods had statistically significantly better diagnostic value than initial 2D US (P <0.001), whereas 3D SIS was the only method that was better than expert 2D US (P <0.001). Although 3D SIS was identical to HL, with the highest accuracy, there was no significant difference in diagnostic value between 3D US with 2D SIS and 3D SIS or between expert 2D US and 3D US with 2D SIS. The high diagnostic value of these ultrasonographic tools

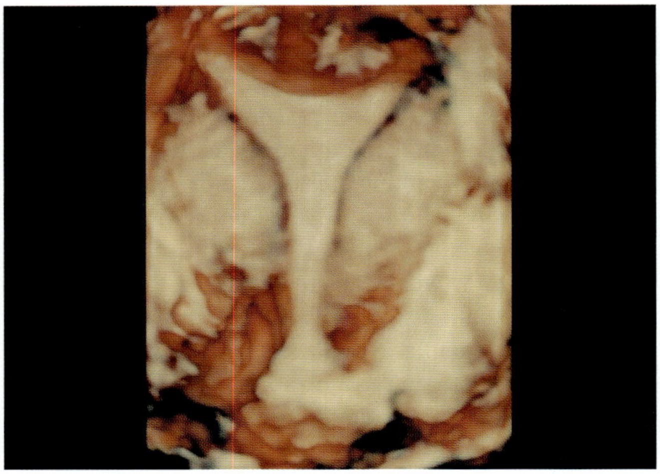

Fig. 11.5: The 3D ultrasound acquired volume of the arcuate uterus, rendered in HD live mode shows a nearly normal shape of the endometrial cavity except concavity at the fundus.

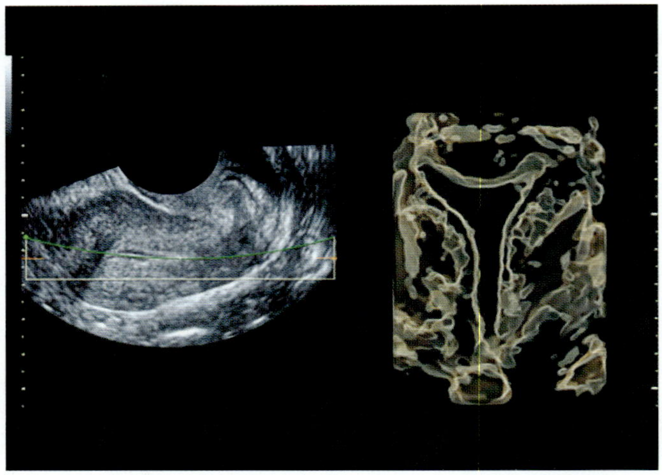

Fig. 11.6: The HD live silhouette mode of an arcuate uterus. Note a typical concave shape of the fundus.

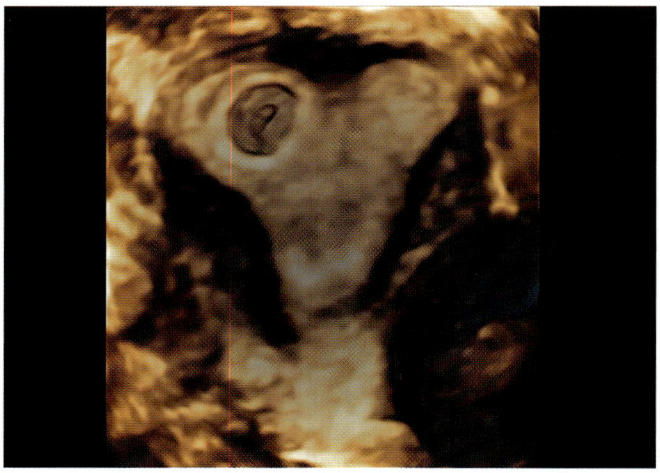

Fig. 11.7: The 3D ultrasound acquired surface mode rendered image of the uterus in coronal plane. Concavity on the fundal surface of the endometrium suggests its arcuate shape. Gestational sac is seen in the endometrial cavity with yolk sac and fetal pole.

questions the need for endoscopy in the differential diagnosis of the most common congenital uterine anomalies.[40]

CONGENITAL UTERINE ANOMALIES: SPECTRUM OF ULTRASOUND FINDINGS

Arcuate Uterus

The arcuate uterus represents the mildest form of resorption failure and is not considered clinically relevant. It is characterized by convex or flat outer surface of the uterus and thickened fundal myometrium, leading to a slight indentation of the uterine cavity by a shallow septum extending less than 10 mm caudally (Figs. 11.5 and 11.6).[33] Clinically, the patient is often asymptomatic with no gynecological complications. Because the arcuate uterus is rarely associated with obstetrical and/or gynecological complications, treatment is not usually indicated (Fig. 11.7). Hysteroscopic metroplasty is not indicated because it does not improve the outcome of pregnancy in women with this diagnosis. If the patient is having trouble with fertility, then she can explore ART treatment options.

Septate Uterus

Uterine septum develops as a result of failure of resorption of the tissue connecting the two paramesonephric (Müllerian) ducts prior to the 20th embryonic week.[12,13] This anomaly may be clinically asymptomatic until pregnancy occurs, or patient may report episodes of dysmenorrhea. It is associated with a high incidence of spontaneous abortion, miscarriages, and premature birth.

The uterus is considered septate, if the septum extends 10 mm or more into the cavity from the midcoronal line, and the serosal surface is convex or flat. Septate uterus has a spectrum of configurations including variations from incomplete or partial septa to a complete septate uterus. A partial septate uterus refers to a single fundus and cervix with a uterine septum extending from the top of the endometrial cavity toward the cervix, partially dividing uterine cavity (Fig. 11.8). The 2D US can demonstrate two separate

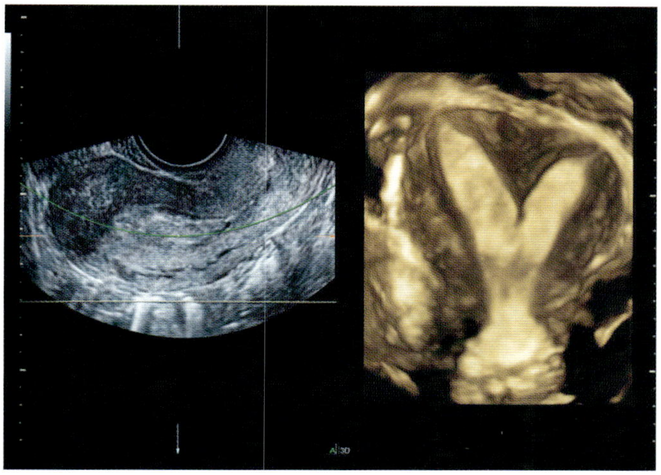

Fig. 11.8: The 2D B mode ultrasound image on the left side is the acquisition plane for the 3D volume of the uterus. This is a sagittal section of the uterus and appears normal. The image on the right side is the rendered image of the same uterus, showing its coronal plane. The endometrial cavity is clearly divided with partial septum, and the outer serosal surface appears smooth and convex. The angle between the two parts of the endometrial cavity is acute, and the septum extends till approximately half of the endometrial cavity. This is an example of incomplete/partial septum or subseptate uterus.

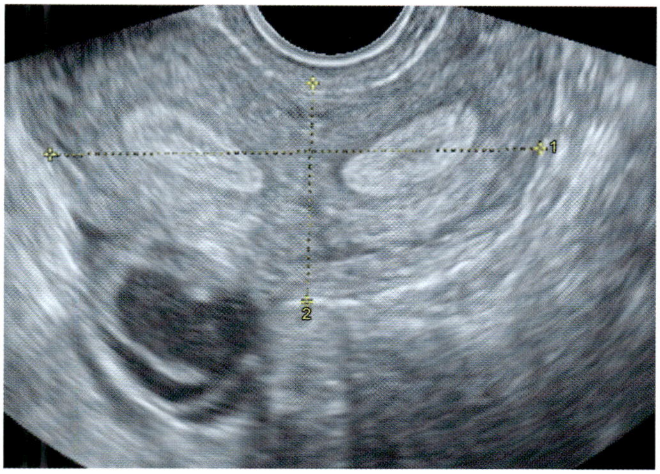

Fig. 11.9: B mode ultrasound image of the transverse section of the uterus showing endometrial cavity divided into two halves, suggesting a duplication abnormality. As no clear indentation is seen on the serosal surface, it is most likely a septate uterus.

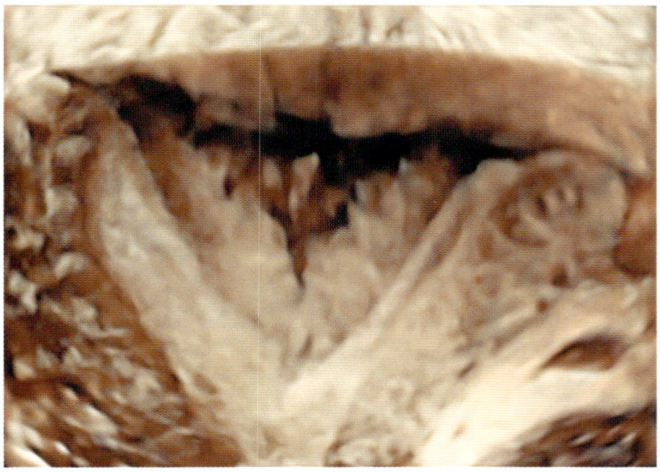

Fig. 11.10: The 3D ultrasound acquired volume rendered in HD live mode shows the same uterus in the coronal plane. The serosal surface is flat, endometrial cavity is partially divided with a thick septum, and angle between two cavities is acute.

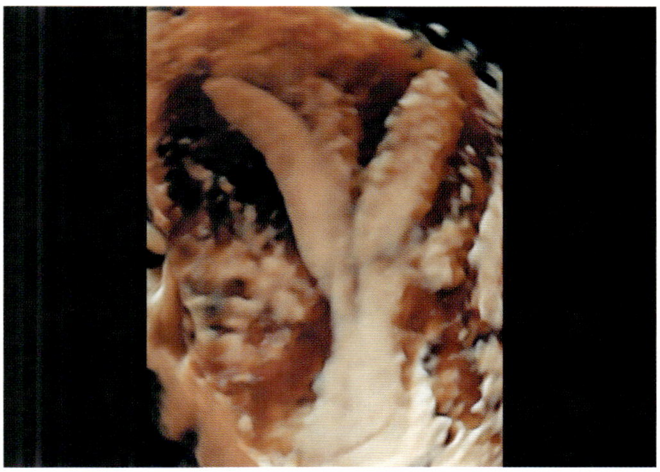

Fig. 11.11: The 3D ultrasound acquired volume of the uterus, rendered in HD live mode shows septate uterus in coronal plane. The serosal surface shows no indentation and endometrial cavity is divided with a complete septum. The angle between the two cavities is acute, and septum extends up to the internal cervical os.

endometrial echoes in transverse or oblique transverse views of the uterus, but the interpretation is operator dependent (Fig. 11.9). Using 3D US, septate uterus is diagnosed in coronal plane, with a septum producing a sagittal notch in the uterine cavity more than equal to 1 cm (Fig. 11.10).

As demonstrated in Figures 11.11 and 11.12, the size and shape of the septum can vary by width and length.

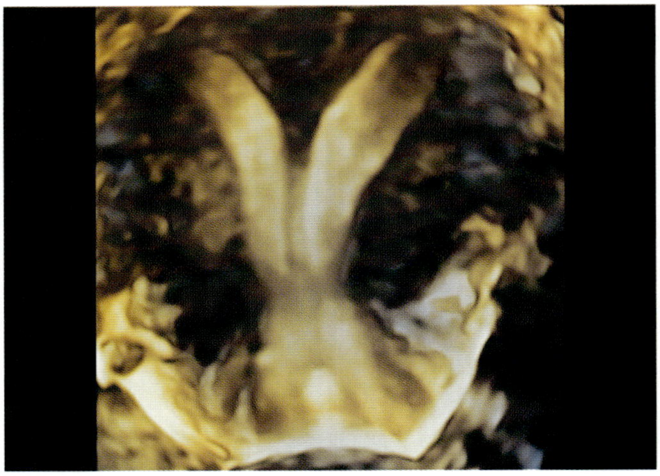

Fig. 11.12A: The 3D ultrasound acquired volume of the uterus, rendered in surface mode shows septate uterus in coronal plane. The serosal surface shows no indentation and endometrial cavity is completely divided with a septum. The angle between the two cavities is acute, and septum is clearly dividing the cervix.

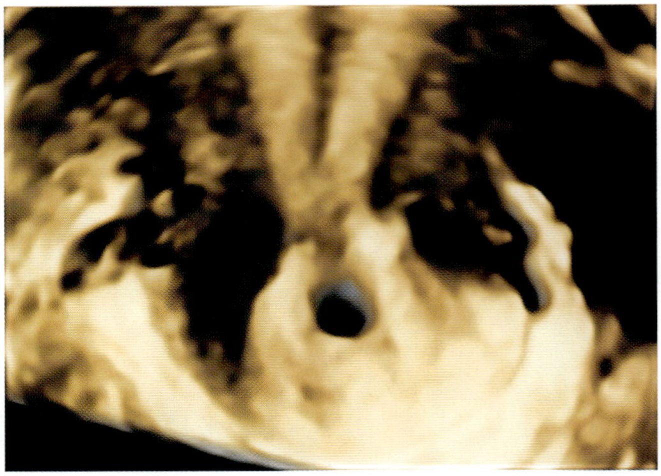

Fig. 11.12B: The same uterus as in Figure 12A. Septum dividing cervical canal into two halves is clearly visualized.

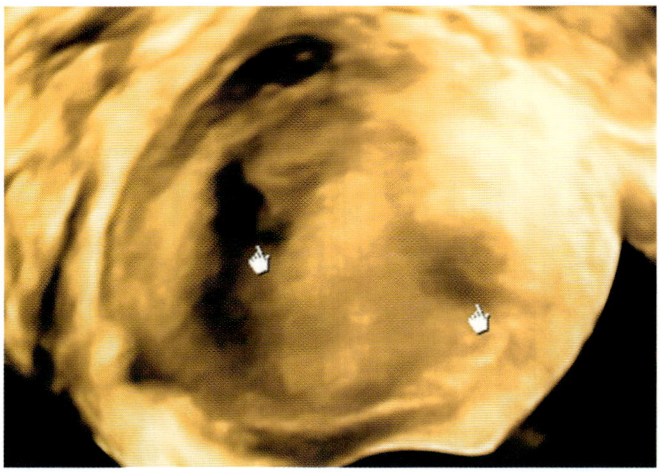

Fig. 11.12C: The same uterus as in Figures 12A and B, showing 3D ultrasound acquired volume of the cervix rendered in transverse section in surface mode. Image shows two cervical canals, but the outer muscular wall and serosa are not divided, favoring the diagnosis of a complete septum, extending into the cervix.

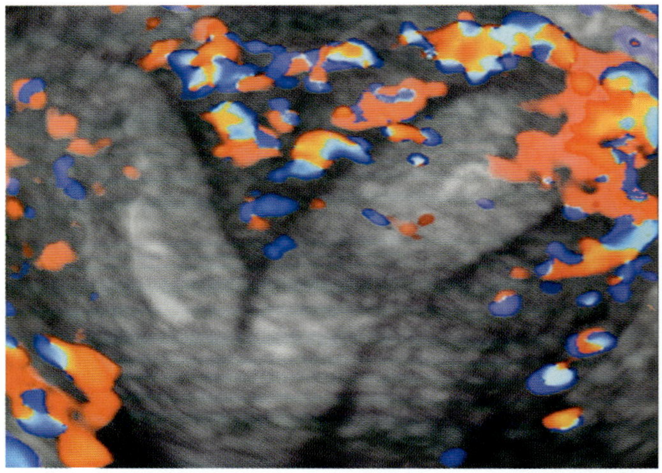

Fig. 11.13: The 3D ultrasound acquired volume of the uterus with color Doppler, rendered in glass body mode, showing a vascularized septum.

Initially, uterine septa were believed to be avascular, consisting of predominantly fibrous tissue. However, biopsy specimens, MRI, and color/power Doppler imaging suggest that septa are composed primarily of muscle fibers and less connective tissue, which could noninvasively be visualized by 3D color and power Doppler ultrasound (Figs. 11.13 and 11.14).[34,36,41,43]

Bicornuate Uterus

Bicornuate uterus (commonly referred as "heart-shaped" uterus) results from a partial nonfusion of the Müllerian ducts (Fig. 11.15).[12,13] This abnormality occurs in the 7th to 9th weeks of embryological development when the paramesonephric ducts fuse to form the uterus in the initial stages. The paramesonephric ducts grow laterally to the

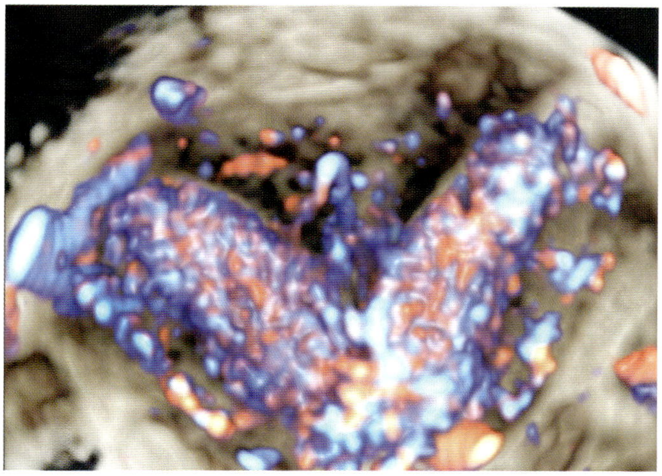

Fig. 11.14: The 3D ultrasound acquired volume of the uterus with HD flow, rendered in glass body mode, showing a septate uterus with abundant vascularity in both halves of the endometrial cavity, marked vascularity in lateral myometrial wall, and scanty vascularity in between the two endometrial cavities, i.e. in the septum.

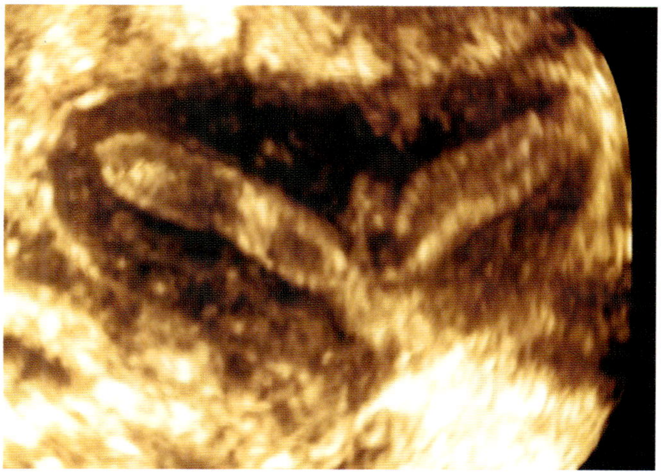

Fig. 11.15: The 3D ultrasound acquired volume of the uterus, rendered in surface mode shows endometrial cavity divided into two parts. The angle between the two cavities is obtuse, and shallow indentation is seen on the external fundal contour. Sonographic findings suggest a bicornuate uterus.

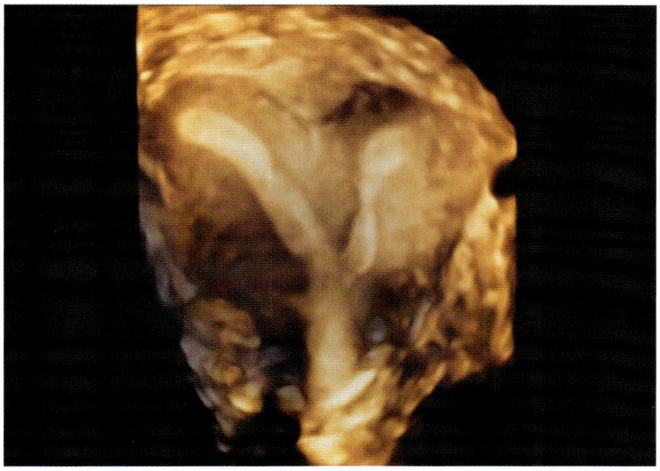

Fig. 11.16: The 3D ultrasound acquired volume of the uterus, rendered in surface mode, showing the uterus in coronal plane, with clear division of the endometrial cavity extending up to the internal cervical os. Angle between the two cavities is acute. These features are suggestive of a septate uterus. Deep indentation on the serosal surface, according to the American Fertility Society classification suggests a bicornuate uterus. This image explains limitations of the existing classification systems to differentiate between different groups of congenital uterine anomalies.

urogenital ridges.[33] In this stage of development, there is lateral fusion of the paramesonephric ducts which ultimately becomes the uterus, cervix, the Fallopian tubes and the upper two-thirds of the vagina. Bicornuate uterus forms as a result of improper fusion of the paramesonephric ducts and the horns of the uterus are not fully developed.[43] A bicornuate uterus has a serosal indentation extending 10 mm or more caudally from the normal serosal surface, creating two horns.[44,45] The obligatory septum or partial septum of bicornuate uterus is called subseptum, and is variable in length and width. The cervix may be single, septate, or duplicated. In complete bicornuate uterus, the central myometrium may extend to the level of the internal cervical os (bicornuate unicollis) or external cervical os (bicornuate bicollis).[33]

A combined bicornuate/septate configuration of the uterus has been described in which the external fundus has an indentation consistent with a bicornuate shape, but at hysteroscopy there is a septum dividing the endometrial cavities (Fig. 11.16).[44] Visualization and differentiation between the variants of bicornuate uterus may be challenged in the presence of uterine fibroids (Figs. 11.17A to C).

Bicornuate uterus may be distinguished from the didelphic because it demonstrates some degree of fusion between the two horns, while in classic didelphic uterus, the two horns and cervices are completely separated. Another difference between didelphic and bicornuate uterus is that the horns of the bicornuate uteri are not fully developed; typically, they are smaller than those of didelphic uteri. Prevalence of bicornuate uterus was reported to be 0.1% of the general population; however, it is highly dependent on the diagnostic method used.[1-10] Clinically, the pregnancy rates of patients with bicornuate uteri are similar to the general population, so surgery is usually

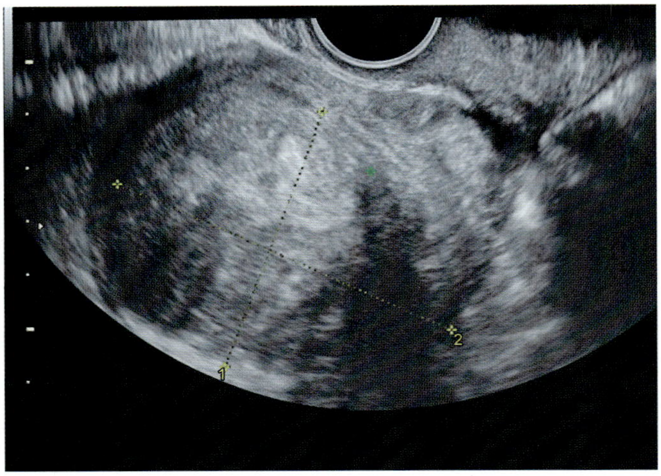

Fig. 11.17A: The B mode ultrasound image of the uterus in a transverse section with a large round, fairly well-defined lesion. The lesion is heterogeneous and displaces the endometrium. Ultrasound findings are suggestive of a fibroid. Patient obstetrical history is significant for recurrent pregnancy loss.

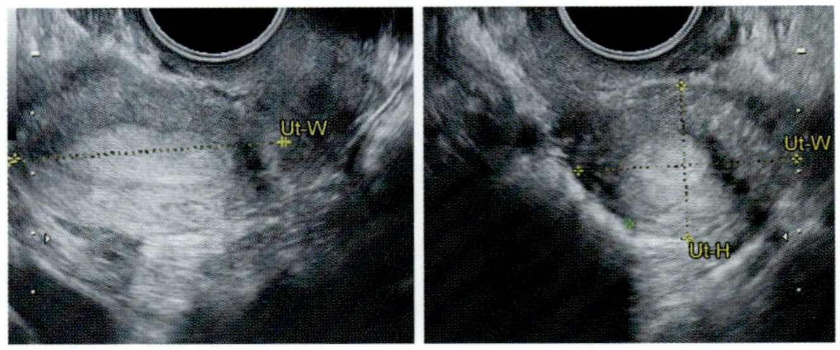

Fig. 11.17B: The B mode ultrasound image of the same patient shows a normal-looking uterus when the probe was spanned toward the left side.

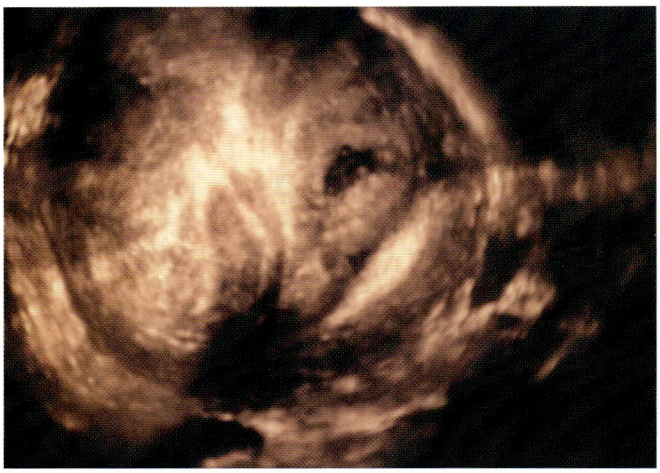

Fig. 11.17C: The 3D ultrasound acquired volume of the same patient. This rendered image shows a large fibroid displacing the endometrial cavity in the right horn, while the left horn appears normal. 3D US suggested bicornuate fibroid uterus, which was confirmed by hysteroscopy with concurrent laparoscopy.

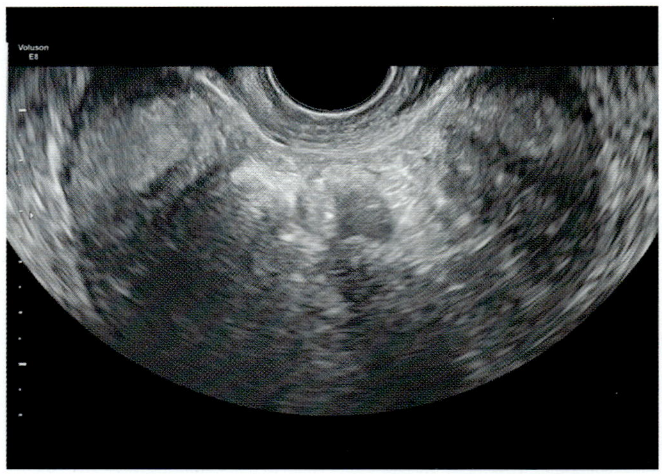

Fig. 11.18A: B mode ultrasound image of the transverse scan of the pelvis. Two hypoechoic well-defined roundish areas are seen on two sides of the image, with central slightly hyperechoic shadow. In this patient, no uterine shadow was seen in the midline. The two shadows on this image appear to be two horns of the uterus. Being placed so widely apart, this is most likely a didelphys uterus.

not indicated. It is an option, if the patient has a history of recurrent pregnancy loss. Reunification of the uterus is an option via laparoscopy or laparotomy.

Didelphys Uterus

Didelphic uterus is comprised of two separate, fully developed uterine horns with two cervices (Figs. 11.18A to E). It has a high association with transverse vaginal septa, which may lead to difficulties in intercourse or vaginal delivery. Embryologically, didelphic uterus has a similar etiology as bicornuate uterus, and is due to failure of fusion of the paramesonephric ducts during the 7th to 9th weeks of development.[9]

Patients with didelphys uterus may have good reproductive outcomes and full-term pregnancies because each

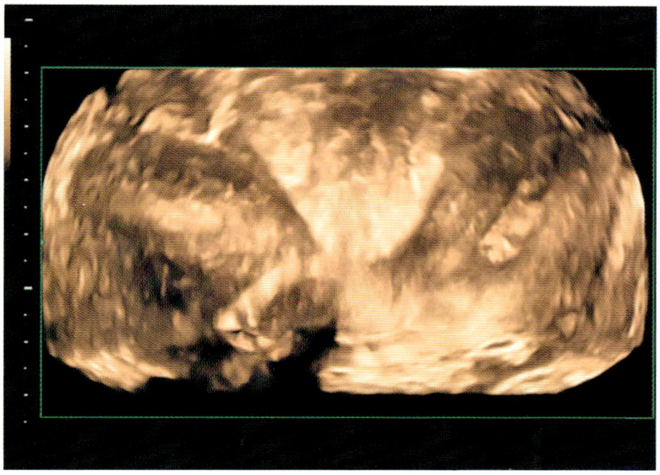

Fig. 11.18B: The 3D ultrasound acquired volume of the same uterus as in Figure 18A, rendered in a surface mode. Note two uterine cornua, placed widely apart. Both cornua show central endometrial shadow.

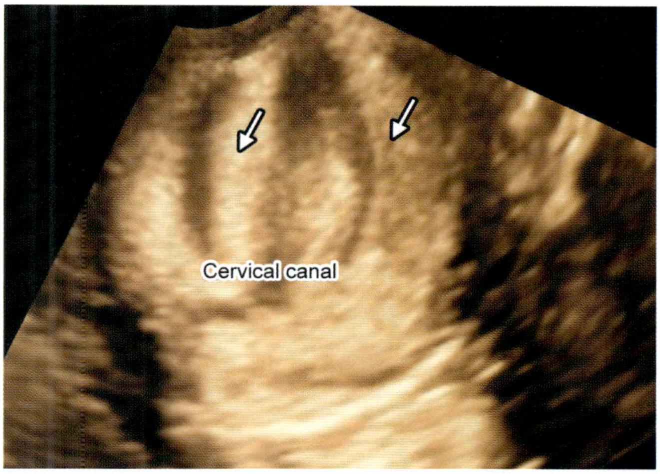

Fig. 11.18C: The 3D ultrasound acquired volume of the cervix of the same uterus as in Figures 18A and B, rendered in a surface mode. Note two separate cervical canals with two separate cervical muscular walls and even a layer of serosa between the two muscular walls. Combining Figures 11.18A to C lead to diagnosis of uterus didelphys.

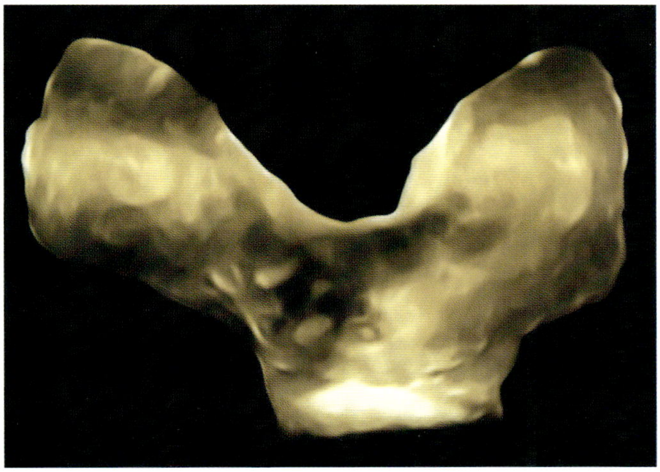

Fig. 11.18D: The same image as in Figure 11.18C, modified by magicut (electronic scalpel). This modality allows extraction of unimportant information from the image, thus highlighting the shape of the didelphys uterus.

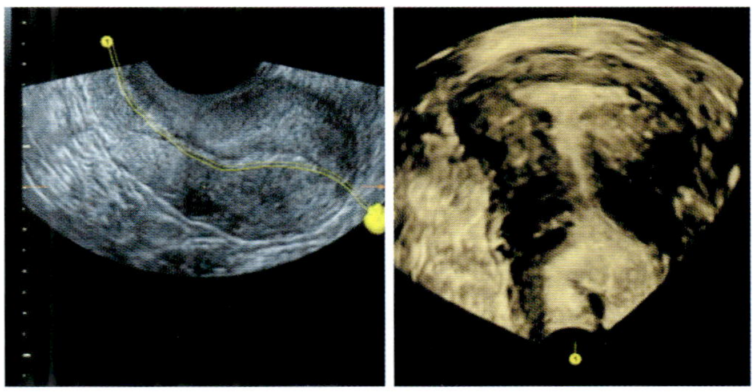

Fig. 11.18E: When the two cornua of the uterus are placed widely apart, or the contrast between the endometrium and the myometrium is week, rendering might not produce the required information to establish the type of duplication defect. In these cases, omniview with volume contrast imaging is beneficial for precise differentiation of the congenital uterine defect.

horn is technically a fully developed uterus. Clinically, some patients may present with preterm births, recurrent pregnancy loss, and pelvic pain. Surgical treatment is not indicated if a patient has recurrent pregnancy loss, because it is generally believed that it would not improve pregnancy outcomes.

Unicornuate Uterus

Unicornuate uterus has a rudimentary horn that may or may not have functioning endometrium; therefore, half of the uterus is not fully developed (Figs. 11.19 and 11.20). It is reported to have a prevalence of 0.4% in the general

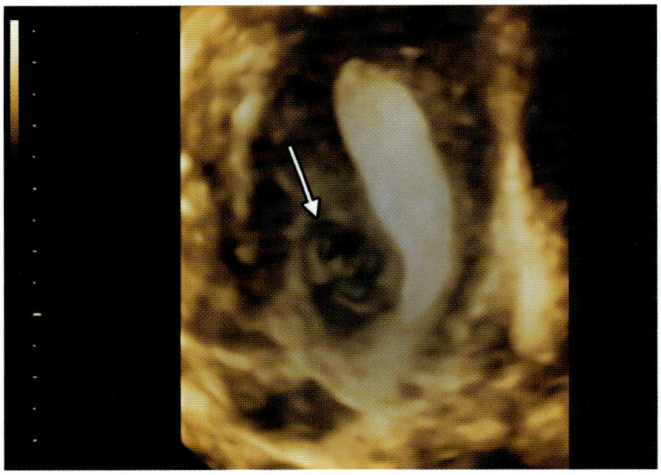

Fig. 11.19: The 3D ultrasound acquired volume of the unicornuate uterus, rendered in a surface mode. Note a banana-shaped endometrial cavity and a well-defined round hypoechoic lesion (intramural/submucous fibroid) seen in the concavity of the endometrial cavity (marked by an arrow).

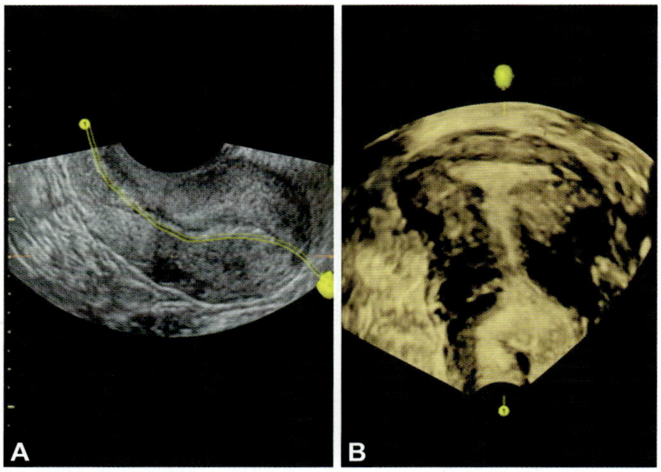

Figs. 11.21A and B: A 3D ultrasound acquired volume of the retroverted uterus on omniview, showing T-shaped endometrial cavity.

population, but it is more common in infertile women.[1-10] Patients with obstruction in the rudimentary horn with functional endometrium may present with a pelvic mass and chronic abdominal/pelvic pain. In these cases surgical excision is imperative, and can be performed laparoscopically.[3] Clinically, unicornuate uterus is associated with spontaneous abortion, ectopic ovaries, endometriosis, preterm delivery, ectopic pregnancy, and kidney abnormalities.[33] Surgery is not indicated for the repair of unicornuate uteri because it is not believed to improve pregnancy outcomes.

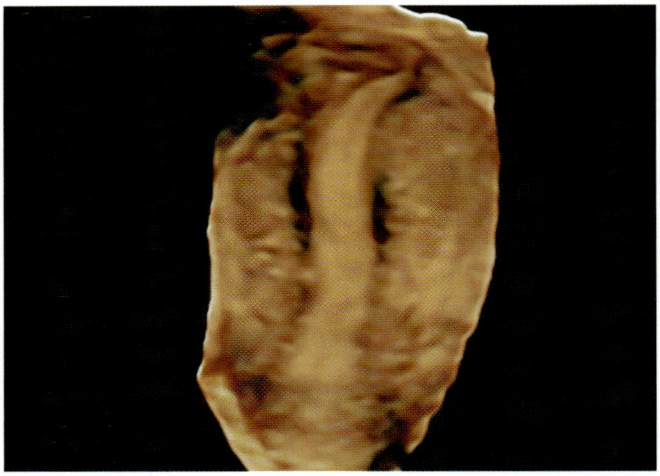

Fig. 11.20: The 3D ultrasound acquired volume of the uterus, rendered in HD live mode shows a sword-shaped endometrial cavity. Sonographic finding indicates unicornuate uterus.

T-shaped Uterus

Diethylstilbestrol (DES) is a synthetic estrogen that was widely prescribed to pregnant women from the late 1940s until 1970 to prevent miscarriage. An estimated 1–1.5 million women received DES during their pregnancies, which affected the reproductive organs of 35–69% of their female offspring.[46] The daughters of women treated with DES developed congenital malformations of the uterus, cervix, and vagina, as well as adenosis and (rarely) clear cell adenocarcinoma of the vagina. This shape of the uterus is a characteristic deformity resulting from the prenatal exposure to DES and is highly associated with infertility and recurrent miscarriage.[46] In an Indian scenario, similar appearance of the uterine cavity may be present in patients with endometrial tuberculosis.

While normal uterine cavity is triangular, a T-shaped uterus is characterized with a waist in the sides of the triangle, such that the corpus of the endometrial cavity is narrowed and takes on a T shape, rather than a V shape (Figs. 11.21 to 11.23). Fernandez et al. evaluated 97 infertile women who had T-shaped uteri, and 49.5% of them became pregnant after metroplasty.[48] For them, the pregnancy rate increased from 0 to 73%, and their miscarriage rate fell from 78 to 27% ($p = 0.05$). For all 57 pregnancies in 48 women, the preterm delivery rate was 14%, the term delivery rate was 49%, and the live birth rate was 63%. This emphasizes the importance that the patients with T-shaped uteri should be managed by infertility specialists with expertise in hysteroscopic surgery.

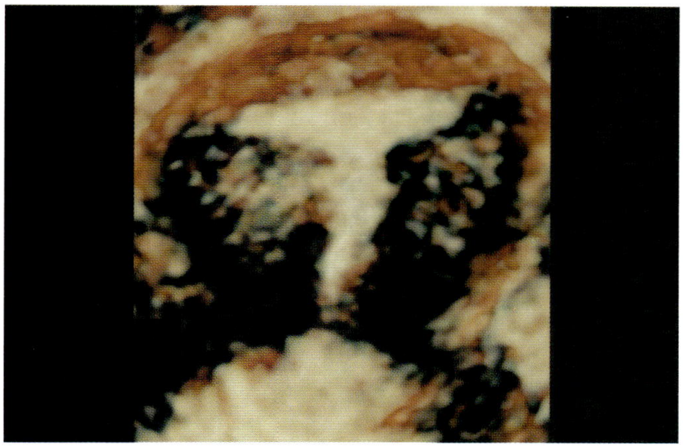

Fig. 11.22: The 3D ultrasound acquired volume of the uterus rendered in HD live mode. It shows normal convex external fundal contour. The endometrial contour shows constriction from both sides converting the triangular endometrial cavity into a T-shaped cavity. In the past, T-shaped uterus was seen in patients exposed to diethylstilbestrol. Today, in Indian scenario, T-shaped uterus is seen in patients with endometrial tuberculosis.

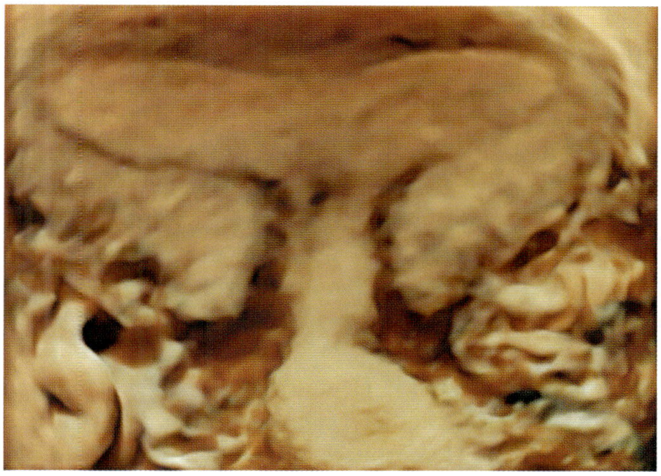

Fig. 11.23: The 3D ultrasound acquired volume of the uterus with flat external fundus. Endometrial cavity shows slight concavity on fundal surface. The cavity generally appears T shaped instead of triangular. Though the endometrial cavity does not appear constricted, horizontal and vertical arms of the endometrial cavity form almost a right angle; this uterus can be categorized as a T-shaped uterus.

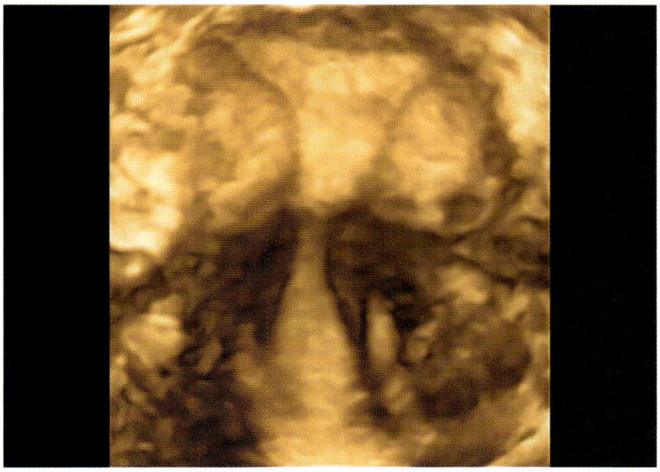

Fig. 11.24: The 3D ultrasound acquired volume of the uterus, rendered in surface mode shows a normal triangular shape of the endometrial cavity and a regular convex contour of the external fundus. Note almost equal length of the endometrial cavity and the cervix, suggesting a hypoplastic uterus.

Hypoplastic Uterus

On ultrasound, hypoplastic uterus is indicated when the distance between the cornua is less than 2 cm, or if the distance from the internal os to the fundus is less than 3–5 cm (Fig. 11.24). Barranger et al. evaluated the reproductive performance after hysteroscopic metroplasty performed for hypoplastic uterus.[48] Twenty-nine women (mean age: 31.4 years; range: 27–38.5 years) with a hypoplastic malformed uterus and a history of primary infertility and/or recurrent abortion and/or preterm delivery were included in this study. Fourteen women suffered from primary infertility and fifteen women had previous pregnancies. Twenty-three women had been exposed to DES in utero. During the follow-up period from 13 to 67 months (the mean was 40 months), 21 women (72.4%) experienced 30 pregnancies. Thirteen women gave birth to 16 live infants. At the time of the follow-up, four women were pregnant in the 2nd trimester. Compared with previous pregnancies, the rate of deliveries increased from 3.8 to 63.2%. No complications occurred during metroplasty, and good hysteroscopic anatomical results were achieved in all cases. Results of this study suggest that hysteroscopic metroplasty, with its simplicity and minimal postoperative complications, seems to be an operation of choice in women with a hypoplastic malformed uterus and a history of severe infertility and/or recurrent pregnancy loss.

REPRODUCTIVE OUTCOMES OF PATIENTS WITH CONGENITAL UTERINE ANOMALIES

Many women with congenital uterine anomalies have normal reproductive history. Obstetrical complications reported to commonly occur in patients with congenital uterine anomalies are 1st and 2nd trimester miscarriages, prematurity, intrauterine growth restriction, antepartum and postpartum hemorrhage, gestational hypertension and preeclampsia, cervical incompetence, premature delivery, malpresentation, and operative delivery.[49-51] In general, obstetrical complications are most common in women with a uterine septum and least common in those with an arcuate uterus.[52,53] Grimbizis et al. reported that septate uterus is the commonest uterine anomaly with a mean incidence of approximately 35%, followed by bicornuate uterus (approximately 25%), and arcuate uterus (approximately 20%).[49] Overall term delivery rates in patients with untreated uterine malformations is reported to be only 50%. Unicornuate and didelphys uterus have term delivery rates of approximately 45%, and the pregnancy outcome of patients with untreated bicornuate and septate uterus is also poor with term delivery rates of only approximately 40%.[49] Arcuate uterus is associated with a slightly better, but still impaired pregnancy outcome with term delivery rates of approximately 65%.

Woelfer et al. studied 1,089 women with no history of infertility or recurrent miscarriage, and used 3D US to determine prevalence of miscarriage and preterm labor in women with normal and abnormal uterine morphology.[54] They found that 983 women had a normally shaped uterine cavity, 72 an arcuate, 29 a subseptate, and 5 a bicornuate uterus. Women with a subseptate uterus had a significantly higher proportion of 1st trimester loss ($P < 0.01$), compared with women with a normal uterus. Women with an arcuate uterus had a significantly greater proportion of 2nd trimester loss ($P < 0.01$) and preterm labor ($P < 0.01$). There were no other significant differences in pregnancy outcomes between women with normal and abnormal uterine morphology. This study confirmed that patients with congenital uterine anomalies were more likely to have adverse pregnancy outcomes than women with a normal uterus, and that 3D US has a potential to be used as a screening tool for congenital uterine anomalies.[54]

Chan et al. performed searches using MEDLINE, EMBASE, the Cochrane Library, and Web of Science.[55] Uterine defects were grouped into arcuate uteri, canalization defects (septate and subseptate uteri), and unification defects (unicornuate, bicornuate, and didelphys uteri). Pooled risk ratios (RR) with 95% confidence intervals (CIs) were computed using random effects models. They identified nine studies comprising 3,805 women. Meta-analysis showed that arcuate uteri were associated with increased rates of 2nd trimester miscarriage (RR, 2.39; 95% CI, 1.33–4.27; $p = 0.003$) and fetal malpresentation at delivery (RR, 2.53; 95% CI, 1.54–4.18; $P < 0.001$). Canalization defects were associated with reduced clinical pregnancy rates (RR, 0.86; 95% CI, 0.77–0.96; $p = 0.009$) and increased rates of 1st trimester miscarriage (RR, 2.89; 95% CI; 2.02–4.14; $P < 0.001$), preterm birth (RR, 2.14; 95% CI, 1.48-3.11; $P < 0.001$), and fetal malpresentation (RR, 6.24; 95% CI, 4.05–9.62; $P < 0.001$). Unification defects were associated with increased rates of preterm birth (RR, 2.97; 95% CI, 2.08–4.23; $P < 0.001$) and fetal malpresentation (RR, 3.87; 95% CI, 2.42–6.18; $P < 0.001$).[55] This systematic review found that canalization defects reduce fertility and increase rates of miscarriage and preterm delivery. None of the unification defects reduces fertility, but some are associated with miscarriage and preterm delivery. Arcuate uteri are specifically associated with 2nd trimester miscarriage.[55] All types of uterine anomalies are associated with renal anomalies. Women with a unicornuate uterus have the highest prevalence of renal anomalies, occurring in approximately 40%.[56]

BENEFITS OF HYSTEROSCOPIC METROPLASTY

As illustrated before, patients with congenital uterine anomalies have decreased reproductive potential and an unfavorable reproductive outcome compared to the population with normal uterine morphology. Although all uterine anomalies are associated with a multitude of reproductive complications, the only type amenable to definitive treatment is the septate uterus.[56] Hysteroscopic metroplasty has replaced the traditional laparotomy approach because of its minimal invasiveness, simplicity, safety, positive and satisfactory outcomes in pregnancy, and live birth rates. The aim of metroplasty is to restore a normal anatomy of the uterine cavity as a prerequisite for a successful implantation and subsequent good obstetrical outcomes. Following hysteroscopic metroplasty, term delivery rate increases from approximately 5 to 75%, and live birth rates increase from approximately 5 to 85%.[49]

Traditionally, hysteroscopy was required in patients with recurrent (≥3) miscarriages. The authors of this chapter believe that this approach should be changed with recent advances made by 3D US. In patients with history of only one or two miscarriages with septate uterus on 3D US, in whom there are no other identifiable causes for pregnancy loss, treatment should be considered at the time of US diagnosis, because endoscopic surgery is low risk and simple to perform.[12] However, septal incision is not always necessary and should be based on the patient's reproductive history and desires, the size of the septum, and consultation with specialists in the field of infertility and hysteroscopy. Decisions on when and whom to treat should be done on individual basis due to the of lack of prospective, randomized controlled trials. In patients with repeated abortions, it is important to rule out other potential causes such as genetic, endocrine, and metabolic abnormalities before proceeding with surgical treatment.

In patients with congenital uterine anomalies and primary infertility, the role of metroplasty continues to be controversial, and although some patients have been treated solely for this reason, the pregnancy rate in this subpopulation has been much lower than when the indication for metroplasty is pregnancy loss and/or other obstetrical complications.

In a study involving hysteroscopic examination of 60 patients after an early miscarriage, uterine anomalies (mainly an incomplete uterine septum) were found in one quarter of the cases.[57] The investigators concluded that a partial uterine septum is a major factor predisposing a patient to missed miscarriage. Thus, a history of missed miscarriage may be considered an indication for intervention. Cararach et al. suggested that coexisting associated features such as dysmenorrhea or abnormal bleeding should prompt earlier intervention.[58] Age is another consideration, because older women may benefit from prompt treatment to optimize outcome. Choe and Baggish suggested that the uterine septum should be corrected as early as possible, especially in patients more than 35 years of age, to increase fecundity.[59] Similar data on the impact of hysteroscopic metroplasty are obtained when analyzing the likelihood of subsequent preterm delivery. In women with a history of preterm delivery, treatment should be offered to reduce the likelihood of a recurrence. Daly et al. pointed out that in their series of patients, metroplasty prolonged the average gestation and improved perinatal outcome.[60]

More recently, Sendag et al. analyzed a total of 74 pregnancies before metroplasty.[61] Of these, 10 (14%) were carried to term, 6 (8%) ended in preterm delivery, and 58 (78%) ended in spontaneous abortion. At least 1 year following hysteroscopic metroplasty, a total of 20 pregnancies occurred. Of these, 11 (55%) were carried to term, 2 (10%) ended in preterm delivery, and 7 (35%) ended in spontaneous abortion. This study illustrated that correction of uterine septum significantly improves the prognosis of the pregnancies in patients with a history of severe obstetrical problems. Another study analyzed 115 patients on whom 129 hysteroscopic metroplasty interventions were performed over a 1 year period.[62] Patients and their reproductive outcome were monitored over a 2-year period and the same group served as a control group, taking into account their previous reproductive history before and after metroplasty. During a follow-up period of 2 years, 31 of 55 patients with previous fetal loss treated by hysteroscopic metroplasty, conceived pregnancy. There was a statistically significant decrease of abortion rate from 88.5 to 19.3%, and a significant increase in term delivery rate from 2.3 to 71%.[62]

Similar results were achieved in a review of 12 published retrospective studies by Homer et al. who compared reproductive outcome before and after hysteroscopic surgery.[63] Their comparative study showed a pooled postoperative pregnancy rate of 80% in women with miscarriage or infertility. In addition, the term birth rate increased from 7 to 73% after hysteroscopic metroplasty. In another systematic review and pooled analysis of 1,501 women in 18 studies, Nouri et al. reported an overall pregnancy rate of 60.1% and a live birth rate of 45% after hysteroscopic metroplasty.[64] A descriptive meta-analysis by Valle and Ekpo, showed a 63.5% pregnancy rate and a 50.2% live birth rate after hysteroscopic metroplasty of septate uterus.[65] These rates may certainly be higher in subjects with exclusive history of recurrent miscarriages in whom hysteroscopic metroplasty was performed. Future studies should focus on specific populations with clear indications with adequate follow-up period to allow accurate calculation of pregnancy and live birth rates.

Because congenital uterine anomalies are associated with certain types of obstetrical complications, these patients require differing degrees of surveillance during pregnancy (Fig. 11.25). Consultation or management by infertility specialist in the 1st trimester, and maternal-fetal medicine experts in the 2nd and 3rd trimesters of pregnancy should be considered. As previously documented, hysteroscopic metroplasty improves reproductive outcomes in women with a history of repeat adverse reproductive events, including fetal loss in the 1st and 2nd trimesters, as well as preterm labor. However, study by Agostini et al. revealed a higher rate of fetal malpresentation and lower birth weight in women who had term pregnancies after septal incision, suggesting that patients following hysteroscopic metroplasty should be appropriately counseled regarding the persisting risk of fetal malpresentation and other obstetrical risks.[66]

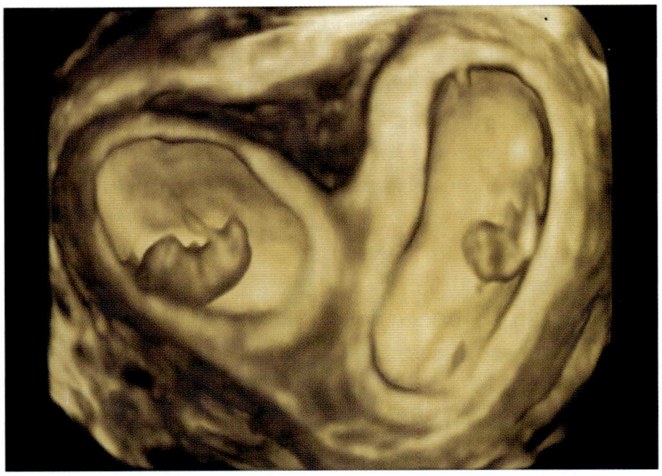

Fig. 11.25: The 3D ultrasound acquired volume of a septate uterus, rendered in surface mode shows twin pregnancy (one gestational sac in each horn of the uterus). Fundal indentation is less than 1 cm.

ROLE OF INTRA- AND POSTOPERATIVE IMAGING

In many institutions, hysteroscopic metroplasty is performed with laparoscopy, and more recently, with ultrasound guidance.[67,68] Unless women need laparoscopy for an associated pathology, ultrasound should be preferred over laparoscopy due to its lower price and no associated risk. Vigoreaux et al. compared the rates of reintervention, and immediate and later complications associated with abdominal ultrasound-guided versus unguided hysteroscopic metroplasty in the surgical repair of intrauterine septa.[68] Forty-six patients underwent abdominal ultrasound-guided metroplasty and sixty-two patients had unguided metroplasty. A persistent septum of more than 10 mm, defined by 3D US hysterosonography, with a need for reintervention, was found in 16 patients (39%) in the unguided group versus 7 patients (18.4%) in the ultrasound guidance group ($p = 0.04$). Results of this study indicate that the risk of a persistent septum after resection (>10 mm) is reduced with ultrasound guidance, as well as the need of reintervention for residual uterine septum.[68] Immediate and late complications (uterine perforation, bleeding, and infection) were also lower for patients with ultrasound guidance, compared to unguided group.

Ghirardi et al. attempted to use 2D and 4D transrectal ultrasonography to monitor hysteroscopic metroplasty and determine the completeness of septum resection.[69] The study group comprised of 27 patients in whom hysteroscopic metroplasty was performed using intraoperative 2D and 4D transrectal US monitoring, while the control group consisted of 18 patients who underwent hysteroscopic metroplasty without intraoperative ultrasound monitoring. During operative procedure of the study group, the ultrasound probe remained in the rectum and the uterus was imaged in sagittal and transverse sections, and the hysteroscopic procedure was continued until a normal uterine fundus was observed. Three months after the procedure, 3D US was performed to identify the number of residual septa. Result of this pilot study indicate that the number of suboptimal resections and incomplete resections was higher in the control group than in the study group ($p = 0.031$).[69]

Muzzii et al. used intraoperative 3D US during hysteroscopic metroplasty on 19 patients, and compared the outcomes of the procedure with 19 age-matched controls undergoing unguided surgeries.[70] In patients who were diagnosed intraoperatively with a residual septum, the procedure was continued until 3D US revealed a normal triangular uterine cavity. The patients were followed with a 3D US 3 months after the procedure. The numbers of complete resections (residual septum absent or <5 mm), of suboptimal resections (residual septum between 5 and 10 mm), and of incomplete resections (residual septum >10 mm) in the intraoperative 3D US group were compared to the numbers in the control group with no intraoperative 3D US. Residual septa of more than 5 mm were not detected in 3D US guidance group, versus 26% of the patients in the control group ($p = 0.04$). Residual septa of more than 10 mm were not detected in the 3D US group, versus 10.5% in the control group ($p = 0.48$). These data clearly indicate that 3D US guidance reduces the incidence of suboptimal septal incision during hysteroscopic metroplasty.

REFERENCES

1. Shipp TD. (2012). Ultrasound examination in obstetrics and gynecology. [online] Available from http://www.uptodate.com/contents/basic-principles-and-safety-of-diagnostic-ultrasound-in-obstetrics-and-gynecology. [Accessed July, 2012].
2. Jayaprakasan J, Chan YY, Sur S, Deb S, Clewes JS, Raine-Fenning NJ. Prevalence of uterine anomalies and their impact on early pregnancy in women conceiving after assisted reproduction treatment. Ultrasound in Obstetrics & Gynecology. 2011;37:727-32.
3. Iverson RE, DeCherney AH, Laufer MR. (2011). Clinical manifestations and diagnosis of congenital anomalies of

the uterus. [online] Available fromhttp://www.uptodate.com/contents/clinical-manifestations-and-diagnosis-of-congenital-anomalies-of-the-uterus.

4. Bermejo C, Martinez TP, Cantarero R, Diaz D, Pérez Pedregosa J, Barròn E, et al. Three-dimensional ultrasound in the diagnosis of Müllerian duct anomalies and concordance with magnetic resonance imaging. Ultrasound Obstet Gynecol. 2010;35:593-601.
5. Maneschi F, Zupi E, Marconi E, Valli E, Romanini C, Mancuso S. Hysteroscopically detected asymptomatic Müllerian anomalies: Prevalence and reproductive implications. J Rerpod Med. 1995;40(10):684-8.
6. Jurkovic D, Grueboeck K, Tailor A, Nicolaides KH. Ultrasound screening for congenital uterine anomalies. Br J Obstet Gyencol. 1997;104(11):1320-1.
7. Saravelos SH, Cocksedge KA. Prevalence and diagnosis of congenital uterine anomalies in women with reproductive failure: a critical appraisal. Hum Reprod Update. 2008;14(5):415-29.
8. Cogendez E, Dolgun ZN, Sanverdi I, Turgut E, Eren S. Post-abortion hysteroscopy: a method for early diagnosis of congenital and acquired intrauterine causes of abortions. Eur J Obstet Gynecol Reprod Biol. 2011;156(1):101-4.
9. Chan YY, Jayaprakasan K, Zamora J, Thornton JG, Raine Fenning N, Coomarasamy A. The prevalence of congenital uterine anomalies in unselected and high risk populations: a systematic review. Hum Reprod Update. 2011;17(6):761-71.
10. Dreisler E, Stampe Sorensen S. Müllerian duct anomalies diagnosed by saline contrast sonohysterography: prevalence in a general population. Fertil Steril. 2014;102(2):525-9.
11. Hassan NA, Lavery SA, Trew GH. Congenital uterine anomalies and their impact on fertility. Women's Health. 2010;6(3):443-61.
12. Kupesic S. Clinical implications of sonographic detection of uterine anomalies for reproductive outcome. Ultrasound Obstet Gynecol. 2001;18:387-400.
13. Lee DM, Osathanondh R, Yeh J. Localization of Bcl-2 in the human fetal Müllerian tract. Fertil Steril. 1998;70:135-40.
14. The American Fertility Society classifications of adnexal adhesions, distal tubal occlusion, tubal occlusion secondary to tubal ligation, tubal pregnancies, Müllerian anomalies, and intrauterine adhesions. Fertil Steril. 1998;49:944-55.
15. Freedman MF. Uterine abnormalities. Semin Reprod Endocrinol. 1986;4:39-54.
16. Buttram VC Jr, Gibbons WE. Müllerian anomalies: a proposed classification (an analysis of 144 cases). Fertil Steril. 1979;32:40-8.
17. Grimbizis G, Camus M, Clasen K, Tournaye H, De Munck L, Devroey P. Hysteroscopic septum resection in patients with recurrent abortions or infertility. Hum Reprod. 1998;13:1188-93.
18. Grimbizis GF, Gordts S, Di Spiezio Sardo A, Brucker S, De Angelis C, et al. The ESHRE-ESGE consensus on the classification of female genital tract congenital anomalies. Gynecol Sur. 2013;10(3):199-212.
19. Di Spiezio Sardo A, Campo R, Gordts S, Spinelli M, Cosimato C, Tanos V, et al. The comprehensiveness of the ESHRE/ESGE classification of female genital tract congenital anomalies: a systematic review of cases not classified by the AFS system. Hum Reprod. 2015;30(5):1046-58.
20. Graupera B, Pascual MA, Hereter L, Browne JL, Ubeda B, Rodriguez I, et al. Accuracy of three-dimensional ultrasound compared with magnetic resonance imaging in diagnosis of Müllerian duct anomalies using ESHRE-ESGE consensus on the classification of congenital anomalies of the female genital tract. Ultrasound Obstet Gynecol. 2015;46(5):616-22.
21. Grimbizis GF, Di Spiezio Sardo A, Saravelos SH, Gordts S, Exacoustos C, Van Schoubroeck D, et al. The Thessaloniki ESHRE/ESGE consensus on diagnosis of female genital anomalies. Hum Reprod. 2016;31(1):2-7.
22. Reichman DE, Laufer MR. Congenital uterine anomalies affecting reproduction. Best Pract Res Clin Obstet Gynaecol. 2010;24(2):193-208.
23. Nicolini U, Bellotti M, Bonazzi B, Zamberletti D, Candiani GB. Can ultrasound be used to screen uterine malformations? Fertil Steril. 1987;47:89-93.
24. Keltz MD, Olive DL, Kim AH, Arici A. Sonohysterography for screening in recurrent pregnancy loss. Fertil Steril. 1997;67:670-4.
25. Soares SR, Barbosa dos Reis MMB, Camargos AF. Diagnostic accuracy of sonohysterography, transvaginal sonography, and hysterosalpingography in patients with uterine cavity diseases. Fertil Steril. 2000;73:406-11.
26. Jurkovic D, Geipel A, Gruboeck K, Jauniaux E, Natucci M, Campbell S. Three-dimensional ultrasound for the assessment of uterine anatomy and detection of congenital anomalies: a comparison with hysterosalpingography and two-dimensional sonography. Ultrasound Obstet Gynecol. 1995;5:233-7.
27. Raga F, Bonilla-Musoles F, Blanes J, Osborne NG. Congenital Müllerian anomalies: diagnostic accuracy of three-dimensional ultrasound. Fertil Steril. 1996;65:523-8.
28. Moini A, Mohammadi S, Hosseini R, Eslami B, Ahmadi F. Accuracy of 3D sonography for diagnosis and classification of congenital uterine anomalies. J Ultrasound Med. 2013;32(6):923-7.
29. Ghi T, Casadio P, Kuleva M, Perrone AM, Savelli L, Giunchi S, et al. Accuracy of three-dimensional ultrasound in diagnosis and classification of congenital uterine anomalies. Fertil Steril. 2009;92(2):808-13.
30. Bocca SM, Oehninger S, Stadtmauer L, Agard J, Duran EH, Sarhan A, et al. A study of the cost, accuracy, and benefits of 3-dimensional sonography compared with hysterosalpingography in women with uterine abnormalities. J Ultrasound Med. 2012;31(1):81-5.
31. Turkgeldi E, Urman B, Ata B. Role of three-dimensional ultrasound in gynecology. J Obstet Gynaecol India. 2015;65(3):146-54.
32. Seshadri S, El-Toukhy T, Douiri A, Jayaprakasan K, Khalaf Y. Diagnostic accuracy of saline infusion sonography in the evaluation of uterine cavity abnormalities prior to assisted

reproductive techniques: a systematic review and meta-analyses. Hum Reprod Update. 2015;21(2):262-74.
33. Tabi S, Kupesic Plavsic S. The role of three-dimensional ultrasound in the assessment of congenital uterine anomalies. Donald School J Ultrasound Ob Gyn. 2012;6(4): 415-23.
34. Kupesic S, Kurjak A. Diagnosis and treatment outcome of the septate uterus. Croatian Med J. 1998;39:185-90.
35. Kupesic S, Kurjak A. Role of three-dimensional ultrasound in diagnosis of congenital uterine anomalies. Ultrasound Rev Obstet Gynecol. 2005;5:194-201.
36. Sparac V, Kurjak A, Kupesic S, Goldenberg M, Ilijas M, Skenderovic S, et al. Histological architecture and vascularization of intrauterine septa excised during hysteroscopic procedure. Gynecol Perinatol. 1996;5:101-3.
37. Kupesic S, Kurjak A, Skenderovic S, Bjelos D. Screening for uterine abnormalities by three-dimensional ultrasound improves perinatal outcome. J Prenat Med. 2002;30:9-17.
38. Nazzaro G, Locci M, Marilena M, Salzano E, Palmieri T, De Placido G. Differentiating between septate and bicornuate uterus: bi-dimensional and 3-dimensional power Doppler findings. J Minim Invasive Surg. 2014;21(5):870-6.
39. Sugiura-Ogasawara M, Ozaki Y, Katano K, Suzumori N, Mizutani E. Uterine anomaly and recurrent pregnancy loss. Semin Reprod Med. 2011;29(6):514-21.
40. Ludwin A, Pityński K, Ludwin I, Banas T, Knafel A. Two- and three-dimensional ultrasonography and sonohysterography versus hysteroscopy with laparoscopy in the differential diagnosis of septate, bicornuate, and arcuate uteri. J Minim Invasive Gynecol. 2013;20(1):90-9.
41. Dabirashrafi H, Bahadori M, Mohammad K, Alavi M, Moghadami-Tabrizi N, Zandinejad K, et al. Septate uterus: new idea on the histologic features of the septum in this abnormal uterus. Am J Obstet Gynecol. 1995;172:105-7.
42. Pellerito JS, McCarthy SM, Doyle MB, Glickman MG, DeCherney AH. Diagnosis of uterine anomalies: 605 relative accuracy of MR imaging, endovaginal sonography, and hysterosalpingography. Radiology. 1992;183:795-800.
43. Kupesic PS. Pelvic ultrasound pearls. In: Kupesic PS (Ed). Color Doppler, 3D and 4D Ultrasound in Obstetrics, Gynecology and Infertility. London, New Delhi, Panama City, St. Louis: Jaypee Publishers; 2011. pp. 256-348.
44. El Saman AM, Shahin AY, Nasr A, Tawfik RM, Saadeldeen HS, Othman ER, et al. Hybrid septate uterus, coexistence of bicornuate and septate varieties A genuine report. J Obstet Gynaecol Res. 2012;38:1308-14.
45. Trioani RN, McCarthy SM. Müllerian duct anomalies: Imaging and clinical issues. Radiology. 2004;233:19-34.
46. Benacerraf B, Goldstein SR, Groszmann YS. T shaped uterus. In: Benacerraf B, Goldstein SR, Groszmann YS (Eds). Gynecologic Ultrasound: A Problem Based Approach. Philadelphia: Elsevier/Saunders; pp. 189-91.
47. Fernandez H, Garbin O, Castaigne V, Gervaise A, Levaillant JM. Surgical approach to and reproductive outcome after surgical correction of a T-shaped uterus. Hum Reprod. 2011;26:1730-4.
48. Barranger E, Gervaise A, Doumerc S, Fernandez H. Reproductive performance after hysteroscopic metroplasty in the hypoplastic uterus: a study of 29 cases. Br J Obstet Gynaecol. 2001;101(12):1331-4.
49. Grimbizis GF, Camus M, Tarlatzis BC, Bontis JN, Devroey P, et al. Clinical implications of uterine malformations and hysteroscopic treatment results. Hum Reprod Update. 2001;7:161.
50. Reichman D, Laufer MR, Robinson BK. Pregnancy outcomes in unicornuate uteri: a review. Fertil Steril. 2009;91:1886.
51. Heinonen PK. Gestational hypertension and preeclampsia associated with unilateral renal agenesis in women with uterine malformations. Eur J Obstet Gynecol Reprod Biol. 2004;114:39.
52. Troiano RN, McCarthy SM. Müllerian duct anomalies: imaging and clinical issues. Radiology. 2004;233:19.
53. Lin PC, Bhatnagar KP, Nettleton GS, Nakajima ST. Female genital anomalies affecting reproduction. Fertil Steril. 2002;78:899.
54. Woelfer B, Salim R, Banerjee S, Elson J, Regan L, Jurkovic D. Reproductive outcomes in women with congenital uterine anomalies detected by three-dimensional ultrasound screening. Obstet Gynecol. 2001;98(6):1099-103.
55. Chan YY, Jayaprakasan K, Tan A, Thornton JG, Coomarasamy A, Raine-Fenning NJ. Reproductive outcomes in women with congenital uterine anomalies: a systematic review. Ultrasound Obstet Gynecol. 2011;38(4);371-82.
56. Benacerraf B, Goldstein SR, Groszmann YS. Müllerian Duct Anomalies. In: Benacerraf B, Goldstein SR, Groszmann YS. (Eds). Gynecologic Ultrasound: A Problem Based Approach. Philadelphia: Elsevier/Saunders; pp. 125-35.
57. Golan A, Schneider D, Avrech O, Raziel A, Bukovsky I, Caspi E. Hysteroscopic findings after missed abortion. Fertil Steril. 1992;58:508-10.
58. Cararach M, Penella J, Ubeda A, Labastida R. Hysteroscopic incision of the septate uterus: scissors versus resectoscope. Hum Reprod. 1994;9:87-97.
59. Choe KJ, Baggish SM. Hysteroscopic treatment of septate uterus with neodymium-YAG laser. Fertil Steril. 1992;57: 81-4.
60. Daly DC, Maier D, Soto-Albers C. Hysteroscopic metroplasty: six years' experience. Obstet Gynecol. 1989;73:201-5.
61. Sendag F, Mermer T, Yucebilgin S, Oztekin K, Bilgin O. Reproductive outcomes after hysteroscopic metroplasty for uterine septum. Clin Exp Obstet Gynecol. 2010;37(4); 287-9.
62. Tofoski G, Antovska V. Influence of hysteroscopic metroplasty on reproductive outcome in patients with infertility and recurrent pregnancy loss. Prilozi. 2014;35(2);95-104.
63. Homer HA, Li TC, Cooke ID. The septate uterus: a review of management and reproductive outcome. Fertil Steril. 2000;73:1-14.
64. Nouri K, Ott J, Huber JC, Fischer E. Reproductive outcome after hysteroscopic septoplasty in patients with septate uterus: a retrospective cohort study and systematic review of the literature. Reprod Biol Endocrinol. 2010;8:52.

65. Valle RF, Ekpo GE. Hysteroscopic metroplasty for the septate uterus: review and meta-analysis. Journal of Minimally Invasive Gynecology. 2013;20(1):22-42.
66. Agostini A, De Guilbert F, Salari K, Crochet P, Bretelle F, Gamerre M. Adverse obstetric outcomes at term after hysteroscopic metroplasty. Journal of Minimally Invasive Gynecology. 2009;16(4):454-7.
67. Garcia-Guzman R, Carasco M, Hernandez J, Puopolo M, Palumbo A. Safety and efficacy of ultrasound guided hysteroscopic metroplasty and subsequent infertility management: an observational study. Fertil Steril. 2013;100(3):S381.
68. Vigoreux S, Fernandeez H, Campas P, Levaillant JM, Legendre JM. Assessment of abdominal ultrasound guidance in hysteroscopic metroplasty. Journal of Minimally Invasive Gynecology. 2016;23(1):78-83.
69. Ghirardi V, Bizzarri N, Venturini P. Intraoperative bidimensional and 4D transrectal ultrasonography for hysteroscopic metroplasty. Journal of Minimally Invasive Surgery. 2014;21(6):S61.
70. Muzii L, Sereni MI, Cafa EV. Intraoperative three-dimensional ultrasound for hysteroscopic metroplasty: a controlled study. Journal of Minimally Invasive Gynecology. 2011;18(6):S80.

CHAPTER

12

Mild Ovarian Hyperstimulation and Intrauterine Insemination

Chaitanya Nagori, Sonal Panchal

INTRODUCTION

Intrauterine insemination (IUI) has attained a wide popularity in management of infertility. However, it is still the least standardized procedure as far as infertility management is concerned. IUI is blamed for low pregnancy rates but primary treatment with IUI is much more cost-effective than IVF.[1]

PRINCIPLE

In IUI, a bolus of potentiated normal motile sperms is placed in the uterus directly, bypassing the vaginal acidity and cervical hostility. This allows a safe quick access of the sperms to ova in the ampullary part of the oviduct.

Optimal guideline adherence has substantial economic benefits when compared with suboptimal guideline adherence.[2] The optimization is important at every step of the entire procedure, which includes patient selection according to correct indications, selection of stimulation (ovulation induction) protocol, ultrasound monitoring and deciding the time of trigger, semen preparation technique, IUI procedure and luteal support. This chapter will discuss each of these individually.

I. INDICATIONS OF IUI

Most Common Indications

- Unexplained infertility: In this group, mild ovarian stimulation with IUI improves the pregnancy rates significantly as compared to natural cycle IUI.[3] A multicentric study revealed that mild ovarian stimulation with IUI achieved pregnancy rate of 27% per cycle as compared to 15.2% with mild ovarian stimulation alone and 11.1% with spontaneous conception.[4]
- Dysovulatory infertility: Absolute pregnancy rate is higher with multifollicular compared to monofollicular growth.[5]
- Male subfertility: When the total motile sperm count before sperm preparation is >10 million, it is called mild male factor subfertility. Mild ovarian hyperstimulation with IUI is done in these cases.[6] Success rate with IUI are highest when 14% or more of the sperms have normal morphology, intermediate with values between 4 and 14% and generally quite poor when fewer than 4% of sperms are normal.[7]
  IUI is less expensive, less invasive, and comparably effective for selected patients as a first-line treatment for couples with unexplained or male factor infertility.[8]
- Mild to moderate endometriosis: These patients must be treated as those with unexplained subfertility and benefit with mild ovarian hyperstimulation with IUI, which results in 2–3 follicles.[9]

Other Uncommon Indications

- Cervical hostility: In these cases, natural cycle IUI may also be tried.[10]
- Immunological infertility: IUI is the first choice before IVF/ICSI.[11] "Cycle low dose prednisolone versus IUI revealed a pregnancy rate of 16.7% in IUI group while 0% in steroid group, in patients with immunological infertility.[12]"
- HIV +ve males with HIV –ve females: There have been no reported cases of HIV seroconversion in either partner or child after IUI in over 3,000 cycles, where male partner was HIV positive and female partner was HIV negative.[13]
- Single patent tube
- Ejaculatory failure
- Failed AID.
- Frozen samples: When husband is absent or on antineoplastic treatment.

II. OVULATION INDUCTION

Ovulation induction is required to improve the results of IUI. The aim here is to produce 2–3 follicles instead of one in natural cycle. This may be called mild ovarian stimulation or superovulation. More number of oocytes is made available for fertilization thus increasing the chances of conception. As several oocytes are released over protracted period, the fertilization window is also lengthened. Because of more oocytes, circulating steroids are increased; subtle hormonal deficiencies are corrected that improve chances of fertilization and implantation. Superovulation with IUI has higher pregnancy rates than after timed intercourse and clomiphene citrate.[14]

No stimulation

Pregnancy rates vary from 2 to 8% per cycle but it is always lower than the stimulated cycle. As stimulated cycles have higher multiple pregnancy rates, many centers including Bourn Hall Clinic, London, offers natural cycle IUI. In couples with cervical factor subfertility, IUI in natural cycles significantly increases the probability of conception.[15]

Clomiphene citrate

It can be given from day 5 to 9 in dosage of 50–100 mg/day. Balasch et al. showed 13% pregnancy rates in IUI cycles with late low dose follicle-stimulating hormone (FSH) as compared to 4% in CC induced cycles with IUI.[16]

Despite being more expensive, existing treatments such as empirical CC and unstimulated IUI do not offer superior birth rates compared with expectant management of unexplained infertility.[3,17] A UK RCT (Scottish unexplained Infertility trial, SUIT) compared the effectiveness of CC and IUI with that of expectant management and concluded that neither showed superior live birth rates compared with expectant management.[18] Higher pregnancy rates are obtained when IUI is combined with gonadotropins than with antiestrogen agents.[19]

Gonadotropins

The pregnancy rates are far better when IUI is combined with gonadotropins as compared to when IUI is combined with natural cycle, CC or CC + HMG.[20]

An analysis of 45 reports have shown that IUI in natural cycles have pregnancy rates of 4%, CC + IUI has a pregnancy rates of 6.7% and hMG + IUI has a pregnancy rate of 18%.[21] Another meta-analysis has clear shown gonadotropins to be more effective compared to CC.[19]

Gonadotropins are especially indicated for ovarian stimulation in IUI cycles in patients with hypogonadotropic hypogonadism as a substitutional therapy and in patients with CC resistance or CC failure. In polycystic ovarian failure (PCOS) patients chronic low dose protocol of gonadotropins with IUI has shown much better results than CC with IUI.[22]

Principles of Gonadotropin Therapy

The basic principles were suggested by Insler and Lunenfield in 1974.[2]

1. Effective dose: ovarian response is seen when certain dose of FSH is given. Below this dose the ovaries do not respond.
2. Latent phase: This phase lasts for 3–7 days. It starts with onset of stimulation, but there is no estrogen rise or ultrasound demonstrable follicular growth during this phase.
3. Active phase: This phase starts with ultrasound demonstrable follicle growth to ovulation and it lasts for 4–6 days.

Understanding of principles is essential to plan the optimal stimulation protocol for each patient. Effective dose for each patient may be different and may depend on ovarian volume, antral follicle count (AFC), ovarian blood flows and also on patients age and body mass index (BMI).[23,24] Having selected the appropriate dose for stimulation, the dose should not be increased during the latent period which may increase the risk of ovarian hyperstimulation.

Different regimes of gonadotropin therapy can be used depending on patient characteristics as discussed above.

1. Step up protocol (conventional protocol)
2. Step down protocol
3. Chronic low-dose protocol

   Though this has been also discussed in Chapters 4 and 5 of this book, a short mention on the same will be done here again.

1. Conventional Protocol

Gonadotropins are started from day 5 in patients with normal reserve normal responding ovaries on baseline scan. About 75 iu FSH is given daily from day 5 to 9. If follicle or endometrium grows, same dose is continued till follicular and endometrial maturity is achieved, otherwise the dose is doubled for 3–5 days. Gonadotropins are continued till you get the mature follicle or endometrium. This protocol has been blamed for higher rates of multiple pregnancies and ovarian hyperstimulation syndrome (OHSS).[25] But the risk of OHSS may be high only when this protocol is used for PCOS patients.

2. Step Down Protocol

If the baseline scan indicates a poor responding ovary, then stimulation is started with 150–225 iu till a follicle of 10 mm or larger appears. Then, the dose is decreased to 75 iu till we get a mature follicle and receptive endometrium.

3. Chronic Low-dose Protocol

This protocol is very useful in PCOS patients. This protocol gives good pregnancy rates with very little risk of OHSS or multiple pregnancies. But it is essential that PCOS is confirmed on baseline ultrasound scan. In this protocol, stimulation is started with 37.5 iu of FSH and same dose is continued for 14 days. If follicle or endometrium grows, the same dose is continued till mature follicle and endometrium are achieved otherwise the dose is increased by 37.5 IU for other 7 days. If follicle or endometrium grows, the same dose is continued till follicular and endometrial maturity otherwise the dose is again increased by 37.5 IU. Almost all the patients develop good follicle and endometrium and incidence of multiple pregnancy and OHSS is extremely low.[26] Majority of the patients develop good follicle within 14 days and dose should not be increased till 14 days even if there is no follicular or endometrial growth. There may be spotting or some bleeding during this period which should be ignored. With chronic low-dose protocol, there is monofollicular development in 70% of cycles, OHSS can be almost totally eliminated and multiple pregnancy rate less than 6% with same pregnancy rate as conventional protocol.[27]

Discussion about FSH and HMG has already been done in Chapters 4 and 5 of this book and Cochrane review in 2009 shows a nonsignificant higher live birth rate with HMG as compared to rFSH.[28] Recombinant products have been claimed to be superior to the urinary products.

Comparison of rFSH with uFSH

The study conducted by Hedan B clearly indicates superiority of rFSH.[29]

	rFSH	uFSH
Higher number of oocytes	10.8	8.9
Lower dose of FSH	2,138 IU	2,385 IU
Shorter period	10.7	11.3
High quality embryos	3.1	2.6
Pregnancy rate with cryopreservation	25.5%	20.4%

The meta-analysis conducted by Daya and Gunby of 12 randomized controlled trials has proved that rFSH is 20% more likely to achieve pregnancy than uFSH. The amount of FSH used was 400 IU less.[30]

Dose adjustability of rFSH and batch to batch consistency are definite advantages above urinary FSH.

4. Letrozole + Gonadotropins

This combination has been proved to be very effective in decreasing the consumption of gonadotropins, monofollicular development and low incidence of multiple pregnancy rates with equally high conception rates as those with only gonadotropins with IUI.

Letrozole is given from day 3 to 7. From day 7, FSH 75 IU is given daily for 5 days. Then, according to the findings on ultrasound monitoring, the dose is adjusted. This is an excellent combination for poor responders.

5. Role of GnRH Agonist and Antagonist in IUI Cycles

GnRH agonist is not used routinely in IUI protocols. It increases the total dose of gonadotropins, increases incidence of OHSS and multiple pregnancy rates. It has no advantage in IUI protocols and we never use them for IUI cycles.

GnRH antagonist may be used in IUI protocols. Adding GnRH antagonist in cycles with mild ovarian hyperstimulation in an IUI program does not increase live birth rate.[31] Though it is very useful in thin lean PCOS patients in whom LH is tonically high. Here antagonists are given when follicle size of 14 mm is reached, till the day of human chorionic gonadotropin (hCG). It prevents premature LH surge and improves the quality of ova and embryo, which in turn gives higher pregnancy rates.

III. ULTRASOUND MONITORING AND TIMING OF OVULATION TRIGGER

It is the key factor for achieving good conception rates with IUI. Using color Doppler in this assessment is mandatory because a large number of biochemical or hormonal changes occur during the cycle, and these reflect as vascular and morphological changes in ovaries and uterus and these vascular changes can be assessed by Doppler.

A follicle that grows to 12 mm is a dominant follicle, it grows at a rate of 2–3 mm/day and ovulation occurs at 18–24 mm size usually. Follicular flow can be first detected when follicular size is 10 mm,[32] and its resistance starts falling 2 days prior to ovulation.

Follicular maturity can be confirmed by following factors.[33]

Optimal Pre-hCG Follicular Parameters (Fig. 12.1)

1. Follicular diameter of at least 16 mm and 3–7 cc volume. The optimal size of the leading follicle in ovulation induction with CC and letrozole is the similar and is closely related to endometrial thickness.[16] The optimal size for the leading follicle has been suggested as 18–22 and 23–27 in different studies.[34,35]
2. Vascularity covering at least 3/4th of follicular circumference.
3. Perifollicular resistance index (RI): 0.4–0.48.[36]
4. Perifollicular PSV >10 cm/second
5. Follicular VI >6, FI >35.[37]
6. Presence of cumulus oophorus.[38]

Optimal Pre-hCG Endometrial Parameters (Fig. 12.2)

1. Endometrial thickness of at least 6 mm, preferably 8 mm.
2. Grade A/B endometrium.[39]
3. Endometrial vascularity in zone 3–4,[40] covering more than 5 mm^2. Endometrial RI: 0.49–0.59, PI: 1.1–2.3.
4. Uterine artery PI <3.2.[40]
5. Endometrial volume >3cc.
6. Endometrial FI >40, VFI >20.[37]

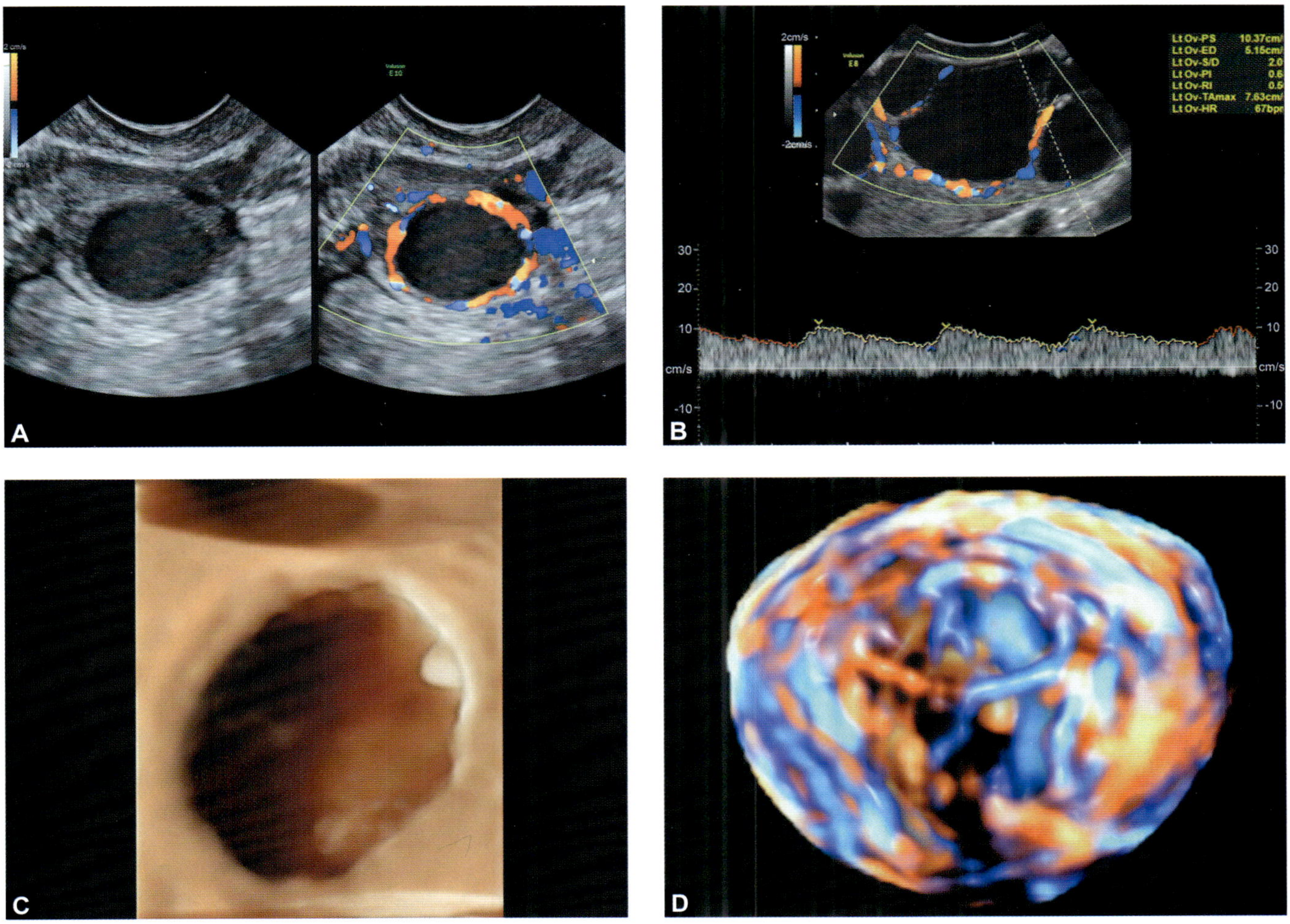

Figs. 12.1A to D: Ultrasound in follicle monitoring–pre-hCG.

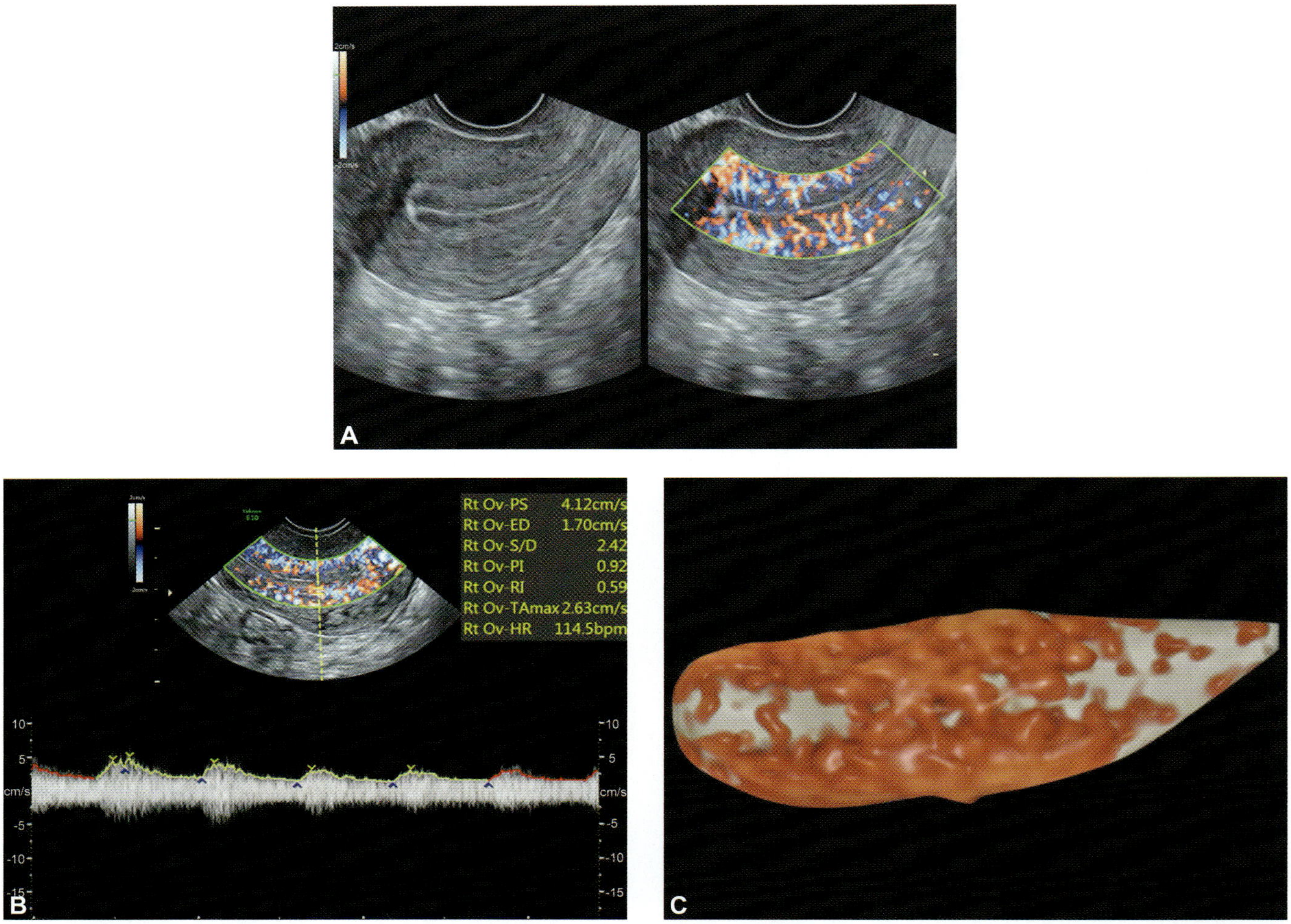

Figs. 12.2A to C: Ultrasound in endometrial monitoring–pre-hCG.

The details about the follicular and endometrial assessments have been mentioned in Chapter 13 of this book.

IV. OVULATION TRIGGER

Appropriate timing, adequate duration and amplitude of the mid-cycle LH surge are prerequisites for female fertility in humans. Ultrasound findings described above confirm follicular and endometrial maturity and also the time when the natural surge may start or when the surrogate surge may be administered. In unstimulated cycles, LH surge is natural and spontaneous. But in gonadotropin stimulated cycles, it is inconsistent both in occurrence and intensity and therefore a surrogate trigger is a must in these cases. And only the follicles in which the LH receptors have developed, will respond to this surrogate surge. The drugs that can be used as trigger are hCG and gonadotropin-releasing hormone agonist.

hCG is available in two forms—recombinant and urinary.

1. rhCG 250 IU is given when follicular and endometrial parameters are satisfied.
2. uhCG 10,000 IU.

hCG leads to high E2 and P because of corpus luteal stimulation and so no luteal phase defect. Effect lasts for 5–8 days and so it maintains corpus luteum more efficiently than endogenous LH. But it should not be forgotten that supraphysiological levels of estrogen and progesterone are detrimental for implantation.[41]

3. GnRH agonist:

   Leuprolide acetate 1 mg.

   Some advocate 1.5 mg 12 hours apart in two doses

   Some centers use 2 mg single dose, or

   Decapeptyl 1 mg.

It produces LH surge as efficiently as hCG. There is no difference in oocyte maturation and ovulation as compared to hCG.[42] Duration of surge is short, 24–36 hours as compared to natural LH surge and hCG. Lower doses of E2 and P and therefore good implantation. Short duration causes less corpus lutea and therefore reduces the risk of OHSS. It causes LPD because of early luteolysis. Additional 600 mg progesterone per day is required to support the luteal phase.[43] GnRH agonist is given in PCOS patients when there are multiple follicles and when OHSS is anticipated.

V. TIMING OF INSEMINATION

Timing of survival of ova is about 8–10 hours, maximum. Therefore, during that time spermatozoa should be surrounding the ovum. Urinary LH kit is useful to decide the LH surge but we have not found it to be useful. After pre-hCG follicular and endometrial maturity is assessed by ultrasound or by serum estradiol levels of more than 150 pg/mL/follicle, the trigger is administered. A prospective study has documented the time of follicular rupture 38.3 hours after the ovulation trigger.[44] Another randomised clinical study has shown a mean ovulation time of 40.4 hours.[45]

Literature shows the following timings of insemination:

1. 36–38 hours (between 32 and 38 hours)[46,47] (18 and 42 hours),
2. 24 hours and 48 hours,
3. 38 hours and 24 hours later if rupture is not seen on US.

A retrospective cohort study by Kucuk showed significantly higher cycle pregnancy rates after follicular rupture 36–38 hours post-hCG compared with that when follicle rupture was not evident.[48] Though another study has compared two different time slots for IUI after the trigger, 32–34 hours and 38–40 hours. The study results have shown no significant difference in the pregnancy rates between these two groups.[49]

Double Intrauterine Insemination

There are various papers that say that double IUI does not increase the pregnancy rates.[50] The Cochrane review also suggests that double IUI adds to cost and inconvenience without improving efficacy.[51] Though double IUI may improve pregnancy rates with double IUI in male factor subfertility.[51] These studies have been all done on unselected population. In a study done at our center in a selected subgroup has shown significantly increased pregnancy rates. This is based on the ultrasound Doppler parameters of follicle and endometrium and following the hormonal changes during ovulation thus.

The LH surge starts when PSV of the follicle is 10 cm/second. It gradually increases and reaches up to 45 cm/second before the rupture.[52] This means that when PSV of the follicle is higher follicle is not 36 hours away from rupture but is closer. This means if hCG is given at this time, follicle will not rupture at 36 hours but will rupture earlier and therefore IUI should be done earlier.

We have done a study of 500 superovulation with IUI cycles[53] with different stimulation protocols, viz. Clomiphene citrate, gonadotropins and letrozole with gonadotropins. We have found that no matter what stimulation protocol is used, if follicular PSV is more than 20 cm/second, double IUI (first one done between 14 and 16 hours after hCG and second done between 34 and 36 hours of hCG) gives significantly higher pregnancy rates as compared to single IUI done between 34 and 36 hours after hCG. This is because higher the PSV, earlier is the follicle likely to rupture.

VI. SEMEN PREPARATION

IUI must be done with the processed semen sample and never with a nit sample of semen. Using unwashed/non-processed semen leads to uterine cramps, infection and collapse. Sperm preparation aids in removing leukocytes, immotile, morphologically abnormal and dead sperms which generate free oxygen radicles and reduce the functional capacity of intact sperm. It removes the seminal plasma containing decapacitation factors and helps capacitation. Semen wash also helps remove pathogenic organisms. All together results in enrichment of functional sperm in terms of motility, DNA integrity, acrosome reaction and normal sperm morphology. Therefore, sperm preparation is an essential step in IUI.

It is essential to remember that before semen collection for IUI, the abstinence should not be more than 3–4 days. This increases the percentage of dead sperms in the sample. It is collected by aseptic technique in sterilized jar. Water or wet hands must not touch semen or inner surface of the jar. Ask the patient to clean and dry parts before collection. Possibly collection should be done in the premises, but if not the case, transport time from collection to incubator should not be more than 30 minutes. During transport semen should not be exposed to direct sunlight. Semen is allowed to stand in the incubator at 37°C temperature for liquefaction for 20–30 minutes. Semen is always analyzed for sperm count, motility and mortality before semen wash is initiated.

The commonly used semen preparation techniques are Swim up technique and gradient technique.

Swim up technique is based on migration principle. The self-propelled movement of sperms is a pre-requisite for this method. It is used for samples with normal count and motility. Swim up can be done from the ejaculate itself or from a pellet after centrifugation of the semen sample.

Gradient method which gives better recovery of sperms for IUI and conversion IVF. It is suitable for viscous samples as well as sample having more debris and WBCs and count is low. Dead and defective sperms and leukocytes produce ROS which cause lipid peroxidation of sperm membrane and decrease motility. These are best removed by gradient method. Debris and immotile sperms are held in between gradient layers. Because of head density sperms swim down and form pellet. Some studies have shown that the method is more useful when percentage of sperms with progressive motility is lower and proportion of sperms with good morphology is lower. Higher centrifugation for shorter interval will give good recovery of motile sperms, than when centrifugation is done at lower speed for longer time.

Whatever the method, there are variations in centrifugation time, speed and also the swim up time to be allowed for each sample depending on the semen parameters and the media used. The ultimate goal should be to achieve 8–10 million/mL post-wash sperm count.

There is a good chance of pregnancy, if 8 million or more motile sperms are available after appropriate selection methods. IUI performed with significantly higher numbers of motile sperms does not lead to a significant increase in pregnancy rates.[54] According to Balasch et al.,[55] minimum post-wash sperm count required for IUI is 2 million with 4% normal spermatozoa. But in our own series, highest pregnancy rates have been achieved when post-wash count is between 6 and 8 million.

VII. INTRAUTERINE INSEMINATION

IUI is done with all aseptic preparations. There is no need to use antiseptics or saline. The patient is in a lithotomy or lithotomy like position. Most literature suggests using Cusco's speculum to visualize the cervix and pass the IUI cannula through the external os, internal os and into the endometrial cavity. Though Sim's speculum may also be used and anterior lip of cervix may be steadied with Alyce's forceps. This helps to straighten the cervicouterine canal. It is easier to achieve the correct uterocervical canal axis and therefore it becomes easy to negotiate the IUI cannula through the cervix and beyond internal os. This also shortens the procedure time and thus also the time taken for the sperms from the incubator to the uterus, which is one of the important factors in deciding the success of IUI. The shorter this time, better are the results. The argument against holding the cervix with Alyce is that it stimulates uterine contractions and may lead to expulsion of the sperms from the endometrial cavity. But manipulation is also equally likely when it is difficult to negotiate through the internal os with Cusco's speculum. In our experience of more than 25 years and with more than 7,500 IUI pregnancies, we have always found Sim's speculum to be more convenient. Do not touch the endometrium with IUI cannula to avoid injury to endometrium. For this purpose, it is best to measure the uterocervical length by ultrasound on the preovulatory scan. This is measured in the midsagittal section of the uterus from the tip of the endometrial cavity to external os. The length of the IUI cannula inserted beyond the external os should be at least 1.5 cm short of this length. Some workers also prefer to place the tip of the IUI cannula just beyond the internal os.

Various IUI cannulas are available in the market and there is no one choice that is claimed to have better results than the others. The selection is up to the clinician's convenience. The cannula is attached to the syringe and then the tip is dipped just below the upper surface of the prepared semen sample and is aspirated to fill up the cannula with an air column between the rubber cock of the syringe and the washed semen sample column. Not more than 0.3–0.7 mL of wash sample is put inside the uterine cavity slowly. Using larger volumes may cause spilling out of the wash sample.

Allow the patient to rest for 15 minutes. About 10–15 minutes of immobilization after IUI significantly improves cumulative ongoing pregnancy rates and live birth rates.[56]

VIII. LUTEAL SUPPORT

Luteal support is an absolute must when ovulation induction is done with gonadotropins. It has been already discussed in Chapters 4 and 5 that when gonadotropins are used for ovulation induction, the progesterone production and corpus luteal function may be inconsistent and therefore in these cases luteal phase support is mandatory. It is usually started on the day following IUI. It is thought that starting progesterone on the day of IUI might quiescent the uterus and may prevent sperm transfer to the tubes for fertilization. The most preferred protocols for luteal support are:

1. 200 mg bd, progesterone effervescent tablets
2. 300–400 mg bd micronized progesterone vaginal pessaries.
3. Luteal phase support with vaginal progesterone significantly improves the live birth rates in IUI cycles with gonadotropins stimulation.[57] But it does not improve pregnancy rates in normo-ovulatory women stimulated with clomiphene citrate for IUI.[58]

But progesterones are available in different forms: synthetic and natural and among the natural also injectable forms (intramuscular-oil-based and subcutaneous water-based formulations), vaginal pessaries, vaginal cream, etc. several products are available and any can be used depending on the convenience of the patient, with almost equal results. Advantages of using vaginal progesterone are that it gives a stable plasma concentration and consistent tissue levels. Its first uterine pass effect facilitates targeted delivery into endometrium and has minimal side effects.

Different progesterones are:

1. Synthetic progesterones:
   - These are medroxy progesterone acetate and dihydrogesterone.
   - Vaginal micronized progesterone is significantly more effective than oral dihydroprogesterone in creating "in-phase secretory endometrium."[59,60]
2. Natural progesterones:
   - Not commonly used routes:
     - Intranasal
     - Sublingual
     - Rectal
   - Commonly used routes:
     - Oral
     - Intramuscular
     - Vaginal routes

Another drug used as a luteal support is human chorionic gonadotropin. The two protocols conventionally used were hCG 5,000 iu on day 5 and day 9 after IUI and hCG 2,000 iu on day 3–7–10 after IUI. It stimulates theca cells to produce more progesterone. It also increases other steroids from corpus luteum and ovary which are helpful for maintenance of pregnancy.[61] It is not preferred lately for the fear of ovarian hyper stimulation syndrome (OHSS). But in IUI with monofollicular development or 2–3 follicles developed the chances of OHSS is almost nil even when hCG is used as a luteal support. Moreover, since agonist can be used for ovulation trigger, hCG in these patients can be used in the dose of 1,500 iu on the day of IUI and then day 5 and 9 of IUI as a luteal phase support.[62] It should not be given when E2 is more than 2,500 pgm/mL in IUI cycles.

Factors that may affect the success rates of IUI:

1. Age: Success rate of IUI sharply decreases after 40 years of age of the female partner.[63] It has been observed that increasing male age seems to be associated with decline in semen volume, sperm motility and sperm morphology but not with sperm concentration.[64] This has a synergistic adverse effect when female partner is also above 35 years.[37] If the morphology score is more than 4%, IUI can be performed with an acceptable success rate even if the IMC (insemination motile count) is more than 1 million.[65] Couples with mild male subfertility, unexplained fertility or mild endometriosis show acceptable cumulative ongoing pregnancy rates after six cycles of IUI with ovarian hyperstimulation.[66]
2. Number of cycles: Pregnancy rate per cycle is highest in the first three treatment cycles.[67] Retrospective analyses of IUI data using life table analysis showed a relatively constant probability of becoming pregnant after each IUI treatment through six cycles which thereafter was hardly increased by continuing longer.[68]

There are very limited studies where more than nine cycles are attempted. Pregnancy rate after six cycles was 30% and after nine cycles it was 41% in this study by Custers et al. They showed a stable pregnancy rate between 6 and 9 months. And finally concluded that if time is not an issue some couples could be offered nine treatment cycles especially couples in which female age is below 35 years.[56]

COMPLICATIONS

Complications are very few and very rare. If at all may occur due to superovulation or incorrect semen wash. Those due to superovulation are OHSS and multiple pregnancy. Those due to incorrect semen wash are infection and pain in abdomen.

CARRY-HOME MESSAGE

1. IUI is the preferred method for dysovulatory infertility, idiopathic infertility or mild male subfertility.
2. Mild ovarian stimulation with gonadotropins is done for best results.
3. Letrozole + FSH give results comparable to gonadotropins alone.

4. Ultrasound monitoring by color Doppler improves results.
5. Ultrasound helps to decide the time of IUI.
6. Semen preparation should be meticulous and should be modified depending on the semen quality.
7. Luteal support is a must in mild ovarian stimulation with IUI.

REFERENCES

1. Goverde AJ, McDonnell J, Vermeiden JP, Schats R, Rutten FF, Schoemaker J. Intrauterine insemination or *in vitro* fertilization in idiopathic subfertility and male subfertility: a randomised trial and cost-effectiveness analysis. Lancet. 2000;355:13-8.
2. Haagen EC, Nelen WLDM, Adang EM, Grol RPTM, Hermens RPMG, Kremer JAM. Guideline adherence is worth the effort: a cost-effectiveness analysis in intrauterine insemination care. Hum Reprod. 2013;28(2):357-66.
3. Verhulst SM, Cohlen BJ, Hughes E, Te VE, Heineman MJ. Intrauterine insemination for unexplained subfertility. Cochrane Database Syst Rev. 2006;(4):CD001838.
4. Crosigani PG, Walters DE, Soliani A. The ESHRE multicentric trial on the treatment of unexplained infertility: a preliminary report. Human Reprod. 1991;6(7):953-8.
5. Van Ruste MM, Custers IM, Van der Veen F, van Wely M, Evers JL, Mol BW. The influence of number of follicles on pregnancy rates in intrauterine insemination with ovarian stimulation: a meta-analysis. Hum Reprod Update. 2008;14: 563-70.
6. Van Weert JM, Repping S, Van Voorhis BJ, Van der Veen F, Bossyut PM, Mol BW. Performance of post wash total motile sperm count as a predictor of pregnancy at the time of intrauterine insemination: a meta-analysis. Fertil Steril. 2004;82(3):612-20.
7. Lee RK, Hou JW, Ho HY, Hwu YM, Lin MH, Tsai YC, et al. Sperm morphology analysis using strict criteria as a prognostic factor in intrauterine insemination. Int J Androl. 2002;25:277
8. Abdelrahman M, Abdelkader M, John Yeh. The potential use of intrauterine insemination as a basic option for infertility: a review for technology limited medical settings. Obstet Gynecol Int. 2009;2009:584837.
9. Werbrouck E, Spiessens C, Meuleman C, D'Hooghe T. No difference in cycle pregnancy rate and in cumulative live-birth rate between women with surgically treatment minimal to mild endometriosis and women with unexplained infertility after controlled ovarian hyperstimulation and intrauterine insemination. Fertil Steril. 2006;86:566-71.
10. Steures P, van der Steeg JW, Verhoeve HR, van Dop PA, Hompes PGA, Bossuyt PMM. Does ovarian hyperstimulation in intrauterine insemination for cervical factor subfertility improve pregnancy rates? Hum Reprod. 2004;19: 2263-66.
11. Ombelet W, Vandeput H, Janssen M, Cox A, Vossen C, Pollet H, et al. Treatment of male infertility due to sperm surface antibodies: IUI or IVF? Hum Reprod. 1997;12(6); 1165-70.
12. Lahteenmaki A, Rasanen M, Hovatta O. Low dose prednisolone does not improve the outcome of *in vitro* fertilization in male immunological infertility. Hum Reprod. 1995;10(12):3124-9.
13. Gilling-Smith C, Almeida P. HIV, hepatitis B and hepatitis C and infertility: Reducing risk. Hum Fertil. 2003;6:106-12.
14. Hughes EG. Stimulated intra-uterine insemination is not a natural choice for the treatment of unexplained subfertility. Hum Reprod. 2003;18(5):912-4.
15. Steures P, Van der Steeg JW, Hopes PG, Bossyut PM, Habbema JD, Eijkmans MJ, et al. Effectiveness of intrauterine insemination in subfertile couples with an isolated cervical factor. A randomised clinical trial. Fertil Steril. 2007;88(6):1692-6.
16. Balasch J, Ballesca JL, Pimentel C, Creus M, Fábregues F, Vanrell JA. Late low dose pure follicle stimulating hormone for ovarian stimulation in intrauterine insemination cycles. Hum Reprod. 1994;9(10):1863-6.
17. Wordsworth S, Buchanan J, Mollison J, Harrild K, Robertson L, Tay C, et al. Clomiphene citrate and intrauterine insemination as first line treatments for unexplained infertility: are they cost-effective? Hum Reprod. 2011;26(2):369-75.
18. Bhattacharya S, Harrild K, Mollison J, Wordsworth S, Tay C, Harrold A, et al. Clomiphene citrate or unstimulated intrauterine insemination compared with expectant management for unexplained infertility: pragmatic randomised controlled trial. BMJ. 2008;337:a716.
19. Cantineau AE, Cohlen BJ, Heineman MJ. Ovarian stimulation protocols (anti-estrogens, gonadotrophins with and without GnRH agonists/antagonists) for intrauterine insemination (IUI) in women with subfertility. Cochrane Database Syst Rev. 2007;(2):CD005356.
20. Mahani IM, Afnan M. The pregnancy rates with intrauterine insemination (IUI) in superovulated cycles employing different protocols (clomiphene citrate (CC), human menopausal gonadotrophin (HMG) and HMG+CC) and in natural ovulatory cycle. J Pak Med Assoc. 2004;54(10):503-5.
21. Guzick DS, Sullivan MW, Adanson GD, Cedars MI, Falk RJ, Peterson EP, et al. Efficacy of treatment for unexplained infertility. Fertil Steril. 1998;70:207-13.
22. Homborg R, Hendriks ML, König TE, Anderson RA, Balen AH, Brincat M, et al. Clomifene citrate or low dose FSH for the first-line treatment of infertile women with anovulation associated with polycystic ovary syndrome: a prospective randomised multinational study. Hum Reprod. 2012;27(2):468-73.
23. Kupesic S, Kurjak A. Predictors of IVF outcome by three-dimensional ultrasound. Hum Reprod. 2002;17(4):950-5.
24. Panchal S, Nagori CB. Ultrasound based decision making on stimulation protocol for superovulated IUI cycles. IJIFM. 2016;7(1):7-13.
25. Westergard LG, Erb K, Laursen SB, Rex S, Rasmussen PE. HMG versus rFSH in normogonadotrophic women down regulated with gonadotrophic releasing hormone agonist who were undergoing IVF and ICSI, a prospective randomised study. Fertil Steril. 2001;76(3):543-9.

26. Homburg R, Levy T, Ben-Rafael Z. A comparative prospective study of conventional regimen with chronic low dos administration of follicle stimulating hormone for anovulation associated with polycystic ovary syndrome. Fertil Steril. 1995;63(4):729-33.
27. Driebergen R, Baer G. Quantification of follicle stimulating hormone (follitropin alpha): is *in vivo* bioassay still relevant in recombinant age? Curr Med Res Opin. 2003;19:41-6.
28. van Wely M, Kwan I, Burt AL, Thomas J, Vail A, Van der Veen F, Al-Inany HG. Recombinant FSH versus urinary gonadotrophins for ovarian hyperstimulation in IVF and ICSI cycles. A systematic review and meta-analysis. Hum Reprod. 2009;24(S1):i134.
29. Hedon B, Out HJ, Hugues JN, Camier B, Cohen J, Lopes P, et al. Efficacy and safety of recombinant follicle stimulating hormone (Puregon) in infertile women pituitary suppressed with triptorelin undergoing in-vitro fertilization: a prospective randomized, assessor-blind, multicentre trial. Hum Reprod. 1995;10:3102-6.
30. Daya S, Gunby. Systematic review and meta-analysis of randomized, controlled trials comparing rFSH and uFSH. Fertil Steril. 2002;77(4):711-4.
31. Cantineau AEP, Cohlen BJ, Klip H, Heineman MJ, the Dutch IUI study Group Collaborators. The addition of GnRH antagonists in intrauterine insemination cycles with mild ovarian hyperstimulation does not increase live birth rates—a randomised, double-blinded, placebo-controlled trial. Hum Repord. 2011;26(5):1104-11.
32. Bourne T, Jurkovic D, Waterstone J, Campbell S, Collins WP. Intrafollicular blood flow during human ovulation. Ultrasound Obstet Gynecol. 1991;1:53-9.
33. Panchal S, Nagori C. Pre-hCG 3D and 3D power Doppler assessment of the follicle for improving pregnancy rates in intrauterine insemination cycles. Journal of Human reproductive sciences. 2009;2(2):62-67.
34. Palatnik A, Strawn E, Szabo A, Robb P. What is the optimal follicular size before triggering ovulation in intrauterine insemination cycles with clomiphene citrate or letrozole? An analysis of 988 cycles. Fertil Steril. 2012;97:1089-94.
35. Farhi J, Orvieto R, Gavish O, Homburg R. The association between follicular size on hCG day and pregnancy rate in clomiphene citrate treated polycystic ovary syndrome patients. Gynecol Endocrinol. 2010;26:546-8.
36. Kupesic S, Kurjak A. Uterine and ovarian perfusion during the periovulatory period assessed by transvaginal colour Dopler. Fertil Steril. 1993;3:439-43.
37. Panchal SY, Nagori CB. Can 3D PD be a better tool for assessing the pre HCG follicle and endometrium? A randomized study of 500 cases. Presented at 16th World Congress on Ultrasound in Obstetrics and Gynecology, 2006, London. J Ultrasound Obstet Gynecol. 2006;28(4):504.
38. Feichtinger W. Transvaginal three dimensional imaging for evaluation and treatment of infertility. In: Merz E (Ed). 3D Ultrasound in Obstetrics and Gynecology. Philadelphia: Lippincott Williams and Wilkins; 1998. pp. 37-43.
39. Gonen Y, Caspers RF. Prediction of implantation by the sonographic appearance of the endometrium during controlled ovarian stimulation for IVF. J *In Vitro* Fertil Embryo Transfer. 1990;7:46.
40. Applebaum M. The 'steel' and 'teflon' endometrium-ultrasound visualization of endometrial vascularity in IVF patients and outcome. Presented at The third World Congress of Ultrasound in Obstetrics and Gynecology. Ultrasound Obstet Gynecol. 1993;3(Suppl 2):10.
41. Gidley-Baird AA, O'Neill C, Sinosich MJ, Porter RN, Pike IL, Saunders DM. Failure of implantation in human in-vitro fertilization and embryo-transfer patients: the effects of altered progesterone/estrogen ratios in human and mice. Fertil Steril. 1986;45:69-74.
42. Iskovitz J, Boldes R, Barlev A, Erlik Y, Kahana L, Brandes JM. The induction of LH surge and oocyte maturation by GnRH analogue (Buserelin) in women undergoing ovarian stimulation for *in vitro* fertilization. Gynecol Endocrinol. 1988;2(Suppl):165.
43. Albano C, Smitz J, Camus M. Comparison of different doses of gonadotrophin-releasing hormone antagonist Cetrorelix during controlled ovarian hyperstimulation. Fertil Steril. 1997;67:917-22.
44. Anderson AG, Als-Neilsen B, Hoennes PJ, Franch Andersen L. Time interval from human chorionic gonadotrophin (hCG) injection to follicular rupture. Hum Reprod. 1995;10:3202-5.
45. Fischer RA, Nakajima ST, Gibson M, Brumsted JR. Ovulation after intravenous and intramuscular human chorionic gonadotrophin. Fertil Steril. 1993;60:418-22.
46. The ESHRE Capri Workshop Group. Intrauterine insemination. Hum Reprod Update. 2009;15:265-77.
47. Ragni G, Somigliana E, Vegetti W. Timing of intrauterine insemination: where are we are? Fertil Steril. 2004:82;25-6.
48. Kucuk T. Intrauterine insemination: is the timing correct? J Assist Reprod Genet. 2008;8:427-30
49. Claman P, Wilkie V, Collins D. Timing intrauterine insemination either 33 or 39 hours after administration of human chorionic gonadotrophin yields the same pregnancy rates as after superovulation therapy. Fertil Steril. 2004;82:13-6.
50. Bagis T, Haydardedeoglu B, Kilicdag EB, Cok T, Simsek E, Parlakgumus AH. Single versus double intrauterine insemination in multi-follicular ovarian hyperstimulation cycles: a randomised trial. Hum Reprod. 2010;25:1684-90.
51. Cantineau AEP, Heineman MJ, Cohlen BJ. Single versus double intrauterine insemination in stimulated cycles for subfertile couples. Cochrane database Syst Rev. 2003;(1):CD003854.
52. Bourne TH. Transvaginal colour Doppler in gynecology. Ultrasound Obstet Gynecol. 1991;1:359-373.
53. Nagori C, Panchal S. Role of double IUI in patients with high perifollicular PSV. 16th World Congress on Ultrasound in Obstetrics and Gynecology, September 2006, London.
54. Van Voorhis BJ, Barnett M, Sparks AE, Syrop CH, Rosenthal G, Dawson J. Effect of total motile sperm count in the efficacy and cost-effectiveness of intrauterine insemination and *in vitro* fertilization. Fertil Steril. 2001;75(4):661-8.
55. Balasch J. Intrauterine insemination. In: Balasch J, Homburg R (Eds). Practical guide to PCOS and IUI. p. 34.

56. Custers IM, Steures P, Hompes P, Flierman P, van Kasteren Y, van Dop PA, et al. Intrauterine insemination: how many cycles should we perform? Hum Reprod. 2008;23(4):885-8.
57. Erem AA, Erdem M, Atmaca S, Guler I. Impact of luteal phase support on pregnancy rates in intrauterine insemination cycles: a prospective randomised study. Fertil Steril. 2009;91:2508-13.
58. Kyrou D, Fatei HM, Tournaye H, Devroey P. Luteal phase support in normo-ovulatory women stimulated with clomiphene citrate for intrauterine insemination: need or habit? Hum Reprod. 2010;25:2501-6.
59. Fatemi HM, Camus M, Kolibianakis EM, Tournaye H, Papanikolaou EG, Donoso P, et al. The luteal phase of recombinant follicle-stimulating hormone/gonadotrophin releasing hormone antagonist *in vitro* fertilization cycles during supplementation with progesterone or progesterone and oestradiol. Fertil Steril. 2007;87:504-8.
60. Fatemi HM, Popovic-Todorovic B, Papanikolaou E, Donoso P, Dervroey P. An update of luteal phase support in stimulated IVF cycles. Hum Reprod Update. 2007;13:581-90.
61. Nosarka S, Kruger T, Seibert I, Grove D. Luteal phase support in *in vitro* fertilization: meta-analysis of randomised trials. Gynecol Obstet Invest. 2005;60:67-74.
62. Humadian P, Ejdrup Bredkjaer H, Westergard LG, Yding Andersen C. 1500 iu human chorionic gonadotrophin administered at oocyte retrieval recues the luteal phase when gonadotrophin-releasing hormone agonist is used for ovulation induction: a prospective, randomized, controlled study. Fertil Steril. 2010;93:847-54.
63. Broekmans FJ, Soules MR, Fauser BC. Ovarian aging: mechanisms and clinical consequences. Endocr Rev. 2009;30(5):465-93.
64. Kidd SA, Eskenazi B, Wyrobak AJ. Effects of male age on semen quality and fertility: a review of literature. Fertil Steril. 2001;75(2):237-48.
65. Mathieu C, Ecochard R, Bied V, Lornage J, Czyba JC. Cumulative conception rate following intrauterine artificial insemination with husband's spermatozoa: influence of husband's age. Hum Reprod. 1995;10(5):1090-7.
66. Aboulghar M, Mansour R, Serour G, Abdrazek A, Amin Y, Rhodes C. Controlled ovarian hyperstimulation and intrauterine insemination for treatment of unexplained infertility should be limited to a maximum of three trials. Fertil Steril. 2001;75(1):88-91.
67. Ombelet W, Vandeput H, Van de Putte G, Cox A, Janssen M, Jacobs P, et al. Intrauterine insemination after ovarian stimulation with clomiphene citrate: predictive potential of inseminating motile count and sperm morphology? Hum Reprod. 1997;12:1458-63.
68. Wallach EE. Gonadotrophin treatment for ovulatory patient: pros and cons of empiric therapy for infertility. Fertil Steril. 1991;55:478-80.

CHAPTER

Ultrasound in a Treatment Cycle

13

Sonal Panchal

INTRODUCTION

Ultrasound has long been considered now to be the modality of choice for monitoring of the patients on treatment for infertility, may it be (IUI) cycles or *in vitro* fertilization (IVF) cycles. The reason for this is that it is patient friendly, easy to use repeatedly, and is financially also viable. Moreover, when used with Doppler, it gives precise idea not only about the morphological changes but also about the hormonal changes occurring during the entire cycle. It is important to mention here that ultrasound is the modality that gives idea about the instantaneous status, unlike the hormonal assessment reports, that take a few hours to give the results.

The discussion about of the role of ultrasound during the entire treatment cycle will be divided into three parts:

1. Baseline scan and deciding the stimulation protocol
2. Preovulatory scan and decision on trigger
3. Luteal phase scan

Baseline Scan and Deciding the Stimulation Protocol

This scan is done when hormonal levels are at baseline on day 2–3 of the menstrual cycle. The ovaries are silent, and have no active follicle or corpus luteum at this stage. Route of scan has to be transvaginal always to allow better resolution and more anatomical details of ovary and endometrium. All the scans are done using B mode ultrasound with color Doppler, pulse Doppler, three-dimensional (3D) ultrasound and 3D power Doppler. Using color Doppler in this assessment is mandatory because a large number of biochemical or hormonal changes occur during the menstrual cycle, which reflect as vascular and morphological changes in the ovaries and uterus and vascular changes can be assessed by Doppler.

One of the earliest studies, by Ravhon et al.[1] has used dynamic assessment of inhibin B and estradiol after buserelin acetate as predictors of ovarian response and have found these to be highly correlating with the ovarian response in IVF patients. The two major drawbacks of this study are that this required several blood tests at different times and the study sample was pretty small (n = 37).

In 2002, Kupesic et al.[2] used 3D ultrasound for assessment of ovarian response in IVF cycles. The antral follicle count (AFC) and ovarian stromal flow parameters on the baseline scan were shown to be most predictive of the ovarian response after pituitary downregulation in this study, followed by total ovarian volume, ovarian stromal area, and age. This study could predict favorable IVF outcome in 50% (11/22) of patients and poor outcome in 85% (29/34) of patients. Though the study results were fairly convincing, the sample volume was only 56 patients. Popovic-Todorovic et al.,[3] in 2003 combined age, body mass index (BMI), cycle length, smoking status, and ultrasound features of the ovaries also to design a dosage nomogram of recombinant follicle-stimulating hormone (rFSH) for IVF/ICSI patients. This was a prospective study and also had a larger sample volume than the previous two studies (n = 145). According to this study, total number of antral follicles and ovarian stromal blood flow were the two most significant predictors of ovarian response, and ovarian volume was highly significant predictor of number of follicles and oocytes retrieved. Using this nomogram for dose calculation was evaluated by the same group in another study. The results of this study were in absolute favor of individualizing dose according to the dosage nomogram proving the reliability of ultrasound parameters, age, and BMI for decision on stimulation doses. Whereas a study by Ng et al.[4] showed basal FSH to be the most reliable parameter for assessment of ovarian response followed by AFC and BMI, where AFC was predictive of number of follicles (S. estradiol level) on the day of hCG, and BMI was predictive of gonadotropins dosage.

Another landmark study by Olivennes and Howles et al.,[5] The CONSORT study, used basal FSH, BMI, age, and AFC for individualizing FSH dose for ovarian stimulation.

A dose calculator was developed using these factors as predictors and was evaluated in a prospective clinical trial.

An ultrasound based study on prediction of ovarian response in 2007 by Merce et al.[6] evaluated ovarian volume, AFC, and 3D power Doppler indices vascularization index (VI), flow index (FI), and vascularity flow index (VFI) for their reliability to calculate the number of follicles grown, oocytes retrieved, and embryos transferred.

This study clearly showed the relevance of ovarian volume and AFC to the number of follicles matured and oocytes retrieved. It also mentioned that 3D power Doppler indices made the assessment of ovarian response to stimulation protocols easier.

The only study that worked on the dose calculations for IUI patients was by Freiesleben NL et al.[7] in 2008 with 159 patients. They evaluated age, spontaneous cycle length, body weight, BMI, smoking status, total ovarian volume, AFC, total Doppler score of ovarian stromal blood flow, baseline FSH, and estradiol as possible predictive factors of ovarian response. This study concluded that body weight and AFC may be used to achieve appropriate ovarian response for IUI in ovulatory patients. Study by the same investigators for IVF and intracytoplasmic sperm injection (ICSI) patients concluded that AFC and age could predict the low response better, whereas to predict hyper-response, AFC and cycle length were better parameters.

The parameters that we have used to calculate the dose for gonadotropins stimulation protocol for IUI cycles in our study are: age, BMI, AFC, ovarian volume, stromal RI, and PSV.

Antral follicle count showed the best correlation with women's age and declines linearly at a rate of 3.8% per year.[8]

Antral follicle count declines at a rate of 4.8% per year before the age of 37 years and declines at rate of 11.7% after 37 years.[9]

Anti-Müllerian hormone (AMH) and AFC both have reflections of primordial follicles and both are stable between cycles.[10]

Linear correlation is seen between AFC and AMH and both help to predict the extremes of response. Therefore, we have included AFC as one of the parameters for ovarian reserve and omitted AMH. Age is known to be one of the most important factors that reduce not only the ovarian reserve but also the oocyte quality. It has been shown in several studies above mentioned that BMI may be an important determinant of the ovarian response. This is because flow in the ovarian stroma is less in obese patients as compared to controls.[10]

A study indicates that AFC is the most useful marker in predicting the ovarian response. Doing AFC assessment alone would be more cost effective for predicting the ovarian response in patients undergoing controlled ovarian stimulation with gonadotropin-releasing hormone (GnRH) antagonist. AFC had the highest accuracy for predicting ovarian response in patients with abnormal ovarian reserve test and was statistically significant (number of oocyte aspirated, $p = <0.001$) than AMH ($p = 0.06$) and FSH ($p = 0.212$) in predicting ovarian response. For prediction of poor ovarian response, a model including AFC + AMH was found to be almost similar to that of ($p = 0.001$) using AFC alone.[11]

Precise calculation of AFC, therefore, can help in predicting the ovarian response. This can be done on 2D ultrasound or by 3D with inversion mode rendering, and Sono-AVC (a specialized 3D ultrasound software for calculation of antral follicle number and volumes). This method is more precise as there is least chance of follicles being missed or being counted twice because of color coding. But postprocessing is required for accurate calculations. It takes longer to perform, because of the need for post-processing, and obtains values that are lower than those obtained by the 2D and 3D-MPV (multiplanar volume) techniques[12,13] (Fig. 13.1).

Ovarian volume less than 3 cc was significantly predictive of higher IVF cancellation rates (> 50%)[14] (Fig. 13.2) *and ovarian volume was also used in decision-making for stimulation protocol for ovarian induction.* AFC and ovarian volume provide direct measurements of ovarian reserve.[15]

Inclusion of stromal blood flows (Fig. 13.3) as one of the decision-making parameters is also considered. It has

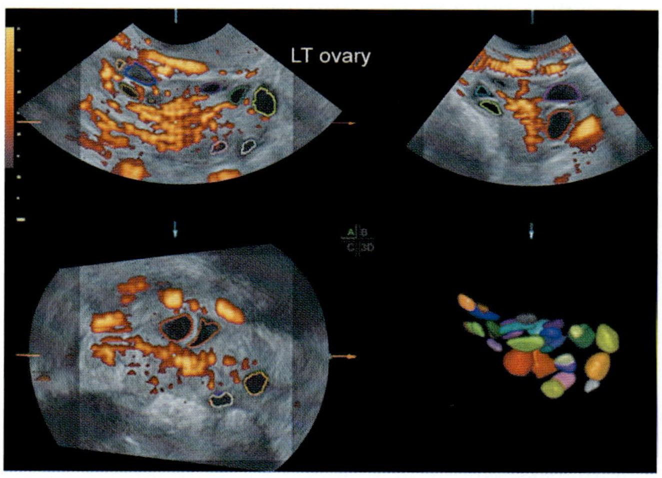

Fig. 13.1: The 3D ultrasound image of the ovary with Sono-AVC for calculating antral follicle counts.

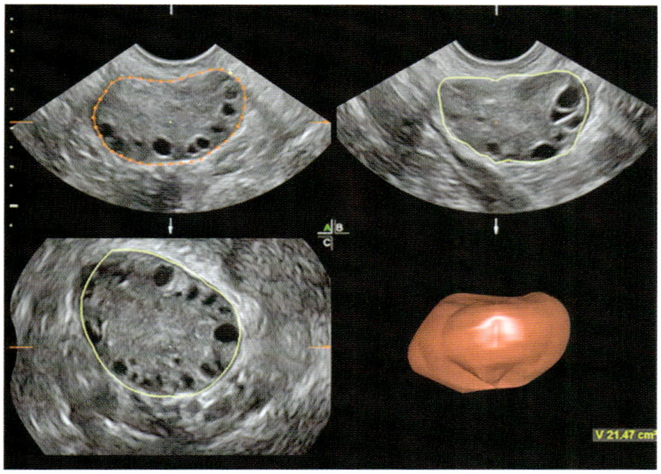

Fig. 13.2: The 3D ultrasound calculated ovarian volume by a software called VOCAL.

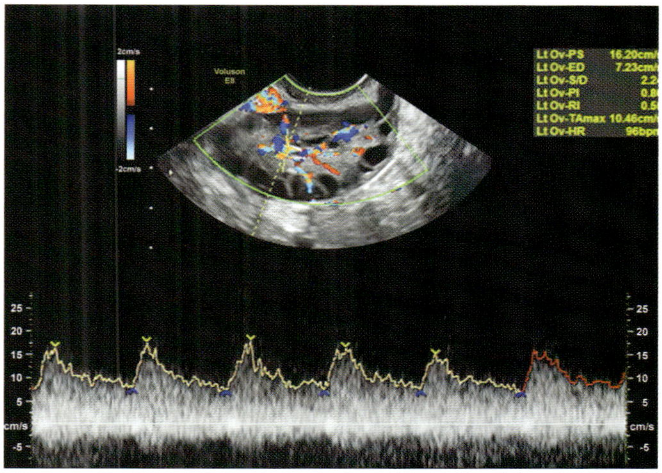

Fig. 13.3: Ovarian stromal flow as seen on color Doppler and pulse Doppler.

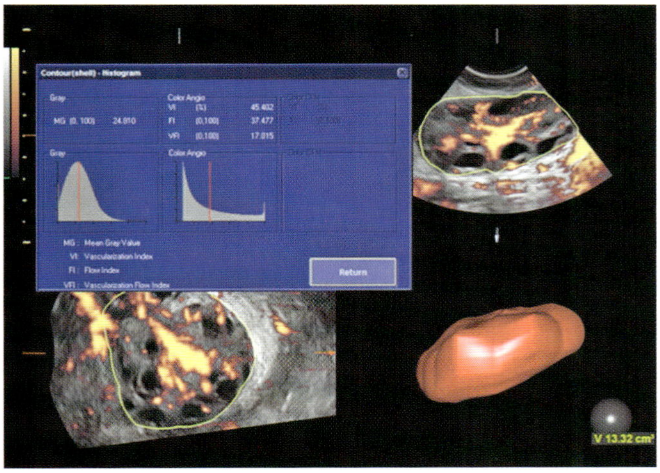

Fig. 13.4: The 3D power Doppler ultrasound image with VOCAL calculated volume with volume histogram (blue box) showing VI, FI, and VFI parameters.

been shown that measurement of ovarian stromal flow in early follicular phase is related to subsequent ovarian response in IVF treatment.[16]

Ovarian stromal PSV after pituitary suppression is predictive of ovarian responsiveness and outcome of IVF treatment.[17] Kupesic has shown correlation between the ovarian stromal flow index and number of mature oocytes retrieved in IVF cycles and pregnancy rates[2] (Fig. 13.4). Stromal FI can define the ovarian response to ovulation induction drugs. [<11, low responder; 11–14, good; >15, risk of ovarian hyperstimulation syndrome (OHSS)].

Table 13.1: Values of different factors that can decide the high or low-dose requirement of gonadotropins for ovulation induction.

	Increase the dose when..	*Decrease the dose when..*
Age	>35 years	<25 years
BMI	>28 kg/m^2	<20 kg/m^2
AFC	<3 (FNPO)	>12 (FNPO)
Stromal RI	>0.7	<0.5
Stromal PSV	<5 cm/sec	>10 cm/sec
Stromal FI	<11	>15
Ovarian Volume	<3 cc	>10 cc

The ovarian stromal blood flow was found to be negatively correlated with age. Ovarian blood flow predicts ovarian responsiveness and hence provides a noninvasive and cost effective prognostic factor of IVF outcome.[18]

Based on all these facts and findings, it is understood that ovaries that have high resistance, low velocity flow require higher doses of gonadotropins for stimulation. Whereas those with low resistance, high velocity flow require lower doses of gonadotropins for stimulation.

The final dose calculation can be based on following factors and we would prefer to simplify it like shown in Table 13.1.

A scoring system, that was developed based on clinical and ultrasound findings, is shown in Table 13.2.

The ovulation induction in all patients was done by rFSH and the stimulation doses were based on the scores of individual patient based on the Table 13.2. The doses

Table 13.2: Nagori's scoring system to decide the starting dose of gonadotropins for ovulation induction.

Score	1	2	3	4	5
Age	>40	35–40	30–35	25–30	<25
BMI	>30	30–28	28–25	25–22	<22
AFC	<5	5–10	10–15	15–20	>20
Ovarian volume	<3	3–5	5–7	7–10	>10
Stromal RI	>0.75	0.75–0.65	0.65–0.55	0.55–0.45	<0.45
Stromal PSV	<3	3–5	5–7	7–10	>10

Table 13.3b: Dose calculation in IVF patients based on Nagori's scoring system

Score	
>23	75 IU
20–22	150 IU
16–20	225 IU
11–15	300 IU
6–10	375 IU
1–5	450 IU

according to the patient's score were decided as shown in Table 13.3(a,b).

The doses for stimulation for IVF cycle according to the patient's score was decided as follows.

As per the results of our study, we believe that the scoring system devised in this study for deciding the stimulation protocol is highly reliable for safe planning of stimulation protocols in assisted reproductive technology (ART) cycles as the OHSS rates and cycle cancellation rates due to poor response are negligible. Multiple pregnancy rates are also acceptable. This study we believe may prove to be an important guide for safe use of gonadotropins for ovulation induction in ART cycles.[19,20]

A follicle that is of more than 10 mm in diameter, grows at a rate of 2–3 mm per day, has no internal echogenicity, and has thin (pencil-line like) walls is not only more likely to become the leading follicle but will also give mature healthy ovum.

B Mode Features of a Mature Follicle

The follicular diameter is measured when the follicle is seen as a rounded structure, or at least three measurements must be taken perpendicular to each other and take

Table 13.3a: Dose calculation in IUI patients based on Nagori's scoring system

Age	*Dose of rFSH*
≥25	25 IU
20–24	37.5
15–20	75 IU
10–15	112.5 IU
6–10	150 IU

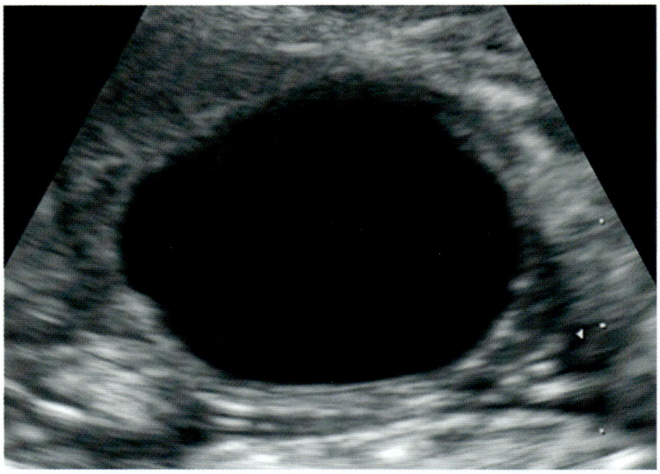

Fig. 13.5: B mode ultrasound image of a mature follicle.

a mean measurement as follicular diameter. A mature follicle is 16–18 mm (Fig. 13.5), has thin walls, regular round shape, and no echogenicity in the lumen and shows a thin hypoechoic rim surrounding the follicle, and sometimes (about 35–40%) cumulus like shadow may be seen. This thin hypoechoic rim and cumulus like shadow develops approximately 36 hours before rupture. A flimsy irregular line is seen inside the follicle parallel to the wall about 6–8 hours before rupture (Fig. 13.6).

Doppler Features of a Good Pre-human Chorionic Gonadotropin Follicle

Increase in perifollicular vascularity of dominant follicle in theca layer starts developing as early as 8th day of the cycle. Fall in perifollicular RI starts 2 days before ovulation, reaches nadir at ovulation, remains low for 4 days, and then with gradual rise reaches 0.5 in midluteal phase.[21]

When functionally mature, on color Doppler, the follicle shows blood vessels covering at least three-fourth of the follicular circumference (Fig. 13.7). Chui et al. graded

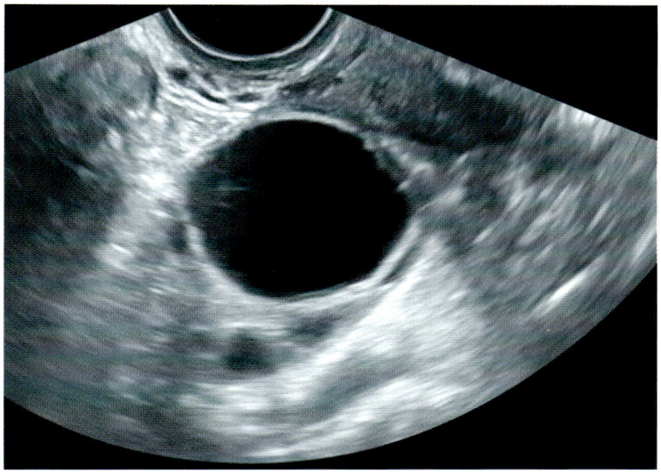

Fig. 13.6: B mode ultrasound image of a follicle of which rupture is impending showing mild separation of inner wall at 2 O'clock and 6 O'clock positions.

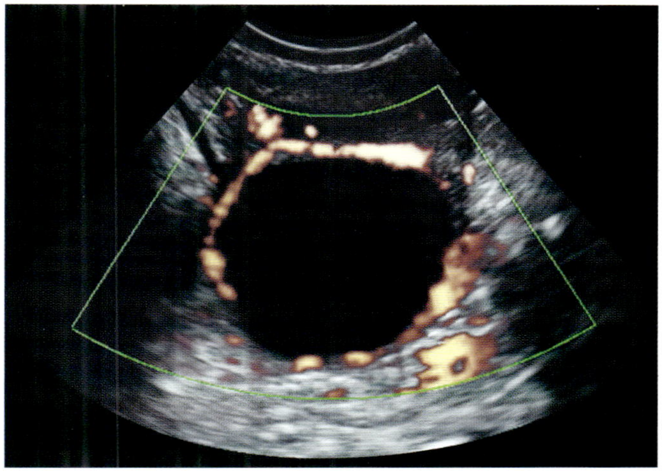

Fig. 13.7: Perifollicular vascularity seen on color Doppler.

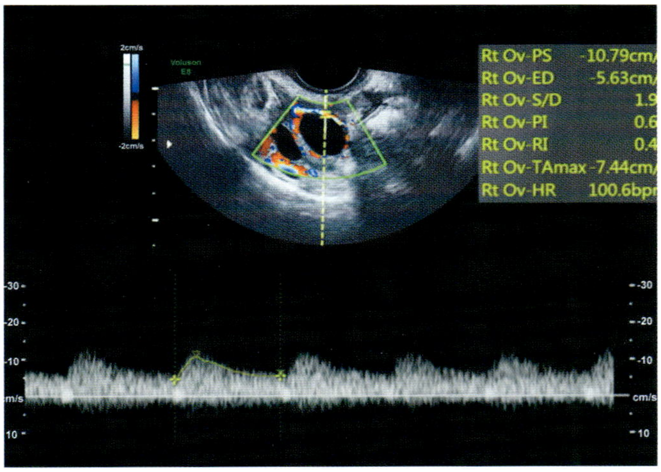

Fig. 13.8: Pulse Doppler image of the low resistance perifollicular flow.

the follicular flow on the day of oocyte collection as grade 1–4, when in a single cross-area slice the flow covered less than 25%, 25–50%, 50–75%, and more than 75% of follicular circumference. The conception was related to grade 3–4 vascularity.[22]

On pulse Doppler, these blood vessels show RI of 0.4–0.48[22] and PSV of more than 10 cm/sec (Fig. 13.8).

The perifollicular flow (PRF) settings for color Doppler are set at 0.3 and wall filter at the lowest. The perifollicular vessels are only those that obliterate the follicular wall with color. If the follicular wall is seen and the vessel is seen just besides it, it is not a perifollicular vessel. Ovarian flow correlates well with oocyte recovery rates and hence may be useful in determining the most appropriate time to administer hCG to optimize recovery rate. It has been quoted in a study by Nargund et al.[22,23] that embryos produced by fertilization of the ova obtained from the follicles, which had a perifollicular PSV of less than 10 cm/sec, are less likely to be grade 1 embryos and also have higher chance of chromosomal malformations. In the same study, it has been shown that the probability of developing a grade 1 or 2 embryo is 75% if PSV was more than 10 cm/sec, 40% if PSV was less than 10 cm/sec, and 24% if there was no perifollicular flow. There is yet another study that supports this finding. Oocytes from severely hypoxic follicles are associated with high frequency of abnormalities of organization of chromosomes on metaphase spindle and may lead to segregation disorders and catastrophic mosaics in embryo.[24]

On 3D ultrasound, the follicular volume of 3–7.5 cc has been found to be optimum in our study.[25] This agrees with the study by Witmack et al.,[26] which says that: in IVF-ET cycles, follicles with mean follicular diameter of 12–24 mm are associated with optimal rates of oocyte recovery, fertilization, and cleavage.[26] This corresponds to the follicular volumes of between 3 and 7 mL. The accuracy of 3D US measurement of follicular volume compared to the standard 2D techniques by comparing the volume of individual follicles estimated by both methods with the corresponding follicular aspirates, using the formula of ellipse, the limits of agreement between aspirates and calculated volume was +3.47 to −2.42 as compared to +0.96 to −0.43 when calculated by 3D US using VOCAL[27] (Fig. 13.9).

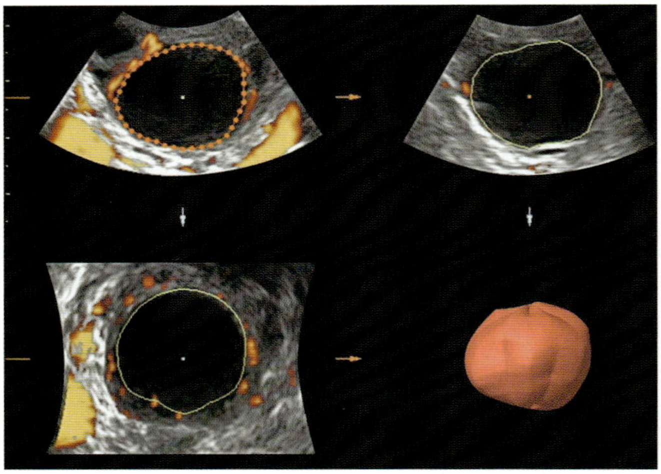

Fig. 13.9: The 3D US acquired, VOCAL calculated volume of follicle.

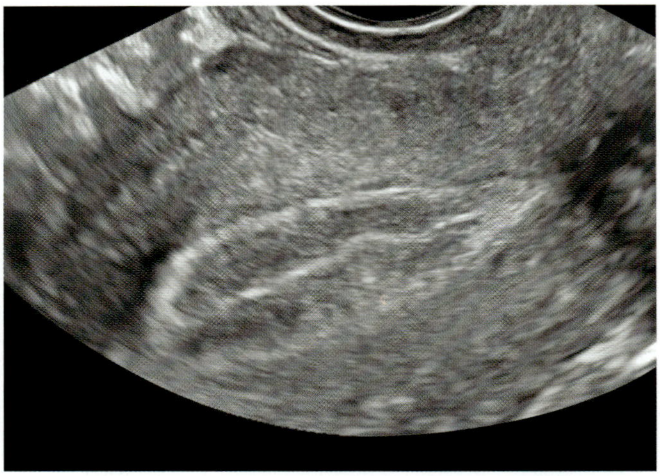

Fig. 13.10: B mode ultrasound image of grade A endometrium.

It has been shown that follicular fluid concentrations of leptin, a follicular angiogenesis related factor, are inversely related to the stromal blood flow index.[28]

It has also been suggested that the follicles containing oocytes capable to produce a pregnancy have a perifollicular vascular network more uniform and distinctive.[29]

In our study,[25] we have found perifollicular VI of between 6 and 20 and perifollicular FI more than 35 as most optimum.

About 68.4% of patients conceived when the VI was between 6 and 18 and 50% when it was between 18 and 20. However, the pregnancy rates were less than 25% when VI was less than 6 and only 7.4% when VI was more than 20. It was only 7.4% of patients with FI less than 27 who conceived, whereas beyond 27, the conception rates rose consistently. It was 50% with FI between 27 and 35, 70% when FI was between 35 and 43, and almost all patients had conceived when FI was more than 43. Although it is possible to assess the follicular flow as expressed by the PSV and perifollicular color map,[30] it is the 3D power Doppler that gives the most precise information about the vascularization and follicular blood flow.[31] hCG plays a major role in inducing influx of blood within follicles. At the LH surge, the perifollicular PSV is 10 cm/sec. This means that if the follicle is said to be functionally mature when PSV is 10 cm/sec, that is the time when the LH surge starts and under the effect of that LH, the perifollicular PSV keeps on rising constantly.[32]

This derives that a rising PSV with steady low RI suggests that the follicle is close to rupture.

Implantation has been the weakest link in the success of infertility treatment. Endometrium is a receptor organ for majority of the hormones involved in fertility and, therefore, study of its morphology and vascularity is thought to explain the mysteries of implantation failure. Therefore, like follicle, endometrium is also assessed by transvaginal 2D US and color Doppler before planning for hCG during any ARTs.

B Mode Features of Endometrium with Good Receptivity

On transvaginal sonography (TVS), an endometrial thickness of minimum 6 mm is required on the day of hCG, but 8–10 mm is optimum. Endometrial thickness has more negative predictive value for implantation. Morphology of the endometrium is as important as thickness of the endometrium. In all the healthy endometria, the endometrio-myometrial interface is always seen as a clear hypoechoic halo surrounding the whole endometrium (Fig. 13.10). Breach or irregularity of endometrio-myometrial junction is an indication of unhealthy endometrium and, therefore, poor receptivity.

Popularly, multilayered endometrium is considered as a desired endometrial pattern. Morphologically, the endometrium is graded as the best grade A, when it is a triple line endometrium with the intervening area as hypoechoic as the anterior myometrium. The echogenicity is attributed to the development of multiple vessels penetrating in the endometrium producing multiple tissue

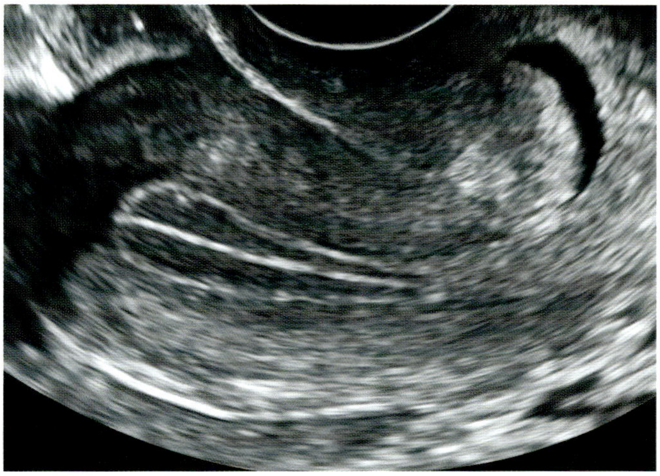

Fig. 13.11: B mode ultrasound image of grade B endometrium.

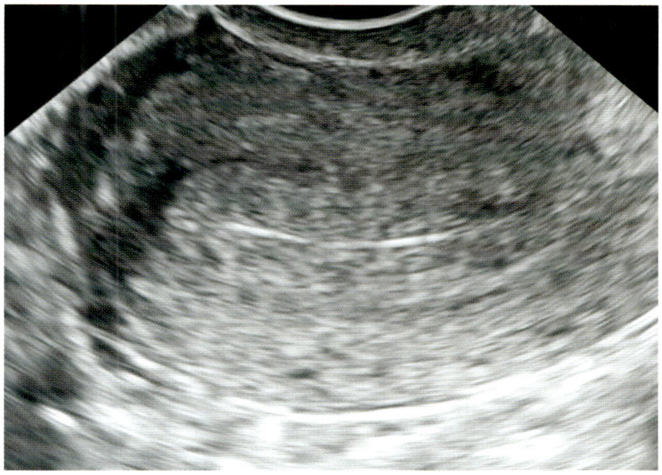

Fig. 13.12: B mode ultrasound image of grade C endometrium.

interfaces and, therefore, causing the echogenicity and due to glycogen storage in the endometrial columnar epithelium (Fig. 13.11). The endometrium is graded as intermediate or grade B (Fig. 13.12) when it is multilayered or triple line with hypoechoic intervening area. In grade C, the most unfavorable endometrium would be a homogeneous isoechoic endometrium,[33] though some studies have shown no significant difference in pregnancy rates amongst different morphological patterns.

Doppler Features of Endometrium with Good Receptivity

There are several reports by different groups[34] that agree on the fact that implantation rates can be more correlated to the vascularity of the endometrium rather than the thickness and morphology of the endometrium.

Segmental uterine artery perfusion demonstrates significant correlation with hormonal and histological markers of uterine receptivity, reaching the highest sensitivity for subendometrial blood flow. The endometrium, that is mature shows vascularity in zone 3 and 4 on colour doppler. This may be called subendometrial and endometrial layers (Figs. 13.13A to D).

The zones of vascularity are defined according to Applebaum[34] as: zone 1, when the vascularity on power Doppler is seen only at endometrio-myometrium junction; zone 2, when vessels penetrate through the hyperechogenic endometrial edge; zone 3, when it reaches intervening hypoechogenic zone; and zone 4, when they reach the endometrial cavity. The pregnancy rates related to the zones of vascular penetration are: 26.7% for zone 1, 36.4% for zone 2, and 37.9% for zone 3.

One more comparison of two studies have also shown similar results:[20]

• Zone 1	3.5–7.5%	5.2%
• Zone 2	15.8–29.7%	28.7%
• Zone 3	24.2–47.8%	52%
• Zone 4	67.3%	74%

Endometrial Vascularity: Its Relation to Implantation Rates[35]

• Vascularity in	Zone 1	Zone 2	Zone 3	Zone 4
• % of patients	6.69%	20.73%	58%	14.47%
• + β-hCG	19%	21.87%	39.77%	70.14
• Gestational sac	9.6%	14.58%	36.8%	68.65%
• Abortions	50%	23.8%	5.6%	1.5%

Zaidi et al. found that absence of flow in the endometrial and subendometrial zones on day of hCG indicate total failure of implantation.[36]

The vessels that reach the endometrium are the spiral arteries. The pulse Doppler of these arteries should have an RI of between 0.6 and 0.8 and PI of between 1.1 and 2.3 for the endometrium to be called mature for implantation.

Moreover, the pulse Doppler analysis of the uterine artery waveform is done and its RI should not be more than 0.9 and PI should be less than 3.2 (Fig. 13.14).

Several authors have shown that the optimum uterine receptivity was obtained when average pulsatility index of the uterine artery was between 2 and 3 on the day of transfer or on the day of hCG.[37,38]

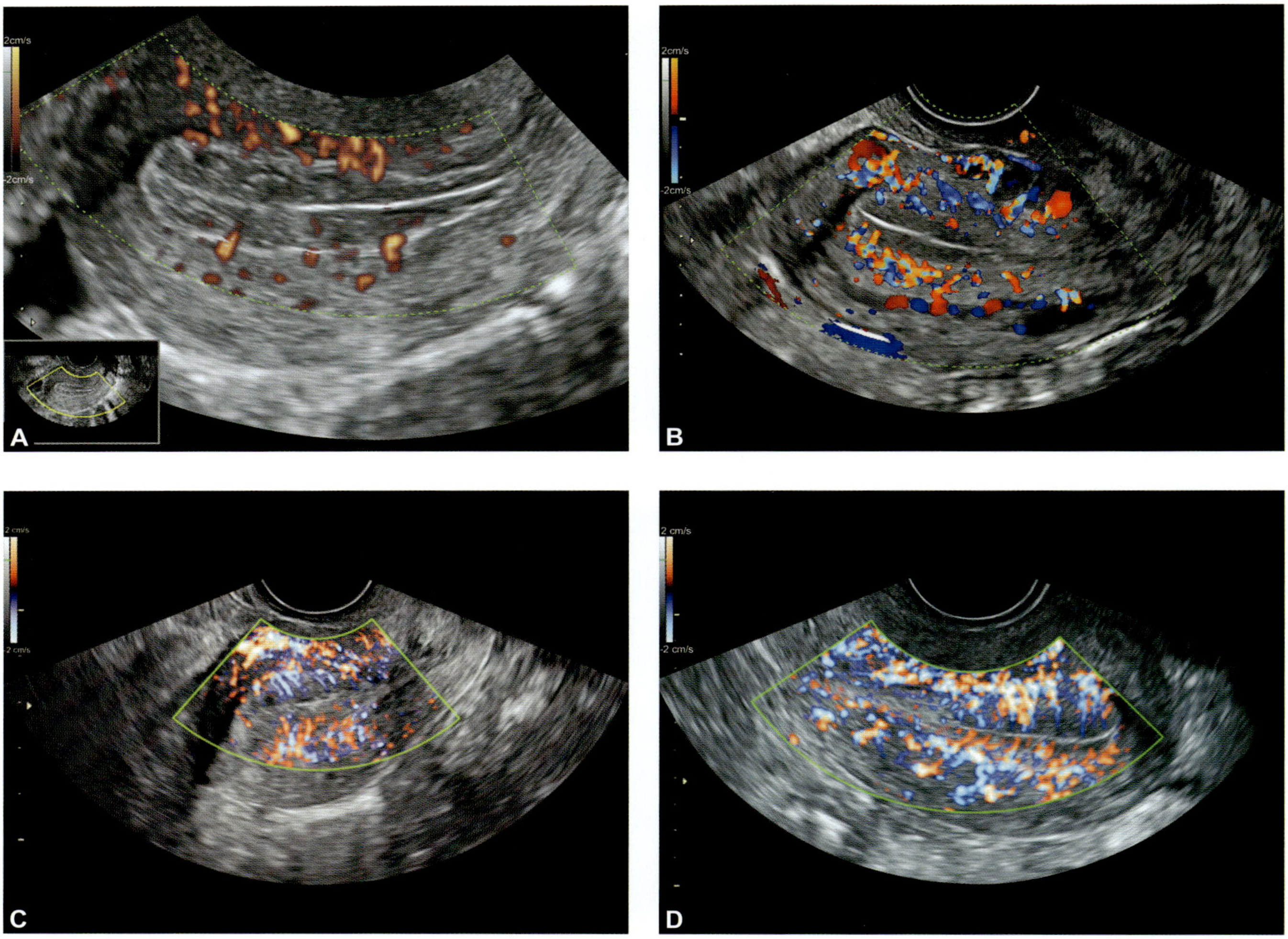

Figs. 13.13A to D: Power Doppler images of the grade 1–4 endometrium.

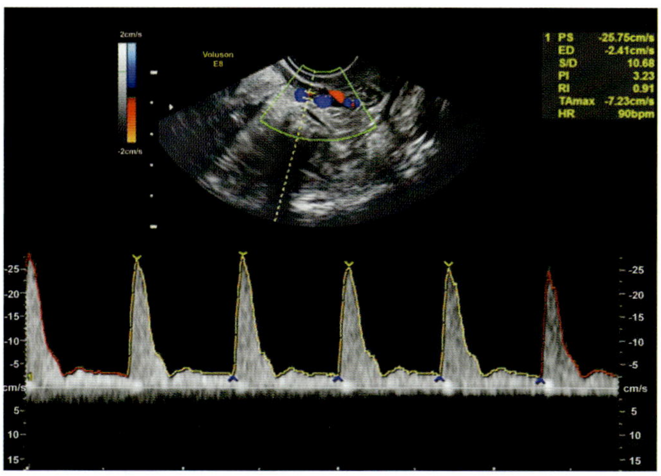

Fig. 13.14: Pulse Doppler image showing high resistance uterine artery flow waveform.

Coulam et al. have also shown that no pregnancy was achieved after embryo transfer, when uterine artery PI was above 3.3 in an IVF program.[39]

Cacciatore et al. suggest that implantation is unlikely when PI is more than 3.3 and RI more than 0.95 or when no velocities are seen at the end of the diastole.[40]

In such cases, therefore, in IUI cycles, hCG is withhold or postponed and in IVF cycles, embryos are frozen for transfer in subsequent cycles.

Endometrial volume by 3D US volume calculation of the endometrium may help to correlate the cycle outcome with quantitative parameter rather than endometrial thickness.[26]

A study by Raga et al.[41] shows pregnancy and implantation rates were significantly lower when endometrial volume was less than 2 mL, while no pregnancy was achieved

Table 13.4: Optimum parameters to define functionally mature follicle and endometrium.

	Follicle	*Endometrium*
Size/thickness	16–18 mm	8–10 mm
Morphology	Thin wall, no internal echoes, halo	Grade A/B
Vascularity	Three-fourth circumference	Zone 3–4
RI	0.4–0.48	<0.5
PSV	>10 cm/sec	-
Uterine Artery PI	-	<3.2
Volume	3–7 cc	3–7 cc
3D Morphology	Cumulus	Intact endo-myo junction
3D PD	More symmetrical, the better	Higher, the better

when endometrial volume was less than 1 mL. Study by Kupesic et al. also shows no pregnancy when endometrial volume was less than 2 mL, or when exceeded 8 mL.[42]

Summary is given in Table 13.4.

Secretory Phase Assessment

Rupture of the follicle leads to formation of corpus luteum. Corpus luteum is responsible for progesterone production. The functional efficacy of the corpus luteum can be assessed by Doppler by assessing the pericorpus luteal vascularity.

Segmental uterine and ovarian artery perfusion demonstrates a significant correlation with histological and hormonal markers of uterine receptivity and may aid in assessment of luteal phase defect.[43] A clear correlation between RI of corpus luteum and plasma progesterone levels has been seen in natural cycle. RI of the corpus luteum can, therefore, be used as an adjunct to plasma progesterone assay as an index of luteal function.[44]

A corpus luteum that is functionally normal and produces adequate amount of progesterone shows corpus luteal flow: RI 0.35–0.50 and PSV 10–15 (Figs. 13.15A and B).

The receptor organ for progesterone also (like estrogen) is endometrium and its vascular studies can be a reliable clue to adequate progesterone production. Though endometrial also becomes hyperechoic as a result of progesterone exposure. But soon after rupture of the follicle, the outer margin of the endometrium starts becoming fluffy and blurred. With adequate progesterone levels, that are achieved in the midluteal phase, the spiral arteries show RI of 0.48–0.52 (low resistance flow) and uterine artery shows PI of 2.0–2.5. This PI is lower than in the preovulatory phase because of smooth muscle relaxing effect of progesterone. Inadequate progesterone production and, therefore, corpus luteal inadequacy is suggested by high resistance flow in corpus luteal vessels.[44]

High spiral artery resistance suggests inadequate response of endometrium to progesterone. This is because of inadequate progesterone receptors in the endometrium or because of local endometrial cause like endometrial injury or chronic endometritis.

In luteal phase defect because of low progesterone levels, the resistance in the pericorpus luteal vessels is high. Because of low progesterone levels, there is inadequate

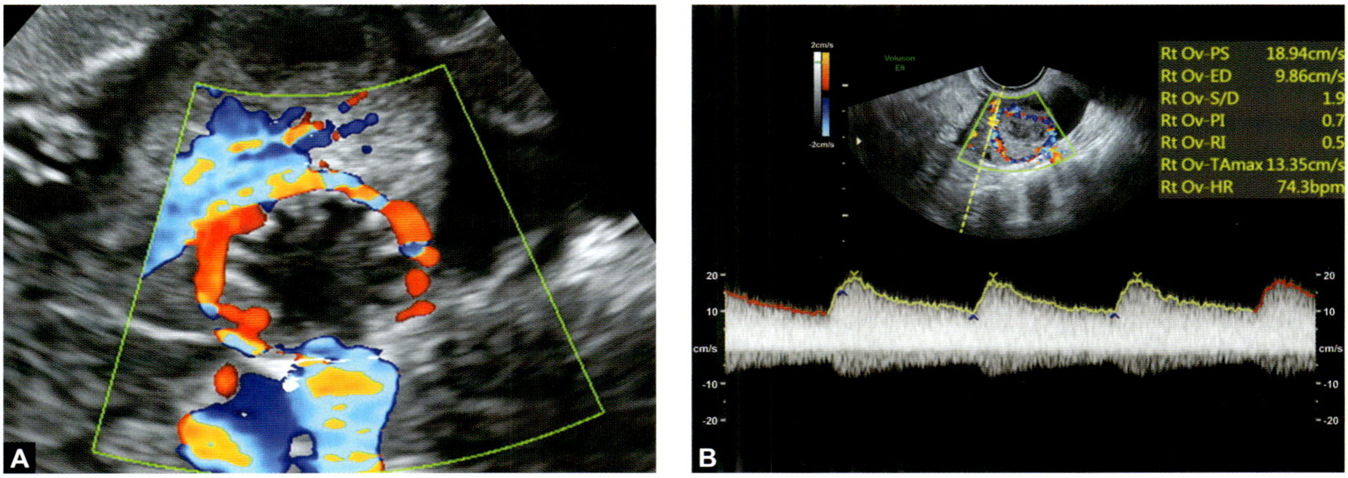

Figs. 13.15A and B: Normal corpus luteal flow seen on color Doppler and pulse Doppler.

Table 13.5: Corpus luteal flow and spiral artery flow in normal cycle and luteal phase defect.[43]

Phase	*Normal*	*Luteal phase defect*
Perifollicular	0.56 ± 0.06	0.58 ± 0.04
LH peak day	0.44 ± 0.04	0.58 ± 0.04
Midluteal phase	0.42 ± 0.06	0.58 ± 0.04
Late luteal phase	0.50 ± 0.04	0.58 ± 0.04

Table 13.6: Endometrial RI in different phases of menstrual cycle in control patients and those with LPD.

Phase	*Control RI*	*LPD RI*
Periovulatory	0.53 ± 0.04	0.70 ± 0.06
Midluteal	0.50 ± 0.02	0.72 ± 0.06
Late luteal	0.51 ± 0.04	0.72 ± 0.04

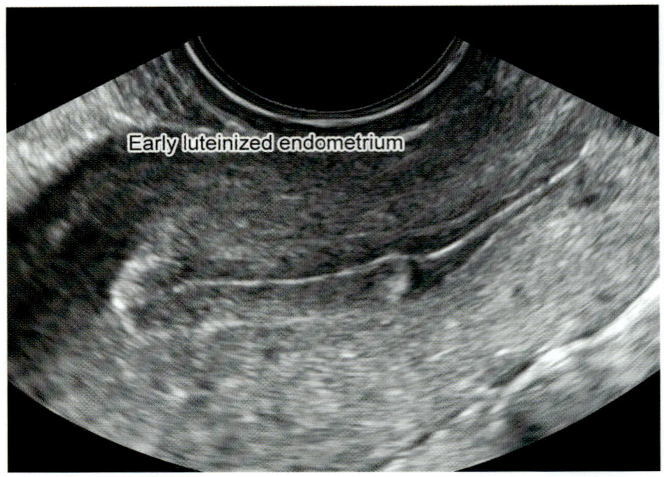

Fig. 13.16: Endometrium of early luteal phase seen on B mode ultrasound. Blurring of outer margins of multilayered endometrium.

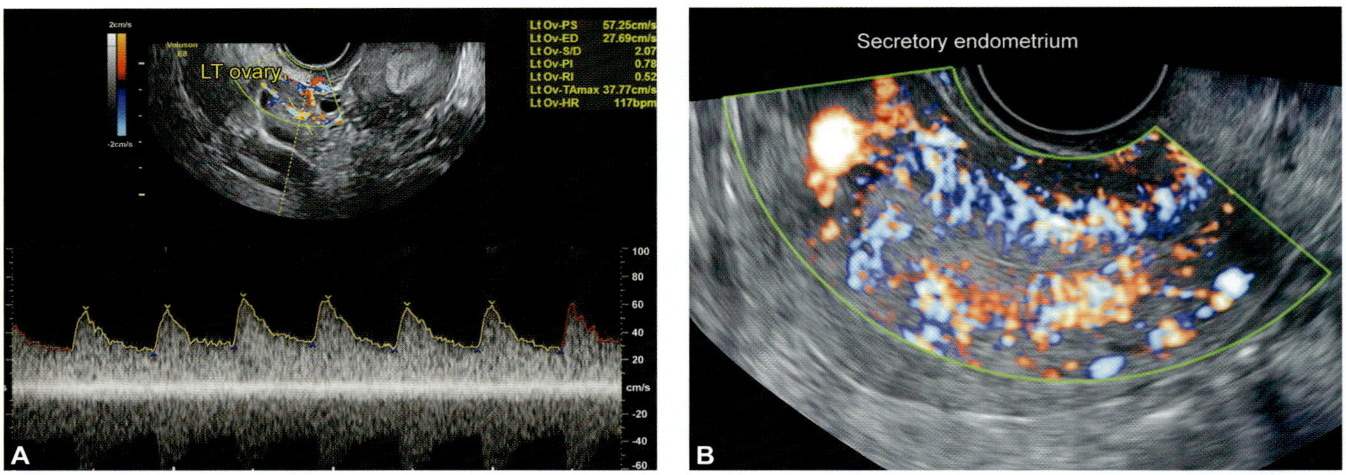

Figs. 13.17A and B: A low resistance blood flow of the corpus luteum demonstrated on pulse Doppler B. High-definition power Doppler showing blood flow in the secretory endometrium.

relaxation of the muscularis of the uterine artery and, therefore, the uterine artery resistance is high along with higher resistance in its branches—the spiral vessels (Tables 13.5 and 13.6).

Correlation of Progesterone to Ultrasound Findings

Blurring of outer margin of multilayered endometrium suggests initiation of progesterone secretion Fig. 13.16).

Low resistance flow in corpus luteum, with echogenic endometrium (Figs. 13.17A and B) and low resistance endometrial vascularity in midluteal phase suggests normal luteal phase.

High resistance corpus luteal flow suggests corpus luteal inadequacy.

High resistance endometrial flow in midluteal phase suggests either inadequate progesterone levels or inadequate progesterone receptors in endometrium.

CONCLUSION

Ultrasound is an excellent tool for assessment of the menstrual cycle. Hormonal changes occurring day to day during the menstrual cycle reflects as morphological and vascular changes in the ovary and the uterus. Assessing these changes by transvaginal ultrasound and Doppler and correctly interpreting can explain the hormonal basis of these changes. Ultrasound with Doppler can thus be used as the only modality for cycle assessment in patients undergoing ART and may be of help to reduce the cost of the cycle by avoiding certain hormonal assessments and still maintaining close and accurate watch on the hormonal changes occurring during treatment cycle.

REFERENCES

1. Ravhon A, Lavery S, Michael S, Donaldson M, Margara R, Trew G, Winston R. Dynamic assays of inhibin B and oestradiol following Buserelin acetate administration as predictors of ovarian response in IVF. Hum Reprod. 2000;15(11):2297-301.
2. Kupesic S, Kurjak A. Predictors of IVF outcome by three-dimensional ultrasound. Hum Reprod. 2002;17(4):950-5.
3. Popovic-Todorovic B, Loft A, Lindhard A, Bangsboll S, Andersson AM, Anderson AN. A prospective study of predictive factors of ovarian response in 'standard' IVF/ICSI patients treated with recombinant FSH. A suggestion for recombinant FSH dosage normogram. Hum Reprod. 2003;18(4):781-7.
4. Ng EH, Tang OS, Chan CC, Ho PC. Ovarian stromal blood flow in the prediction of ovarian response during *in vitro* fertilization treatment. Hum Reprod. 2005;0(11): 31147-51.
5. Oliveness F, Howles CM, Borini A, Germond M, Trew G, Wikland M, et al. Individualizing FSH dose for assisted reproduction using a novel algorithm: the CONSORT study. Reproductive Bio Medicine Online. 2009;18(2):195-204.
6. Merce LT, Barco MJ, Bau S, Troyano JM. Prediction of ovarian response and IVF/ICSI outcome by three dimensional ultrasonography and power Doppler angiography. Eur J Obstet Gynecol Reprod Biol. 2007;132(1):93-100.
7. Freiesleben NL, Lossl K, Bogstad J, Bredkjaer HE, Toft B, Loft A, et al. Predictors of ovarian response in intrauterine insemination patients and development of a dosage nomogram. Reprod Biomed Online. 2008;17(5):632-41.
8. Ernest Hung Yu Ng, William Shu Biu Yeung. Reproductive age can be assessed by a number of ovarian reserve tests. Human Reproduction. 2003;18(10):2169-74.
9. Scheffer GJ, Broekmans FJ, Dorland M, Habbema JD, Looman CW, te Velde ER. Antral follicle counts by TVS are related to age in women with proven natural fertility. Fertil Steril. 1999;72:845-51.
10. Lam PM, Johnson IR, Rainne-Fenning NJ. Three dimensional ultrasound features of the polycystic ovary and the effect of different phenotypic expressions on these parameters. Hum Reprod. 2007;22(12):3116-23.
11. Jayakrishnan Krishnakumar, Akansha Agarwal, Akansha Agarwal, Divya Nambiar, Shankar Radhakrishnan. Comparison of antral follicle count, antiMullerian hormone and day 2 follicle stimulating hormone as predictor of ovarian response and clinical pregnancy rate in patient with an abnormal ovarian reserve test. Int J Reprod Contracept Obstet Gynecol. 2016;5(8):2762-7.
12. Rainne-Fenning NJ. What is in a number? The polycystic ovary revisited. Hum Reprod. 2011;26(11);3118-22.
13. Deb S, Jayaprakasan K, Campbell BK, Clewes JS, Johnson IR, Raine-Fenning NJ. Ultrasound in Obstetrics and Gynecology. 2009;33(4):477-83.
14. Lass A, Skull J, McVeigh E, Margara R, Winston RM. Measurement of ovarian volume by transvaginal sonography before ovulation induction with human menopausal gonadotrophin for *in vitro* fertilization can predict poor response. Hum Reprod. 1992;12(2):294-7.
15. ER teVelde. Advances in fertility studies and reproductive medicine. IFFS. 2007;306.
16. Zaidi J, Barber J, Kyei-Mensah A, Zaidi J, Barber J, Kyei-Mensah A. Relationship of ovarian stromal blood flow at baseline ultrasound to subsequent follicular response in an *in vitro* fertilization program. Obstet Gynecol. 1996;88:779-84.
17. Engmann L, Saldkevicius P, Agrawal R, Bekir JS, Campbell S, Tan S. Value of ovarian stromal blood flow velocity measurement after pituitary suppression in the prediction of ovarian responsiveness and outcome of *in vitro* fertilization treatment. Fertil Steril. 1999;71(1):22-9.
18. Arora A, Gainder S, Dhaliwal L, Suri V. Clinical significance of ovarian stromal blood flow in assessment of ovarian response in stimulated cycle for *in vitro* fertilization. Int J Reprod Contracept Obstet Gynecol. 2015;4(5):1380-83.
19. Panchal S, Nagori CB. Ultrasound based decision making on stimulation protocol for superovulated IUI cycles. IJIFM. 2016;7(1):7-13.
20. Panchal S, Nagori CB. Ultrasound Based decision making on stimulation protocol in IVF. DSJUOG. 2016;10(3):330-7.
21. Jokubkeine L, Sladkevicius P, Rovas L, Valentine L. Assessment of changes in volume and vascularity of ovaries during the normal menstrual cycle using three dimensional power Doppler ultrasound. Hum Reprod. 2006;21(10):2661-8.
22. Nargund G, Doyle PE, Bourne TH, Parsons JH, Cheng WC, Campbell S, et al. Ultrasound-deviced indices of follicular blood flow before HCG administration and prediction of oocyte recovery and preimplantation embryo quality. Hum Reprod. 1996;11:2512-17.
23. Nargund G, Bourne TH, Doyle PE, Parsons J, Cheng W, Campbell S, et al. Association between ultrasound indices of follicular blood flow, oocyte recovery and preimplantation embryo quality. Hum Reprod. 1996;11:109-13.
24. Van Blerkom, Antezak M, Schrader R. The developmental potential of human oocyte is related to the dissolved oxygen content of follicular fluid: association with vascular endothelial growth factor levels and perifollicular blood flow characteristics. Hum Reprod. 1997;12(5):1047-55.
25. Panchal SY, Nagori CB. Can 3D PD be a better tool for assessing the pre HCG follicle and endometrium? A randomized study of 500 cases. Presented at 16th World Congress on Ultrasound in Obstetrics and Gynecology, 2006, London. J Ultrasound Obstet Gynecol. 2006;28(4):504.
26. Wittmack FM, Kreger DO, Blasco L, Tureck RW, Mastroianni L Jr Lessey BA. Effect of follicular size on oocyte retrieval, fertilization, cleavage and embryo quality in *in vitro* fertilization cycles: a 6 year data collection. Fertil Steril. 1994;62:1205-10.

27. Kyei-Mensah A, Zaidi J, Pittrof R, Shaker A, Campbell S, Tan SL. Transvaginal three dimensional ultrasound reproducibility of ovarian and endometrial volume measurements. Fertil Steril. 1996;66:718-22.
28. Wu MH, Tsai SJ, Pan HA, Hsiao KY, Chang FM. Three dimensional power Doppler imaging of ovarian stromal blood flow in women with endometriosis undergoing *in vitro* fertilization. Ultrasound Obstet Gynecol. 2003;21:480-5.
29. Vlaisavljevic V, Reljic M, GavricLovrec V, ZazulaD, Sergent N. Measurement of perifollicular blood flow of the dominant preovulatory follicle using three dimensional power Doppler. Ultrasound Obstet Gynecol. 2003;22:520-6.
30. Merce LT. Ultrasound markers of implantation. Ultrasound Rev Obstet Gynecol. 2002;2:110-23.
31. Merce LT, Barco MJ, Kupesic S, Kurjak A. 2D and 3D power Doppler ultrasound from ovulation to implantation. In: Kurjak A, Chervenak F (Eds). Textbook of Perinatal Medicine. London: Parthenon Publishing; 2005.
32. Bourne TH, Jurkovic D, WaterstoneJ, Campbell S, Collins WP. Intrafollicular blood flow during human ovulation. Ultrasound Obstet Gynecol. 1991;1:53-9.
33. Smith, Porter R, Ahuja K, Craft I. Ultrasonic assessment of endometrial changes in stimulated cycles in an *in vitro* fertilization and embryo transfer program. J *In Vitro* Fertil Embryo Transf. 1984;1:233-8.
34. Applebaum M. The 'steel' or 'teflon' endometrium—ultrasound visualization of endometrial vascularity in IVF patients and outcome. Presented at The Third World Congress of Ultrasound in Obstetrics and Gynaecology. Ultrasound Obstet Gynecol. 1993;3(Suppl 2):10.
35. Nagori C, Panchal S. Endometrial vascularity: Its relation to implantation rates. International Journal of Infertility and Fetal Medicine. 2012;3(2):48-50.
36. Zaidi J, Campbell S, Pittrof R, Tan SL. Endometrial thickness, morphology, vascular penetration and velocimetry in predicting implantation in an *in vitro* fertilization program. Ultrasound ObstetGynecol. 1995;6:191-8.
37. Steer CV, Campbell S, Tan SL, et al. The use of transvaginal colour flow imaging after *in vitro* fertilization to identify optimum uterine conditions before embryo transfer. Fertil Steril. 1992;57:372-6.
38. Zaidi J, Pittrof R, Shaker A, Kyei-Mensah A, Campbell S, Tan SL. Assessment of uterine artery blood flow on the day of human chorionic gonadotrophin administration by transvaginal colour Doppler ultrasound in an *in vitro* fertilization program. Fertil Steril. 1996;65:377-81.
39. Coulam CB, Stern JJ, Soenksen DM, Britten S, Bustillo M. Comparison of pulsatility indexes on the day of oocyte retrieval and embryo transfer. Hum Reprod. 1995;10: 82-4.
40. Cacciatore B, Simberg N, Fusaro P, Tiitinen A. Transvaginal Doppler study of uterine artery blood flow in *in vitro* fertilization embryo transfer cycles. Fertil Steril. 1996;66: 130-4.
41. Raga F, Bonilla-Musoles F, Casan EM, Klein O, Bonilla F. Assessment of endometrial volume by three dimensional ultrasound prior to embryo transfer: clues to endometrial receptivity. Hum Reprod. 1999;14:2851-4.
42. Kupesic S, Bekavac I, Bjelos D, Kurjak A. Assessment of endometrial receptivity by transvaginal colour Doppler and three dimensional power Doppler ultrasonography in patients undergoing *in vitro* fertilization procedures. J Ultrasound Med. 2001;20:125-34.
43. Kupesić S, Kurjak A, Vujisić S, Petrović Z. Luteal phase defect: comparison between Doppler velocimetry, histological and hormonal markers. Ultrasound Obstet Gynecol. 1997;9(2):105-12.
44. Glock JL, Brumsted JR. Colour flow pulsed Doppler ultrasound in diagnosing luteal phase defect. Fertil Steril. 1995;64:500-4.

CHAPTER 14

Assisted Reproduction Treatments

Francis A Tharakan, Kanna M Jayaprakasan

INTRODUCTION

The current prevalence of infertility lasting for at least 12 months is estimated to be around 9% worldwide for women aged 20–44 years. About 20–30% of infertility cases are explained by physiological causes in men, 20–35% by physiological causes in women, and 25–40% of cases are because of a problem in both partners. In 10–20% cases, no cause is found. Infertility is also associated with lifestyle factors such as smoking, body weight, and stress. Increasing age in the female partner is one of the most common explanations today.

Regardless of the cause of infertility, assisted reproduction treatment (ART) offers the highest pregnancy rates per cycle among all the fertility treatment options and is therefore being increasingly used worldwide. Assisted reproductive technique (ART) involve interventions manipulating gametes to enhance fertilization and subsequent occurrence of pregnancy and include *in vitro* fertilization (IVF), intracytoplasmic sperm injection (ICSI), gamete intrafallopian transfer (GIFT), zygote intrafallopian transfer (ZIFT), transfer of cryopreserved embryos (frozen embryo replacement, FER), and treatment using donor gametes and embryos. More recently GIFT and ZIFT have become less popular as the success rates are inferior to IVF and more invasive.

Since the first successful birth following IVF in 1978, there have been considerable advances in the field of ART. One in six couples worldwide experience some form of infertility problem at least once during their reproductive lifetime (Fig. 14.1). It is now estimated that more than 5 million babies have been born worldwide since the first IVF baby was born in 1978. Most ART treatments take place in women aged between 30 and 39. Europe leads the world in ART, initiating approximately 55% of all reported ART cycles. In 2011, the latest year for which figures are available, 588,629 treatment cycles were reported from 33 European countries. This compares globally (in 2011) with 151,923 cycles from the United States and 66,347 cycles from Australia and New Zealand. The number of cycles performed in many developed countries has grown by 5–10% per annum over the last few years, but that growth is now showing signs of slowing.

The most common treatment technique is ICSI. Overall, ICSI accounts for around two-thirds of all treatments worldwide, and conventional IVF around one third. However, these proportions vary greatly between countries, even though outcome rates with each technique are comparable. Success rates from frozen embryo transfer (ET) are increasing, as are the number of FER cycles. Vitrification, as an efficient cryopreservation technique, has improved the outcome of both embryo and oocyte freezing.

Ovarian hyperstimulation syndrome (OHSS) is a complication related to ART. In 2011, there were 1,683 OHSS cases recorded in 28 out of 33 European countries reporting to ESHRE, making up 0.6% of cycles. Russia (520), Italy (189), and Spain (184) reported the highest number of patients with OHSS.

The Human Fertilization and Embryology Authority (HFEA) was established in 1991 by the Human Fertilization

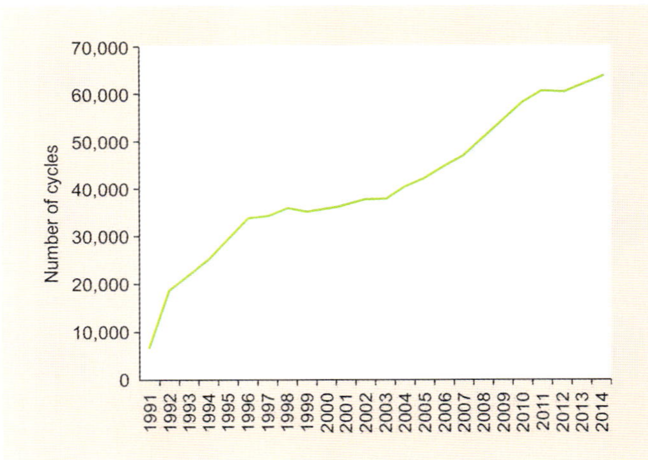

Fig. 14.1: Number of treatment cycles (1991–2014) (HFEA 2014).

and Embryology Act 1990 (HFE Act) in the United Kingdom and was the first statutory body of its kind in the world. The introduction of guidelines into clinical practice in general and in assisted reproduction in particular has led to an ever-increasing role for an evidence-based approach to the provision of these services. Clinical guidelines for the assessment and treatment for people with fertility problems were published by the National Institute for Clinical Excellence in 2004 and later updated in Feb 2013 to streamline services and avoid unnecessary waste of resources. In this chapter, we will review the current status of conventional IVF, ICSI and other treatments, new developments in ART, as well as the clinical risks associated with these techniques. The obstetric and neonatal consequences of these treatments and in particular the impact of the number of embryos transferred on the outcome will be discussed.

SELECTION AND PREPARATION OF PATIENTS

Although IVF was initially introduced to bypass tubal blockage, the currently available techniques enable the treatment of various causes of infertility. The current indications are:

- Tubal disease
- Unexplained infertility
- Treated endometriosis
- Male factor infertility
- Failed artificial insemination by donor (AID)
- Failed ovulation induction
- Absent or inappropriate ovaries
- IVF in association with preimplantation genetic diagnosis (PGD)
- Fertility preservation for cancer patients and social reasons
- Treatment of single women and same sex couples

Emphasis should be placed on the pretreatment evaluation of the individual or couple both medically and psychologically. The assessment of the welfare of the child that may result from ART, including its need for a positive male role model, has become central to the provision of treatment in the eyes of the HFEA. With that in mind there should be careful consideration of the duration and stability of the couple's relationship, their medical and social backgrounds, and other relevant issues. In addition, information-giving and decision-making aspects of counseling should be made available by a specially trained counselor as a matter of routine, to all couples. Any couple should be interviewed together and appropriate history and clinical examination are undertaken for both. For the female partner, baseline hormone profile, midluteal phase progesterone assay, and rubella status must be determined. Additional tests such as thyroid function, high vaginal or endocervical swabs, and cytomegalovirus (CMV) status are carried out where necessary. Hepatitis B and C and human immunodeficiency virus (HIV) screening are mandatory in the United Kingdom before ART for both partners.

EVALUATION OF PELVIS

Ultrasound evaluation of the pelvis is often performed prior to ART to rule out any adnexal and uterine pathologies such as polycystic ovarian disease, endometriosis, tubal disease, fibroids, and endometrial polyps, that are clearly associated with aberrant and compromised outcomes during IVF.

Polycystic ovary syndrome (PCOS) is recognized as the most common endocrine disorder of reproductive-aged women around the world. The diagnosis of polycystic ovarian disease was based on the definition derived by Rotterdam consensus workshop, which suggested the presence of 12 or more follicles measuring 2–9 mm in diameter and/or an ovarian volume of more than 10 cm^3 for the ultrasound diagnosis,[1] but that now seems obsolete. Stromal vascularity and blood flow velocities are higher in women with polycystic ovaries[2] and this may account for their tendency toward ovarian hyperstimulation in response to gonadotropin therapy. The Androgen Excess and Polycystic Ovarian Syndrome Society Task Force recommends using follicle number per ovary (FNPO) for the definition of PCOM setting the threshold at more than or equal to 25, but only when using newer technology that affords maximal resolution of ovarian follicles (i.e. transducer frequency ≥8 MHz). If such technology is not available, we recommend using ovarian volume (OV) rather than FNPO for the diagnosis of PCOM for routine daily practice but not for research studies that require the precise full characterization of patients.[3]

Endometriosis is defined as the presence of endometrial-like tissue outside the uterus, which induces a chronic, inflammatory reaction.[4] The exact prevalence of endometriosis is unknown but estimates range from 2 to 10% of women of reproductive age, to 50% of infertile women.[5,6] Clinicians are recommended to perform

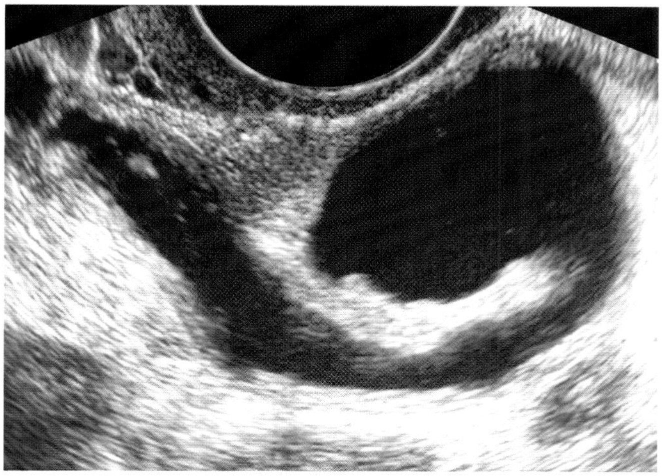

Fig. 14.2: Hydrosalpinx.

transvaginal sonography (TVS) to diagnose or to exclude an ovarian endometrioma.[7] The ESHRE Guideline Developing Group recommends that clinicians should consider the diagnosis of endometriosis in the presence of gynecological symptoms such as dysmenorrhea, noncyclical pelvic pain, deep dyspareunia, infertility, and fatigue in the presence of any of the above. The diagnosis should also be considered in women of reproductive age with nongynecological cyclical symptoms (dyschezia, dysuria, hematuria and rectal bleeding, and shoulder pain).

The presence of a hydrosalpinx is associated with poor implantation and pregnancy rates and early pregnancy loss (Fig. 14.2). The exact mechanism is unknown but substances toxic to the endometrium are thought to be produced that negatively affect endometrial receptivity.[8] Salpingectomy, ideally performed laparoscopically, prior to IVF has been shown to be beneficial and is recommended. The diagnosis of hydrosalpinx can generally be made using transvaginal ultrasound with a high degree of confidence. The diagnosis of hydrosalpinx can generally be made using transvaginal ultrasound with a high degree of confidence.[8] Surgical treatment should be considered for all women with hydrosalpinges prior to IVF treatment. Salpingectomy, ideally performed laparoscopically, prior to IVF has been shown to be beneficial and is recommended. Previous evidence supported only unilateral salpingectomy for a unilateral hydrosalpinx (bilateral salpingectomy for bilateral hydrosalpinges). Laparoscopic tubal occlusion is an alternative to laparoscopic salpingectomy in improving IVF pregnancy rates in women with hydrosalpinges. Laparoscopic procedures are often contraindicated in women with dense pelvic adhesions. Hysteroscopic sterilization (Essure) appears to be an effective option for management of hydrosalpinx in women before IVF although evidence from a randomized controlled clinical trial is lacking.[9]

Ultrasound assessment of the uterus is generally restricted to measurement of the endometrial thickness and a description of the locality and size of any fibroids. Conventional ultrasound may also detect uterine anomalies although these are more readily identified and correctly qualified with three-dimensional ultrasound. The diagnosis of uterine anomalies is important as they are associated with lower implantation rates and increased rates of early miscarriage, preterm labor, and malpresentations.[10] The outcome appears to relate more to the length of the remaining uterine cavity than the degree of septum and this may be measured reliably with three-dimensional ultrasound.[11]

The diagnosis and classification of fibroids into subserosal, intramural, and submucosal is usually straightforward and important as these progressively exert a negative effect on pregnancy rates respectively. Whilst intramural fibroids measuring more than 4 cm in diameter and submucous fibroids of any size are thought to negatively affect the outcome of fertility treatment and to be associated with lower pregnancy rates, the effect that smaller intramural fibroids have on reproductive outcome is unclear.[12] Systematic review and meta-analysis[13] suggested the adverse effect of intramural fibroids without uterine cavity involvement on the outcome of IVF treatment. There is also doubt about the exact impact of endometrial polyps, the other commonly encountered intrauterine pathology, have on treatment outcome and early pregnancy. Some authors suggest conservative management especially if it is small[14] but this can be difficult in patients undergoing fertility treatment or with a history of miscarriage when a polyp is identified before treatment begins. Polyps are usually evident with conventional transvaginal imaging, although false positive diagnoses are common. Saline infusion sonohysterography (SISH) can reduce this and facilitate appropriate operative planning.[15] Delineation of the polyp with saline ensures that the size and position of the polyp can be accurately defined allowing surgeons to modify their approach and resect the larger, more broad-based polyps rather than planning for simple polypectomy. Hysteroscopy is the gold standard technique for uterine cavity assessment and may be necessary, if diagnosis of intrauterine pathologies is in doubt.

Assessment of Ovarian Reserve

Evaluation of ovarian reserve has become an integral part of the pretreatment assessment of a woman about to undergo ART and is recommended for all women planning ART.[16] The aim is to identify women likely to respond poorly, who have a low chance of success and are more likely to have their treatment cycle cancelled, and those prone to ovarian hyperstimulation which is associated with significant morbidity and even mortality. Accurate assessment of ovarian reserve and prediction of response therefore facilitates pretreatment counseling of couples of their potential risks and allows treatment to be tailored to the individual potentially increasing the number of oocytes retrieved without risking an exaggerated response. Ovarian reserve, defined by the size and quality of the remaining ovarian follicular pool at any given time, reflects the fertility potential of a woman.[17]

Although women's age is an important predictor of ovarian reserve and response, a great deal of interindividual variation exists even at same age.[18] This is indicative of a wide variation in the rate of age related decline in the ovarian follicle population. Several endocrine and ultrasound markers have been reported with an aim to estimate the number of gonadotropin-responsive or "selectable follicles" more accurately. The endocrine markers include factors produced by the developing follicles [estradiol, inhibin B, and anti-Müllerian hormone (AMH)] or the hormones under the inhibitory control of these factors [follicle-stimulating hormone (FSH)]. The ultrasound markers are antral follicle count (AFC), ovarian volume, and ovarian vascularity. The sensitivities, specificities, and predictive values of these tests have been evaluated in many studies by correlating the test results with the number of oocytes retrieved, poor or exaggerated ovarian response, and pregnancy or live birth rates during ART.[17]

Early follicular FSH is the most widely used marker of ovarian reserve worldwide and women with raised FSH levels (above 10–15 IU/L) are more likely to have reduced ovarian response and poor ART outcome.[19,20] A meta-analysis of 21 studies looking at the value of basal FSH in the prediction of IVF outcome has concluded that the performance of basal FSH as a screening test is limited in predicting poor ovarian response and nonpregnancy. Predictions with a substantial shift from pre-FSH test probability to post-FSH test probability are only achieved at an extremely high cut-off levels.[21] Moreover the cycle-to-cycle variability of basal FSH levels limits the reliability of a single measurement for the assessment of ovarian reserve. However, it is important to note that the ovarian response and the pregnancy rates during IVF are low in women with high intercycle variability[22] or who demonstrate an abnormal FSH levels in any menstrual cycle.[23]

Measurement of basal estradiol along with FSH level is recommended to improve the predictive accuracy. A premature elevation of estradiol level due to advanced follicular development and early selection of a dominant follicle may tend to suppress the FSH levels thus masking a rise that might otherwise reflect a low ovarian reserve.[24] Elevated level of basal estradiol (≥60 pg/mL) even in the presence of normal FSH levels are reported to be at an increased risk of cycle cancellation due to poor ovarian response.[25] However, the use of serum estradiol estimation for ovarian reserve assessment is limited by the fact that some women in the presence of normal ovarian reserve may have an occasional accelerated cycle with FSH levels of mid-follicular range in their true early follicular phase.[24] Furthermore, elevated estrogen may simply reflect the presence of functional ovarian cyst.

Inhibin-B is principally produced by the granulosa cells of the developing cohort of antral follicles during the luteal-follicular transition and, therefore, its levels in the early follicular phase are considered as an indicator of quantity or quality of developing follicles.[26] A low level (<45 pg/mL) of early follicular phase inhibin-B may predict poor ovarian response.[27] However, the reliability of its measurement has been questioned because of a significant intercycle variability.[28]

Studies have shown AMH to be a promising serum marker of ovarian reserve.[29] AMH, a member of the transforming growth factor β family of growth and differentiation factors are primarily produced by the preantral and small antral follicles in women of reproductive age and, therefore, its levels in the serum are indicative of growing follicle pool.[30] In the female fetus it is expressed by the granulosa cells of the ovary from as early as 36 weeks of gestation and production continues until the menopause. While AMH has a high degree of predictive ability to identify potential poor or exaggerated responders to ovarian stimulation during ART, its accuracy to predict the occurrence of pregnancy after one cycle of ART is only marginal.[31]

Recent studies have suggested that AMH levels vary minimally between menstrual cycles and are cycle independent.[32,33] Therefore, AMH measurement could be undertaken at any cycle and at any time of the cycle for the prediction of ovarian response adequately and this makes it an attractive marker for routine use. There is also a nonsignificant variation in AMH levels during short-term oral contraceptive use and short-term gonadotropin-releasing hormone analogue administration. Long-term use (for >1 year) of oral contraceptives and gonadotropin releasing hormone (GnRH) analogues can reversibly reduce AMH concentrations.

The lack of a single standardized assay for the measurement of AMH has led to much confusion over interpretation and comparison of results. There are two assays that have been used for AMH, with differing values and units. These are:

1. The Diagnostic Systems Laboratories (DSL)
2. The Immunotech–Beckman.

Studies comparing the two assays showed AMH levels to be five to seven times lower with the DSL assay than with the Immunotech-Beckman assay. Beckman Coulter has developed a new assay for AMH (AMH Gen II A79765) and was introduced to replace earlier DSL and Immunotech assays, which uses the DSL antibodies but is standardized to the Immunotech calibration. AMH is shown to be comparable to AFC as a marker of ovarian reserve, but is superior to FSH and inhibin B.

Dynamic ovarian reserve tests have also been reported for the assessment of ovarian reserve. Dynamic testing is a provocative test of ovarian reserve that examines the endocrine dynamics of the menstrual cycle which changes with the functional activity of the remaining follicles within the ovary. This involves the measurement of an endocrine marker of ovarian reserve (FSH or estradiol) both before and after ovarian stimulation using clomiphene [clomiphene citrate challenge test (CCCT)], GnRH agonist [gonadotropin releasing hormone agonist test (GAST)] or FSH [exogenous FSH ovarian reserve test (EFFORT)]. The literature suggests that none of these tests offer any more predictive information than the previously described tests. Moreover, the inconvenience, the expenses, and the potential side effects associated with the use of the additional pharmacological agents limit its use for pretreatment assessment of ovarian reserve.

Antral follicle count is the most significant predictor of ovarian response among the ultrasound markers,[34,35] although decreased ovarian volume (<3 cm^3) and stromal blood flow are also implicated for poor treatment outcome during ART. The number of gonadotropin-responsive antral follicles measuring 2–10 mm can be measured using 2D or 3D ultrasound with an acceptably high level of agreement both between and within observers.[36] A total follicle count of 7 and 22 is generally considered as the optimum cut-off levels for the prediction of poor and exaggerated ovarian response, respectively. The AFC measurement can be performed either in the early follicular phase of the cycle before treatment begins or after downregulation with similar predictive accuracy.[37] However, assessment prior to treatment has an additional advantage in that it provides an opportunity for a pretreatment evaluation of pelvis to screen for pathology. AFC and AMH are currently the best two predictors of ovarian reserve among all the endocrine and ultrasound markers and are equally predictive of poor ovarian response during ART.[38] AFC is currently the ovarian reserve test of choice as it is easy to perform while there is no international assay standard for AMH measurement.

Ovarian reserve tests including AFC and AMH have limited value in the prediction of nonconception despite its adequate capacity to predict ovarian response during ART.[17] Pregnancy may occur even at extreme cut-offs for an abnormal test result and, therefore, IVF treatment cannot be denied based on these tests especially in participants who are seeking first cycle of treatment.[39] However, the identification of participants who are likely to respond poorly during IVF treatment is clinically relevant as a couple could be counseled accordingly. They can be made aware that they have an increased chance of cycle cancellation and a significantly lower chance of success allowing an informed decision to be taken. Such prediction also allows clinicians to formulate individualized treatment protocols to improve or at least maximize ovarian response.

EVALUATION OF MALE PARTNER

The male partner should be evaluated carefully. Clinical examination, semen analysis including sperm function tests, genetic assessment, and biochemical tests show that the etiology of male subfertility can be divided into four main groups as follows.

1. Primary spermatogenic failure, which is a testicular disorder, resulting in the reduction of sperm count and abnormal sperm function. A number of different factors can induce this condition including testicular maldescent, trauma, karyotype abnormalities, severe infection, and antimitotic therapy, but in many patients a cause cannot be ascertained.
2. Congenital or acquired obstructive lesions: Men with failed reversal of vasectomy are increasingly seen in

infertility clinics and at present constitute up to 10% of all male problems.

3. Disturbances of erection or ejaculatory disorders including those following spinal injuries.
4. Endocrine disorders such as Cushing disease, thyroid disorders, and androgen receptor abnormalities.

Many causes of male infertility may have considerable congenital implications for the children of such patients. About 60% of men with congenital bilateral absence of the vas deferens (CBAVD) were shown to have one or more of the cystic fibrosis (CF) genes. The use of ICSI in these circumstances should be carefully considered and men must be screened with the CF gene mutation before their treatment.

Genetic tests before, during, or after ART should be done to give adequate counseling to couples and their families in cases such as women with Turner syndrome, men with 47XXY, men or women with structural chromosomal aberrations, and men with either Yq11 deletion or CBAVD (ESHRE Capri Workshop Group 2000).

The couple must be well informed about the treatment options that are suitable for them, the indications for the tests they have to undergo, details of the proposed treatment, and its success rate, risks, and complications.

CLINICAL MANAGEMENT OF THE TREATMENT CYCLE

The first successful birth from IVF ET in 1978 resulted from a single oocyte obtained from the dominant follicle in a natural ovarian cycle. Success rates were found to be improved when multiple embryos were available, allowing competitive selection of the best quality embryos for transfer; thus at present, the majority of assisted reproduction programs undertake controlled ovarian stimulation to induce multiple follicular development and subsequently to obtain many fertilizable oocytes.

The main components of a typical conventional ART include:

- Pituitary downregulation using GnRH analogues
- Controlled ovarian stimulation using gonadotropins
- Monitoring follicular development using transvaginal ultrasound with or without serum estradiol levels
- Oocyte maturation using human chorionic gonadotropin (hCG)
- Egg collection and sperm production or sperm recovery
- Fertilization (IVF/ICSI) and subsequent embryo culture
- Fresh ET into the uterus and cryopreservation of surplus good quality embryos
- Luteal support by progesterone administration

Normal Folliculogenesis

This involves several important and inter-related steps.

1. Follicular recruitment: This occupies the first few days of the ovarian cycle and allows the follicle to continue to mature in the correct gonadotropic environment and to progress toward ovulation.
2. Selection: The mechanism whereby a single follicle is chosen and ultimately achieves ovulation.
3. Dominance: The selected follicle maintains its preeminence over all other follicles and occupies days 8–12 of the primate ovarian cycle.

Follicular development beyond the antral stage depends on the concentration of FSH in the circulation. Once a threshold level has been attained, follicular growth beyond 4 mm occurs. The interval during which FSH remains elevated above threshold level can be regarded as a window through which a follicle must pass to avoid atresia. The width of the window will therefore determine the number of follicles that can be selected for ovulation. The preovulatory luteinizing hormone (LH) surge is triggered by the positive feedback of estradiol (E_2) from the dominant follicle as well as other follicular contributory factors. Ovulation occurs between 24 and 36 hours after the onset of the LH surge.

Pituitary Downregulation

In the conventional ART protocol, it is a standard practice to use a continuous and supraphysiological dose of GnRH agonist to obtain control over the hypothalamic-pituitary-ovarian axis. GnRH agonist causes an initial flare response, characterized by increased gonadotropin secretion, due to upregulation of GnRH receptors. However, prolonged administration of GnRH agonists induces downregulation of GnRH receptors. This prevents a premature surge in LH and subsequent spontaneous ovulation with luteinization, which occurs in up to 23% of cycles when gonadotropins alone are used and facilitates the timing of oocyte retrieval. The use of GnRH agonists in ART has been shown to increase the number of oocytes retrieved, to improve pregnancy rates, and to significantly reduce the chance of cancellation.[40]

The two different GnRH agonist protocols used in most assisted conception units are long and short protocols.

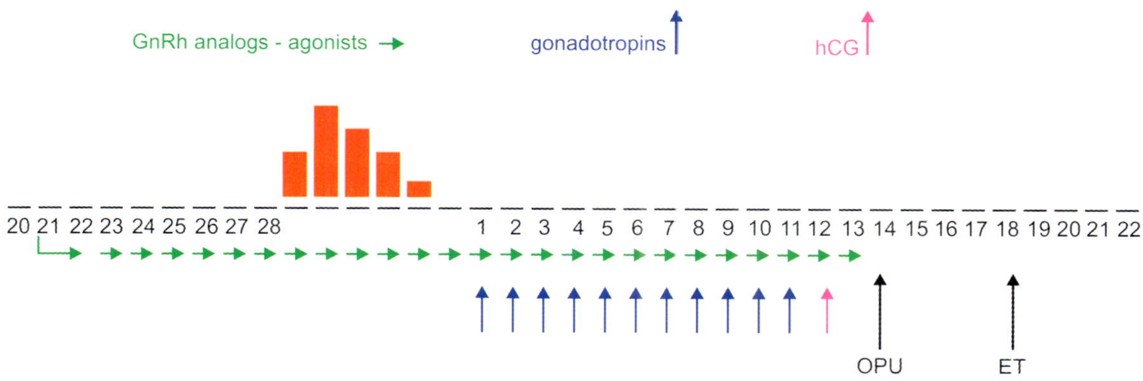

Fig. 14.3: Long GnRH agonist protocol.

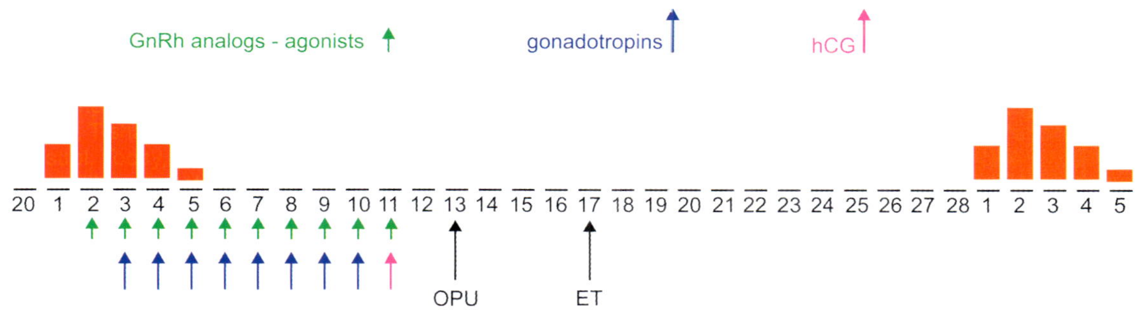

Fig. 14.4: Short GnRH agonist protocol.

In long protocols, GnRH agonists, buserelin or nafarelin are started in the midluteal phase (day 21) of the previous menstrual cycle to achieve pituitary downregulation in about 8–21 days after which gonadotropins are commenced (Fig. 14.3). The duration of GnRH agonist administration is about 10–14 days in a short protocol (Fig. 14.4). In both regimens GnRH agonists are administered daily until the day of hCG or LH injection, which is used to trigger oocyte maturation. Short protocol takes advantage of the initial flare effect which can be utilized to augment the ovarian response to gonadotropin stimulation. However, a systematic review of 26 randomized control trials found increased clinical pregnancy rate per cycle and fewer cycle cancellations with long GnRH agonist protocol when compared with short GnRH agonist protocols.[41] Therefore, the long GnRH agonist protocol is generally recommended in most ART cycles. The pregnancy rate was found to be higher when GnRHa was used in a long protocol as compared to a short or ultrashort protocol, Cochrane Database Systematic Reviews.[42]

The use of long GnRH agonist protocol often prolongs the stimulation phase resulting in increased requirement of gonadotropins and increased treatment cost in addition to causing undesirable side effects of hypoestrogenism. It may also be associated with poor response in some patients as well as introducing a higher risk of OHSS. Some of the disadvantages can be obviated with the use of GnRH antagonists such as cetrorelix and ganirelix. GnRH antagonists induce immediate pituitary downregulation by competitively binding to GnRH receptors and avoid the flare effects or the need for prolonged treatment associated with GnRH agonist protocols. Two different regimes have been described. The multiple-dose protocol involves the administration of 0.25 mg cetrorelix or ganirelix daily from day 5 to 7 of stimulation, or when the leading follicle is 12–14 mm, until hCG/LH administration. The single-dose protocol involves the single administration of 3 mg cetrorelix on day 5–7 of stimulation. GnRH antagonist protocols are therefore short and simple, but more importantly reduces the incidence of severe OHSS. While the clinical pregnancy rates following IVF treatment were reported significantly lower with GnRH antagonist use when compared with long downregulation GnRH agonist protocol (OR 0.82, 95% CI 0.68–0.97) based on review of older studies,[43] the recent data from the units with experience with the use of antagonist protocol are encouraging.

More recent trials of GnRH antagonists have reported better pregnancy rates than earlier trials, which used antagonist protocols that would now be recognized as suboptimal. The recent Cochrane review comparing the antagonist and long agonist protocols have reported similar live birth rates (OR 1.02, 95% CI 0.85–1.23; 12 RCTs) but significantly reduced OHSS in the antagonist group (OR 0.61, 95% C 0.51–0.72).[44] The use of a protocol consisting of GnRH agonist trigger after GnRH antagonist co-treatment combined with adequate luteal phase and early pregnancy estrogen and progesterone supplementation reduces the risk of OHSS in high-risk patients undergoing IVF without affecting implantation rate. The use of low doses of hCG in the luteal phase postagonist trigger is associated with normalization of pregnancy rates and also supports the concept of its effectiveness for high responders reducing OHSS risk.[45,46] Cochrane database systematic review in 2011 suggested that GnRH agonists should not be routinely used as a final oocyte maturation trigger in fresh autologous cycles because of lowered live birth rates, a lower ongoing pregnancy rate (pregnancy beyond 12 weeks), and a higher rate of early miscarriage (<12 weeks). Cochrane database systematic review in 2014 suggested that in donor-recipient cycles, use of GnRH agonists instead of hCG resulted in a lower incidence of OHSS, with no evidence of a difference in live birth rate. GnRH agonist as an oocyte maturation trigger could be useful for women who choose to avoid fresh transfers (for whatever reason), women who donate oocytes to recipients, or women who wish to freeze their eggs for later use in the context of fertility preservation

Controlled Ovarian Stimulation

Pregnancy rate with unstimulated IVF remains much lower than in stimulated cycles, achieving a live birth rate of 2.3% per initiated cycle and 4.7% per ET (HFEA 2000). These results have remained low over the past decade. Although an unstimulated cycle is simpler, faster, less painful or expensive, and with no risk of ovarian hyperstimulation, it requires relatively extensive monitoring which increases the cost and results in inconvenience in the timing of the oocyte retrieval. Additionally, women with irregular cycles and/or hormonal imbalance or couples with male factor infertility, where fertilization may be a problem, are not suitable for natural cycle IVF. The aims of superovulation regimens in assisted reproduction are to maximize the number of follicles which mature to minimize the degree of asynchrony amongst developing follicles and to minimize the deleterious effects of the abnormal follicular environment on luteal function and endometrial receptivity. Multiple follicular development and ovulation can be achieved by widening the FSH window. Several drug combinations have been used to achieve this.

Oocyte retrieval may be programmed to coincide with a working day by manipulating the onset of the menstrual cycle using norethisterone tablets, the combined oral contraceptive pill, or utilizing the hypogonadotropic effect of GnRH agonists prior to commencing gonadotropins on a predetermined day of the week. The downregulatory phase may be prolonged to allow a fixed number of patients to be treated each week. In long downregulation protocol, gonadotropins are commenced following the confirmation of ovarian suppression, characterized by a thin endometrium of 5 mm or less on transvaginal scan and serum estradiol level of 200 pmol/L.

The first commercially available gonadotropin preparations used in superovulation protocols, human menopausal gonadotropin (HMG), were extracted from the urine of menopausal women. The initial preparations had been shown to be of low purity with the major protein components not being gonadotropins, with only 5% of them constituted FSH and LH activity. The repeated injection of nongonadotropin proteins may be the cause of unwanted effects, such as pain and allergic reactions. The desirability of having high-purity preparations led to the development of an immunopurified FSH product of more than 95% purity following the removal of LH activity from HMG. The introduction of highly purified urinary FSH (u-FSH HP) was associated with much reduced hypersensitivity allowing subcutaneous route for administration. The currently available commercial preparation of HMG is also highly purified and contains both FSH and LH activity at a ratio of 1:1. The LH activity in HMG is partly due to the presence of exogenous hCG, which is being added to correct imbalances in the FSH/LH ratio.

Genetic and molecular engineering has led to the production of recombinant human FSH (rFSH) with high purity (>99%), high specific bioactivity (>10,000 IU/mg protein), and absent intrinsic LH activity which is suitable for intramuscular or subcutaneous administration.[47] Two different rFSH preparations are commercially available: follitropin alpha (Gonal-F) and follitropin beta (Puregon). These two rFSH preparations differ in that follitropin alpha has a more acidic isoform profile than follitropin beta due to a slight difference in its carbohydrate component. Consequently they differ in metabolic clearance, half-life, and biologic activity, but both are equally effective during ART cycles in terms of live birth rates. A number of well-designed randomized controlled trials have compared both preparations of rFSH against HMG in their clinical effectiveness during conventional IVF with long GnRH agonist protocol. While none of them individually showed any statistically significant difference in live birth rates between the two treatment arms, two recent systematic reviews have demonstrated a significant 4% increase in live birth rate in the HMG arm.[48,49] However, the results of the meta-analysis needs to be interpreted with caution because of the clinical heterogeneity of the trials and, therefore, a large multicenter randomized double blind trial is warranted. Moreover, such studies should consider reporting the more clinically relevant cumulative live birth rates as primary outcome.

Recombinant DNA technologies have made it possible to produce LH (rLH) also. Because of the potential role of LH in follicular development according to the two-cell theory of gonadotropin system, supplemental rLH has been suggested to improve the IVF outcome if rFSH is used for ovarian stimulation. However, a recent systematic review of randomized trials failed to demonstrate any difference in live birth rates with adding rLH to rFSH protocol.[50] Although it is possible that rLH supplementation may be beneficial in a subset of IVF population, e.g. poor responders,[51] its generalized use is currently limited.

The collective evidence from many studies suggests that 150–225 IU/day of gonadotropins is the appropriate starting dose for most women undergoing conventional IVF treatment. Majority of the units use a daily dose according to women's age and presence or absence of PCO: 150 IU in women under the age of 30 years or having PCO, 225 IU for those between 30 and 39 years, and 300 IU for those aged 40 years or over. The lowest possible dose to achieve the optimum ovarian response should be used to reduce the risks of ovarian hyperstimulation. Although there is no consensus on what constitute optimum ovarian stimulation, a recent study has reported the implantation rate is maximum when 10 oocytes are retrieved following conventional IVF using long downregulation protocol.[52]

Recently, mild ovarian stimulation protocols have gained a lot of interest in the field of ART with the current trend of limiting the number of embryos to be transferred reducing the need for large numbers of oocytes. The principal aim with this approach is to reduce the number of developing follicles and thereby minimizing the adverse effects of ovarian stimulation particularly OHSS and multiple pregnancies. Three reported mild stimulation protocols include clomiphene citrate alone or in combination with gonadotropins, delayed commencement (day 5 of the cycle) of gonadotropins with GnRH antagonist comedication, and late follicular replacement of FSH with administration LH/hCG.[53] All these protocols have shown to reduce the gonadotropin dosage and have the potential to reduce the cost of the treatment and patient distress associated with conventional ART. As expected, the ongoing pregnancy rates/live birth rates per cycle have been lower when compared with conventional protocol, but similar effectiveness could be achieved with more treatment cycles.

Monitoring Follicular Development

The purpose of monitoring ovarian response is to ensure safe practice in reducing the incidence and severity of OHSS and also to optimize the timing of luteinization before oocyte retrieval. Ultrasound monitoring forms the integral part of monitoring. Follicular response together with endometrial thickness is monitored by ultrasound scans commencing on the 6th to 8th day of the treatment cycle. Some units measure serum estradiol levels in addition. However, current evidence does not support the adjuvant use of estradiol for monitoring as it does not give additional information with regard to live birth rate or OHSS rate. The gonadotropin dosage is adjusted according to ovarian response, although the evidence for this practice is limited. Typically, follicles are noted to grow at a rate of 2–3 mm/day accompanied by a steady increase in serum E_2 levels. When three or more follicles are greater than 18 mm in diameter, 5,000–10,000 U of hCG or 250 μg of choriogonadotropin alfa (recombinant preparation) are given subcutaneously to induce oocyte maturation before oocyte retrieval.

Ovarian response is poor when no or less than three follicles develop after 14 days of gonadotropin treatment and generally results in cancellation of the stimulation cycle. This problem is frequently encountered in women with reduced predicted ovarian reserve. Conversely, excessive ovarian response may result in OHSS, which will be discussed later. Other problems such as premature LH surge or preoperative ovulation have been largely eliminated by the introduction of GnRH analogues in superovulation protocols.

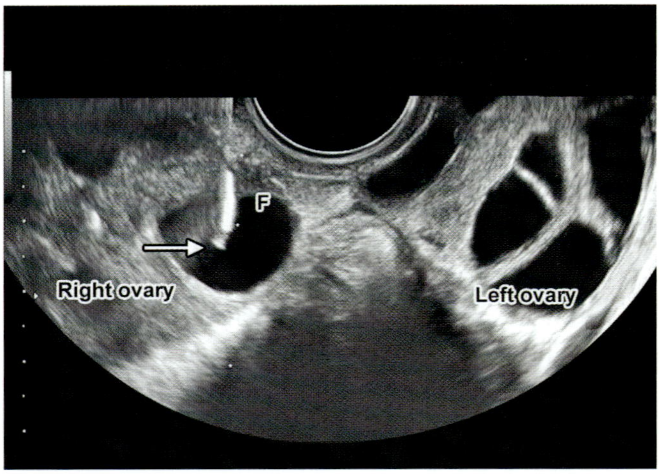

Fig. 14.5: Ultrasound picture during vaginal egg recovery. The tip of the needle (arrow) is seen within the follicle (F).

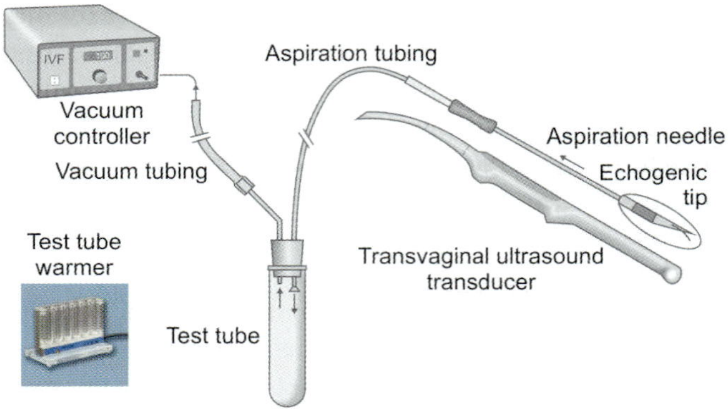

Fig. 14.6: Follicle aspiration equipment: an assembled follicle aspiration single lumen needle connected to a test tube. The test tube is in turn connected to a suction pump. The needle is attached to the transvaginal ultrasound transducer through needle guide and bracket.

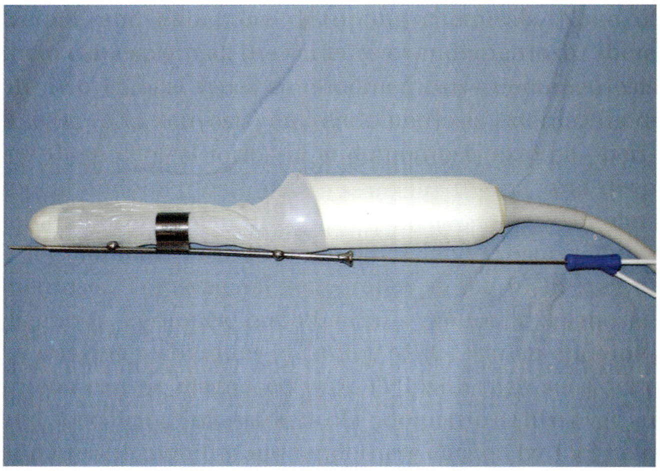

Fig. 14.7: Vaginal ultrasound transducer enclosed in a sterile condom with needle guide attached. The needle tip is protruding from the proximal end of the probe.

OOCYTE RETRIEVAL

It is important to provide effective anesthesia and analgesia for transvaginal oocyte recovery as they are painful. No technique of anesthesia, analgesia or sedation is free from side effects. Whatever technique is used, recognized standards of practice should be adhered to and all IVF professionals should follow the safe practice of administering sedative drugs published by the Academy of Medical Royal Colleges. Conscious sedation should be offered to all women having the procedure as it is safe and acceptable method of providing analgesia.

Oocyte retrieval is performed 36 hours after the trigger injection of hCG/LH. Methods of egg collection have improved considerably since the introduction of ART. At first, all egg collections were performed laparoscopically. This is now rarely used and is reserved for women if their ovaries are inaccessible through the transvaginal route. With the introduction of endovaginal transducers, the transvaginal ultrasound guided approach became the predominant method for egg collection. In this, the specially designed transducer is used to visualize the follicles and the aspirating needle is passed alongside it. This method is generally well tolerated when carried out under light intravenous sedation, can be learnt very quickly, and is associated with minimal morbidity.

Several designs of aspiration needles are available. They may have a single or double lumen to enable aspiration and flushing through different routes. The needle is usually 16-guage and must have a very sharp tip to enable easy puncture of mobile ovaries and its distal 2 cm should be roughened to enhance ultrasound visualization (Fig. 14.5). The needle is connected to a test tube by tubing and suction is applied either from a foot-operated pump (Fig. 14.6) or manually. The ultrasound transducer (Fig. 14.7) is enclosed in a special sterile condom and plastic sleeve prior to insertion into the vagina and should be thoroughly cleaned with a damp cloth after each procedure.

Generally, very few technical difficulties are encountered during vaginal egg collections. The main risks of transvaginal oocyte recovery are pelvic infection (0.6%) and bleeding (>100 mL in 0.8% cases),[54] which may be serious, sometimes even fatal. Appropriate preoperative vaginal preparation and minimizing the number of repeated vaginal penetrations may serve to lower the risk of infection. While there is no evidence that routine antibiotics reduce the risk of infection, the administration of an intravenous bolus of antibiotics is generally recommended to women with history of severe pelvic inflammatory disease or if an endometrioma is punctured. Intestinal, vascular, uterine, and tubal injuries with the aspiration needle have also been reported. Bleeding and infections may be serious, sometimes even fatal, complications.

LABORATORY TECHNIQUES

The oocytes obtained are fertilized by conventional IVF or ICSI treatment dependent on the quality of the sperm obtained on the day of oocyte retrieval. ICSI is indicated, if there is a severe deficit in sperm quality, obstructive or nonobstructive azoospermia, and for couples in whom a previous IVF treatment cycle has resulted in failed or very poor fertilization. Sperm utilized for conventional IVF/ICSI is obtained by masturbation. When there is azoospermia, it is aspirated from the epididymis [percutaneous epididymal sperm aspiration (PESA), testicular sperm aspiration (TESA)] or extracted from the testes [testicular sperm extraction (TESE)]. Mirco TESE has a better success rate in extracting sperm when compared with standard single biopsy.

There are numerous techniques for performing the insemination of oocytes that vary from laboratory to laboratory. Differences in culture systems can be: the quantity and volume of sperm added to oocytes, the oocytes can be cultured either singly or in groups, and an open or oil covered culture system can be employed.

In cases of ICSI, the meiotic maturity is assessed after denudation and only mature oocytes are injected with sperm following its immobilization. Fertilization as determined by the presence of two pro nuclei (2 PN) is assessed at 18–20 hours postinsemination. On day 2 or 3, based on the cleavage rate, the size, shape, symmetry and cytoplasmic appearance of the blastomeres, and the presence or absence of nucleus, embryo quality was graded by the embryologists as grade 1, 2, 3, or 4.[55] Grade 1 and 2 embryos were considered to be of high quality. While ET is performed with one or two best available embryo/s, regardless of their grading, only top quality, grade 1 and 2 embryos were considered eligible for freezing and this option was then offered to the couple.

Embryo Transfer

Embryo transfer is a critical step in determining the final outcome of the treatment. The convention has been to replace embryos on the 2nd or 3rd day postinsemination, when the embryos are usually two to eight cell stage of cleavage. With improvements in culture media, there is an increasing tendency for delaying ET with an aim to improve the implantation rates. While there is no improvement in live birth rates (1.07, 95% CI 0.84–1.37) with delaying ET from day 2 to day 3,[56] transfer of embryos at blastocyst stage (day 5/6) has shown significant increase in live birth rate (OR 1.35, 95% CI 1.05–1.74) when compared with day 2 to 3 transfers.[57] It is a more physiological approach, allowing synchronization of the embryo with the endometrium and the selection of viable embryos for transfer will be more efficient. However, the rates of embryos freezing are lower and the treatment cancellation rates are higher with blastocyst transfer. But in selected group of couples, the practice of blastocyst transfer has the potential to favor single ET without compromising the overall success rates but can significantly reduce the occurrence of multiple pregnancies. The most favored group for blastocyst transfer are those having high numbers of eight cell embryos on day 3, in whom the cycle cancellation is not increased.

Transcervical embryo replacement into the uterine cavity is a relatively simple procedure, which must be carried out meticulously to ensure appropriate placement of the embryos (Fig. 14.8). Variations among clinicians in the technique of ET may influence the pregnancy rate. Avoidance of blood, mucus, bacterial contamination, excessive

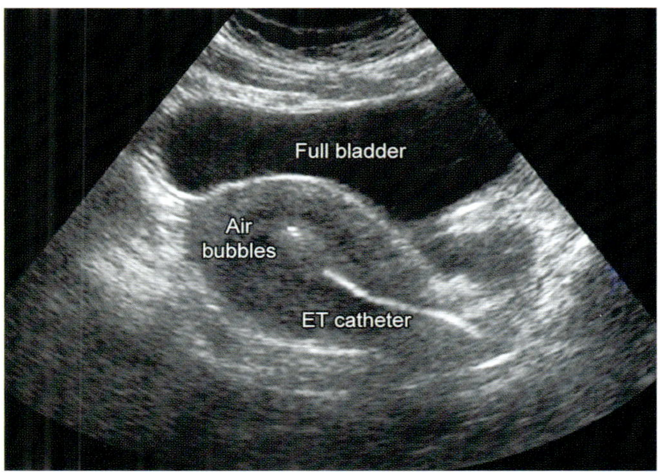

Fig. 14.8: Transcervical embryo transfer.

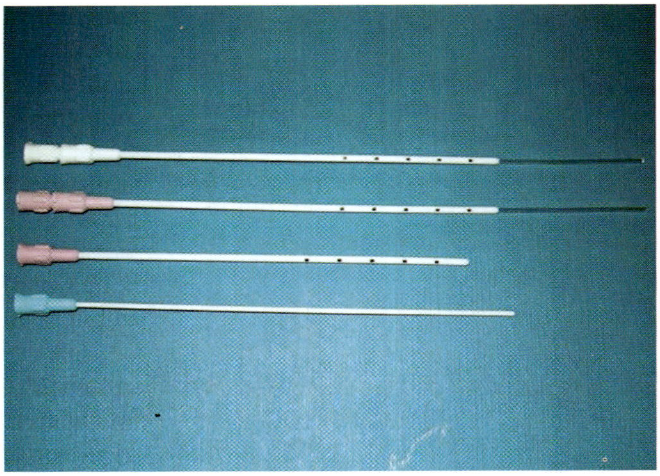

Fig. 14.9: Embryo transfer catheters. From top to bottom: Trial Wallace (no lumen), Wallace, Outer sheath and Stylet of Malleable Catheter.

uterine contractions, and trauma to the endometrium is associated with optimal pregnancy and implantation rates after transcervical ET. Transabdominal ultrasonographic guidance to determine the precise depth of embryo placement within the uterus appear to facilitate successful ET and is preferred, therefore,[58] although a recent large randomized trial from a single center did not show any benefit over "clinical touch" transfer.[59] The full bladder required for abdominal ultrasound also helps to straighten the cervicouterine angle and facilitate entry of the catheter, particularly for the strongly anteverted uterus. Since first described by Strickler et al. in 1985, numerous studies evaluating the effect of ultrasound guidance in ET on PRs have been published. A 2010 Cochrane review of 17 RCTs comparing ultrasound versus clinical touch concluded that ultrasound did increase ongoing clinical PRs over clinical touch. Three other recent meta-analyses of RCTs have had similar conclusions. Disadvantages with ultrasound may include the need for a second operator, a longer procedure time, and the inconvenience of filling the patient's bladder. Patients also seem to take great comfort in visualizing this final step of an often long and difficult process.

Soft catheters are preferred over rigid ones as they are less likely to traumatize the cervix and endometrium and to invoke any uterine contractions. The commonly used soft catheters (Wallace) (Fig. 14.9) have a softer inner cannula and a stiffer outer sheath. In two recent meta-analyses of RCTs, the use of soft catheters was associated with a higher PR than firm catheters.[60,61] Alternatively, the outer sheath from this trial catheter can be left in place, either routinely or with difficult cases, while the soft inner catheter is loaded with the embryos and advanced through the sheath to the correct placement. This method, sometimes referred to as the afterloading technique, may also decrease mucus contamination of the catheter. Occasionally, resistance to pass the soft inner cannula into the uterus usually at the level of internal os is encountered and in these cases the stiffer outer sheath is advanced in the cervical canal to negotiate the resistance with the inner cannula, which can now be advanced into the uterine cavity. A malleable stylet device can be used with some soft catheters to negotiate a difficult internal os.[62] It was demonstrated that the use of this device compared with a soft catheter alone did not decrease clinical pregnancy or implantation rates. The inner stylet is then removed and the softer cannula with embryos loaded in it is fed through the outer sheath to advance into the uterine cavity for transfer. When using the malleable stylet, it is important to leave the outer sheath just proximal to the internal os. Keeping it in this location before inserting the inner soft catheter was found to significantly improve clinical pregnancy rates.[63] In some cases, insertion of the catheter is difficult owing to cervical stenosis. Different approaches have been undertaken to alleviate this issue, including cervical dilation at the time of retrieval.[64] However, this was found to lower subsequent pregnancy rates. Dilation has also been accomplished several weeks before ET and was found to improve outcomes.[65]

Contamination of the catheter with blood may be a marker for difficult ET and has also been linked to poor ET outcomes. When retrospectively assessing outcomes, Goudas et al. demonstrated a clinical pregnancy rate of 50% with no blood, and this rate fell by half when a small amount of blood was noted on the catheter tip. Pregnancy rates fell even further, to 10%, when there was a significant amount of blood. Similarly, in a preliminary study, blood or mucus on the tip was associated with a significantly lower pregnancy outcome. Blood was associated with a lowered odds ratio for pregnancy of 1.9 and for mucus the odds ratio for pregnancy was lowered by 1.8.

In a RCT performed in patients undergoing ultrasound-guided ET, a higher PR (60% vs. 39.3%) was achieved when the distance was 15–20 mm compared with 10 mm. Other studies have shown that embryos deposited less than 5 mm from the fundus have a decreased PR and an increased rate of ectopic pregnancy. The preponderance of data in the literature supports ET in the mid to lower-mid portion of the uterus, avoiding transfers high in the fundus. Lambers et al. assessed the position of the air bubble transferred at the time of ET and its relation to pregnancy rate. When the relative position of the air bubbles was in the fundal half of the endometrial cavity, pregnancy rates were significantly higher, at 43% (this compared with when the bubble was in the lower half of the cavity, 24.4%). More recently, it was demonstrated that pregnancy and implantation rates among subjects with air bubble flashes located 15 mm from the fundus.[66]

After injection of the embryos, pressure on the plunger of the syringe should be maintained until the catheter is completely withdrawn from the uterus. Furthermore, the outer sheath should be completely retracted and removed simultaneously with the inner catheter to avoid a "plunger" effect. Withdrawing the catheter slowly will also minimize negative pressure. Another concern with ET is the possibility of expelled embryos. Knutzen et al. found that using a radio-opaque dye to mimic ET contrast after ET remained primarily in the uterine cavity in only 68% of cases.

The influence of the time interval before withdrawal of the catheter after ultrasound-guided ET was also investigated, comparing an immediate withdrawal versus a 30-second delay.[67] No difference in clinical outcome was seen between these two options.

The embryo trauma may be related to the rapidity of injection, and care should be taken to inject the fluid as slowly as possible. Additionally, *in vitro* modeling suggests that rapid injection may lead to embryo placement issues and possibly promote ectopic pregnancies.[68]

A recent meta-analysis examining 16 studies concluded that although the existing quality of data is moderate, there does seem to be a benefit of hyaluronan inclusion in transfer media.[69]

Historically patients have been placed on bed rest for varied amounts of time after the transfer, as decreased physical activity was thought to improve embryo retention within the uterine cavity. ET subsequently became an outpatient procedure, as prolonged bed rest was shown not to improve pregnancy rates. Even brief bed rest (30 minutes) has since been shown to offer no benefit over immediate ambulation. So following ET, women are often advised to continue their normal daily activities. Luteal support is usually required as ART is associated with inadequate luteal function, possibly because of the removal of the granulosa cells surrounding the oocytes while performing the oocyte retrieval and of the use of GnRH agonists. hCG or progesterone is traditionally used to provide luteal support during conventional IVF cycles. However, the routine use of hCG is not recommended because of the increased likelihood of OHSS and no benefit over progesterone in terms of IVF success. The progesterone can be administered either 200–800 mg/day vaginally or 50–100 mg/day intramuscularly and is continued for 14–16 days, when pregnancy test is performed.

OUTCOME MEASURES AND FACTORS AFFECTING SUCCESS RATE

Pregnancy and live birth rates per treatment cycle for IVF and ICSI have steadily improved worldwide over the past decade. Figure 14.10 shows the improvement in the live birth rate per treatment cycle in the United Kingdom between 1991 and 2005 (HFEA 2008). It is now widely accepted that when attempting to ascertain whether or not a treatment is required, it is essential that the time-specific or cycle-specific conception rate is used. Crude pregnancy rate per couple is almost meaningless. Pregnancy rate per cycle can also be misleading if limited to the first cycle or two because the rate may fall in subsequent cycles. Thus, cumulative conception or cumulative live birth rates have been increasingly used in reporting conventional and ART outcomes. Cumulative conception rates for some of the most common causes of infertility in the untreated population were compared to those in couples following treatment with conventional methods.[70] The results showed that in some conditions such as ovulatory dysfunction, or in those being treated with donor insemination, the cumulative conception rate following conventional therapy is

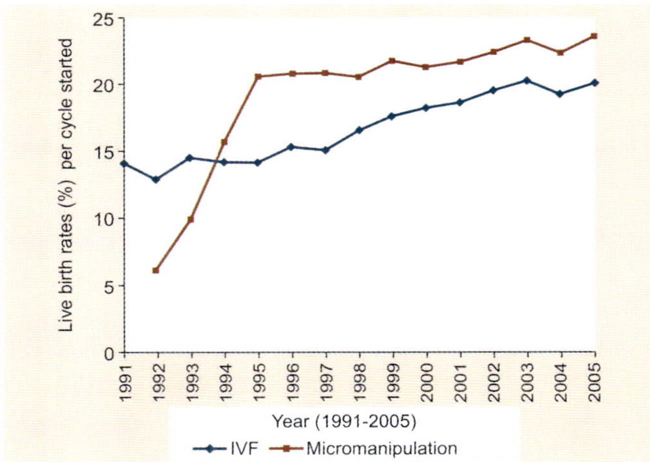

Fig. 14.10: Live birth rates per treatment cycle (1991–2005) (HFEA 2008).

almost the same as in normal women. However, in other circumstances, such as salpingostomy for distal tubal occlusion, or the use of high-dose glucocorticosteroids for seminal antisperm antibodies, the prognosis is worse and the cumulative conception rates are lower than that which can now be expected in a single cycle of IVF treatment.

The effectiveness of infertility treatments (IVF, ICSI, egg and sperm donation, embryo donation) is dependent on a reasonable likelihood that embryos can be created *in vitro* and then placed in the uterus with a reasonable expectation that implantation will occur. Many factors determine the outcome of treatment, such as patient selection, age, cause and duration of infertility, and the number of attempts that couples undergo. The decision to recommend ART should be based on the likelihood that a pregnancy will occur without treatment, the possibility that a less invasive form of treatment might be effective and the likely outcome of IVF treatment.[71] The likelihood of treatment-independent pregnancy depends on the woman's age, cause and duration of infertility, and history of previous pregnancy. In a retrospective study,[72] the incidence of spontaneous treatment-independent pregnancy in couples enlisted on an IVF program was reported to be 11% of couples with low fertility. The main difference from those in whom pregnancy did not occur was a shorter duration of infertility.

Success of ART is also dependent on where the provision of service takes place. It is clear from the HFEA annual reports that the outcome of treatment varies between small and large centers. When discussing the likelihood of birth following IVF treatment with any couple, it is essential to consider the factors that can significantly affect the outcome. These include female age, cause and duration of infertility, previous pregnancy history, number of embryos replaced, availability of surplus embryos for cryopreservation, and the number of any previous treatment cycles. Such advice is particularly relevant and important in women over the age of 40 in whom success rates are considerably reduced and the risk of miscarriage is increased.

Female Age

The woman's age at the time of treatment is an important prognostic factor when the success of IVF is discussed with any couple. The number of oocytes and consequently the number of embryos decline with age. However, the cleavage rate does not seem to alter in the same manner. The number of embryos replaced compounds the effect of age and embryo implantation rates on pregnancy rate. The total number of embryos available for replacement further influences this. When a larger number of embryos are available for replacement, the selection of the most appropriate embryos for transfer would improve the implantation and pregnancy rates.

Indeed, when women over the age of 40 had four or more embryos transferred, their pregnancy rate was not significantly different from younger women, whether following IVF[72] or ICSI.[73] Hence, it may be concluded that older women with good ovarian response, producing three or more embryos suitable for transfer, have similar prospects to establishing a pregnancy to younger patients. However, there are other data, which supported reduced implantation rates in older women regardless of the number of embryos transferred.[74] Younger women, even if their ovarian response is poor, have a better implantation rate than women older than 40 experiencing a normal ovarian response.[75] This indicates that age is the major determinant of the implantation potential of oocytes. However, the reported finding of similar pregnancy rates in older women having treatment using donor eggs compared to younger women indicates that the oocyte quality or its implantation potential rather than the endometrial receptivity declines with women's age.[76]

Age and Pregnancy, Live Birth, and Miscarriage Rates

Although live birth rates per treatment cycle following IVF and ICSI have increased consistently over the past decade, they decline with advancing age of women when using their own eggs (Fig. 14.11). A number of investigators have examined different age cut-offs such as 40 years[72,20] or 35 years.[77]. Mardesic et al. reported that the cut-off point of effectiveness for an IVF program was 36–37 years, with marked decline in pregnancy rate per ET in women over the age of 38.[78]

In an attempt to identify factors that affect the outcome of treatment, Templeton and colleagues analyzed the HFEA database between 1991 and 1994.[79] The authors reported that the overall live birth rate per cycle of treatment was 13.9%. The highest live birth rates were in the 25–30 years age group, with younger women (under 25 years) having lower rates, while a sharp decline was noted in older women. At all ages over 30 years, the use of donor eggs was associated with significantly higher live birth rates compared with the use of women's own eggs,

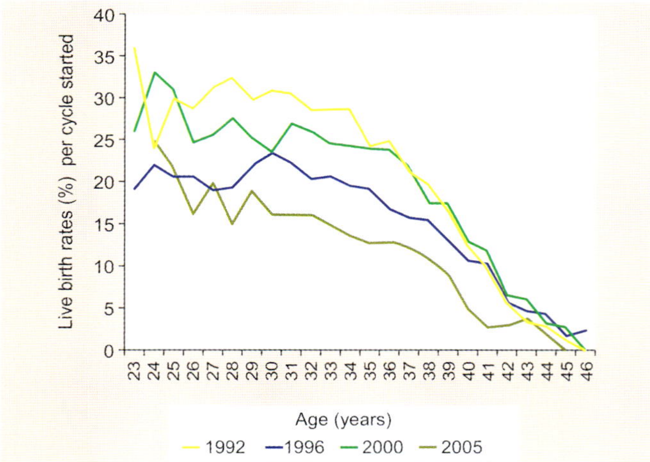

Fig. 14.11: Live birth rates by age of women who have IVF or ICSI. Success rates have improved over the years for all ages (HFEA 2008).

though there was equally a downward trend in success rates with age. After adjustment for age, increasing duration of infertility was associated with a significant decrease in live birth rates. The indications for treatment had no significant effect on the outcome, while previous pregnancy and live birth significantly increased treatment success.

Miscarriage rates have been reported to be higher in all the women following IVF and there is a twofold to threefold increase in the rate of spontaneous abortion in women aged 40 or more.[80] It is more likely that embryo quality is the main factor influencing the poor reproductive performance of women with advancing age rather than defective response of uterine vasculature to steroids or uterine ageing. Increasing maternal age correlates with a higher risk of fetal chromosomal aneuploidy, which results in an increased miscarriage rate.[81] A large prospective register linkage study reported the age-related risk of miscarriage in recognized pregnancies to be: 12–19 years (13%); 20–24 years (11%); 25–29 years (12%); 30–34 years (15%); 35–39 years (25%); 40–44 years (51%); and elder than or equal to 45 years (93%). Advanced paternal age has also been identified as a risk factor for miscarriage. The risk of miscarriage is highest among couples where the woman is elder than or equal to 35 years of age and the man elder than or equal to 40 years of age. The risk of a further miscarriage increases after each successive pregnancy loss, reaching approximately 40% after three consecutive pregnancy losses, and the prognosis worsens with increasing maternal age. A previous live birth does not preclude a woman developing recurrent miscarriage.

Obesity

Although the consequences of obesity in women's fertility are well known, there is controversy regarding the effect of obesity on the outcome of IVF treatment. Many obese women and men are fertile. Obesity in women is associated with ovulatory dysfunction, reduced ovarian responsiveness to agents that induce ovulation, altered oocyte as well as endometrial functions, and lower birth rates. Lower rates of embryo transfer, pregnancy, and live birth have also been reported, as have higher miscarriage rates.[82] Other studies have been unable to find any negative impact of obesity on ART outcome[83,84] However, a recent systematic review of all the reported studies has confirmed the adverse effect of obesity on the success of IVF[85] and, therefore, obese women should be advised to lose weight before commencing ART to improve their chances of success. A meta-analysis of 33 IVF studies including 47,967 cycles concluded that overweight or obese women have a higher rate of miscarriage (RR 1.31, $P < 0.0001$) compared with normal-weight women (BMI <25).[86] Obese women are at increased risk of developing maternal and fetal complications during pregnancy. A meta-analysis of 18 observational studies confirms the associations between maternal obesity and obese mothers were at increased odds of pregnancies affected by neural tube defects, spina bifida, cardiovascular anomalies, cardiac septal anomalies, cleft palate, cleft lip and palate, anorectal atresia, hydrocephaly, and limb reduction anomalies.[87] These fetal abnormalities are linked with maternal metabolic dysfunction, which also promotes in the offspring an increased risk for obesity in later life, thereby perpetuating obesity in subsequent generations. Recent retrospective studies have reported that obesity increases the risk of both sporadic and recurrent miscarriage. Obesity in men may be associated with impaired reproductive function.

Lifestyle modification in women and men is the first-line treatment for obesity, followed by adjunctive medical therapy. Overweight (BMI ≥25) and obesity (BMI ≥30) have been associated with the need for higher doses of gonadotropins, increased cycle cancellation rates, and fewer oocytes retrieved.

Cause of Infertility

Reports have differed in their analysis of the impact of infertility factors on the cumulative conception and live birth rates. While some have found significant differences, with the lowest rates being reported in patients with male

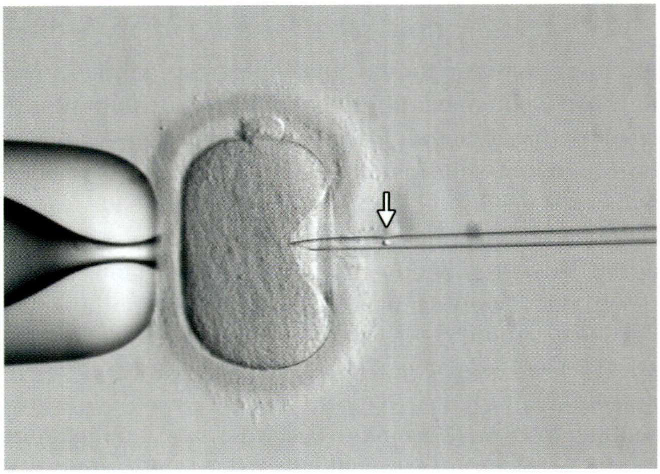

Fig. 14.12: Intracytoplasmic injection of a single sperm (arrow) into the egg.

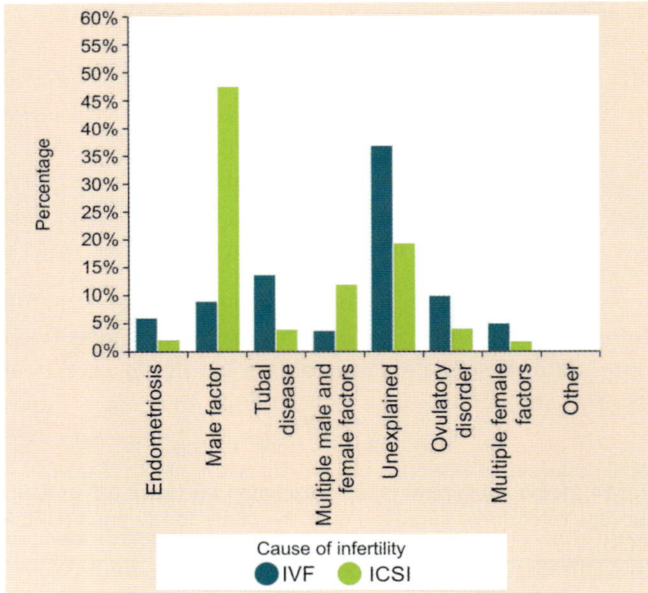

Fig. 14.13: Percentage of couple seeking standard IVF or ICSI, by the reason they sought treatment in 2014 (HFEA Data).

infertility or multiple infertility factors,[88] others found no significant effect on the outcome.[79] However, history of previous pregnancy and live birth significantly increased treatment success. The IVF clinical pregnancy and live birth rates in the HFEA report of 2,000 show similar results for tubal disease, endometriosis, and unexplained infertility (Figs. 14.12 and 14.13). Reports of higher fertilization rates after ICSI suggested that this technique may be better than the conventional method for all couples seeking IVF. A multicenter randomized controlled trial comparing clinical outcome after ICSI or conventional IVF in couples with nonmale factor infertility showed higher implantation and pregnancy rates per cycle after IVF, hence supporting the practice of reserving ICSI for severe male factor infertility.[89]

All stages of endometriosis are viewed as suitable indications for ART. The timing of treatment is dependent on the severity of the disease, previous therapy, and other factors, such as female age and duration of infertility. In women with severe endometriosis with mechanical tubal blockage and where surgery is inappropriate, IVF should be expedited. IVF should also be recommended 1–2 years after previous unsuccessful medical or surgical therapy, while in minimal or mild endometriosis, the balance of choice seems to be in favor of IVF after more than 2 years of expectant management. Initially, poor results were reported in women with severe disease.[90] The introduction of ultrasound-guided techniques for oocyte collection resulted in retrieving larger number of oocytes and hence achieving higher pregnancy and implantation rates in advanced-stage disease.[91] The use of GnRH agonists in stimulation protocols or as a pretreatment of women with endometriosis has also resulted in a higher number of preovulatory oocytes retrieved and transferred, lower cancellation of treatment cycles, and a higher pregnancy rate, especially in women with advanced-stage disease. A recent meta-analysis has indicated that presence of ovarian endometrioma does not affect the quality of the oocytes as the pregnancy rates were similar to that of controls, although ovarian response to gonadotropins was reduced.[92] While prospective randomized controlled trials are lacking, the evidence based on the case-control studies suggest that surgeries for bilateral endometrioma could significantly impair IVF outcome possibly due to damage to the remaining healthy ovarian follicles.[93]

For male factor infertility, ICSI was successfully introduced in 1992[94] and since then, the annual number of treatment cycles has increased steadily. Previous techniques such as partial zona dissection (PZD) and subzonal insemination (SUZI) were very disappointing[95] and comparative studies indicated that ICSI was a much more efficient technique than either of the others.[96] It gave men who had previously been diagnosed with severe male factor infertility the chance to have their own genetic children. The sperm may be obtained either by ejaculation, percutaneous aspiration from the epididymis (PESA) or testis (TESA), or testicular extraction (TESE), resulting in equally high fertilization, pregnancy, and implantation rates, especially in men with borderline or very poor sperm quality. Recognized indications for ICSI include:

1) Very poor sperm quality
2) Both obstructive and nonobstructive azoospermia
3) Prolonged unexplained infertility
4) Previously failed or very poor fertilization

A remarkable change in fertilization rate with a significant increase in the percentage of two pronuclei oocytes occurred when the technique was slightly modified by breaking the sperm tail before injection.[97] The technique requires a high-quality inverted microscope and special equipment with holding and injection pipettes being used to stabilize and inject the oocyte, respectively. The injecting pipette is pushed almost entirely through the ooplasm before the spermatozoon is deposited inside the oocyte.

The Duration of Infertility

The duration of infertility remains one of the most important variables that influence the outcome of assisted reproduction, with lower pregnancy and live birth rates associated with a longer period of infertility. Analysis of the HFEA database between 1991 and 1994 showed that, even with adjustment for age, there was a significant decrease in live birth rate with increasing duration of infertility from 1 to 12 years.[79]

Endometrial Thickness

Endometrial thickness on its own is a poor predictor for pregnancy. However, no conception was recorded when endometrial thickness was below 5 mm on the day of transfer and hence it is recommended that consideration should be given to cryopreserving all embryos and preparing the endometrium with exogenous hormones at a subsequent cycle.[98]

Number of Embryos Transferred

Regarding the optimum number of embryos to be transferred, there is a great deal of debate and a wide variation in practice across the world. Unarguably, ART is the single most important cause of increase in multiple pregnancies over the last 2 decades, which is a direct consequence of the number of embryos transferred. Retrospective studies, as early as 1985, had argued that multiple pregnancies and births increased with the increase in the number of embryos replaced.[99] Randomized studies comparing two- with three-embryo transfers[100] or four-embryo transfers[101] reported similar pregnancy rates as long as there were sufficient morphologically regular embryos available for transfer. Analysis of the HFEA database of more than 44,000 cycles[102] and the HFEA reports (1999, 2000) showed that when four or more fertilized eggs were available, the transfer of three embryos did not result in improved pregnancy rates compared to the elective transfer of two embryos only. However, the incidence of triplets or higher order multiple births decreased considerably when two embryos were replaced.

Despite transferring only two embryos during most IVF cycles, 40% of all IVF babies are twins (HFEA 2008). In order to deal with the unacceptably high multiple birth rates following ART, there is a recent move from the IVF community particularly in the Europe to limit the number of embryos transferred to one in carefully selected patients. HFEA has set a target of bringing down the multiple pregnancy rates to 10% in the United Kingdom over a period of about 3 years and has urged the fertility clinics to devise a "multiple pregnancy minimization strategy" to achieve the agreed target. To facilitate this, the British Fertility Society in unison with Association of Clinical Embryologists in the United Kingdom has produced a guideline for practice, which focuses on the effectiveness of eSET and patient selection for eSET.[103] The two most important criteria to choose the couple for eSET are the women's age and the quality of embryos available (Fig. 14.14 and Table 14.1). Twin pregnancy causes increased risks to the fetus and the mother. Given the higher risks of premature delivery (threefold), perinatal mortality (sixfold), cerebral palsy (fourfold to sixfold), and pregnancy complications (hypertension, pre-eclampsia, gestational diabetes, etc.) and the consequent resource implications for the health service with twin births as compared to singleton deliveries, HFEA in the UK has urged to re-define the success after IVF as "full term singletons with a normal birth weight" in order to promote single ET and thereby reducing multiple births.[103] A Cochrane review comparing the outcome of double ET in a single cycle versus eSET (combined with transfer of a single frozen-thawed embryo in a subsequent cycle if needed), identified similar pregnancy rates in both groups (odds ratio 1.19, 95% CI 0.87–1.62) with substantially greater multiple pregnancy rates following double ET (odds ratio 62.83, 95% CI 8.52–463.57).[104] Several European countries have now adopted eSET coupled with effective cryopreservation programs in good prognosis patients and have reported no significant difference in pregnancy rates but a significant reduction in twin rates (Fig. 14.15). In carefully selected patients (e.g., women below 37 years of age, undergoing first IVF cycle and having more than one top quality embryos), eSET plus subsequent FER can be as effective as double ET.

HFEA report in 2016 suggest overall success rates continue to rise: the IVF birth rate increased slightly, to 26.5% in 2013 from 25.9% the year before. Importantly, this increase in the birth rate has happened as the multiple birth rate has fallen. Multiple births have dropped from one in four IVF births in 2008 to one in six in 2013, showing that our "One at a time" campaign to reduce multiple births without harming success rates continues to be successful (Tables 14.2 and 14.3) (Fig. 14.16).

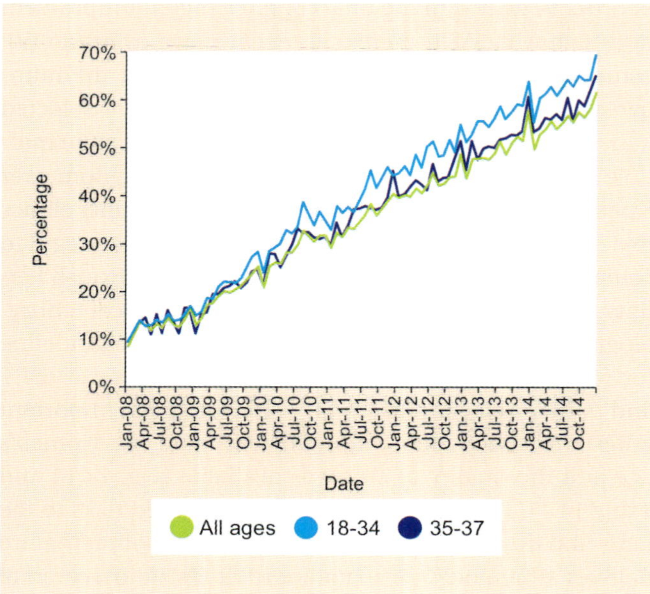

Fig. 14.14: Proportion of blastocyst transfer since 2008 (HFEA Data).

Number of Assisted Reproductive Technique Attempts

The literature appears to be somewhat divided when the pregnancy and live birth rates in relation to the number of ART attempts are examined. In one study,[105] the pregnancy rate per ET was similar for at least seven attempts, while other studies,[88,79] reported decline in the chances of pregnancy and live birth rates with successive treatment cycles. The data from the HFEA 1998 annual report showed a steady decline after the fifth attempt with pregnancy and live birth rates per cycle, being 11.1% and 8.6%, respectively at the eleventh attempt.

When IVF cumulative pregnancy rates were estimated for a cohort of women, the rates showed a constant rise during the six initial IVF treatments and plateaued subsequently.[106] Similarly, the rates were reported to be as high as 80% after seven cycles and a history of previous pregnancy significantly improved a couple's probability of conception.[107]

Embryo Cryopreservation

The ability to cryopreserve embryos enables any supernumerary embryos to be stored for some time before subsequent replacement when fresh ET has failed or if further children are desired. Additionally, cryopreservation has the added benefit of increasing the number of potential embryo replacement cycles without the need to undergo

Table 14.1: Pregnancy rate per embryo transfer by stage and number of embryo transferred in 2014 in UK (HFEA Data).

No.of embryos	*eSET*		*DET*	
Stage	*Cleavage (%)*	*Blastocyst (%)*	*Cleavage (%)*	*Blastocyst (%)*
Age				
18-34	36.9	50.7	38.3	50.7
35-37	31.4	47.4	33.5	49.3
38-39	23.6	40.9	25.7	41.6
40-42			17.7	32.8
43-44	6.8	30.0	7.3	19.3
45+				
All ages	**32.6**	**48.5**	**30.5**	**45.2**

superovulation and oocyte retrieval, hence reducing the risk of OHSS. Embryo quality has the most significant impact on post-thaw survival and ultimately pregnancy and implantation rates. As with fresh embryos, factors such as patient's age, the number of embryos transferred, and whether a pregnancy resulted from the original stimulation cycle will affect the outcome of the FER cycle.

The clinical value of embryo cryopreservation has steadily increased over the decades with significant technological advances made in our ability to freeze cleavage-stage and blastocyst-stage embryos. The first success in cryopreservation was achieved with slow-freezing methods and for the past 2 decades slow freezing has been the method of choice for embryo cryopreservation. More recently, optimized vitrification methods, with the use of cryoprotectant and rapid freezing, have become more widely utilized. When implemented correctly, vitrified embryos have excellent survival rates following thawing. Indeed, a 95% survival rate has been reported in a large cohort of vitrified blastocysts.[108] Recent systematic reviews and meta-analyses have compared the outcomes of vitrification versus slow-freezing methods.[109,110] Vitrification has higher post-thaw survival rates compared with slow freezing both for cleavage stage [OR 15.57; 95% confidence interval (95% CI) 3.68–65.82] and blastocyst-stage embryos (OR 2.2; 95% CI 1.53–3.16) (four studies).[109] Furthermore, assessment of embryo vitrification by clinical outcomes

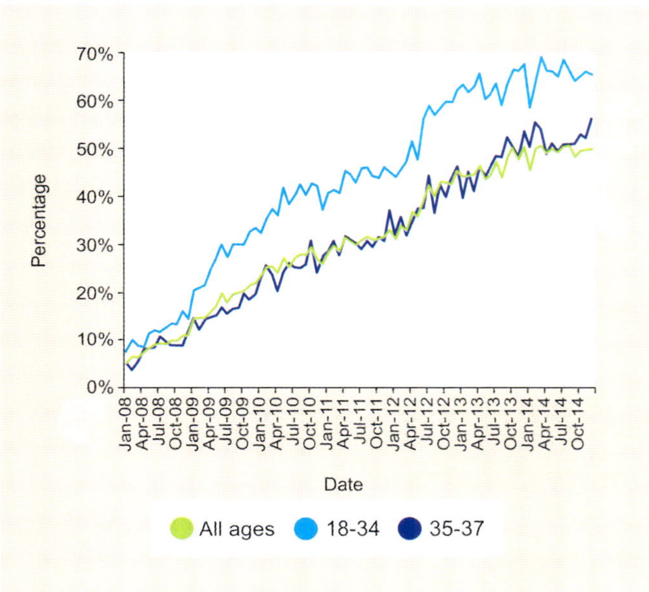

Fig. 14.15: Trend of ESET on all embryo transfer since 2008 (HFEA Data).

Table 14.2: Multiple birth rate (% of live birth) using own fresh eggs (HFEA Data).

Age	*2012 (%)*	*2013 (%)*
18-34	16.9	15.0
35-37	18.8	16.2
38-39	16.4	15.4
40-42	12.4	14.9
43+	6.7	9.3
All ages	**16.9**	**15.3**

Table 14.3: Multiple pregnancy rate (% of pregnancies) fresh own eggs, by Stage and by Number embryos transferred, 2014 (HFEA Data).

<table>
<tr><th>Stage</th><th colspan="2">Cleavage stage embryo</th><th colspan="2">Blastocyst stage embryo</th></tr>
<tr><th>Transfer type</th><th>eSET (%)</th><th>Double (%)</th><th>eSET (%)</th><th>Double (%)</th></tr>
<tr><td>Age</td><td></td><td></td><td></td><td></td></tr>
<tr><td>18-34</td><td rowspan="6">0.6</td><td>29.5</td><td>2.1</td><td>41.5</td></tr>
<tr><td>35-37</td><td>21.3</td><td>1.3</td><td>38.7</td></tr>
<tr><td>38-39</td><td>17.9</td><td rowspan="4">1.7</td><td>30.1</td></tr>
<tr><td>40-42</td><td rowspan="3">9.0</td><td rowspan="3">21.1</td></tr>
<tr><td>43-44</td></tr>
<tr><td>45+</td></tr>
<tr><td>All ages</td><td>0.6</td><td>23.5</td><td>1.9</td><td>36.4</td></tr>
</table>

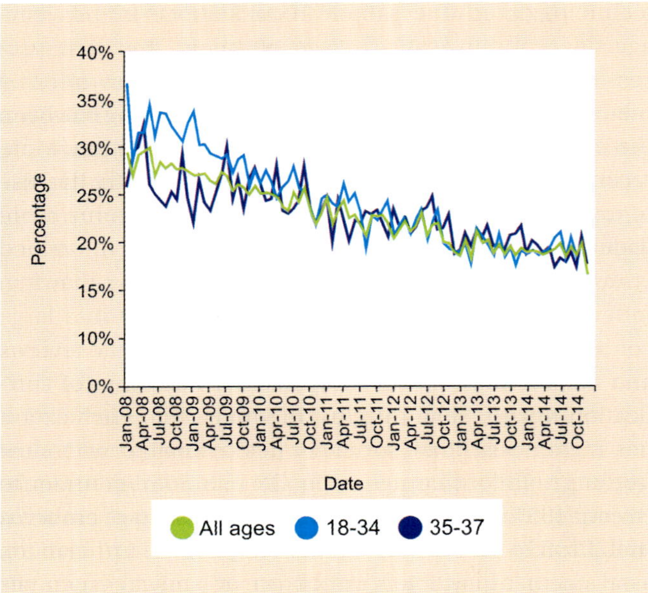

Fig. 14.16: Trends in multiple pregnancy rates from 2008–2014 (HFEA Data).

(six studies)[110] showed that CPRs were more than 50% higher in the vitrification groups compared with slow frozen embryos (OR 1.55, 95% CI 1.03–2.32), with similar results seen in ongoing pregnancy and implantation rates.

Overall, the findings indicate that birth outcomes after FET are better compared with fresh ETs. It should also be emphasized that these studies were all observational in nature, and that the frozen/thawed embryos available for transfer were therefore inevitably "second choice" as the best embryos would have been transferred in the preceding fresh transfer. It is thus highly conceivable that the obstetrical and neonatal outcomes following elective FET, which also includes the best embryos, may be even further improved, but such studies have yet to be performed.

A stronger argument in favor of adopting elective FET (eFET) as the default IVF protocol is the potential for higher pregnancy rates. A recent systematic review and meta-analysis of three randomized controlled trials including 633 women assessed clinical and ongoing CPRs and miscarriage rates following eFET and fresh ETs.[111] The overall conclusions were that eFET resulted in an increase in the CPR (RR 1.31; 95% CI 1.10–1.56) and the ongoing pregnancy rate (RR 1.32; 95% CI 1.10–1.59), with no difference in the miscarriage rate (RR 0.83; 95% CI 0.43–1.60). Randomized patients were high responders in two studies[112,113] and normal responders in the other study,[114] but all showed the same trend. The observed effect was also similar in those studies that transferred day 5[113,114] and day 2 embryos.[112]

Frozen thawed embryos can be replaced in natural or hormonally adjusted cycles utilizing GnRH agonist and estrogen/progestogen preparations with comparable results. The use of GnRH agonist is useful in anovulatory or irregular cycles and the use of different progestogens for luteal phase support is equally effective. The cost per delivery for an FER cycle has been estimated to be between 25 and 45% of a fresh cycle. In view of these advantages, cryopreservation should be accessible and discussed with all couples where surplus good quality embryos are available.

Some clinical studies suggest that hormonal intervention can be detrimental to endometrial receptivity and pregnancy success[115-118] and it is therefore plausible that the true effect size of elective FET in natural cycles may well be higher in the absence of hormonal intervention. Importantly, over 1,000 patients have already been recruited for a new multicenter randomized trial (The ANTARCTICA trial) to assess the effect of natural and artificial FET cycles on numerous outcomes such as live birth rate, health costs, adverse events, and patient burden[119] and its outcomes are keenly awaited.

Oocyte Donation

Oocyte donation is an effective treatment for women with premature ovarian failure, Turner syndrome, following oophorectomy, chemotherapy- or radiotherapy-related ovarian failure, in certain cases where there is a high risk of transmitting a genetic disorder to the child and where repeated failure of fertilization is attributed to poor oocyte quality. High pregnancy rates have been reported following oocyte donation for Turner syndrome patients.[120] However, Turner's patients were reported to have significantly higher biochemical pregnancy rates and early miscarriages, lower clinical pregnancy and delivery rates when compared to other women with premature ovarian failure.[121] An important factor in the establishment of pregnancy is an endometrial thickness of greater than 6.5 mm. Other factors include the number of previous natural conceptions and live births and the fertilization rate, while increasing female age does not affect the outcome.[122]

The HFEA recommends the age limit for the egg donors should be 35 years except in exceptional circumstances. This is because there is an increased pregnancy rate and reduced risk of aneuploidy in the offspring, if the treatment is performed using eggs from young donors. Oocyte donors are screened for infections [HIV, hepatitis B, hepatitis C, CMV, and venereal disease research laboratory (VDRL) tests for syphilis] as well as for genetic diseases such as CF and for major chromosomal anomalies. Targeted screening based on the ethnic background is also recommended, e.g. Tay-Sachs disease for Jewish population, sickle cell screening in Afro-Caribbean population and thalassemia in Asian population. If the prospective donor is found to be heterozygous for CF, the partner of the recipient should also be screened for CF.

Oocyte donation has considerable emotional and social effects on both the donor and recipient, more so if the donor is undergoing IVF treatment herself. Both the recipients and the donors should have counseling from someone who is independent of the treatment unit regarding the physical and psychological implications of treatment for themselves and their genetic children, including any potential children resulting from donated oocytes. Apart from anonymous and known oocyte donation, an egg share scheme is an efficient use of resource of oocytes. This aims to reduce the imbalance between the large number of potential recipients and the small number of available donors. This also allows women requiring IVF and having insufficient funds for her own treatment to access IVF treatment for either free or at a significantly reduced cost. Many studies have reported a safe "cut-off" number of oocytes that have to be collected from the egg share donor to share with the recipient.

The live birth rates following treatment using oocyte donation is excellent. Pregnancy and live birth rates per treatment cycle following oocyte donation in comparison with other treatments are depicted in Table 14.4, where fresh embryos are replaced. Neither recipient's age nor the indication of treatment affects the success of oocyte donation substantially. However, pregnancy resulted from oocyte donation should be considered as high risk especially in those with ovarian failure, because of an increased incidence of small for gestational age. Oocyte recipients should also be counseled regarding their increased risk for pregnancy induced hypertension and postpartum hemorrhage.

Table 14.4: Live birth rate per IVF treatment cycle started using fresh donor eggs and partner sperm (HFEA Data).

Age	*2012 (%)*	*2013 (%)*
18-34	35.1	30.7
35-37	40.8	34.4
38-39	39.3	32.7
40-42	40.3	32.3
43-44	33.0	34.8
45+	35.3	29.3
All ages	**37.1**	**32.0**

HEALTH RISKS ASSOCIATED WITH ASSISTED REPRODUCTIVE TECHNOLOGY

Ectopic Pregnancy

The first pregnancy following IVF was an ectopic pregnancy. There is a higher rate of ectopic pregnancies after IVF/ICSI treatment principally due to the high prevalence of tubal factor infertility. The obstetric risks and outcome of ARTs have always been the subject of considerable debate. About 2–5% of ART pregnancies have been reported to be ectopic and 0.1–0.3% heterotopic.[123] For comparison, the prevalence of ectopic pregnancy and heterotopic pregnancy following natural conception is approximately 1 in 100 and 1 in 30,000, respectively. The overall ectopic pregnancy rates per treatment cycle was 0.3% of over 467,778 IVF/ICSI cycles performed in the United Kingdom from 1991 to 2005 (HFEA register data 2008).

Ovarian Hyperstimulation Syndrome

The OHSS remains the most serious and potentially lethal complication of ovarian hyperstimulation, correlates positively with conceptual cycles, and is almost exclusively related to either exogenous or endogenous hCG stimulation. The pathophysiology of OHSS is characterized by increased capillary permeability, mediated by the vasoactive substances released from the hyperstimulated ovaries. Fluid leaks from the intravascular compartment into the third space causing intravascular dehydration and in severe cases, multisystem dysfunction. Young age, presence of PCOS, lean body mass, and previous history of OHSS have all been reported to be risk factors for the development of OHSS. The risk increases with excessive ovarian response to gonadotropins, characterized by the development of a large numbers of follicles including immature and intermediate follicles and/or high serum estradiol levels. Mild forms are common affecting up to 33% of IVF cycles. The overall prevalence of moderate to severe OHSS varies from 3 to 8% of IVF/ICSI cycles.[124]

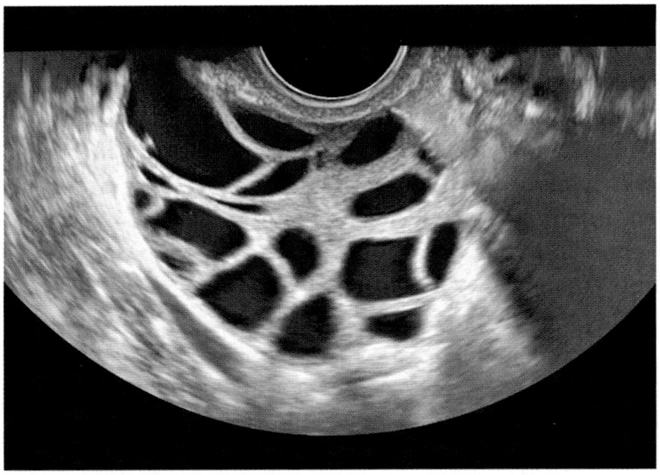

Fig. 14.17: Vaginal ultrasound appearance of the hyperstimulated ovary. The enlarged ovary contains excessive number of large, intermediate and small follicles.

The time of onset of OHSS may determine the prognosis with late onset OHSS is likely to be severe and to last longer than early onset OHSS. Early onset OHSS is due to the effects of exogenous hCG and present within 9 days after the ovulatory trigger hCG. Endogenous hCG from an early pregnancy triggers the development of late onset OHSS, which develop 9 days after the ovulatory hCG.

Prevention and early recognition are the two most important components in the management of OHSS. The key to prevention is proper identification of the population at risk before treatment and close monitoring of hormone levels as well as follicular response on ultrasound (Fig. 14.17). When a high-risk situation is recognized, withholding the ovulatory dose of hCG injection and cancellation of the treatment cycle will almost certainly prevent OHSS. The couple should be advised to avoid intercourse as spontaneous ovulation may occur up to 11 days after discontinuing gonadotropin treatment, resulting in conception and development of severe OHSS.

Alternative strategies have been attempted and when effective, they usually ameliorate the severity of OHSS rather than prevent it absolutely. They include:

1. Low starting dose of gonadotropin in high risk women has been attempted with varying degrees of success.
2. Use of GnRH antagonist for pituitary downregulation
3. Reduction of the ovulatory hCG dose and avoiding its use in the luteal phase
4. Triggering ovulation with GnRH agonist instead of hCG in GnRH antagonist cycles
5. Metformin co-treatment during gonadotropin stimulation in women having PCOS
6. Cabergoline has prophylactic role in reducing risk of moderate-severe OHSS
7. Segmentation of the treatment cycle with freezing the embryos and avoiding fresh embryo transfer will invariably avoid the risk of late onset OHSS. Frozen ET can subsequently be planned once OHSS symptoms are settled.

Among all the methods described, cancelling the cycle by withholding hCG can only prevent OHSS completely. The preventive roles of all the other strategies are still debated and, therefore, continued research is needed in this area.

A diagnosis of OHSS is usually straightforward, with typical symptoms of abdominal distension, abdominal pain, nausea and vomiting, reduced urine output, and breathing difficulties. Women with OHSS should have the severity of their condition assessed (RCOG Green-top guideline No.5 2006). Treatment of established OHSS depends on its severity, the stage at which the diagnosis is made and whether the patient is pregnant or not. In mild/most cases of moderate OHSS (hematocrit <45%), bed rest, simple analgesia, increased fluid intake, and close monitoring of electrolyte balance may be sufficient. Women should be encouraged to drink to thirst, rather than to excess. The patient's progress can be supervised on an outpatient basis. Hospital admission should be recommended to some women with moderate OHSS and all those with severe OHSS (hematocrit ≥45%, massive ascites). Women should be kept under review until resolution of the condition. The inpatient management is mainly aimed toward preventing or alleviating hemoconcentration, renal hypoperfusion, and thromboembolic phenomena. Initiation of intravenous fluid is not always necessary unless oral intake cannot maintain renal perfusion and function. Analgesics and antiemetics for symptomatic relief and subcutaneous heparin for antithrombotic prophylaxis should be instituted. Diuretics should not be used in women with oliguria secondary to a reduced blood volume and decreased renal perfusion, as they may worsen intravascular dehydration. Paracentesis, for symptomatic relief or failing renal function, may be necessary as it result in dramatic improvement in clinical symptoms and, diuresis and improved creatinine clearance.[125] Multidisciplinary input including critical care may be required for women who develop severe complications like severe ascites, liver or renal dysfunction, thromboembolism, and adult respiratory distress syndrome (ARDS).

Risk of Genital and Breast Cancer

The potential risk of genital cancer from follicular stimulation has initiated considerable debate.[126] While the results of earlier studies were alarming, subsequent studies with much longer follow-up period and better design showed reassuring results. In a cohort study of 12,193 women, Brinton et al. (2004) reported no increased risk associated with clomiphene or gonadotropin use among subjects, who have been followed up for a median of 18.8 years. Subsequent larger studies concentrating on the effect of exposure to drugs used during IVF rather than those prescribed in earlier times also reported reassuring results[127,128] However, the average follow-up period in these studies were only 6–7 years. Therefore, long-term follow-up data are needed to fully evaluate the risk of exposure to gonadotropins during IVF. Moreover, appropriate control groups should be used to determine whether the link is causal as it is hard to distinguish the effect of fertility treatment from that of infertility per se on the development of malignancies.

It is well established that endometrial cancer are sensitive to estrogen, which is excessively produced during ovarian hyperstimulation. Most smaller cohort studies have not found any association between the fertility drugs and endometrial cancer, but the follow-up period in these studies has been less than 10 years.[126] In a larger series with an average of over 20 years of follow-up, a significant twofold increase in endometrial cancer was associated with ovulation induction agents.[129] However, this study evaluated women undergone fertility treatment between 1964 and 1974 and, therefore, these results cannot be extrapolated to the modern day IVF treatment.

Concerns relating to the effect of high estrogen and progesterone levels on the potential risk for the development of breast cancer have also been expressed. A large cohort study of over 90,000 subjects has shown no association between the exposure to ART and breast cancer.[130]

In summary, the knowledge on the effect of ovulation induction agents currently used in ART on genital cancer risk is confusing. Considering the treatment protocols, preparations, and their dosages used during IVF are relatively new and women exposed to IVF are only beginning to reach the cancer age range, further follow-up studies are required in this area.

Risk of Congenital Anomalies and Malignancy in the Newborn

Since IVF and ICSI became a common fertility treatment modality, concerns have been raised regarding the risk of major congenital malformations in children born following these treatments. While majority of studies have shown an increased risk of major anomalies when compared with spontaneously conceived pregnancies, some studies have been reassuring. A recent meta-analysis of 25 studies has concluded a statistically significant 30–40% increase in birth defect over that of a background risk.[131] The authors have expressed this results in terms of the number needed to harm (NNTH), which in this case equates to the number of children that need to be conceived by ART for one additional child to be born with a birth defect. Therefore, for an underlying prevalence of birth defects between 1 and 4% of all births, the NNTH is between 250 and 62 treatments. ICSI enabled men with severe oligospermia or azoospermia to pass their genes on to their own progeny, an event that may not have been possible a few years ago. This raised certain questions about the genetic constitution of any resulting pregnancies after ICSI. A 1.2-fold increased risk of major birth defect in children born after ICSI (95% CI: 0.97–1.28) over that of IVF babies was noted on a systematic review of the reported studies.[132] Sons of infertile males with Y chromosome microdeletions and born following ICSI treatment may inherit the same abnormality and are likely to become infertile.

The increased risk of congenital malformations in ART children may largely be due to the underlying parental background, rather than the treatment techniques themselves. In a recent comparative study of malformation in children born to fertile (time to pregnancy interval of ≤12 months), and subfertile parents (time to pregnancy interval of >12 months), the overall prevalence increased with increasing time to pregnancy. Compared to children in the fertile group, singletons born to infertile couples had a higher rate of congenital malformations regardless of whether they were conceived naturally (OR 1.20, 95% CI 1.07–1.35) or after infertility treatment (OR 1.39, 95% CI 1.23–1.57).[133]

There have been concerns with increased risks of rare imprinting disorders such as of Beckwith-Wiedemann syndrome and Angelman syndrome in children following ART. However, the data are inconsistent with some reporting increased frequency in ART children[134] while others not finding any association.[135] Due to the rarity of these conditions, much larger studies are required to reliably detect such associations. A Netherland registry-based study included live births, stillbirths, and terminated pregnancies with congenital anomalies without a known cause that had a birth year between 1997 and 2010 (N=4,525). A total of 4,185 malformed cases were born to fertile couples and 340 to subfertile couples, of whom 139 had conceived after IVF/ICSI and 201 had conceived naturally after more than 12 months. Parental subfertility was associated with an increase in abdominal wall defects, penoscrotal hypospadia, right ventricular outflow tract obstruction, and methylation defects causing imprinting disorders. IVF/ICSI was associated with an increase in polydactyly, mainly of the hands.

On the basis of the current literature, it is not possible to distinguish the effect of parental subfertility, the effect of ovarian stimulation, and the ART laboratory techniques on the risk of congenital anomalies, but it has clearly been shown that children conceived without fertility treatment in subfertile couples also carry a higher risk of congenital anomalies compared with singletons conceived by fertile couples. Future research should be devoted to finding the mechanisms of the association between ART and congenital anomalies.

Risk of Malignancy in Children

The issue of childhood cancer among children born after ART has been addressed in a few studies. An increased prevalence of retinoblastoma and Langerhan histiocytosis among children born after ART in comparison to general population have been reported in two separate studies.[136,137] However, the overall risk of cancer, and the individual incidence of all other recorded cancers, was not greater than that expected from rates in the general population.[137] As childhood cancers are rare, larger studies are required for reliable evaluation of any increase in their risk amongst ART children.

In the context of pregnancy outcomes, the aim of ART should be a healthy singleton delivery at term. However, infertile couples may not share this target. They do not appreciate the risks associated with multiple pregnancy and indeed, between 67 and 90% of couples may desire a twin birth, while less than a third regard a single child as an ideal outcome. Increasing age or duration of infertility has been associated with greater desire for multiple births.[138] As discussed earlier in this chapter, increased multiple pregnancy rates is a major reason for the increased adverse obstetric and perinatal outcome associated with ART

OBSTETRIC AND PERINATAL OUTCOMES OF ASSISTED REPRODUCTION TECHNIQUE

Antenatal and Intrapartum Complications Following Assisted Reproduction

Many studies have examined the obstetric outcome after fertility treatments. The risk of spontaneous miscarriage appears to be higher among ART pregnancies than that reported in the general population. This comparison can be misleading sometimes as ART pregnancies are commonly under intense surveillance, so losses from a very early stage of the pregnancy are often carefully documented and reported in contrast to miscarriage rates among natural conceptions, which are extremely difficult to measure and can be easily underestimated by ART standards. However, a large prospective study with a meticulously chosen control group concluded that the risk of spontaneous abortion may be increased by 20–34% in the cohort of ART pregnancies than in the natural pregnancies after adjusting for differences in maternal age and previous spontaneous abortion.[139] However, this increased risk may be as a result of infertility itself rather than due to the ART as there was no difference in miscarriage rate between patients who achieved pregnancy following any fertility treatment including ART and those who conceived naturally while waiting for fertility treatment.[140]

Comparison of the obstetric outcome of IVF/ICSI pregnancies with matched normally conceived pregnancies showed a significantly increased incidence of premature delivery, intrauterine growth restriction, vaginal bleeding and hypertension requiring hospitalization, pre-eclampsia, and caesarean births.[141] The increased obstetric risk can be attributed to the high rate of multiple pregnancies in most cases. However, the risk of a more complicated pregnancies were found to be increased even when the ART twin and singleton pregnancies were compared with spontaneously conceived twins and singletons, respectively in two separate meta-analyses even after matched for maternal age.[142,143] A similar conclusion was drawn in another systematic review with similar objectives.[144]

Pregnancy following ICSI treatment has generated interest due to the additional risks involved with these pregnancies, such as the microinjection technique and the use of testicular or epididymal sperm. However, no significant difference in obstetrical outcome between IVF and

ICSI pregnancies was noted except for prematurity, which was higher in IVF singletons.[145] Couples undergoing ICSI for severe male infertility (oligoasthenoteratozoospermia) have slightly reduced fertilization rates but have similar pregnancy loss and other obstetric outcome as compared to other couples undergoing ICSI and IVF for non-male factor infertility.[146]

Women who conceive following oocyte donation, especially with a history of ovarian failure, should be considered as "high risk". While the majority of oocyte recipients experience a favorable outcome, an increased rate of obstetric complications in these pregnancies have been reported by many investigators.[147] Pregnancy-induced hypertension appears to occur more often than expected even among young recipients,[148] and the caesarean section rate is high.

Embryo Cryopreservation and Obstetric Outcome

There is a large body of evidence showing that a freeze-all strategy would lead to greatly improved birth outcomes. First, a population study in Victoria, Australia, showed that a specific group of birth defects linked to abnormal blastogenesis were increased more than threefold in fresh ETs but not in FETs, when both were compared with spontaneously conceived babies.[149]

Secondly, a recent systematic review and meta-analysis[150] analyzed data from 11 observational studies on obstetric and perinatal outcomes. The authors concluded that singleton pregnancies following frozen versus fresh ETs were significantly less likely to be complicated by perinatal mortality, small for gestational age, preterm birth, low birth weight, and antepartum hemorrhage. Although the evidence from this meta-analysis appears to favor FET, there was heterogeneity between the 11 studies at the level of design, population and also the freezing, thawing, and transfer protocols: subsequent inclusions and analysis of a greater number of studies could further strengthen these conclusions.

A large and more recent study from the Nordic countries[151] has since largely corroborated the above findings. It also showed that compared with singletons born after fresh IVF and ICSI, singletons born after FET had a higher risk of being large for gestational age and having macrosomia, which is in line with findings from other large population-based studies.[152-154] However, another large population-based study (of 56,792 infants) found that fresh transfers result in low birth weight rather than FET offspring necessarily being larger.[155]

Further recent evidence from a large observational study by[156] reports on clinical pregnancy and neonatal outcomes of 1,157 fresh and 645 vitrified-warmed single embryo blastocyst transfers. The blastocyst thaw survival rate was 94.4% and similar clinical outcomes were achieved for fresh and vitrified-warmed blastocyst transfers with live birth rates of 52.8% versus 55.3%, respectively, for grade I blastocysts. Babies conceived following single embryo transfer (SET) with vitrified warmed blastocysts were born on average 0.3 weeks later and had a birth weight that was 145 gm heavier compared with fresh transfers.

Perinatal Outcome of Assisted Reproduction Pregnancies

It is widely accepted that the increased incidence of multiple pregnancies following ART account for a disproportionately large share of adverse perinatal outcomes including increased incidence of very low birth weight, low birth weight, perinatal and neonatal mortality, as well as infant death. The increased incidence of death and morbidity in twin as compared to singleton pregnancy has been attributed mainly to prematurity and to adverse outcomes associated with premature delivery such as hyaline membrane disease, hypocalcaemia, hypoglycemia, hyperbilirubinemia, small for dates, and low Apgar scores. In one report,[157] it was suggested that monoamniotic multiple gestations may be increased in zona-manipulated cycles (ICSI, zona drilling, assisted hatching) and although all resulting monoamniotic pregnancies ended in live births, there was high incidence of intrauterine discordance in fetal growth. Even when compared to matched control spontaneous twin pregnancies, ART twin pregnancies have low birth weight and need more neonatal intensive care.[144] However, twins conceived with IVF/ICSI have comparable perinatal mortality and morbidity rates to spontaneously conceived controls.[142]

Elimination of multiple pregnancies will not eliminate the increased risk of adverse perinatal outcome in ART. While the twins born from assisted conception are not significantly disadvantaged when compared to spontaneous twin pregnancies, ART singletons have worse perinatal outcome compared to other singletons.[144] Singletons born from ART are at risk for lower mean birth weight and small for gestational age. Perinatal mortality appears to be significantly higher even after matching for maternal age, parity, and infant sex. ICSI treatment does not appear to differ from conventional IVF when the perinatal outcomes are compared. Retrospective comparison of births resulting from cryopreserved embryos with those after conventional IVF and fresh ET showed no difference in the perinatal mortality between the two groups.[157]A systematic review and meta-analysis[150] suggested singletons pregnancies after IVF/ICSI are associated with higher risks of obstetric and perinatal complications when compared with those from spontaneous conceptions, and should be managed as high-risk pregnancies. The increased risk is persistent even with frozen ETs and with single elective ETs (removing the effect of vanishing twins that could be present double ET).

PREIMPLANTATION GENETIC DIAGNOSIS/SCREENING

Preimplantation genetic diagnosis has been developed as an alternative to prenatal diagnosis of chromosomal or sex-linked disorders in embryos formed through ART procedures. Preimplantation genetic screening (PGS) is the term, which commonly refers to the application of PGD technique in infertile couples undergoing conventional ART as an alternative to the traditional selection of embryos based on morphological criteria, which do not detect aneuploidy embryo that are nonviable or could give rise to viable, but disabled child.[158] Aneuploid embryos are most commonly resulting from fertilization of oocytes that affected with meiotic nondisjunction, a common reason for age related decline in oocyte quality. By detecting and avoiding transfer of aneuploidy embryos and selecting only the euploid embryos for transfer, the success of ART cycles could potentially be improved. The application of PGD has also been extended to preimplantation HLA matching to ensure the birth of HLA-identical offspring for stem cell transplantation therapy to siblings.

The procedure involves biopsy of a single cell from the human cleavage stage embryo at around the eight-cell stage or from the blastocyst followed by the application of a sensitive diagnostic technique to that cell. At present, biopsied polar body and/or blastomeres and/ or trophoblast cells biopsied from blastocyst have been used and pregnancies as well as healthy babies have resulted from such biopsied and diagnosed embryos. The diagnostic technique, specific for the disorder being tested, may be analysis of enzymes, chromosomes or specific mutation in the DNA. If the cell shows no abnormality in the course of this analysis, the embryo is judged to be normal and transferred to the mother to initiate pregnancy.

The enzyme approach has been disregarded, for the few genes studied, as it has been difficult to differentiate between maternal gene expression (mRNA inherited in the egg cytoplasm) and embryonic gene expression in the early embryo.[159] However, the analysis of chromosomes using fluorescent in-situ hybridization (FISH) and the analysis of specific gene sequences using sensitive polymerase chain reaction (PCR) for sexing or detection of a specific gene mutation such as CF have been used successfully.

Analysis of the first and second polar bodies is an alternative to embryonic biopsy. As the polar bodies contain the genetic information from the oocyte, it is possible to diagnose maternally derived mutations, translocations, and aneuploidy. Paternally derived chromosomal abnormalities will be missed by polar body biopsies. In cases of recessive disorders, polar body biopsies are helpful as it can provide information about the maternal contribution to the embryo. It may be difficult to achieve a reliable diagnosis even with embryo biopsy, with which mosaicism and/or uniparental disomies deriving from trisomies originating from female meiotic errors will be missed. With the expanding range of PGD indications, combined testing is required when testing for causative gene, linked markers, HLA typing, and aneuploidy in the same case. Therefore, single, double, or even triple biopsy may be required in order to establish an accurate PGD.[160] Sequential or simultaneous additional biopsy procedures have been shown to have no detrimental effect on embryo development.[161]

The PGS has been proposed to improve the IVF outcome in women of advanced age, and in those with a history of recurrent miscarriage, repeated implantation failure, or severe male infertility, who are at risk for having increased proportions of aneuploidy embryos. Most commonly nine chromosomes (13, 14, 15, 16, 18, 21, 22, X, and Y) are screened for aneuploidy.

A meta-analysis of five prospective randomized controlled trials evaluating the effect of PGS for the indication of advanced women's age has reported a significant reduction in ongoing pregnancy rates (OR: 0.56, 95% CI: 0.42–0.76) compared to controls.[162] While the studies evaluating the use of PGS for other indications mentioned above is limited, the early evidence suggest that PGS does not improve the outcome even in good prognosis patients (young age) who are undergoing single ET.[100]

The increased use of PGS for aneuploidy has been reinforced by recent data suggesting that PGS increases IVF efficiency. PGS is an excellent tool to increase IVF efficiency in appropriately selected couples. PGS takes a biopsy cell(s) sample from embryos obtained through IVF and evaluates the chromosomal status of this sample. Embryos that test chromosomally normal (euploid) are then considered for ET. Importantly, PGS is only a testing strategy; it in no way changes the genetic composition of the embryos. Therefore, PGS may improve the chance of achieving pregnancy per ET. However, PGS does not improve the chances of achieving pregnancy per retrieval.

In other words, multiple frozen ETs from a single oocyte retrieval will ultimately result, in theory, in the same ultimate live birth rate as a PGS cycle. Therefore, it is inaccurate to counsel patients that PGS will improve their chances of live birth per retrieval.

However, PGS does increase the efficiency of IVF by improving embryo selection, thereby increasing the implantation rate and reducing the rate of miscarriage per ET. When considering IVF alone or IVF and PGS, the majority of couples undergoing IVF and PGS will achieve their goal of having a healthy baby in as short a period as possible.

Preimplantation genetic screening is not perfect in its diagnostic accuracy. This chance of misdiagnosis results from both biological and technical limitations. One chief limitation of PGS is the presence of chromosomal mosaicism within the developing embryo, a phenomenon in which different chromosomal cell lines reside within a single embryo. The percentage of embryos with mosaicism at the cleavage stage is by some reports as high as 50%.The obvious concern for misdiagnosis associated with embryonic mosaicism is that the cells biopsied may not reflect the chromosomal status of the resulting embryo. In other words, even if the technical diagnostic process is flawless, the clinical outcome may be different from the PGS result.

Mosaicism is thought to be less common in blastocyst stage embryos. Current data strongly support obtaining embryo biopsy at the blastocyst stage over the cleavage stage. However, discordance in the ploidy status between the inner cell mass and the trophectoderm is still relatively common at approximately 3–5%. This mosaicism between the placenta and fetus has been well documented for decades before PGS, with data showing discordance in the ploidy status between chorionic villus sampling of placental DNA and subsequent amniocentesis (fetal DNA) in approximately 2–3% of samples, a condition known as confined placental mosaicism.

Therefore, PGS at the trophectoderm stage still has a chance of misdiagnosis based purely on the biology of the developing embryo. This represents a biological limitation that is not possible to overcome even with the best diagnostic techniques. The diagnostic platforms used to perform PGS have improved considerably in recent years. Current data strongly support the utilization of technologies that are capable of simultaneously evaluating the ploidy status of all 23 chromosome pairs. Therefore, other more limited technologies, including fluorescence in situ hybridization, are discouraged. At this time, there are not conclusive data that definitively demonstrate one technology superior to another according to outcomes.

Examples of technical errors include the following: methodologic misdiagnosis, allele drop-out, amplification errors, hybridization errors, technological misdiagnosis, DNA contamination, and human error. Some platforms may be able to limit the impact of some of these problems, such as contamination, through allele mapping. However, no diagnostic platform will ever be able to ensure 100% accuracy. This must be acknowledged and discussed with patients during the counseling process for PGS. In the opinion of these authors, such claims are clinically inaccurate and further the misunderstanding held by clinicians and patients regarding PGS. These high estimates are often taken from clinical validation studies and are not necessarily reflective of true clinical outcomes.

The true error rate of PGS in a clinical context is difficult to determine. In many cases in which a normal result is given and the embryo is aneuploid, the pregnancy will either not implant or fail to develop to a point at which clinical testing on the products of conception could be performed. In other cases in which an abnormal result is given in a euploid embryo, no pregnancy will be attempted and the embryo will likely be discarded. In both of these circumstances, errors will not be clinically apparent or reported.

Another risk that must be understood by patients is the chance of physical damage to the embryo incurred at the time of biopsy. Current data show that embryos biopsied at the cleavage stage lag developmentally compared with controls, implying a significant level of damage incurred with PGS. Although available data do not imply such damage with blastocyst-stage biopsy, the possibility of embryo damage with PGS must still be addressed during patient counseling.

Additionally, because PGS is a relatively new and emerging technology, the detrimental effects of embryo biopsy, especially those related to late-onset disorders, may not be evident until children born as a result of this technology become older. Therefore, there may be unidentified risks associated with PGS. The true rate of all-cause clinical misdiagnosis with PGS using current genetic platforms testing for aneuploidy in all 23 chromosome pairs is approximately 5% per embryo.

Furthermore, clinical outcome data is insufficient to define this limitation due to the lack of pregnancy progression in embryos with a normal PGS result but aneuploid cell populations. The reasons for this misdiagnosis rate are both biological, resulting from mosaicism within developing embryos, and technical, resulting from other sources of diagnostic laboratory error. Therefore, a PGS result can never be used to definitively predict the chromosomal status of the fetus. At present, amniocentesis is the only technology capable of testing the chromosomal status of the fetus rather than the placenta. The act of embryo biopsy may incur damage to embryos, especially at the cleavage stage, and the long-term effects of embryo biopsy are not defined at this time. It is important that patients understand these points during the counseling and consenting process. Once these limitations are understood and accepted, however, PGS is a useful tool that may dramatically improve the efficiency of IVF cycles for many patients.

LOOKING INTO THE FUTURE

Assisted reproduction technologies have improved substantially over the last 3 decades and many subfertile couples are now able to have children through its application. However, clinicians and researchers continue to strive to achieve the desired outcome, i.e. single healthy baby, with minimal side effects and this poses new challenges. It is tempting to speculate on the areas that are most likely to witness such developments over the next few years.

Recombinant gonadotropin preparations are now well established in superovulation protocols. While these compounds are well tolerated and as effective as the urinary products, the associated risks of OHSS and of multiple pregnancies and the need for daily parenteral administration of medications do not constitute the features of a patient-friendly procedure. Active investigations are ongoing to develop a number of molecules with gonadotropin-like activity. Longer acting forms and orally bioactive preparations may revolutionize IVF treatment in the near future. Additionally, the use of mild ovarian stimulation protocols with single ET policy may become a norm leading to a less drug orientated IVF treatment.

Improving pregnancy and live birth rates will remain a challenge for the future. Molecular cytogenetic procedures on polar bodies or blastomeres have indicated that more than 50% of the embryos derived after ART are aneuploidy. Elective transfer of euploid or highest quality embryo(s) increases the chances of successful outcome. Currently, the embryos are scored based on its morphology, but this is notoriously difficult and often subjective. Available evidence does not support the use of more invasive PGS techniques to improve the live birth rates following ART and, therefore, more accurate assessment methods are needed. A number of noninvasive tests embryo viability, assessment of metabolomic profile, or amino acid turn over in the embryo culture media, are being evaluated in many studies and have the potential to predict the embryos that have the highest implantation potential.[163,164]

The unraveling of the human genome and the increase in our knowledge of the genetic basis for many more diseases that we had ever imagined previously will lead to a greater understanding of the factors involved in male infertility and how to increase fecundity. This, coupled with advances in PGD, will enable accurate screening of parents for specific genes before treatment, biopsied embryos before replacement, and the resulting child afterward. Additionally, these advances will permit rapid progress in gene therapy for single or multiple gene disorders where a normal cloned gene(s) is used to replace the faulty genome.

Another challenging area for research is that of preserving fertility in children or young adults treated for cancer. As survival rates continue to improve more young people want to know if they will be fertile, if their children will have a greater risk of developing cancer and what alternatives exist should pelvic irradiation or chemotherapy adversely affect their fertility permanently. Sperm banking is a well-recognized preservation technique for pubertal males and adults. In women, several approaches are being explored but none is yet clinically established.

The recent introduction of oocyte vitrification has significantly advanced the outcome of oocyte cryopreservation, leading to clinical results comparable to those achieved in IVF using fresh oocytes, as reported by experienced centers. This has led to new debate, both in the professional community and in society at large, about the acceptability of offering this technology to reproductively healthy women who want to cryopreserve their oocytes against the threat of time. The mature oocyte is extremely fragile due to intracellular ice formation during the freezing or thawing process. There is potentially an increased risk of damage to the meiotic spindle apparatus and of hardening of the zona pellucida leading to reduced post-thaw survival, fertilization, and pregnancy rates. Improvements in both advanced vitrification and slow-freezing methods have recently resulted in an increase in the efficiency of using human cryopreserved oocytes in assisted reproduction. It is reassuring that there is no increased chromosomal abnormalities, birth defects, or developmental delay in children born from cryopreserved oocytes based on the limited number of pregnancies and deliveries reported to date.

Ovarian cryopreservation has been regarded as a potential method of fertility preservation for more than a decade.[165] This method has the potential advantages of preservation of a large number of oocytes within primordial follicles, it does not require hormonal stimulation when time is short, and indeed may be appropriate for the prepubertal. The ovarian tissues can subsequently be auto-transplanted either at orthotopic (at or around the ovarian fossa) or at heterotopic locations (subcutaneously at various locations including the forearm and abdominal wall) after the patient has completed the treatment. Although few live births following either spontaneous or IVF conceptions are reported, more research is needed in order to enhance the revascularization process with the goal of reducing the follicular loss that takes place after tissue grafting. These technologies are still experimental, although tremendous progress has been made recently. There are many ethical concerns with these interventions, particularly their experimental nature in emotionally vulnerable patients, who often present to ART units with unrealistic expectations, the possibility of harvesting malignant cells with the germ cells, and the potential for continued transmission of germ-line mutations in cancer predisposition genes. All these highlight the need for further research and well-designed controlled clinical trials.

REFERENCES

1. Balen AH, Laven JS, Tan SL, Dewailly D. Ultrasound assessment of the polycystic ovary: international consensus definitions. Hum Reprod Update. 2003;9:505-14.
2. Agrawal R, Conway G, Sladkevicius P, Tan SL, Engmann L, Payne N, et al. Serum vascular endothelial growth factor and Doppler blood flow velocities in *in vitro* fertilization: relevance to ovarian hyperstimulation syndrome and polycystic ovaries. Fertil Steril. 1998;70:651-8.
3. Dewailly D, Lujan ME, Carmina E, Cedars MI, Laven J, Norman RJ, et al. Definition and significance of polycystic ovarian morphology: a task force report from the Androgen Excess and Polycystic Ovary Syndrome Society. Hum Reprod Update. 2014;20(3):334-52.
4. Kennedy S, Bergqvist A, Chapron C, D'Hooghe T, Dunselman G, Greb R, et al. ESHRE guideline for the diagnosis and treatment of endometriosis. Hum Reprod. 2005;20: 2698-704.
5. Eskenazi B, Warner ML. Epidemiology of endometriosis. Obstet Gynecol Clin North Am. 1997;24:235-58.
6. Meuleman, Tondreau T, Ahmad I, Kwan J, Crokaert F, Delforge A, et al. Infusion of mesenchymal stromal cells can aid hematopoietic recovery following allogeneic hematopoietic stem cell myeloablative transplant: a pilot study. Stem Cells Dev. 2009;18(9):1247-52.
7. Moore J, Copley S, Morris J, Lindsell D, Golding S, Kennedy S. A systematic review of the accuracy of ultrasound in the diagnosis of endometriosis. Ultrasound Obstet Gynecol. 2002;20:630-4.
8. Strandell A. Treatment of hydrosalpinx in the patient undergoing assisted reproduction. Curr Opin Obstet Gynecol. 2007;19:360-5.
9. Arora P, Arora RS, Cahill D. Essure for management of hydrosalpinx prior to *in vitro* fertilisation-a systematic review and pooled analysis. BJOG. 2014;121(5):527-36.
10. Lin PC. Reproductive outcomes in women with uterine anomalies. J Womens Health (Larchmt). 2004;13:33-9.
11. Salim R, Woelfer B, Backos M, Regan L, Jurkovic D. Reproducibility of three-dimensional ultrasound diagnosis of congenital uterine anomalies. Ultrasound Obstet Gynecol. 2003;21:578-82.
12. Oliveira FG, Abdelmassih VG, Diamond MP, Dozortsev D, Melo NR, Abdelmassih R. Impact of subserosal and intramural uterine fibroids that do not distort the endometrial cavity on the outcome of *in vitro* fertilization-intracytoplasmic sperm injection. Fertil Steril. 2004;81:582-7.
13. Sunkara SK, Khairy M, El-Toukhy T, Khalaf Y, Coomarasamy A. The effect of intramural fibroids without uterine cavity involvement on the outcome of IVF treatment: a systematic review and meta-analysis. Human Reproduction. 2010;25(2):418-29.
14. Isikoglu M, Berkkanoglu M, Senturk Z, Coetzee K, Ozgur K. Endometrial polyps smaller than 1.5 cm do not affect ICSI outcome. Reprod Biomed Online. 2006;12:199-204.
15. Bartkowiak R, Kaminski P, Wielgos M, Bobrowska K. The evaluation of uterine cavity with saline infusion sonohysterography and hysteroscopy in infertile patients. Neuro Endocrinol Lett. 2006;27:523-8.
16. Speroff L, Fritz MA. Assisted reproductive technologies. In: Clinical Gynecologic Endocrinology and Infertility, 6th edition. 2005.
17. Broekmans FJ, Kwee J, Hendriks DJ, Mol BW, Lambalk CB. A systematic review of tests predicting ovarian reserve and IVF outcome. Hum Reprod Update. 2006;12:685-718.

18. te Velde ER, Pearson PL. The variability of female reproductive ageing. Hum Reprod Update. 2002;8:141-54.
19. Scott RT, Toner JP, Muasher SJ, Oehninger S, Robinson S, Rosenwaks Z. Follicle-stimulating hormone levels on cycle day 3 are predictive of *in vitro* fertilization outcome. Fertil Steril. 1989;51:651-4.
20. Sharif K, Elgendy M, Lashen H, Afnan M. Age and basal follicle stimulating hormone as predictors of *in vitro* fertilisation outcome. Br J Obstet Gynaecol. 1998;105:107-12.
21. Bancsi LF, Broekmans FJ, Mol BW, Habbema JD, te Velde ER. Performance of basal follicle-stimulating hormone in the prediction of poor ovarian response and failure to become pregnant after *in vitro* fertilization: a meta-analysis. Fertil Steril. 2003;79:1091-100.
22. Scott RT Jr, Hofmann GE, Oehninger S, Muasher SJ. Intercycle variability of day 3 follicle-stimulating hormone levels and its effect on stimulation quality in *in vitro* fertilization. Fertil Steril. 1990;54:297-302.
23. Abdalla H, Thum MY. Repeated testing of basal FSH levels has no predictive value for IVF outcome in women with elevated basal FSH. Hum Reprod. 2006;21:171-4.
24. Frattarelli JL, Bergh PA, Drews MR, Sharara FI, Scott RT. Evaluation of basal estradiol levels in assisted reproductive technology cycles. Fertil Steril. 2000;74:518-24.
25. Evers JL, Slaats P, Land JA, Dumoulin JC, Dunselman GA. Elevated levels of basal estradiol-17beta predict poor response in patients with normal basal levels of follicle-stimulating hormone undergoing *in vitro* fertilization. Fertil Steril. 1998;69:1010-4.
26. Hall JE, Welt CK, Cramer DW. Inhibin A and inhibin B reflect ovarian function in assisted reproduction but are less useful at predicting outcome. Hum Reprod. 1999;14:409-15.
27. Seifer DB, Lambert-Messerlian G, Hogan JW, Gardiner AC, Blazar AS, Berk CA. Day 3 serum inhibin-B is predictive of assisted reproductive technologies outcome. Fertil Steril. 1997;67:110-4.
28. McIlveen M, Skull JD, Ledger WL. Evaluation of the utility of multiple endocrine and ultrasound measures of ovarian reserve in the prediction of cycle cancellation in a high-risk IVF population. Hum Reprod. 2007;22:778-85.
29. van Rooij IA, Broekmans FJ, te Velde ER, Fauser BC, Bancsi LF, de Jong FH, et al. Serum anti-Müllerian hormone levels: a novel measure of ovarian reserve. Hum Reprod. 2002;17:3065-71.
30. de Vet A, Laven JS, de Jong FH, Themmen AP, Fauser BC. Anti-Müllerian hormone serum levels: a putative marker for ovarian aging. Fertil Steril. 2002;77:357-62.
31. Broekmans FJ, Visser JA, Laven JS, Broer SL, Themmen AP, Fauser BC. Anti-Müllerian hormone and ovarian dysfunction. Trends Endocrinol Metab. 2008;19:340-7.
32. Fanchin R, Taieb J, Lozano DH, Ducot B, Frydman R, Bouyer J. High reproducibility of serum anti-Müllerian hormone measurements suggests a multi-staged follicular secretion and strengthens its role in the assessment of ovarian follicular status. Hum Reprod. 2005;20:923-7.
33. La Marca A, Stabile G, Artenisio AC, Volpe A. Serum anti-Müllerian hormone throughout the human menstrual cycle. Hum Reprod. 2006;21:3103-7.
34. Kwee JJ, Elting MM, Schats RR, McDonnell JJ, Lambalk NC. Ovarian volume and antral follicle count for the prediction of low and hyper responders with *in vitro* fertilization. Reprod Biol Endocrinol. 2007;5:9.
35. Jayaprakasan K, Al-Hasie H, Jayaprakasan R, Campbell B, Hopkisson J, Johnson I, et al. The three-dimensional ultrasonographic ovarian vascularity of women developing poor ovarian response during assisted reproduction treatment and its predictive value. Fertil Steril. 2008a.
36. Jayaprakasan K, Campbell BK, Clewes JS, Johnson IR, Raine-Fenning NJ. Three-dimensional ultrasound improves the interobserver reliability of antral follicle counts and facilitates increased clinical work flow. Ultrasound Obstet Gynecol. 2008c;31:439-44.
37. Jayaprakasan K, Hopkisson JF, Campbell BK, Clewes J, Johnson IR, Raine-Fenning NJ. Quantification of the effect of pituitary down-regulation on 3D ultrasound predictors of ovarian response. Hum Reprod. 2008d;23:1538-44.
38. Jayaprakasan K, Campbell B, Hopkisson J, Johnson I, Raine-Fenning N. A prospective, comparative analysis of anti-Müllerian hormone, inhibin-B, and three-dimensional ultrasound determinants of ovarian reserve in the prediction of poor response to controlled ovarian stimulation. Fertil Steril. 2008b.
39. Broekmans FJ, Knauff EA, te Velde ER, Macklon NS, Fauser BC. Female reproductive ageing: current knowledge and future trends. Trends Endocrinol Metab. 2007;18:58-65.
40. Hughes EG, Fedorkow DM, Daya S, Sagle MA, Van de Koppel P, Collins JA. The routine use of gonadotropin-releasing hormone agonists prior to *in vitro* fertilization and gamete intrafallopian transfer: a meta-analysis of randomized controlled trials. Fertil Steril. 1992;58:888-96.
41. Daya S. Gonadotropin releasing hormone agonist protocols for pituitary desensitization in *in vitro* fertilization and gamete intrafallopian transfer cycles. Cochrane Database Syst Rev. 2000;CD001299.
42. Maheshwari A, Gibreel A, Siristatidis CS, Bhattacharya S. Gonadotrophin-releasing hormone agonist protocols for pituitary suppression in assisted reproduction. Cochrane Database Syst Rev. 2011;(8):CD006919.
43. Al-Inany HG, Abou-Setta AM, Aboulghar M. Gonadotrophin-releasing hormone antagonists for assisted conception: a Cochrane review. Reprod Biomed Online. 2007;14:640-9.
44. Youssef MA, Van der Veen F, Al-Inany HG, Mochtar MH, Griesinger G, Nagi Mohesen M, et al. Gonadotropin-releasing hormone agonist versus HCG for oocyte triggering in antagonist-assisted reproductive technology. Cochrane Database Syst Rev. 2014;(10):CD008046.
45. Shapiro BS, Daneshmand ST, Garner FC, Aguirre M, Thomas S. Gonadotropin-releasing hormone agonist combined with a reduced dose of human chorionic gonadotropin for final oocyte maturation in fresh autologous cycles of in vitro fertilization. Fertil Steril. 2008;90(1):231-3.
46. Castillo JC, Dolz M, Bienvenido E, Abad L, Casañ EM, Bonilla-Musoles F. Cycles triggered with GnRH agonist: exploring low-dose HCG for luteal support. Reprod Biomed Online. 2010;20(2):175-81.

47. Mannaerts B, de Leeuw R, Geelen J, Van Ravestein A, Van Wezenbeek P, Schuurs A, Kloosterboer H. Comparative in vitro and in vivo studies on the biological characteristics of recombinant human follicle-stimulating hormone. Endocrinology. 1991;129(5):2623-30.
48. Al-Inany HG, Abou-Setta AM, Aboulghar MA, Mansour RT, Serour GI. Efficacy and safety of human menopausal gonadotrophins versus recombinant FSH: a meta-analysis. Reprod Biomed Online. 2008;16:81-8.
49. Coomarasamy A, Afnan M, Cheema D, van der Veen F, Bossuyt PM, van Wely M. Urinary hMG versus recombinant FSH for controlled ovarian hyperstimulation following an agonist long down-regulation protocol in IVF or ICSI treatment: a systematic review and meta-analysis. Hum Reprod. 2008;23:310-5.
50. Kolibianakis EM, Kalogeropoulou L, Griesinger G, Papanikolaou EG, Papadimas J, Bontis J, et al. Among patients treated with FSH and GnRH analogues for *in vitro* fertilization, is the addition of recombinant LH associated with the probability of live birth? A systematic review and meta-analysis. Hum Reprod Update. 2007;13:445-52.
51. Mochtar MH, Van der V, Ziech M, van Wely M. Recombinant Luteinizing Hormone (rLH) for controlled ovarian hyperstimulation in assisted reproductive cycles. Cochrane Database Syst Rev. 2007;CD005070.
52. Verberg MF, Eijkemans MJ, Macklon NS, Heijnen EM, Baart EB, Hohmann FP, et al. The clinical significance of the retrieval of a low number of oocytes following mild ovarian stimulation for IVF: a meta-analysis. Hum Reprod Update. 2009a;15:5-12.
53. Verberg MF, Macklon NS, Nargund G, Frydman R, Devroey P, Broekmans FJ, et al. Mild ovarian stimulation for IVF. Hum Reprod Update. 2009b;15:13-29.
54. Bennett SJ, Waterstone JJ, Cheng WC, Parsons J. Complications of transvaginal ultrasound-directed follicle aspiration: a review of 2670 consecutive procedures. J Assist Reprod Genet. 1993;10:72-7.
55. Van Royen E, Mangelschots K, De Neubourg D, Valkenburg M, Van de Meerssche M, Ryckaert G, et al. Characterization of a top quality embryo, a step towards single-embryo transfer. Hum Reprod. 1999;14:2345-9.
56. Oatway C, Gunby J, Daya S. Day three versus day two embryo transfer following *in vitro* fertilization or intracytoplasmic sperm injection. Cochrane Database Syst Rev. 2004;CD004378.
57. Blake DA, Farquhar CM, Johnson N, Proctor M. Cleavage stage versus blastocyst stage embryo transfer in assisted conception. Cochrane Database Syst Rev. 2007;CD002118.
58. Brown JA, Buckingham K, Abou-Setta A, Buckett W. Ultrasound versus 'clinical touch' for catheter guidance during embryo transfer in women. Cochrane Database Syst Rev. 2007;CD006107.
59. Drakeley AJ, Jorgensen A, Sklavounos J, Aust T, Gazvani R, Williamson P, et al. A randomized controlled clinical trial of 2295 ultrasound-guided embryo transfers. Hum Reprod. 2008;23:1101-6.
60. Abou-Setta AM, Al-Inany HG, Mansour RT, Serour GI, Aboulghar MA. Soft versus firm embryo transfer catheters for assisted reproduction: a systematic review and meta-analysis. Hum Reprod. 2005;20:3114-55.
61. Buckett W. A review and meta-analysis of prospective trials comparing different catheters used for embryo transfer. Fertil Steril. 2006;85:728-34.
62. Silberstein T, Weitzen S, Frankfurter D, Trimarchi JR, Keefe DL, Plosker SM. Cannulation of a resistant internal os with the malleable outer sheath of a coaxial soft embryo transfer catheter does not affect in vitro fertilization-embryo transfer outcome. Fertil Steril. 2004;82(5):1402-6.
63. Abdelmassih VG, Neme RM, Dozortsev D, Abdelmassih S, Diamond MP, Abdelmassih R. Location of the embryo-transfer catheter guide before the internal uterine os improves the outcome of in vitro fertilization. Fertil Steril. 2007;88(2):499-503. [Epub 2007 May 16]
64. Groutz A, Lessing JB, Wolf Y, Yovel I, Azem F, Amit A. Cervical dilatation during ovum pick-up in patients with cervical stenosis: effect on pregnancy outcome in an in vitro fertilization-embryo transfer program. Fertil Steril. 1997;67(5):909-11.
65. Glatstein IZ, Pang SC, McShane PM. Successful pregnancies with the use of laminaria tents before embryo transfer for refractory cervical stenosis. Fertil Steril. 1997;67(6):1172-4.
66. Saravelos SH, Wong AW, Chan CP, Kong GW, Cheung LP, Chung CH, et al. Assessment of the embryo flash position and migration with 3D ultrasound within 60 min of embryo transfer. Hum Reprod. 2016;31(3):591-6. [Epub 2016 Jan 11]
67. Devranoğlu B, Özdamar Ö, Çakıroğlu Y, Küçükbaş M, Eken MK, Doğer E. The timing of embryo transfer catheter removal: should it be delayed or done immediately? A Prospective Randomized Trial. Gynecol Obstet Invest. 2017 Feb 22. [Epub ahead of print]
68. Eytan O, Elad D, Jaffa AJ. Evaluation of the embryo transfer protocol by a laboratory model of the uterus. Fertil Steril. 2007;88(2):485-93. [Epub 2007 Apr 20]
69. Bontekoe S, Heineman MJ, Johnson N, Blake D. Adherence compounds in embryo transfer media for assisted reproductive technologies. Cochrane Database Syst Rev. 2014;(2):CD007421.
70. Hull MG. Infertility treatment: relative effectiveness of conventional and assisted conception methods. Hum Reprod. 1992;7:785-96.
71. NICE. Fertility: Assessment and Treatment for People with Fertility Problems. National Collaborating Centre for Women's and Children's Health for the National Institute for Clinical Excellence. London: RCOG Press; 2004. p. 33.
72. Widra EA, Gindoff PR, Smotrich DB, Stillman RJ. Achieving multiple-order embryo transfer identifies women over 40 years of age with improved *in vitro* fertilization outcome. Fertil Steril. 1996;65:103-8.
73. Alrayyes S, Fakih H, Khan I. Effect of age and cycle responsiveness in patients undergoing intracytoplasmic sperm injection. Fertil Steril. 1997;68:123-7.
74. Piette C, de Mouzon J, Bachelot A, Spira A. In-vitro fertilization: influence of women's age on pregnancy rates. Hum Reprod. 1990;5:56-9.
75. van Rooij IA, Bancsi LF, Broekmans FJ, Looman CW, Habbema JD, te Velde ER. Women older than 40 years of age and those with elevated follicle-stimulating hormone levels

differ in poor response rate and embryo quality in *in vitro* fertilization. Fertil Steril. 2003;79:482-8.
76. Van Voorhis BJ. Clinical practice. *In vitro* fertilization. N Engl J Med. 2007;356:379-86.
77. Preutthipan S, Amso N, Curtis P, Shaw RW. The influence of number of embryos transferred on pregnancy outcome in women undergoing *in vitro* fertilization and embryo transfer (IVF-ET). J Med Assoc Thai. 1996;79:613-7.
78. Mardesic T, Muller P, Zetova L, Mikova M. Factors affecting the results of *in vitro* fertilization-I. The effect of age. Ceska Gynekol. 1994;59:259-61.
79. Templeton A, Morris JK, Parslow W. Factors that affect outcome of in-vitro fertilisation treatment. Lancet. 1996;348:1402-6.
80. Toner JP, Flood JT. Fertility after the age of 40. Obstet Gynecol Clin North Am. 1993;20:261-72.
81. Spandorfer SD, Davis OK, Barmat LI, Chung PH, Rosenwaks Z. Relationship between maternal age and aneuploidy in *in vitro* fertilization pregnancy loss. Fertil Steril. 2004;81:1265-9.
82. Fedorcsak P, Dale PO, Storeng R, Ertzeid G, Bjercke S, Oldereid N, et al. Impact of overweight and underweight on assisted reproduction treatment. Hum Reprod. 2004;19:2523-8.
83. Dechaud H, Anahory T, Reyftmann L, Loup V, Hamamah S, Hedon B. Obesity does not adversely affect results in patients who are undergoing *in vitro* fertilization and embryo transfer. Eur J Obstet Gynecol Reprod Biol. 2006;127:88-93.
84. Sneed ML, Uhler ML, Grotjan HE, Rapisarda JJ, Lederer KJ, Beltsos AN. Body mass index: impact on IVF success appears age-related. Hum Reprod. 2008;23:1835-9.
85. Maheshwari A, Stofberg L, Bhattacharya S. Effect of overweight and obesity on assisted reproductive technology—a systematic review. Hum Reprod Update. 2007;13:433-44.
86. Rittenberg V, Seshadri S, Sunkara SK, Sobaleva S, Oteng-Ntim E, El Toukhy T. Effect of body mass index on IVF treatment outcome: an updated systematic review and meta-analysis. Reprod Biomed Online. 2011;23:421-39.
87. Stothard KJ, Tennant PWG, Bell R, Rankin J. Maternal overweight and obesity and the risk of congenital anomalies: a systematic review and meta-analysis. JAMA. 2009;301:636-50.
88. Tan SL, Royston P, Campbell S, Jacobs HS, Betts J, Mason B, et al. Cumulative conception and livebirth rates after in-vitro fertilisation. Lancet. 1992;339:1390-4.
89. Bhattacharya S, Hamilton MP, Shaaban M, Khalaf Y, Seddler M, Ghobara T, et al. Conventional in-vitro fertilisation versus intracytoplasmic sperm injection for the treatment of non-male-factor infertility: a randomised controlled trial. Lancet. 2001;357:2075-9.
90. Matson PL, Yovich JL. The treatment of infertility associated with endometriosis by *in vitro* fertilization. Fertil Steril. 1986;46:432-4.
91. Geber S, Paraschos T, Atkinson G, Margara R, Winston RM. Results of IVF in patients with endometriosis: the severity of the disease does not affect outcome, or the incidence of miscarriage. Hum Reprod. 1995;10:1507-11.
92. Gupta S, Agarwal A, Agarwal R, Loret de Mola JR. Impact of ovarian endometrioma on assisted reproduction outcomes. Reprod Biomed Online. 2006;13:349-60.
93. Somigliana E, Arnoldi M, Benaglia L, Iemmello R, Nicolosi AE, Ragni G. IVF-ICSI outcome in women operated on for bilateral endometriomas. Hum Reprod. 2008;23:1526-30.
94. Palermo G, Joris H, Devroey P, Van Steirteghem AC. Pregnancies after intracytoplasmic injection of single spermatozoon into an oocyte. Lancet. 1992;340:17-8.
95. Cohen J, Alikani M, Malter HE, Adler A, Talansky BE, Rosenwaks Z. Partial zona dissection or subzonal sperm insertion: microsurgical fertilization alternatives based on evaluation of sperm and embryo morphology. Fertil Steril. 1991;56:696-706.
96. Tarin JJ. Subzonal insemination, partial zona dissection or intracytoplasmic sperm injection? An easy decision? Hum Reprod. 1995;10:165-70.
97. Fishel S, Lisi F, Rinaldi L, Green S, Hunter A, Dowell K, et al. Systematic examination of immobilizing spermatozoa before intracytoplasmic sperm injection in the human. Hum Reprod. 1995;10:497-500.
98. Friedler S, Schenker JG, Herman A, Lewin A. The role of ultrasonography in the evaluation of endometrial receptivity following assisted reproductive treatments: a critical review. Hum Reprod Update. 1996;2:323-35.
99. Wood C, McMaster R, Rennie G, Trounson A, Leeton J. Factors influencing pregnancy rates following *in vitro* fertilization and embryo transfer. Fertil Steril. 1985;43:245-50.
100. Staessen C, Verpoest W, Donoso P, Haentjens P, Van der Elst J, Liebaers I, et al. Preimplantation genetic screening does not improve delivery rate in women under the age of 36 following single-embryo transfer. Hum Reprod. 2008;23:2818-25.
101. Vauthier-Brouzes D, Lefebvre G, Lesourd S, Gonzales J, Darbois Y. How many embryos should be transferred in *in vitro* fertilization? A prospective randomized study. Fertil Steril. 1994;62:339-42.
102. Templeton A, Morris JK. Reducing the risk of multiple births by transfer of two embryos after *in vitro* fertilization. N Engl J Med. 1998;339:573-7.
103. Cutting R, Morroll D, Roberts SA, Pickering S, Rutherford A. Elective single embryo transfer: Guidelines for Practice British Fertility Society and Association of Clinical Embryologists. Hum Fertil (Camb). 2008;1-16.
104. Pandian Z, Templeton A, Serour G, Bhattacharya S. Number of embryos for transfer after IVF and ICSI: a Cochrane review. Hum Reprod. 2005;20:2681-7.
105. Padilla SL, Garcia JE. Effect of maternal age and number of *in vitro* fertilization procedures on pregnancy outcome. Fertil Steril. 1989;52:270-3.
106. Dor J, Seidman DS, Ben-Shlomo I, Levran D, Ben-Rafael Z, Mashiach S. Cumulative pregnancy rate following in-vitro fertilization: the significance of age and infertility aetiology. Hum Reprod. 1996;11:425-8.
107. Croucher CA, Lass A, Margara R, Winston RM. Predictive value of the results of a first in-vitro fertilization cycle on the outcome of subsequent cycles. Hum Reprod. 1998;13:403-8.
108. Cobo A, de los Santos MJ, Castello D, Gamiz P, Campos P, Remohi J. Outcomes of vitrified early cleavage-stage and blastocyst-stage embryos in a cryopreservation program: evaluation of 3,150 warming cycles. Fertil Steril. 2012;98:1138-46. e1131.

109. Loutradi KE, Kolibianakis EM, Venetis CA, Papanikolaou EG, Pados G, Bontis I, et al. Cryopreservation of human embryos by vitrification or slow freezing: a systematic review and meta-analysis. Fertil Steril. 2008;90:186-93.
110. Abdel Hafez FF, Desai N, Abou-Setta AM, Falcone T, Goldfarb J. Slow freezing, vitrification and ultra-rapid freezing of human embryos: a systematic review and meta-analysis. Reprod Biomed Online. 2010;20:209-22.
111. Roque M, Lattes K, Serra S, Sola I, Geber S, Carreras R, et al. Fresh embryo transfer versus frozen embryo transfer in *in vitro* fertilization cycles: a systematic review and meta-analysis. Fertil Steril. 2013;99:156-62.
112. Aflatoonian A, Oskouian H, Ahmadi S, Oskouian L. Can fresh embryo transfers be replaced by cryopreserved-thawed embryo transfers in assisted reproductive cycles? A randomized controlled trial. J Assist Reprod Genet. 2010;27: 357-63.
113. Shapiro BS, Daneshmand ST, Garner FC, Aguirre M, Hudson C, Thomas S. Evidence of impaired endometrial receptivity after ovarian stimulation for *in vitro* fertilization: a prospective randomized trial comparing fresh and frozen thawed embryo transfer in normal responders. Fertil Steril. 2011a;96:344-8.
114. Shapiro BS, Daneshmand ST, Garner FC, Aguirre M, Hudson C, Thomas S. Evidence of impaired endometrial receptivity after ovarian stimulation for *in vitro* fertilization: a prospective randomized trial comparing fresh and frozen-thawed embryo transfers in high responders. Fertil Steril. 2011b;96:516-8.
115. Fatemi HM, Kyrou D, Bourgain C, Van den Abbeel E, Griesinger G, Devroey P. Cryopreserved-thawed human embryo transfer: spontaneous natural cycle is superior to human chorionic gonadotropin-induced natural cycle. Fertil Steril. 2010.
116. Chang EM, Han JE, Won HJ, Kim YS, Yoon TK, Lee WS. Effect of estrogen priming through luteal phase and stimulation phase in poor responders in in-vitro fertilization. J Assist Reprod Genet. 2011;29:225-30.
117. El Bahja D, Hertz P, Schweitzer T, Lestrade F, Ragage JP. Frozen embryo transfer protocol: does spontaneous cycle give good results? Gynecol Obstet Fertil. 2013;41: 648-52.
118. Xiao Z, Zhou X, Xu W, Yang J, Xie Q. Natural cycle is superior to hormone replacement therapy cycle for vitrificated-preserved frozen-thawed embryo transfer. Syst Biol Reprod Med. 2012;58:107-12
119. Groenewoud ER, Cantineau AE, Kollen BJ, Macklon NS, Cohlen BJ. What is the optimal means of preparing the endometrium in frozen-thawed embryo transfer cycles? A systematic review and meta-analysis. Hum Reprod Update. 2013;19:458-70.
120. Khastgir G, Abdalla H, Thomas A, Korea L, Latarche L, Studd J. Oocyte donation in Turner's syndrome: an analysis of the factors affecting the outcome. Hum Reprod. 1997;12:279-85.
121. Yaron Y, Ochshorn Y, Amit A, Yovel I, Kogosowki A, Lessing JB. Patients with Turner's syndrome may have an inherent endometrial abnormality affecting receptivity in oocyte donation. Fertil Steril. 1996;65:1249-52.
122. Burton G, Abdalla HI, Kirkland A, Studd JW. The role of oocyte donation in women who are unsuccessful with in-vitro fertilization treatment. Hum Reprod. 1992;7:1103-5.
123. Clayton HB, Schieve LA, Peterson HB, Jamieson DJ, Reynolds MA, Wright VC. Ectopic pregnancy risk with assisted reproductive technology procedures. Obstet Gynecol. 2006;107:595-604.
124. Mathur R, Kailasam C, Jenkins J. Review of the evidence base of strategies to prevent ovarian hyperstimulation syndrome. Hum Fertil (Camb). 2007;10:75-85.
125. Navot D, Bergh PA, Laufer N. Ovarian hyperstimulation syndrome in novel reproductive technologies: prevention and treatment. Fertil Steril. 1992;58(2):249-61.
126. Brinton L. Long-term effects of ovulation-stimulating drugs on cancer risk. Reprod Biomed Online. 2007;15:38-44.
127. Venn A, Jones P, Quinn M, Healy D. Characteristics of ovarian and uterine cancers in a cohort of in vitro fertilization patients. Gynecol Oncol. 2001;82(1):64-8.
128. Klip H, van Leeuwen FE, Schats R, Burger CW; OMEGA Project Group. Risk of benign gynaecological diseases and hormonal disorders according to responsiveness to ovarian stimulation in IVF: a follow-up study of 8714 women. Hum Reprod. 2003;18(9):1951-8.
129. Modan B, Ron E, Lerner-Geva L, Blumstein T, Menczer J, Rabinovici J, et al. Cancer incidence in a cohort of infertile women. Am J Epidemiol. 1998;147:1038-42.
130. Gauthier E, Paoletti X, Clavel-Chapelon F. Breast cancer risk associated with being treated for infertility: results from the French E3N cohort study. Hum Reprod. 2004;19:2216-21.
131. Hansen M, Bower C, Milne E, de Klerk N, Kurinczuk JJ. Assisted reproductive technologies and the risk of birth defects—a systematic review. Hum Reprod. 2005;20:328-38.
132. Lie RT, Lyngstadaas A, Orstavik KH, Bakketeig LS, Jacobsen G, Tanbo T. Birth defects in children conceived by ICSI compared with children conceived by other IVF-methods; a meta-analysis. Int J Epidemiol. 2005;34:696-701.
133. Zhu JL, Basso O, Obel C, Bille C, Olsen J. Infertility, infertility treatment, and congenital malformations: Danish national birth cohort. BMJ. 2006;333:679.
134. Sutcliffe AG, Peters CJ, Bowdin S, Temple K, Reardon W, Wilson L, et al. Assisted reproductive therapies and imprinting disorders—a preliminary British survey. Hum Reprod. 2006;21:1009-11.
135. Bowdin S, Allen C, Kirby G, Brueton L, Afnan M, Barratt C, et al. A survey of assisted reproductive technology births and imprinting disorders. Hum Reprod. 2007;22:3237-40.
136. Moll AC, Imhof SM, Cruysberg JR, Schouten-van Meeteren AY, Boers M, van Leeuwen FE. Incidence of retinoblastoma in children born after in-vitro fertilisation. Lancet. 2003;361:309-10.
137. Kallen B, Finnstrom O, Nygren KG, Olausson PO. *In vitro* fertilization in Sweden: child morbidity including cancer risk. Fertil Steril. 2005;84:605-10.
138. Murdoch A. Triplets and embryo transfer policy. Hum Reprod. 1997;12:88-92.
139. Wang JX, Norman RJ, Wilcox AJ. Incidence of spontaneous abortion among pregnancies produced by assisted reproductive technology. Hum Reprod. 2004;19:272-7.

140. Pezeshki K, Feldman J, Stein DE, Lobel SM, Grazi RV. Bleeding and spontaneous abortion after therapy for infertility. Fertil Steril. 2000;74:504-8.
141. Halliday J. Outcomes of IVF conceptions: are they different? Best Pract Res Clin Obstet Gynaecol. 2007;21:67-81.
142. McDonald S, Murphy K, Beyene J, Ohlsson A. Perinatal outcomes of *in vitro* fertilization twins: a systematic review and meta-analyses. Am J Obstet Gynecol. 2005a;193:141-52.
143. McDonald SD, Murphy K, Beyene J, Ohlsson A. Perinatal outcomes of singleton pregnancies achieved by *in vitro* fertilization: a systematic review and meta-analysis. J Obstet Gynaecol Can. 2005b;27:449-59.
144. Helmerhorst FM, Perquin DA, Donker D, Keirse MJ. Perinatal outcome of singletons and twins after assisted conception: a systematic review of controlled studies. BMJ. 2004; 328:261.
145. Ombelet W, Cadron I, Gerris J, De Sutter P, Bosmans E, Martens G, et al. Obstetric and perinatal outcome of 1655 ICSI and 3974 IVF singleton and 1102 ICSI and 2901 IVF twin births: a comparative analysis. Reprod Biomed Online. 2005;11:76-85.
146. Mercan R, Lanzendorf SE, Mayer J Jr, Nassar A, Muasher SJ, Oehninger S. The outcome of clinical pregnancies following intracytoplasmic sperm injection is not affected by semen quality. Andrologia. 1998;30(2):91-5.
147. Soderstrom-Anttila V. Pregnancy and child outcome after oocyte donation. Hum Reprod Update. 2001;7:28-32.
148. Wiggins DA, Main E. Outcomes of pregnancies achieved by donor egg *in vitro* fertilization—a comparison with standard *in vitro* fertilization pregnancies. Am J Obstet Gynecol. 2005;192:2002-6; discussion 2006-8.
149. Halliday JL, Ukoumunne OC, Baker HW, Breheny S, Jaques AM, Garrett C, et al. Increased risk of blastogenesis birth defects, arising in the first 4 weeks of pregnancy, after assisted reproductive technologies. Hum Reprod. 2010.
150. Maheshwari A, Pandey S, Shetty A, Hamilton M, Bhattacharya S. Obstetric and perinatal outcomes in singleton pregnancies resulting from the transfer of frozen thawed versus fresh embryos generated through *in vitro* fertilization treatment: a systematic review and meta-analysis. Fertil Steril. 2012;98:368-77.
151. Wennerholm UB, Henningsen AK, Romundstad LB, Bergh C, Pinborg A, Skjaerven R, et al. Perinatal outcomes of children born after frozen-thawed embryo transfer: a Nordic cohort study from the CoNARTaS group. Hum Reprod. 2013;28(9):2545-53.
152. Pelkonen S, Koivunen R, Gissler M, Nuojua-Huttunen S, Suikkari AM, Hyden-Granskog C, et al. Perinatal outcome of children born after frozen and fresh embryo transfer: the Finnish cohort study 1995–2006. Hum Reprod. 2010;25:914-23.
153. Pinborg A, Wennerholm UB, Romundstad LB, Loft A, Aittomaki K, Soderstrom-Anttila V, et al. Why do singletons conceived after assisted reproduction technology have adverse perinatal outcome? Systematic review and meta-analysis. Hum Reprod Update. 2010;19:87-104.
154. Sazonova A, Kallen K, Thurin-Kjellberg A, Wennerholm UB, Bergh C. Neonatal and maternal outcomes comparing women undergoing two *in vitro* fertilization (IVF) singleton pregnancies and women undergoing one IVF twin pregnancy. Fertil Steril. 2012;99:731-7.
155. Kalra SK, Ratcliffe SJ, Coutifaris C, Molinaro T, Barnhart KT. Ovarian stimulation and low birth weight in newborns conceived through in vitro fertilization. Obstet Gynecol. 2011;118(4):863-71.
156. Roy TK, Bradley CK, Bowman MC, McArthur SJ. Single-embryo transfer of vitrified-warmed blastocysts yields equivalent live-birth rates and improved neonatal outcomes compared with fresh transfers. Fertil Steril. 2014;101:1294-301.
157. Wada I, Macnamee MC, Wick K, Bradfield JM, Brinsden PR. Birth characteristics and perinatal outcome of babies conceived from cryopreserved embryos. Hum Reprod. 1994;9:543-6.
158. Anderson RA, Pickering S. The current status of preimplantation genetic screening: British Fertility Society Policy and Practice Guidelines. Hum Fertil (Camb). 2008;11:71-5.
159. Braude PR, Regan L, Trembath PL. Influence of past reproductive performance on risk of spontaneous abortion. BMJ. 1989;299:541-5.
160. Kuliev A, Verlinsky Y. Preimplantation genetic diagnosis: technological advances to improve accuracy and range of applications. Reprod Biomed Online. 2008;16:532-8.
161. Cieslak-Janzen J, Tur-Kaspa I, Ilkevitch Y, Bernal A, Morris R, Verlinsky Y. Multiple micromanipulations for preimplantation genetic diagnosis do not affect embryo development to the blastocyst stage. Fertil Steril. 2006;85:1826-9.
162. Mastenbroek S, Scriven P, Twisk M, Viville S, Van der Veen F, Repping S. What next for preimplantation genetic screening? More randomized controlled trials needed? Hum Reprod. 2008;23:2626-8.
163. Nagy ZP, Sakkas D, Behr B. Symposium: innovative techniques in human embryo viability assessment. Non-invasive assessment of embryo viability by metabolomic profiling of culture media ('metabolomics'). Reprod Biomed Online. 2008;17:502-7.
164. Sturmey RG, Brison DR, Leese HJ. Symposium: innovative techniques in human embryo viability assessment. Assessing embryo viability by measurement of amino acid turnover. Reprod Biomed Online. 2008;17:486-96.
165. Anderson RA, Wallace WH, Baird DT. Ovarian cryopreservation for fertility preservation: indications and outcomes. Reproduction. 2008;136:681-9.

CHAPTER

Laboratory Aspects of *In Vitro* Fertilization and Intracytoplasmic Sperm Injection

15

Jayant G Mehta

INTRODUCTION

In vitro fertilization (IVF) and intracytoplasmic sperm injection (ICSI) are two most distinct assisted reproductive technology (ART) procedures frequently practiced in achieving pregnancy in subfertile couples. While IVF interventions have resulted in significant success for patients with tubal infertility,[1] unexplained infertility, and patients with endometriosis,[2] the introduction of ICSI in early1990s revolutionized the male factor treatment. Palermo and colleagues[3] accidently injected a single sperm into the oocyte through the zona pellucida and advanced the injection needle by breaking the membrane of the oocyte (oolemma), achieving fertilization and a subsequent viable pregnancy. Currently, this technique is offered to most couples without a diagnosis of a severe male factor, including mild and borderline male factor infertility, unexplained infertility, and women of advanced age.[4-7] Moreover, the last 4 decades have also seen advances in newer laboratory techniques requiring the use of micromanipulation of gametes—oocytes and sperm, and embryos. The benefits and safety of these newer techniques still need validation.[5]

Scientific evidence, mainly from studies in animals, have demonstrated the need and the importance of a better physiological understanding of gametes and embryos in culture conditions impacting on pre- and postimplantation development and the health of the newborn.[8-12]

One major advantage IVF laboratories now enjoy is a selection of commercially prepared scientifically formulated quality-assured culture media. Although these media are based on data from animal studies raising doubts to the validity of its use in human embryology, what is reassuring is that the preparation and up-scaling of these culture media follow "good manufacturing conditions" (GMP) and quality assurance ensuring improved batch-to-batch consistency and evidence of no contamination.[13,14] However, due to the lack of transparency about formulations, it has not been possible to refine the existing IVF culture media for culturing human gametes.[15,16] As a consequence, various regulatory bodies now require IVF media to be classified as Class III medical devices. Medicines and Healthcare products Regulatory Agency (MHRA) oversees this classification. All media used in the IVF laboratories in the EU are now CE (Conformité Européene) class III marked.

Furthermore, the influence of air quality on the oocytes and embryos within the ART laboratories has extensively been addressed within the EU directives for the ART laboratories. All the tissue culture laboratories should maintain a grade D air quality within the laboratory and grade C in the areas where gametes are manipulated. The fact that less than 40% of the ART laboratories worldwide do not have their ICSI setup within an air-flow cabinet, it becomes mandatory to ensure grade C air quality in the laboratory.[17-27]

Moreover, to ensure continuous good results and safety of the gametes and patients, it is necessary that all Art laboratory procedures are monitored under "Quality Control (QC) and Quality Management (QM) system", allowing corrective actions to be implemented during a regular review of the IVF and ICSI processes.[23-27]

This chapter reviews all the laboratory aspects of human IVF and ICSI that influence the outcome and helps to understand how to improve methods that lead to step limited failures, the timing of various phases, and procedures that will enhance the success rates.

IN VITRO FERTILIZATION

Birth of Louise Brown in July 1978, confirmed the possibility of achieving fertilization *in vitro* by mixing sperms and oocyte collected in a natural cycle and co-culturing them in a desiccator placed in an incubator at 37°C.[1]

Availability of gonadotropins resulted in the development of controlled ovarian stimulation protocols and aspiration of more than one oocyte. Currently, on average ten mature (MII) oocytes are aspirated under the influence of various stimulations protocols, which include agonist and antagonist regimes.[26]

Oocyte Collection

The gametes culturing techniques and conditions have evolved over the last 4 decades. Due to regulatory requirements, currently, EU directives require all laboratories to use embryo toxic tested, sterilized, and CE marked disposable consumables for all their ART treatment cycles.[27] As a consequence, laboratories now have an extensive choice of various consumables from different manufacturers, to the extent that some companies have focused purely on supplying consumables for ART-related cycles only.

The aspirated follicular fluid is examined under a stereo zoom microscope mounted in a class two cabinet. On identification of the oocyte cumulus complex (OCC), it is removed from the follicular fluid, gently agitated in a buffered media covered with liquid paraffin using a sterile flamed glass pipettes. This process removes any red blood cells surrounding the OCC. Once cleaned, OCCs are placed in a 60-mm circular holding dish (CHD) containing the same buffered media, normally MOPS or HEPES-based or one containing both MOPS and HEPES. The CHD with the oocytes remains under gas bell jar at 37°C for the entire period of egg collection. At the end of the collection, all the oocytes are transferred to a four well dish containing 500 μL of bicarbonate buffered culture media covered with 500 μL of liquid paraffin. The oocytes are cultured in groups of three per well, and only three wells are used leaving the fourth well for storing the denuded eggs for fertilization check 18 hours, postinsemination. The four well dishes are then placed in the incubator which allows the oocytes to equilibrate with the culture media and the incubator environment. Liquid paraffin acts as a barrier between the media interface and the incubator environment, thus avoiding any damage to the oocyte or embryos in culture due to pH or osmotic stress and also briefly protects the oocytes from the laboratory environment.[28]

Insemination and Fertilization Check

A freshly prepared semen sample is preferred for IVF. The partner of the patient is asked to produce a sample once the oocytes are collected. On liquefaction, the sample is processed as described elsewhere.[29] On occasions, the patient would have his semen sample cryopreserved due to the anxiety of producing on the day of egg collection. It is always advisable that all patients undergoing IVF/ICSI cycles should be recommended to have their semen preserved. The oocytes in the four well dish(s) are inseminated 40 hours, post-human chorionic gonadotropin (hCG) trigger with a concentration of 10,000 prepared motile sperms per oocyte and the dish is returned to the humidified incubator for a further 18 hours.

Using stereo zoom microscope mounted in a class two cabinet, the oocytes are denuded one at a time, 18 hours, postinsemination using a 135–140 μm denuding pipette. Fertilization is confirmed when two pronuclei and expulsion of the second polar body is observed. Zygotes (fertilized oocyte) are transferred into a 30 μL droplet of culture media under liquid paraffin in a 60-mm circular dish containing nine drops of buffered culture media, prepared the night before. After gentle agitation in the successive droplets, three washed zygotes are placed into one droplet. Those oocytes not fertilized are kept in a separate dish. On occasions, more than two pronuclei are observed, suggestive of polyspermy. These zygotes are also transferred into the same dish as the unfertilized oocytes and identified by circles them at the bottom of the dish. For sequential culture protocols, the dish with fertilized oocytes is placed in a humidified incubator at 37°C for a further 48 hours, when the zygotes are scored as cleaved embryos and transferred into fresh 30μL drops of pre-equilibrated media, three per drop, in a fresh dish for blastocyst culture. When using single continuous culture media, some laboratories do not change the cleaved embryos into fresh drops. However, to avoid detrimental effects of ammonium build-up in the droplets, some laboratories prefer to change the cleaved embryos into fresh continuous media on day 3 (48 hours, postinsemination or injection). The bench top incubators are gassed with premixed gasses of 6% CO_2, 5% O_2, and balanced with nitrogen.[30]

In both IVF and ICSI cycles, 15–20% of oocytes collected are not at MII stage, 10–15% remaining at prophase I, and 5% at MI stage. It is therefore not surprising that in IVF a small percentage of the oocytes fail to fertilize. These oocytes are scored for the extrusion of the polar bodies, or the presence of sperm bound to the zona pellucida. When a total fertilization is observed in the presence of a single polar body, some laboratories have attempted rescue ICSI by injecting these oocytes. This is suggestive of the fact that the oocyte matured overnight. If ICSI rescue is considered, one should always use the freshly prepared sample.

Unfortunately, the results from rescue ICSI are not very encouraging. Although *in vitro maturation* (IVM) is not normally considered for failed IVF oocytes, their potential clinical use may be an option to consider in cycles with no MII oocytes at the time of fertilization check, followed by ICSI.[31-33]

INTRACYTOPLASMIC SPERM INJECTION

Similar to IVF, oocyte aspiration, identification, washing of OCC, and storing them in a holding dish before transferring into a four well dish and placing them in the incubator is the same for ICSI.

However, unlike IVF, where the oocytes are denuded for checking fertilization, in ICSI, the denuding of the OCC is done 30 minutes before the injection and normally 38 hours post-hCG trigger. Although the OCC denuding protocol first described by Mahadevan and Trounson[34] remains the generic protocol used by most of the ART laboratories worldwide, studies have looked into the use of recombinant hyaluronidase,[35] and most recently the effect of reducing the concentration of hyaluronidase by tenfolds[36] concluded improved fertilization rates and embryo quality. Once denuded, mature (MII) oocytes, with first polar body expelled are placed in a 30 μL droplet of culture media after gently washing through successive droplets. Those oocytes which are immature either MI or showing germinal vesicle (GV) are placed in two separate droplets, respectively. Unlike IVF where all the oocytes are inseminated, in ICSI only MII oocytes are injected with a single morphologically normal sperm.

Failed fertilization in ICSI can be attributed either to dysfunctional gametes or to potential weaknesses during micromanipulation due to lack of attention to finer details.[37]

When is the Best Time to Inject?

Although studies have concluded that the fertilization and pregnancy rates improve when oocytes are incubated for 2–6 hours before insemination in IVF,[38-44] the timing of injection postoocyte retrieval is still being debated. As mentioned earlier, only MII oocytes are injected in ICSI ensuring that both nuclear and cytoplasmic maturity is synchronized and normal fertilization can occur.

As stimulated cycles demonstrate delayed synchronization of nuclear and cytoplasmic maturity,[42-44] it is not surprising that the preincubation of oocytes before IVF or ICSI may influence the cytoplasmic maturation resulting in a possible increase in fertilization and pregnancy rates.

Based on the evidence presented, human oocytes progressively develop the ability for normal activation when arrested at MII stage.[44] Moreover, unless the ovulated oocytes have been fertilized, they undergo a time-dependent process of aging and can influence the embryonic development and pregnancy rates following *in vitro* procedures.[45,46] The timing of injection in ICSI, therefore, represents a critical step in the overall procedure.

Furthermore, studies looking at the timing of preincubation of oocytes with cumulus-corona cells before denudation and injection have reported no statistical differences in survival, fertilization, cleavage, and pregnancy rates. The preincubation time of 2–3 hours has resulted in higher fertilization rates, higher good quality embryo development rates, and a significantly higher clinical pregnancy rates.[47-51]

When cumulus and corona cells were removed within 1 hour from oocyte retrieval[52] and after 2 hours,[53] there was no effect on the outcome. In my laboratory, we denude the oocytes for ICSI after 2 hours of preincubation and inject only MII oocytes within 30 minutes of denuding them. Dozortsev and colleagues[54] have demonstrated that when ICSI is performed between 37 and 39 hours after hCG administration, the highest level of implantation and ongoing pregnancies were observed, suggestive of the fact that a very narrow sensitive time window exists during which injection should be completed. However, the most recent report by Garor and colleagues[55] concluded that there was no effect on the incubation time.

Although studies reported here are concordant with the observations that a preincubation time with cumulus-corona cells may influence the optimization of nuclear and cytoplasmic maturation for ICSI, data are non-concordant when this time was extended.

Is there a Role of *In Vitro* Maturation as an Adjunct to IVF/ICSI?

To answer this question, it is necessary to review the biological process of maturation. Briefly, it has been established that the development of the oocyte within the follicle is under the influence of a highly coordinated signaling mechanism between the follicle cells and the oocyte. These signals initiate the resumption of meiotic division, chromatin condensation, organelle redistribution, and cytoskeletal changes resulting in the oocyte acquiring nuclear and developmental competency. This signaling further ensures the relocation and reorganization of ribosomes, mitochondria, and endoplasmic reticulum (ER). Moreover, the ability to modulate calcium release, an essential process during fertilization is also developed.[56-60] It has been reported that when comparing *in vivo* maturation and development, IVM oocytes have a reduced potential for fertilization and development to blastocysts.[57]

Chromosome condensation and spindle formation after GV breakdown is critical for oocyte maturation. The homologous chromosomes align on the metaphase spindle and enter into the meiotic exit process. The entire event is dependent on cyclin-dependent protein kinase 1 (CDK1) and is controlled by the ligase-promoting complex (APC). The extrusion of the first polar body is signaled by the decrease in CDK1 activity as a result of degradation of cyclin B1. Simultaneously, the cytoplasmic maturation is initiated and is completed when the oocyte reaches MII stage. The expulsion of the first polar body confirms the nuclear maturity.[60]

Synthesis of various maternal mRNAs and proteins constitute cytoplasmic maturity process. These proteins have very specific and precise mechanisms in the organization of the cytoplasmic organelles within the cytoskeleton and influence the full complement of Ca^{2+} signaling molecules.[58] As reported, defects in the organization of the spindles or chromosomal aberrations represent the most significant intervention preventing synchronization of nuclear and cytoplasmic maturation.[56,59]

Considering the complexity of the maturation process, it is customary only to inject MII oocytes. However, the use of immature oocytes can increase the number of embryos available. Maturation of MI oocytes to MII varies between clinical laboratories with no single protocol. Availability of preimplantation genetic screening (PGS) has renewed interest in a short-term (8 hours) *in vitro* cultured of MI oocytes matured to MII.

Although studies have reported higher than 60% fertilization for *in vitro* matured MI oocytes, they remain significantly lower when compared to *in vivo* retrieved MII oocytes.[32,44,60-68] Cleavage rates in some studies reported were not different, while the pregnancy outcomes in rescue MI oocytes were poor.[32,61,63,66] Shin and colleagues[68] reported no pregnancies when they reduced the IVM culture time to 3–4 hours. Fluorescence in situ hybridization (FISH) study reported a 100% aneuploidy for oocytes when incubated for 24 hours, however, reducing to 40% after a short incubation period of 2 hours.[65]

Even though IVM of MI to MII will increase the number of embryos available for transfer, given the evidence presented here, it is not advisable to recommend it for widespread clinical use. However, those clinics proposing to follow this path should offer aneuploidy screening and counseling to their patients, ensuring the safety of the patient and the resulting pregnancy.

Intracytoplasmic Sperm Injection and Degeneration of Oocytes

The ICSI technicians have reported degeneration rate of 5–19% during ICSI. Leakage of cytoplasm at the site of injection on withdrawal of the injecting needle is a common observation. In some cases formation of retracted and darkened ooplasm, 18 hours after injection is also suggestive of oocyte degeneration.[3,69-73] Furthermore, stimulation protocols affect the quality of the oocytes collected as does the amount of cytoplasm aspirated, excessive manipulation inside the oocyte, or inadvertent damage to the oolemma at the opposite site of the injection hole due to a too deep penetration by the injection pipette.[70,71,73,74]

The process of denudation of the oocyte can also influence the degeneration, if the diameter of the pipette used for removal of the cumulus is very small. This indirectly damages the cytoskeleton creating strong compression resulting in leakage of cytoplasm and sudden breakage of oolemma at the time of injection.[70] Incomplete removal of cumulus and corona cells also hinders the injection procedure and can lead to degeneration.[71,75]

Yavas and colleagues,[72] in a retrospective study, reported a significant decrease in the degeneration and recommended the use of injection pipette with a smaller inner diameter and a longer taper: 3–5 mm inner diameter instead of 5–7 mm. They found three positive benefits of a thinner injection pipette. Firstly, it reduced the degree of mechanical trauma that is exerted on the oolemma. It further reduced the volume of cytoplasm aspirated into the injection pipette avoiding disturbing the cytoskeleton and also reduced the amount of polyvinylpyrrolidone (PVP) injected into the oocyte with the sperm.

The thickness of zona pellucida can also offer considerable resistance to injection and can lead to degeneration of oocyte. To overcome the problems with resistance, laser-mediated ICSI has been proposed. In this technique, a micro-hole of 5–10 mm diameter is created in the zona pellucida by a laser beam just before introducing the injecting pipette with the sperm.[76-80] This technique reduced the percentage of degenerated oocyte, increased fertilization rate, and better quality of day 3 embryos was observed, suggesting that reduction in the cytoplasmic disturbance and damage to subcellular components is critical for the better developmental potential of the embryos and subsequent pregnancies. However, this technique lost favor when it was realized that the small hole created may be associated with embryo trapping leading to degeneration of blastocysts and monozygotic twinning due to the restriction to hatching and subsequent splitting.[81]

An alternate approach devoid of the risk discussed was to thin the zona immediately before injection thus reducing the resistance. A higher fertilization, higher blastulation, and clinical pregnancies have been reported with this technique.[82] This technique is currently used to prevent oocyte damage in patients with a history of poor oocyte quality and history of higher degeneration rates with a sudden breakage feature in previous ICSI cycles.

Significance of Polar Body Positioning during Injection

Based on our physiological understandings,[83-86] it has been assumed that the second meiotic MII spindle resides in the proximity to the first polar body. The position of the polar body at the time of injection should either be at 12 or 6 o'clock position with the injecting pipette with the sperm in it at 3 o'clock position. This will prevent any possible damage to MII plate and the spindle.[87-92] Partial or total disruption of the MII spindle will lead to perturbation of chromosomal segregation resulting in an aneuploidy with a possibility of cell death. Although the orientation of a polar body at 12 or 6 o'clock would avoid damage to the MII spindles, studies had reported better outcomes when the polar body was position at 6 o'clock instead of 12 o'clock.[93,94] Further studies have also looked at different orientation at 7 or 11 o'clock with no different outcomes.[95,96] These studies, however, confirmed the importance of delivering the sperm as close to the spindle as possible, ensuring fertilization and cleavage of the resulting embryos.

Use of imaging polarization microscopy has helped with our knowledge of the positioning of the MII spindle demonstrating that it may not be located below the first polar body but could be anywhere and in some cases by more than 90° from the polar body.[77,97] This discrepancy observed may be due to the manipulation and stress generated during the denuding of the oocyte. Also, polar body displacement may also be influenced by intrinsic factors such as oocyte aging, as seen in mouse.[98,99] Moreover, the orientation of the spindle away from the polar body has caused an alteration in the position of the polarized molecules within the cytoplasm influencing embryo development and consequent clinical pregnancy.[100]

Given this discrepancy, in the absence of the polarization microscopy, the optimal polar body or spindle position during ICSI remains unclear, and care should be taken. Furthermore, competency of the ICSI technician will influence the outcome in so much as to the amount of cytoplasm aspirated into the injection pipette or the force with which the injection pipette is introduced through the zona pellucida.

Intracytoplasmic Sperm Injection and Fertilization Failure

Unlike IVF, complete fertilization failure is a rare occurrence in ICSI cycles. However, studies had reported 1–3% complete failures even when morphologically normal sperms were used.[101-104] Montag and colleagues[105] have observed up to 30% fertilization failure in repeated ICSI cycles of some their patients.

It is well documented that in the conventional IVF, 60–90% of the oocytes fail to fertilize as sperm penetration is not possible or sperm ejection is considered to be the main cause resulting in no presence of sperm nuclei within the cytoplasm.[106] However, in ICSI, 40–70% of oocytes present a swollen sperm head confirming that the oocyte was properly injected but it failed to be activated.[107-111] It is also likely that fertilization failure could be due to failed sperm decondensation, premature sperm chromatin condensation, spindle defects, sperm aster defects, or incorrect ICSI procedure.[112]

Oocyte activation initiates the cortical granule exocytosis, expulsion of the second polar body, recruitment of maternal RNA and formation of pronuclei, and finally the activation of the embryonic gene expression.[113] Furthermore, it is the fusion of the spermatozoon and oocyte that initiates the rise in the intracellular Ca^{2+}, leading to cytological changes in fertilized oocytes.[114,115] The Ca^{2+}signals are species-specific; in mammals, these oscillations last for hours and may affect embryo development.[116] Neri and colleagues[117] have reported that the physical contact of sperm and egg plasma membranes is not critical for the egg activation; however, post ICSI development is sperm-specific. The phospholipase Cz (PLCz), a sperm factor, has been identified to be responsible for oocyte activation trigger. The absence of this factor results in failure to activate the oocyte and fertilization.[116,118]

Those patients, with total or low fertilization failure, should be offered mouse oocyte-activation test (MOAT).[119-121] In the MOAT test, patient's sperm should be tested against heterologous sperm (with proven activation capacity) and depending on the percentage of mouse oocyte being activated, patient can be divided into three groups: low-activation group (≤20%); intermediate-activation group (21–84%); and high-activation group (≥85%). Patients in low-activation group reflect the failure of the sperm to activate the oocyte, while those in intermediate group reflect inconclusive results suggestive of the possible contribution of both the egg and the sperm. In the case of globozoospermia, MOAT test would indicate a deficiency of sperm oocyte-activating ability. Moreover, those patients with poor or no fertilization and identified by MOAT to be in a high-activation group would benefit from assessing likely transient biological reasons, possibly technical imperfection. Review of the test should allow different options to be considered and artificial oocyte activation (AOA) using mechanical, physical, or chemical stimuli should be considered and offered.

In mechanical method, ICSI technique is slightly modified in that, the cytoplasm is vigorously aspirated from the central area of the oocyte and is reinjected along with the spermatozoa as close to the oocyte periphery on the opposite side of the injection puncture site. This vigorous aspiration increases the influx of Ca^{2+} from the surrounding culture media.[122,123] Furthermore, it is likely that this vigorous aspiration will disrupt the ER organelle resulting in the release of Ca^{2+}. This action also allows the collection of more mitochondria from the periphery, and when deposited at the site of fertilization, collectively they generate extra energy in the form of ATP aiding fertilization. Ebner and colleagues[123] observed fertilization rate of 53% and pregnancy rate of 33.3% in 14 previously failed ICSI cycles using this mechanical technique.

Physically, application of an electric pulse leads to the charged proteins present in the cell membrane of gametes and somatic cells to move. As a consequence, the cytoplasm gets activated; Ca^{2+} levels are increased and returning to their original values within minutes. In all ICSI failed patients, on the application of the electric pulse 20–30 minutes after ICSI procedure, good fertilization rates, better quality embryos, and clinical pregnancies were reported procedures.[124-128]

Of the chemical stimulants, strontium chloride ($SrCl_2$) is preferred over Ca^{2+} ionophore treatment by many ART clinics for AOA. $SrCl_2$ mediates its action via IP3 receptors when activated by PLCz and moves down a concentration gradient to release Ca^{2+} from ER. Although no continuous influxes of Ca^{2+} are observed in human oocytes, studies in mice have shown patterns similar to those observed during spontaneous fertilization.[129,130] AOA is carried out by incubating the oocytes for 30 minutes after ICSI procedure, in a solution containing 10 mM $SrCl_2$ for 60 minutes. The oocytes are gently agitated in fresh 30 μL droplets of the culture media under oil and moved to a fresh drop.

Based on the MOAT test results, those patients exhibiting globozoospermia, asthenozoospermia (AA), and teratoasthenozoospermia including testicular aspirated sperm will benefit from AOA.[131-141] Even though no one single protocol exists, ionophores such as ionomycin calservedmicyn (A23187) are preferred for use in AOA; most ART laboratories use a single exposure of oocytes to ionophore within 30–60 minutes of ICSI procedure for anywhere between 5 and 10 minutes. The most preferred concentration is 5–10 mM of Ca^{2+} ionophore. One group has reported incubation with puromycin 10 mg/mL for 4–5 hours. No significant differences were observed in fertilization rates, embryo development rates, and clinical pregnancies when the results from all different protocols were compared.[142-162]

Although the neurodevelopmental outcomes in children between the ages of 3 and 10 years are reassuring, the standardization of the procedure is still not established. As most of the evidence presented here represents small studies with few patients in the study arms, it is mandatory that long-term RCT should be carried out to evaluate the physiological safety of AOA.[163,164] For now, ICSI with AOA should be considered experimental. However, PLCz is now recognized as an essential component in the activation of the oocyte because of its physiological action.[116]

Advance Sperm Selection

Over the years, ICSI has been established as the only treatment option for male factor. However, a higher rate of miscarriages among the ICSI patients has also been associated with DNA fragmented sperm.[165]

Globozoospermia, characterized by an absence of acrosome and aberrant nuclear membrane, associated midpiece defects was first reported in 1971.[166-168] This condition, observed in 0.1% of infertile males is described as a rare type of monomorphic teratozoospermia and is inherited as an autosomal recessive trait of three genes, PICK1 (protein interacting with PRKCA 1), SPATA16 (spermatogenesis associated 16), and DPY19L2 (one of a transmembrane gene family).[166-175]

Although, the number of studies has described the lack of normal morphological development of the sperm in globozoospermia,[176-178] the inability of the acrosome less spermatozoon to penetrate the zona pellucida and failure to fuse with the oolemma of the oocyte has generated a lot of interest for this group of patients.[179-181] Moreover, Perrin and colleagues[175] have reported significantly higher sperm fragmentation index with increased aneuploidy rates in globozoospermia men compared to fertile men. As discussed earlier, AOA will aid fertilization when globozoospermia is the only sperm available for ICSI.

Absolute asthenozoospermia (AA) is a condition in which no motile sperms are reported and has a frequency of 1 in 5,000, in the infertile male population. Due to the inability to identify immotile viable spermatozoa, fertility prognosis remains very poor. Genetic syndromes such as Kartagener syndrome,[182] Klinefelter syndrome,[183] and primary ciliary dyskinesia[184] are typical AA cases, as is necrozoospermia.[185]

In AA, the only option of selecting a viable sperm for ICSI is to use chemical substances added to the semen sample before the procedure. Moreover, when 100% necrozoospermia is observed, the patients would benefit from TESE,[186] as it is likely that TESE may show some motile sperms.

Treatment with Chemical Substances

Pentoxifylline

Until recently, pentoxifylline, a methylxanthine derivative has been used to increase the sperm motility in a prepared sample. It causes a nonselective inhibition of phosphodiesterase (PDE), acting via the cyclic AMP pathway and leads to sperm tail protein phosphorylation stimulating the motility.[187] Concentrations between 1.5 and 3.6 mM and incubation times between 10 and 20 minutes have resulted in good fertilization rates, embryo development, and clinical pregnancies.[188-190] Due to the potential embryo toxicity observed in animal embryo development and in the absence of safety evidence in the children born using pentoxifylline treated sperm, Human Fertilisation and Embryology Authority (HFEA), in the United Kingdom have recommended that pentoxifylline should not be used clinically.[191,192]

Theophylline

Theophylline, a weak nonselective inhibitor of PDE isoenzymes appears to be a superior agent to pentoxifylline because of its increased half-life. Like pentoxifylline, it increases the intracellular concentrations of cAMP and cyclic 3′,5′ guanosine monophosphate. Ebner and colleagues,[193] in a prospective study, using ready-to-use theophylline commercial solution instead of pentoxifylline reported taking less time to identify a motile sperm for ICSI. Fertilization and blastulation rates were higher when compared with nontreated sperm. Moreover, in the treated group, higher implantation and clinical pregnancies were also documented. In a separate case report, theophylline was found to be an efficient stimulating agent for retrograde sample and total AA.[194] However, like pentoxifylline, theophylline has been reported to have the teratogenic effect in the rodents, and extensive reproductive studies have been recommended.[195]

How to Identify a Viable Sperm?

Different techniques are currently used in ART laboratories to identify immotile viable sperm. All of them utilize the inherent physiological properties of the sperm tail. There are three popular techniques, namely sperm tail flexible test (STFT), hypo-osmotic swelling test (HOS), and laser contact test.

Sperm Tail Flexible Test

Soares and collegues[196] have demonstrated that immotile viable sperms have a flexible tail which bends and recovers to its original position when touched with ICSI injecting needle. This sperm is considered to be viable and can be used for ICSI. Other groups have defined "viability" when both the head and tail move when touched. Identification of viable sperm remains subjective and is highly dependent on the expertise of ICSI technician and has steep learning curve. Although one retrospective study,[197] using motile versus nonmotile STFT selected sperm has reported significant differences in fertilization, pregnancy, and take home baby rates, concerns have been raised that when cryopreserved and thawed sperm are subjected to STFT, sperm tails spontaneous curl but fail to return to their original position.[198] The technique remains to be validated as no prospective randomized studies exist which compares other ICSI technique with STFT.

Hypo-osmotic Swelling Test

When nonmotile sperms are exposed to the hypo-osmotic solution, 75 mM fructose and 25 mM sodium citrate dehydrate, seven different sperm tail swelling patterns (a-g)[199-202] are observed mainly due to the influx of water into the cells. This test is commonly known as "hypo-osmotic sperm swelling test". In this test, the pattern "a" is considered nonviable and nonfunctional as there is no swelling observed indicative of the sperm being nonviable.[201,202] However, in the remaining patterns, swelling of the tail is observed confirming a viable sperm as per the WHO criteria[200] and can be used for ICSI.

Although a popular test, steric problems due to hypo-osmotic exposure have resulted in both false-positive and false-negative observations.[203,204] Moreover, when this technique was used to identify viable sperms from testicular biopsies,[204,205] cells spontaneously develop tail swelling[206] making it difficult to identify a viable sperm.

Furthermore, reports on the effectiveness of this technique have demonstrated a mixed bag of results, some positive, others showing no difference.[199,203-205,207-210] However, in Kartagener and immotile cilia syndrome and also in TESE samples, HOS test has been successful.[211-213]

Non-contact Laser

Finally, the use of noncontact 1.48 mm diode laser shot to the tip of the flagellum to identify viable sperms has resulted in similar results to those as HOS test. In this technique, if the laser shot causes coiling of the tail at the site of impact, the sperm is considered to be viable.[214,215]

Influence of DNA-fragmented Sperm

Muratori and colleagues[216] have suggested that the process of apoptosis triggered by testicular conditions and oxidative stress leads to sperm DNA damage, as it transits in the male genital tract. Other causes of DNA fragmentations have extensively been reviewed elsewhere.[217-219]

The influence of sperm DNA fragmentation is more evident in ICSI as sperm is injected directly into the ooplasm avoiding zona binding as observed in IVF. The paternal pronucleus is formed once the condensed nucleus rapidly undergoes decondensation to release the DNA within the ooplasm. Minor or single DNA strand breaks are normally repaired by the processes in the ooplasm. However, the risk of repair decreases with increasing strand breaks leading to severe delay in replication of paternal pronucleus, embryo development, implantation, birth defects in the offspring, and early pregnancy loss by arresting.[220-227]

In an attempt to increase DNA intact spermatozoa, various methods of sperm preparation have been reported.[228-229]

The most popular and currently favored method for selecting sperm during ICSI procedure is hyaluronic acid binding technique. This is based on the fact that, as sperm negotiate their way toward the zona pellucida through cumulus cells surrounding the oocyte, a specific protein PH20 located on the sperm head binds to hyaluronic acid present in the cumulus cells. Percentage of sperm with apoptotic marker proteins was significantly lower in hyaluronan-bound spermatozoa suggestive of the fact that bound sperm had an intact DNA.[226,230-235] This observation has allowed scientists to develop methods which select good quality spermatozoa capable of binding to hyaluronan.[230-234]

Of the two protocols that have been reported in the literature, the first one utilized a drop of diluted hyaluronic acid, spread and allowed to dry at the bottom of the ICSI dish. An amount of 5μL of sperm preparation, prepared by density gradient (40%/80%) followed by swim-up is added to this area. Sperms that bind to the hyaluronic acid are then selected for injection.[236] Availability of ready-to-use dishes "PICSI" has made it easier for the laboratories to accept this protocol.[237]

The second protocol also utilizes ready-to-use hyaluronic acid media, the only difference being a 10 μL of sperm suspension is added to 10 μL of ready-to-use hyaluronic acid solution. The entire volume is then transferred to the bottom of the ICSI dish. The sperm that is bound show a considerably lower progressive motility; this additionally allows the sperm to be picked up for ICSI, without the use of PVP medium.[237]

Our observations (Mehta J. unpublished data) using ready-to-use, "PICSI'" dishes show a significant inverse correlation between DNA fragmentation and hyaluronic acid bound sperm. A significantly higher fertilization and blastocyst formation were observed. However, there was no difference noted with the implantation rates and on-going clinical pregnancies. Our findings compliment those reported by Nasr-Esfahani and collegues[236] (2008b). A recent study[238] has concluded that use of PICSI technique had a considerable higher chance almost fivefold to achieve pregnancy when compared with the no-PICSI selection. In their study, teratozoospermia patients benefited the most.

Moreover, in a prospective study, normal morphology selected sperm using PVP showed a higher DNA fragmentation levels, higher nuclear abnormalities, and poor embryo development when compared with hyaluronan-selected sperm cells.[234]

Several studies have reported the use of Annexin V-magnetic activated cell sorting (MACS) technique to identify sperm with less or no DNA fragmented sperm.[239-247] Annexin V is a major cell membrane component of macrophages that selectively binds with the phospholipid phosphatidylserine (PS). It becomes accessible when it is relocated from the inner to the outer cytosolic leaf when the plasma membrane gets disrupted.[248] On density gradient centrifugation, PS exposed cells bind with the magnetically labeled Annexin V-conjugated microbeads and are retained under the influence of a magnetic field, as they pass through a MACS column, while nonexposed sperm cells pass through and are collected as a pellet.[249,250] Prospective studies comparing density gradient separation with Annexin-V labeled beads, and those without the presence of labeled beads have reported controversial results. [242,251-254]

However, concerns have been raised because of the lack of safety using this technique. There is a possibility that the microbeads may be present on the surface of the sperm used for injection. It is, therefore, essential that before Annexin-V technique is recommended for general clinical use, prospective randomized clinical trials need to be conducted.

Electrostatic Surface Charge

Although Chan and colleagues[254] reported an inexpensive technique utilizing electrostatic surface charge to immobilize the sperm, it was Focarelli and coworkers[256] who demonstrated the existence of a static electric charge of 216–220 mV on the surface of a mature sperm and named the charge a zeta potential. Chan[255] placed a glass centrifuge tube inside a latex glove and generated an electrostatic surface charge by rotating the tube three to four times at room temperature for 1 minute. This allowed the charged sperm to adhere to the tube wall. That sperm with low or no charge did not adhere to the wall and was washed away by centrifugation. The bound sperm was detached from the tube wall using serum supplemented medium which neutralized the charge. They further demonstrated the high level of DNA integrity and low histone content in highly charged sperm. Only one prospective randomize study exists that has reported higher fertilization rates when compared with sperm from density gradient separation only.[257] A comparative study, using this technique and hyaluronic acid binding has reported a higher percentage of spermatozoa with intact DNA.[258]

Extension of the zeta potential concept was applied to electrophoretic separation. As the highest quality spermatozoa within the ejaculate carry the greatest negative charge,[259,260] Ainsworth and colleagues[260] applied an electric field that forced the spermatozoa to pass through a polycarbonated filter containing 5 mm pores. Using sperm separated in this manner, they reported the first human pregnancy and the prospective randomized controlled clinical trial has also reported three normal deliveries when compared with simple density gradient separation.[261]

As no more studies have been reported confirming the safety of this procedure to validate it for general clinical use, for now, it should be considered experimental. Moreover, there are no studies which examine its usefulness for testicular or epididymal biopsies.

Based on author's unpublished data and other studies reported here, hyaluronan-selected sperm appears to be most favored technique. However, in the absence of comprehensive evidence of clinical outcomes such as miscarriage, fetal abnormalities, and safety of these techniques, it is difficult to recommend one specific method of sperm selection when high sperm DNA fragmentation is suspected.

Other Aspects of the Laboratory that Influence the IVF and ICSI Outcome

A well-established robust quality management system (QMS) provides an environment of quality and safety for gametes and embryos and has three arms to it, quality control (QC, quality assurance (QA) and quality improvement or quality audit (QI), which will benefit all the patients attending ART clinic, ART professionals, and the embryologists.

Although all the three arms of QMS are important, QC alone allows you to ensure that correct monitoring of each occurrence in the laboratory is recorded correctly on a regular basis allowing the opportunity to correct any deviation from set expected values. QC follows a set regime of monitoring all essential equipment within the laboratory, culture media and contact materials and the outcome. It also addresses the importance of maintaining correct culture environment inside and outside of the incubator. Through this chapter, it is hoped that the reader will benefit from suggestions made here and improve their ART outcomes.

QUALITY CONTROL

Quality control can be attributed to all the activities carried out to ensure a specific procedure or a piece of equipment operates correctly as stipulated by the standard operating procedure (SOP) or as specified by the manufacturer. This action allows correcting any deviation of the observation from the established standards. In practice, internal quality control (IQC) ensures that a given laboratory procedure will have the same result or outcome all the time it is carried out).[25] Briefly, the QC parameters that influence the outcome and require to be monitored include:

1. Appropriately educated and trained laboratory personnel[24,262]
2. Correct use of calibrated laboratory instruments: It is essential that all laboratory equipment are annually calibrated, validated against a standard norm and maintained in optimum working conditions as per the manufacturer's recommendation. Instruments used for calibration also require being calibrated against a known standard and a validation certificate to be available for audit purposes. Any laboratories registered for ISO certification like ISO9001(2012), soon to be updated to ISO9001(2015), will require all standards to be "UKAS" or similar agency certified and the importance on uncertainties and risk assessment has been stressed in the 2015 standards.
3. Use of only embryo toxicity tested chemicals, reagents, and culture media, all of which should be CE marked as medical devices Class II or III: as most of the laboratories now use commercially prepared media, laboratory personnel have to ensure that the manufacture provides a validation certificate of the steps taken in producing the media including results of mouse embryo toxicity and limulus amebocyte lysate (LAL) tests. When medium contains protein, the source of protein and certification indicating that no infection was detected, should also be available.[16,22]
4. To ensure that proper execution of appropriate techniques and methods as written in each of the SOPs for all of the laboratory occurrences are performed in achieving a safe, viable pregnancy: In addition to the IVF and ICSI procedures, this would include vitrification, thawing, extended cultures, co-cultures, preimplantation genetic diagnosis (PGD) and screening (PGS).
5. Acceptance of media delivery in a cold chain condition and the testing of the culture media: Transportation and storage temperatures of all media used should always be 4–8°C and at no time should the cold chain be broken during its transport from the manufacturer to the end user. Osmolality and pH of the media should be checked on receipt. Embryologists/technicians should familiarize themselves with the product information and follow the recommended storage conditions.
6. All the procedure and policy manuals including forms used for record keeping have to be "date and version" controlled: Date and version control documents allow the laboratory to edit any documents in use ensuring that only the most recent corrected documents are used. The documents have to be reviewed annually and the old copies destroyed to avoid confusion. The date when the use of new documents was implemented should also be recorded. This will serve as an audit trail for all the incidents which require changes.
7. Documentation and record keeping: All occurrences and steps involved in the outcomes of the steps should be recorded meticulously as this acts as a record of delivery of patient care. The records should also demonstrate traceability, batch numbers, and expiry dates of all the disposable consumables, equipment, media used for the culture, and the witnessing steps in any given procedure. The details in the documents should allow an audit of the entire pathway followed for the delivery of any IVF treatment, and this should be risk assessed. In the United Kingdom, HFEA requires each event of gamete manipulation to be witnessed by an independent witness.[27]
8. Air quality in the laboratory and the incubators also influence the outcome: This should be monitored on a weekly basis to ensure that the air in the laboratory is Grade D. Minimum of Grade C should be available in those areas where the gametes are manipulated. The bench top incubators are normally connected to set value Trigas mixture cylinders (5% O_2, 6% CO_2 balanced by nitrogen). This mixture should be certified as medical gas and a validation certification to be obtained from the supplier of the gases.[17-21,30]

Quality assurance and QI utilize the data collected from QC parameters to carry out the monthly and annual audits of the essential parameters. This further allows corrective actions to be implemented when deviations in the observations have been reported. Following this exercise, patients can be reassured that their gametes are manipulated by trained embryologist in a safe and controlled environment.

CONCLUSION

Laboratory and clinical aspects of IVF and ICSI have evolved over the last 4 decades. Basic research and laboratory practices continue to add to our understanding of molecular processes at the cellular level. Although protocols of every step involved in the ART have been established, it is time to revisit them to consider how safely they can be changed to adapt the new molecular-based knowledge.[5]

The appreciation of the outcome of any given technique discussed here allows the embryologist to be extra vigilant when performing the procedure and to trouble shoot. Although there is no one single way of performing a procedure, the outcome will certainly depend on the expertise of the operator, and therefore, the chapter deals with various aspects of how to trouble shoot a poor outcome in IVF and ICSI, and it is hoped that the reader will benefit from the suggested tips.

In any ART laboratory, several factors influence the outcome. However, the existence of a well-established QMS will most certainly help with auditing the results. Moreover, laboratory environment such as the air quality and humidity influence the outcome. Controlling these parameters is an essential aspect of the overall laboratory conditions. Use of correct gas mixture for culture conditions within an incubator and the sensitivity of the temperature prone oocyte should not be ignored.

Finally, it rests upon the embryologist to ensure the safety of the oocytes and the sperm entrusted to them by patients. They should be responsible for the ethical and regulatory aspects when creating embryos using IVF and ICSI techniques.[263] As sperm selection using ultra-high magnification (IMSI) has extensively been reviewed elsewhere, the topic has not been discussed.[266,267] Furthermore, each and every embryologist should ensure that they are competent in their knowledge of cellular physiology and molecular events, understanding that an oocyte and sperm are single cells that need to be manipulated safely.

REFERENCES

1. Edwards RG, Steptoe PC, Purdy JM. Establishing full-term human pregnancies using cleaving embryos grown *in vitro*. Br J Obstet Gynecol. 1980;87:737-56.
2. Mahadevan MM, Trounson A, Leeton JF. The relationship of tubal blockage, infertility of unknown cause, suspect male infertility, and endometriosis to success of *in vitro* fertilization and embryo transfer. Fertil Steril. 1983;40:755-62.
3. Palermo G, Joris H, Devroey P, Van Steirteghem AC. Pregnancies after intracytoplasmic injection of single spermatozoon into an oocyte. Lancet. 1992;340:17-8.
4. Nyboe Andersen A, Carlsen E, Loft A. Trends in the use of intracytoplasmaic sperm injection marked variability between countries. Hum Reprod Update. 2008;14:593-604.
5. Harper J, Cristina Magli M, Lundin K, Barratt CLR, Brison D. When and how should new technology be introduced into the IVF laboratory? Hum Reprod. 2012;27:303-13.
6. Babayev SN, Park CW, Bukulmez O. Intracytoplasmic sperm injection indications: how rigorous? Semin Reprod Med. 2014;32:283-90.
7. Sanchez-Calabuig MJ, Lopez-Cardona AP, Fernandez-Gonzalez R, Ramos-Ibeas P, Fonseca Balvis N, Laguna-Barraza R, et al. Potential health risks associated to ICSI: insights from animal models and strategies for a safe procedure. Front Public Health. 2014;2:241.
8. Dumoulin J, Land J, Van Montfoort A, Nelissen E, Coonen E, Derhaag J, et al. Effect of *in vitro* culture of human embryos on birthweight of newborns. Hum Reprod. 2010;25:605-12.
9. Nelissen E, Van Montfoort A, Coonen E, Derhaag J, Geraedts J, Smits L, et al. Further evidence that culture media affect perinatal outcome: findings after transfer of fresh and cryopreserved embryos. Hum Reprod. 2012;27:1966-76.
10. Nelissen ECM, Van Montfoort APA, Smits LJM, Menheere PPCA, Evers JLH, Coonen E, et al. IVF culture medium affects human intrauterine growth as early as the second trimester of pregnancy. Hum Reprod. 2013;28:2067-74.
11. El Hajj N, Haaf T. Epigenetic disturbances in *in vitro* cultured gametes and embryos: implications for human assisted reproduction. Fertil Steril. 2013;99:632-41.
12. Mantikou E, Youssef MAFM, van Wely M, van der Veen F, Al-Inany HG, Repping S, et al. Embryo culture media and IVF/ICSI success rates: a systematic review. Hum Reprod Update. 2013;19:210-20.
13. Karamalegos C, Bolton VN. A prospective comparison of 'in house' and commercially prepared Earle's balanced salt solution in human in-vitro fertilization. Hum Reprod 1999;14:1842-6.
14. Quinn P. The development and impact of culture media for assisted reproductive technologies. Fertil Steril. 2004;81:27-9.
15. Biggers JD. Ethical issues and the commercialization of embryo culture media. Reprod Biomed Online. 2000;1:74-6.
16. Wale PL, Gardner D. The effects of chemical and physical factors on mammalian embryo culture and their importance for practice of assisted human reproduction. Hum Reprod Update. 2016:22:2-22.
17. Hall J, Gilligan A, Schimmel T, Cecchi M, Cohen J. The origin, effects and control of air pollution in laboratories used for human embryo culture. Human Reprod. 1998;13(Suppl 4):146-55.

18. Cohen J, Gilligan A, Esposito W, Schimmel T, Dale B. Ambient air and its potential effects on conception *in vitro*. Hum Reprod. 1997;12(8):1742-9.
19. Brown RH. Monitoring VOCs in air—the development of ISO standards and a critical appraisal of the methods. J Environ Monit. 2002;4(6):112N-8N.
20. Boone WR, Johnson JE, Locke AJ, Crane MM 4th, Price TM. Control of air quality in an ART lab. Fertil Steril. 1999;71(1):150-4.
21. Cutting R, Pritchard J, Clarke H, Martin K. Establishing quality control in the new IVF laboratory. Hum Fertil. 2004;7(2):119-25.
22. Cohen J, Gilligan A, Willadsen S. Culture and quality control of embryos. Hum Reprod. 1998;13(Suppl 3):137-44.
23. Magli MC, Van den Abbeel E, Lundin K, Royere D, Van der Elst J, Gianaroli L. Revised guidelines for good practice in IVF laboratories. Hum. Reprod. 2008;23:1253-62.
24. Mayer JF, Jones EL, Dowling-Lacey D, Nehchiri F, Muasher SJ, Gibbons WE, et al. Total quality improvement in the IVF laboratory: choosing indicators of quality. Reprod Biomed Online. 2003;7(6):695-9.
25. Mehta J. Media and quality control in IVF laboratory. In: Jain K, Talwar P (Eds). IVF Techniques for the Beginners. ISBN 9789380903599. New Delhi: Jaypee Publishers; 2013. p. 36.
26. Alper MM, Fauser BC. Ovarian stimulation protoocls for IVF is more better than less? Reprod Biomed Online. 2017;34:345-53.
27. HFEA Code of Practice. [online] Available from www.hfea.gov.uk/docs/Code_of_Practice_8. [Accessed October, 2013].
28. Mehta J. Culture media constituents. In: Mehta J, Woodward B. Male Infertility, Sperm Diagnosis, Management and Delivery. New Delhi: JP Medical Ltd. pp. 25-35.
29. Mehta J. Intrauterine insemination with special reference to density gradient centrifugation. J Reprod Ste Cell Biotechnol. 2012;3(1):9-21.
30. Mehta J, Varghese A. Gases for embryo culture and volatile organic compounds in the incubator. In: Esteves SG, Varghese AC, Worrilow KC (Eds). Clean Room Technology in ART Clinics—A Practical Guide. CRC Press; 2016.
31. Cha KY, Chian RC. Maturation *in vitro* of immature human oocytes for clinical use. Hum Reprod Update. 1998;4:103-20.
32. De Vos A, Van de Velde H, Joris H, Van Steirteghem A. In-vitro matured metaphase-I oocytes have a lower fertilization rate but similar embryo quality as mature metaphase-II oocytes after intracytoplasmic sperm injection. Hum Reprod. 1999;14:1859-63.
33. Nogueira D, Romero S, Vanhoutte L, deMatos DG, Smitz J. In: Gardner DK, Weissman A, Howles C, Shoham Z (Eds). Textbook of Assisted Reproductive Techniques: Laboratory and Clinical Perspectives, 2nd edition. London: Taylor and Francis; 2004.
34. Mahadevan MM, Trounson AO. Removal of the cumulus oophorus from the human oocyte for *in vitro* fertilization. Fertil Steril. 1985;43:263-7.
35. De Vos A, Van Landuyt L, Van Ranst H, Vandermonde A, D'Haese V, Sterckx J, et al. Randomised sibling-oocyte study using recombinant human hyaluronidase versus bovine derived sigma hyaluronidase in ICSI patients. Hum Reprod. 2008;23:1815-9.
36. De Moura BRL, Gurgel MCA, Machado SPP, Marques PA, Rolim JR, De Lima MC, et al. Low concentration of hyaluronidase for oocyte denudation can improve fertilization rates and embryo quality. JBRA Assist Reprod. 2017;21(1):27-30.
37. Meerschaut FV, Nikiforaki D, Heindryckx B, De Sutter P. Assisted oocyte activation following ICSI fertilisation failure. Reprod Biomed Online. 2014;28:560-71.
38. Trounson AO, Mohr LR, Wood C, Leeton JF. Effect of delayed insemination on in-vitro fertilization, culture and transfer of human embryos. J Reprod Fertil. 1982;64:285-94.
39. Harrison KL, Wilson LM, Breen TM, Pope AK, Cummins JM, Hennessey JF. Fertilization of human oocytes in relation to varying delay before insemination. Fertil Steril. 1988;50:294-7.
40. Veeck LL. Oocyte assessment and biological performance. Ann N Y Acad Sci. 1988;541:259-74.
41. Khan I, Staessen C, Van den Abbeel E, Camus M, Wisanto A, Smitz J, et al. Time of insemination and its effect on in-vitro fertilization, cleavage and pregnancy rates in GnRH agonist/HMG-stimulated cycles. Hum Reprod. 1989;4:921-6.
42. Sundstrom P, Nilsson BO. Meiotic and cytoplasmic maturation of oocytes collected in stimulated cycles is asynchronous. Hum Reprod. 1988;3:613-9.
43. Eppig JJ, Schultz RM, O'Brien M, Chesnel F. Relationship between the developmental programs controlling nuclear and cytoplasmic maturation of mouse oocytes. Dev Biol. 1994;164:1-9.
44. Balakier H, Sojecki A, Motamedi G, Librach C. Time-dependent capability of human oocytes for activation and pronuclear formation during metaphase II arrest. Hum Reprod. 2004;19:982-7.
45. Miao YL, Kikuchi K, Sun QY, Schatten H. Oocyte aging: cellular and molecular changes, developmental potential and reversal possibility. Hum Reprod Update. 2009;15:573-85.
46. Zhu J, Zhang J, Li H, Wang TY, Zhang CX, Luo MJ, et al. Cumulus oocyte aging by releasing soluble Fas ligand in mice. Sci Rep. 2015;5:8683.
47. Rienzi L, Ubaldi F, Anniballo R, Cerulo G, Greco E. Preincubation of human oocytes may improve fertilization and embryo quality after intracytoplasmic sperm injection. Hum Reprod. 1998;13:1014-9.
48. Yanagida K, Yazawa H, Katayose H, Suzuki K, Hoshi K, Sato A. Influence of oocyte preincubation time on fertilization after intracytoplasmic sperm injection. Hum Reprod. 1998;13:2223-6.
49. Hassan HA. Cumulus cell contribution to cytoplasmic maturation and oocyte developmental competence *in vitro*. J Assist Reprod Genet. 2001;18:539-43.
50. Ho JY, Chen MJ, Yi YC, Guu HF, Ho ES. The effect of preincubation period of oocytes on nuclear maturity, fertilization rate, embryo quality, and pregnancy outcome in IVF and ICSI. J Assist Reprod Genet. 2003;20:358-64.
51. Aletebi F. Denudation and sperm injection interval timing: impact on outcome of intracytoplasmic sperm injection. Int J Womens Health. 2011;3:99-103.

52. Andrews MM, Fishel SB, Rowe PH, Berry JA, Lisi F, Rinaldi L. Analysis of intracytoplasmic sperm injection procedures related to delayed insemination and ejaculated, epididymal and testicular spermatozoa. Reprod Biomed Online. 2001;2:89-97.
53. Falcone P, Gambera L, Pisoni M, Lofiego V, De Leo V, Mencaglia L, et al. Correlation between oocyte preincubation time and pregnancy rate after intracytoplasmic sperm injection. Gynecol Endocrinol. 2008;24:295-9.
54. Dozortsev D, Nagy P, Abdelmassih S, Oliveira F, Brasil A, Abdelmassih V, et al. The optimal time for intracytoplasmic sperm injection in the human is from 37 to 41 hours after administration of human chorionic gonadotropin. Fertil Steril. 2004;82:1492-6.
55. Garor R, Shufaro Y, Kotler N, Shefer D, Krasilnikov N, Ben-Haroush A, et al. Prolonging oocyte *in vitro* culture and handling time does not compensate for a shorter interval from human chorionic gonadotropin administration to oocyte pickup. Fertil Steril. 2015;103:72-5.
56. Coticchio G, Brambillasca F. The choreography of fertilization. In: Coticchio G, Albertini DF, De Santis L (Eds). Oogenesis. London, UK: Springer-Verlag; 2013. pp. 289-306.
57. Coticchio G, Dal-Canto M, Guglielmo MC, Mignini-Renzini M, Fadini R. Human oocyte maturation *in vitro*. Int J Dev Biol. 2012;56:909-18.
58. Coticchio G, Dal Canto M, Mignini Renzini M, Guglielmo MC, Brambillasca F, Turchi D, et al. Oocyte maturation: gamete-somatic cells interactions, meiotic resumption, cytoskeletal dynamics and cytoplasmic reorganization. Hum Reprod Update. 2015;21:427-54.
59. Jones KT, Lane SIR, Holt JE. Start and stop signals of oocyte meiotic maturation. In: Coticchio G, Albertini DF, De Santis L (Eds). Oogenesis. London, UK: Springer-Verlag; 2013. pp. 183-93.
60. Mehta JG. *In vitro* maturation. Fertil Sci Res. 2014;1:7-15.
61. Huang FJ, Chang SY, Tsai MY, Lin YC, Kung FT, Wu JF, et al. Relationship of the human cumulus-free oocyte maturational profile with *in vitro* outcome parameters after intracytoplasmic sperm injection. J Assist Reprod Genet. 1999;16:483-7.
62. Vanhoutte L, De Sutter P, Van der Elst J, Dhont M. Clinical benefit of metaphase I oocytes. Reprod Biol Endocrinol. 2005;3:71.
63. Shu Y, Gebhardt J, Watt J, Lyon J, Dasig D, Behr B. Fertilization, embryo development, and clinical outcome of immature oocytes from stimulated intracytoplasmic sperm injection cycles. Fertil Steril. 2007;87:1022-7.
64. Strassburger D, Friedler S, Raziel A, Kasterstein E, Schachter M, Ron-El R. The outcome of ICSI of immature MI oocytes and rescued *in vitro* matured MII oocytes. Hum Reprod. 2004;19:1587-90.
65. Strassburger D, Goldstein A, Friedler S, Raziel A, Kasterstein E, Mashevich M, et al. The cytogenetic constitution of embryos derived from immature (metaphase I) oocytes obtained after ovarian hyperstimulation. Fertil Steril. 2010;94:971-8.
66. Li M, Li Y, Ma SY, Feng HL, Yang HJ, Wu KL, et al. Evaluation of the developmental potential of metaphase I oocytes from stimulated intracytoplasmic sperm injection cycles. Reprod Fertil Dev. 2011;23:433-7.
67. De Vincentiis S, De Martino E, Buffone MG, Brugo-Olmedo S. Use of metaphase I oocytes matured *in vitro* is associated with embryo multinucleation. Fertil Steril. 2013;99:414-21.
68. Shin SB, Cho JW, Lee SH, Yang KM, Lim CK, Lee HS. Fertilization and pregnancy potential of immature oocytes from stimulated intracytoplasmic sperm injection cycles. Clin Exp Reprod Med. 2013;40:7-11.
69. Van Steirteghem AC, Nagy Z, Joris H, Liu J, Staessen C, Smitz J, et al. High fertilization and implantation rates after intracytoplasmic sperm injection. Hum Reprod. 1993;8:1061-6.
70. Nagy ZP, Liu J, Joris H, Bocken G, Desmet B, Van Ranst H, et al. The influence of the site of sperm deposition and mode of oolemma breakage at intracytoplasmic sperm injection on fertilization and embryo development rates. Hum Reprod. 1995;10:3171-7.
71. Ebner T, Yaman C, Moser M, Sommergruber M, Jesacher K, Tews G. A prospective study on oocyte survival rate after ICSI: influence of injection technique and morphological features. J Assist Reprod Genet. 2001;18:623-8.
72. Yavas Y, Roberge S, Khamsi F, Shirazi P, Endman MW, Wong JC. Performing ICSI using an injection pipette with the smallest possible inner diameter and a long taper increases normal fertilization rate, decreases incidence of degeneration and tripronuclear zygotes, and enhances embryo development. J Assist Reprod Genet. 2001;18:426-35.
73. Rosen MP, Shen S, Dobson AT, Fujimoto VY, McCulloch CE, Cedars MI. Oocyte degeneration after intracytoplasmic sperm injection: a multivariate analysis to assess its importance as a laboratory or clinical marker. Fertil Steril. 2006;85:1736-43.
74. Palermo GD, Alikani M, Bertoli M, Colombero LT, Moy F, Cohen J, et al. Oolemma characteristics in relation to survival and fertilization patterns of oocytes treated by intracytoplasmic sperm injection. Hum Reprod. 1996;11:172-6.
75. Ebner T, Moser M, Sommergruber M, Shebl O, Tews G. Incomplete denudation of oocytes prior to ICSI enhances embryo quality and blastocyst development. Hum Reprod. 2006;21:2972-7.
76. Rienzi L, Greco E, Ubaldi F, Iacobelli M, Martinez F, Tesarik J. Laser-assisted intracytoplasmic sperm injection. Fertil Steril. 2001;76:1045-7.
77. Rienzi L, Ubaldi F, Martinez F, Iacobelli M, Minasi MG, Ferrero S, et al. Relationship between meiotic spindle location with regard to the polar body position and oocyte developmental potential after ICSI. Hum Reprod. 2003;18:1289-93.
78. Rienzi L, Ubaldi F, Martinez F, Minasi MG, Iacobelli M, Ferrero S, et al. Clinical application of laser-assisted ICSI: a pilot study. Eur J Obstet Gynecol Reprod Biol. 2004;115(Suppl. 1):S77-9.
79. Nagy ZP, Oliveira SA, Abdelmassih V, Abdelmassih R. Novel use of laser to assist ICSI for patients with fragile oocytes: a case report. Reprod Biomed Online. 2002;4:27-31.

80. Demirol A, Benkhalifa M, SariT, Gurgan T. Use of laser-assisted intracytoplasmic sperm injection (ICSI) in patients with a history of poor ICSI outcome and limited metaphase II oocytes. Fertil Steril. 2006;86:256-8.
81. Mantoudis E, Podsiadly BT, Gorgy A, Venkat G, Craft IL. A comparison between quarter, partial and total laser assisted hatching in selected infertility patients. Hum Reprod. 2001;16:2182-6.
82. Choi KH, Lee JH, Yang YH, Yoon TK, Lee DR, Lee WS. Efficiency of laser-assisted intracytoplasmic sperm injection in a human assisted reproductive techniques program. Clin Exp Reprod Med. 2011;38:148-52.
83. Gitlin SA, Gibbons WE, Gosden RG. Oocyte biology and genetics revelations from polar bodies. Reprod Biomed Online. 2003;6:403-9.
84. Brunet S, Verlhac MH. Positioning to get out of meiosis: the asymmetry of division. Hum Reprod Update. 2011;17: 68-75.
85. Chaigne A, Verlhac MH, Terret ME. Spindle positioning in mammalian oocytes. Exp Cell Res. 2012;318:1442-7.
86. Li R. The art of choreographing asymmetric cell division. Dev Cell. 2013;25:439-50.
87. Maro B, Johnson MH, Webb M, Flach G. Mechanism of polar body formation in the mouse oocyte: an interaction between the chromosomes, the cytoskeleton and the plasma membrane. J Embryol Exp Morphol. 1986;92:11-32.
88. Deng M, Suraneni P, Schultz RM, Li R. The Ran GTPase mediates chromatin signaling to control cortical polarity during polar body extrusion in mouse oocytes. Dev Cell. 2007;12:301-8.
89. Azoury J, Verlhac MH, Dumont J. Actin filaments: key players in the control of asymmetric divisions in mouse oocytes. Biol Cell. 2009;101:69-76.
90. Larson SM, Lee HJ, Hung PH, Matthews LM, Robinson DN, Evans JP. Cortical mechanics and meiosis II completion in mammalian oocytes are mediated by myosin-II and Ezrin-Radixin-Moesin (ERM) proteins. Mol Biol Cell. 2010;21:3182-92.
91. Maddox AS, Azoury J, Dumont J. Polar body cytokinesis. Cytoskeleton (Hoboken). 2012;69:855-68.
92. Yi K, Li R. Actin cytoskeleton in cell polarity and asymmetric division during mouse oocyte maturation. Cytoskeleton (Hoboken). 2012;69:727-37.
93. Van Der Westerlaken LA, Helmerhorst FM, Hermans J, Naaktgeboren N. Intracytoplasmic sperm injection: position of the polar body affects pregnancy rate. Hum Reprod. 1999;14:2565-9.
94. Stoddart NR, Fleming SD. Orientation of the first polar body of the oocyte at 6 or 12 o'clock during ICSI does not affect clinical outcome. Hum Reprod. 2000;15:1580-5.
95. Blake M, Garrisi J, Tomkin G, Cohen J. Sperm deposition site during ICSI affects fertilization and development. Fertil Steril. 2000;73:31-7.
96. Dumoulin JM, Coonen E, Bras M, Bergers-Janssen JM, Ignoul-Vanvuchelen RC, van Wissen LC, et al. Embryo development and chromosomal anomalies after ICSI: effect of the injection procedure. Hum Reprod. 2001;16:306-12.
97. Hardarson T, Lundin K, Hamberger L. The position of the metaphase II spindle cannot be predicted by the location of the first polar body in the human oocyte. Hum Reprod. 2000;15:1372-6.
98. Eichenlaub-Ritter U, Chandley AC, Gosden RG. Alterations to the microtubular cytoskeleton and increased disorder of chromosome alignment in spontaneously ovulated mouse oocytes aged *in vivo*: an immunofluorescence study. Chromosoma. 1986;94:337-45.
99. Taylor TH, Chang CC, Elliott T, Colturato LF, Kort HI, Nagy ZP. Effect of denuding on polar body position in in-vitro matured oocytes. Reprod Biomed Online. 2008;17:515-9.
100. Cooke S, Tyler JP, Driscoll GL. Meiotic spindle location and identification and its effect on embryonic cleavage plane and early development. Hum Reprod. 2003;18:2397-405.
101. Sousa M, Tesarik J. Ultrastructural analysis of fertilization failure after intracytoplasmic sperm injection. Hum Reprod. 1994;9:2374-80.
102. Liu J, Nagy Z, Joris H, Tournaye H, Smitz J, Camus M, et al. Analysis of 76 total fertilization failure cycles out of 2732 intracytoplasmic sperm injection cycles. Hum Reprod. 1995;10:2630-6.
103. Ludwig M, Strik D, Al-Hasani S, Diedrich K. No transfer in a planned ICSI cycle: we cannot overcome some basic rules of human reproduction. Eur J Obstet Gynecol Reprod Biol. 1999;87:3-11.
104. Esfandiari N, Javed MH, Gotlieb L, Casper RF. Complete failed fertilization after intracytoplasmic sperm injection—analysis of 10 years' data. Int J Fertil Womens Med. 2005;50: 187-92.
105. Montag M, Koster M, van der Ven K, Bohlen U, van der Ven H. The benefit of artificial oocyte activation is dependent on the fertilization rate in a previous treatment cycle. Reprod Biomed Online. 2012;24:521-6.
106. Mahutte NG, Arici A. Failed fertilization: is it predictable? Curr Opin Obstet Gynecol. 2003;15:211-8.
107. Flaherty SP, Payne D, Swann NJ, Mattews CD. Aetiology of failed and abnormal fertilization after intracytoplasmic sperm injection. Hum Reprod. 1995;10:2623-9.
108. Flaherty SP, Payne D, Matthews CD. Fertilization failures and abnormal fertilization after intracytoplasmic sperm injection. Hum Reprod. 1998;13(Suppl 1):155-64.
109. Rawe VY, Olmedo SB, Nodar FN, Doncel GD, Acosta AA, Vitullo AD. Cytoskeletal organization defects and abortive activation in human oocytes after IVF and ICSI failure. Mol Hum Reprod. 2000;6:510-6.
110. Yamano S, Nakagawa K, Nakasaka H, Aono T. Fertilization failure and oocyte activation. J Med Invest. 2000;47:1-8.
111. Yanagida K. Complete fertilization failure in ICSI. Hum Cell. 2004;17:187-93.
112. Swain JE, Pool TB. ART failure: oocyte contributions to unsuccessful fertilization. Hum Reprod Update. 2008;14:431-46.
113. Horner VL, Wolfner MF. Transitioning from egg to embryo: triggers and mechanisms of egg activation. Dev Dyn. 2008;237:527-44.
114. Miyazaki S, Ito M. Calcium signals for egg activation in mammals. J Pharmacol Sci. 2006;100:545-52.

115. Ramadan WM, Kashir J, Jones C, Coward K. Oocyte activation and phospholipase C zeta (PLCzeta): diagnostic and therapeutic implications for assisted reproductive technology. Cell Commun Signal. 2012;10:12.
116. Amdani SN, Jones C, Coward K. Phospholipase C zeta (PLCzeta): oocyte activation and clinical links to male factor infertility. Adv Biol Regul. 2013;53:292-308.
117. Neri QV, Lee B, Rosenwaks Z, Machaca K, Palermo GD. Understanding fertilization through intracytoplasmic sperm injection (ICSI). Cell Calcium. 2014;55:24-37.
118. Kashir J, Heindryckx B, Jones C, DeSutter P, Parrington J, Coward K. Oocyte activation, phospholipase C zeta and human infertility. Hum Reprod Update. 2010;16: 690-703.
119. Heindryckx B, De Gheselle S, Gerris J, Dhont M, De Sutter P. Efficiency of assisted oocyte activation as a solution for failed intracytoplasmic sperm injection. Reprod Biomed Online. 2008;17:662-8.
120. Rybouchkin A, Dozortsev D, Pelinck MJ, De Sutter P, Dhont M. Analysis of the oocyte activating capacity and chromosomal complement of round-headed human spermatozoa by their injection into mouse oocytes. Hum Reprod. 1996;11:2170-5.
121. Heindryckx B, Van der Elst J, De Sutter P, Dhont M. Treatment option for sperm- or oocyte-related fertilization failure: assisted oocyte activation following diagnostic heterologous ICSI. Hum Reprod. 2005;20:2237-41.
122. Tesarik J, Rienzi L, Ubaldi F, Mendoza C, Greco E. Use of a modified intracytoplasmic sperm injection technique to overcome sperm-borne and oocyte-borne oocyte activation failures. Fertil Steril. 2002;78:619-24.
123. Ebner T, Moser M, Sommergruber M, Jesacher K, Tews G. Complete oocyte activation failure after ICSI can be overcome by a modified injection technique. Hum Reprod. 2004;19:1837-41.
124. Yanagida K, Katayose H, Yazawa H, Kimura Y, Sato A, Yanagimachi H, et al. Successful fertilization and pregnancy following ICSI and electrical oocyte activation. Hum Reprod. 1999;14:1307-11.
125. Zhang J, Wang CW, Blaszcyzk A, Grifo JA, Ozil J, Haberman E, et al. Electrical activation and *in vitro* development of human oocytes that fail to fertilize after intracytoplasmic sperm injection. Fertil Steril. 1999;72:509-12.
126. Egashira A, Murakami M, Haigo K, Horiuchi T, Kuramoto T. A successful pregnancy and live birth after intracytoplasmic sperm injection with globozoospermic sperm and electrical oocyte activation. Fertil Steril. 2009;92:2037.e5-9.
127. Mansour R, Fahmy I, Tawab NA, Kamal A, El-Demery Y, Aboulghar M, et al. Electrical activation of oocytes after intracytoplasmic sperm injection: a controlled randomized study. Fertil Steril. 2009;91:133-9.
128. Baltaci V, Ayvaz OU, Unsal E, Aktas Y, Baltaci A, Turhan F, et al. The effectiveness of intracytoplasmic sperm injection combined with piezoelectric stimulation in infertile couples with total fertilization failure. Fertil Steril. 2010;94:900-4.
129. Yanagida K, Morozumi K, Katayose H, Hayashi S, Sato A. Successful pregnancy after ICSI with strontium oocyte activation in low rates of fertilization. Reprod Biomed Online. 2006;13:801-6.
130. Kyono K, Kumagai S, Nishinaka C, Nakajo Y, Uto H, Toya M, et al. Birth and follow-up of babies born following ICSI using SrCl2 oocyte activation. Reprod Biomed Online. 2008;17:53-8.
131. Tejera A, Molla M, Muriel L, Remohi J, Pellicer A, De Pablo JL. Successful pregnancy and childbirth after intracytoplasmic sperm injection with calcium ionophore oocyte activation in a globozoospermic patient. Fertil Steril. 2008;90:1202.e1-e5.
132. Lundin K, Sjogren A, Nilsson L, Hamberger L. Fertilization and pregnancy after intracytoplasmic microinjection of acrosome less spermatozoa. Fertil Steril. 1994;62:1266-7.
133. Kilani ZM, Shaban MA, Ghunaim SD, Keilani SS, Dakkak AI. Triplet pregnancy and delivery after intracytoplasmic injection of round-headed spermatozoa. Hum Reprod. 1998;13:2177-9.
134. Stone S, O'Mahony F, Khalaf Y, Taylor A, Braude P. A normal live birth after intracytoplasmic sperm injection for globozoospermia without assisted oocyte activation: case report. Hum Reprod. 2000;15:139-41.
135. Nardo LG, Sinatra F, Bartoloni G, Zafarana S, Nardo F. Ultrastructural features and ICSI treatment of severe teratozoospermia: report of two human cases of globozoospermia. Eur J Obstet Gynecol Reprod Biol. 2002;104:40-2.
136. Zeyneloglu HB, Baltaci V, Duran HE, Erdemli E, Batioglu S. Achievement of pregnancy in globozoospermia with Y chromosome microdeletion after ICSI. Hum Reprod. 2002;17:1833-6.
137. Banker MR, Patel PM, Joshi BV, Shah PB, Goyal R. Successful pregnancies and a live birth after intracytoplasmic sperm injection in globozoospermia. J Hum Reprod Sci. 2009;2: 81-2.
138. Bechoua S, Chiron A, Delcleve-Paulhac S, Sagot P, Jimenez C. Fertilisation and pregnancy outcome after ICSI in globozoospermic patients without assisted oocyte activation. Andrologia. 2009;41:55-8.
139. Shu Y, Peng W, Zhang J. Pregnancy and live birth following the transfer of vitrified warmed blastocysts derived from zona- and corona-cell-free oocytes. Reprod Biomed Online. 2010;21:527-32.
140. Sermondade N, Hafhouf E, Dupont C, Bechoua S, Palacios C, Eustache F, et al. Successful childbirth after intracytoplasmic morphologically selected sperm injection without assisted oocyte activation in a patient with globozoospermia. Hum Reprod. 2011;26:2944-9.
141. Zhang ZQ, Long SG, Huang ZH, Xin CL, Wu QF. Different outcomes after intracytoplasmic sperm injection without oocyte activation in two patients with different types of globozoospermia. Andrologia. 2016;48:116-20.
142. Borges E Jr, de Almeida Ferreira Braga DP, de Sousa Bonetti TC, Iaconelli A Jr, Franco JG Jr. Artificial oocyte activation using calcium ionophore in ICSI cycles with spermatozoa from different sources. Reprod Biomed Online. 2009a;18:45-52.
143. Borges E Jr, de Almeida Ferreira Braga DP, de Sousa Bonetti TC, Iaconelli A Jr, Franco JG Jr. Artificial oocyte activation

with calcium ionophore A23187 in intracytoplasmic sperm injection cycles using surgically retrieved spermatozoa. Fertil Steril. 2009b;92:131-6.
144. Ebner T, Koster M, Shebl O, Moser M, Van der Ven H, Tews G, et al. Application of a ready-to-use calcium ionophore increases rates of fertilization and pregnancy in severe male factor infertility. Fertil Steril. 2012;98:1432-7.
145. Ebner T, Montag M, Van der Ven K, Van der Ven H, Shebl O, Oppelt P, et al. Live birth after artificial oocyte activation using a ready-to-use ionophore: a prospective multicentre study. Reprod Biomed Online. 2015;30:359-65.
146. Battaglia DE, Koehler JK, Klein NA, Tucker MJ. Failure of oocyte activation after intracytoplasmic sperm injection using round-headed sperm. Fertil Steril. 1997;68:118-22.
147. Kim ST, Cha YB, Park JM, Gye MC. Successful pregnancy and delivery from frozen-thawed embryos after intracytoplasmic sperm injection using round headed spermatozoa and assisted oocyte activation in a globozoospermic patient with mosaic Down syndrome. Fertil Steril. 2001;75:445-7.
148. Kyono K, Nakajo Y, Nishinaka C, Hattori H, Kyoya T, Ishikawa T, et al. A birth from the transfer of a single vitrified-warmed blastocyst using intracytoplasmic sperm injection with calcium ionophore oocyte activation in a globozoospermic patient. Fertil Steril. 2009;91:931.7-e11.
149. Taylor SL, Yoon SY, Morshedi MS, Lacey DR, Jellerette T, Fissore RA, et al. Complete globozoospermia associated with PLC zeta deficiency treated with calcium ionophore and ICSI results in pregnancy. Reprod Biomed Online. 2010;20:559-64.
150. Eldar-Geva T, Brooks B, Margalioth EJ, Zylber-Haran E, Gal M, Silber SJ. Successful pregnancy and delivery after calcium ionophore oocyte activation in a normozoospermic patient with previous repeated failed fertilization after intracytoplasmic sperm injection. Fertil Steril. 2003;79(Suppl 3): 1656-8.
151. Chi HJ, Koo JJ, Song SJ, Lee JY, Chang SS. Successful fertilization and pregnancy after intracytoplasmic sperm injection and oocyte activation with calcium ionophore in a normozoospermic patient with extremely low fertilization rates in intracytoplasmic sperm injection cycles. Fertil Steril. 2004;82:475-7.
152. Isachenko E, Isachenko V, Todorov P, Ostashko V, Kreienberg R, Kaufmann M, et al. Pregnancy after the calcium ionophore correction of pronuclei position in oocytes after intracytoplasmic sperm injection. Fertil Steril. 2010;94:2770.e3-5.
153. Ahmady A, Michael E. Successful pregnancy and delivery following intracytoplasmic injection of frozen-thawed nonviable testicular sperm and oocyte activation with calcium ionophore. J Androl. 2007;28:13-4.
154. Kim JW, Yang SH, Yoon SH, Kim SD, Jung JH, Lim JH. Successful pregnancy and delivery after ICSI with artificial oocyte activation by calcium ionophore in in-vitro matured oocytes: a case report. Reprod Biomed Online. 2015;30:373-7.
155. Nasr-Esfahani MH, Razavi S, Javdan Z, Tavalaee M. Artificial oocyte activation in severe teratozoospermia undergoing intracytoplasmic sperm injection. Fertil Steril. 2008a;90:2231-7.
156. Terada Y, Hasegawa H, Takahashi A, Ugajin T, Yaegashi N, Okamura K. Successful pregnancy after oocyte activation by a calcium ionophore for a patient with recurrent intracytoplasmic sperm injection failure, with an assessment of oocyte activation and sperm centrosomal function using bovine eggs. Fertil Steril. 2009;91:935.e11-4.
157. Check JH, Levito MC, Summers-Chase D, Marmar J, Barci H. A comparison of the efficacy of intracytoplasmic sperm injection (ICSI) using ejaculated sperm selected by high magnification versus ICSI with testicular sperm both followed by oocyte activation with calcium ionophore. Clin Exp Obstet Gynecol. 2007;34:111-2.
158. Moaz MN, Khattab S, Foutouh IA, Mohsen EA. Chemical activation of oocytes in different types of sperm abnormalities in cases of low or failed fertilization after ICSI: a prospective pilot study. Reprod Biomed Online. 2006;13:791-4.
159. Tesarik J, Mendoza C, Greco E. The activity (calcium oscillator?) responsible for human oocyte activation after injection with round spermatids is associated with spermatid nuclei. Fertil Steril. 2000;74:1245-7.
160. Combelles CM, Morozumi K, Yanagimachi R, Zhu L, Fox JH, Racowsky C. Diagnosing cellular defects in an unexplained case of total fertilization failure. Hum Reprod. 2010;25:1666-71.
161. Vanden Meerschaut F, Nikiforaki D, De Gheselle S, Dullaerts V, Van den Abbeel E, Gerris J, et al. Assisted oocyte activation is not beneficial for all patients with a suspected oocyte-related activation deficiency. Hum Reprod. 2012;27:1977-84.
162. Kuentz P, Vanden Meerschaut F, Elinati E, Nasr-Esfahani MH, Gurgan T, Iqbal N, et al. Assisted oocyte activation overcomes fertilization failure in globozoospermic patients regardless of the DPY19L2 status. Hum Reprod. 2013;28:1054-61.
163. Vanden Meerschaut F, D'Haeseleer E, Gysels H, Thienpont Y, Dewitte G, Heindryckx B, et al. Neonatal and neurodevelopmental outcome of children aged 3–10 years born following assisted oocyte activation. Reprod Biomed Online. 2014;28:54-63.
164. van Blerkom J, Cohen J, Johnson M. A plea for caution and more research in the 'experimental' use of ionophores in ICSI. Reprod Biomed Online. 2015;30:323-4.
165. Oehninger S. Clinical management of male infertility in assisted reproduction: ICSI and beyond. Int J Androl. 2011;34:319-29.
166. Dam AH, Feenstra I, Westphal JR, Ramos L, van Golde RJ, Kremer JA. Globozoospermia revisited. Hum Reprod Update. 2007a;13:63-75
167. Dam AH, Koscinski I, Kremer JA, Moutou C, Jaeger AS, Oudakker AR, et al. Homozygous mutation in SPATA16 is associated with male infertility in human globozoospermia. Am J Hum Genet. 2007b;81:813-20.
168. Singh G. Ultrastructural features of round-headed human spermatozoa. Int J Fertil. 1992;37:99-102.
169. Florke-Gerloff S, Topfer-Petersen E, Muller-Esterl W, Mansouri A, Schatz R, Schirren C, et al. Biochemical and genetic investigation of round-headed spermatozoa in infertile men including two brothers and their father. Andrologia. 1984;16:187-202.

170. Carrell DT, Emery BR, Liu L. Characterization of aneuploidy rates, protamine levels, ultrastructure, and functional ability of round-headed sperm from two siblings and implications for intracytoplasmic sperm injection. Fertil Steril. 1999;71:511-6.
171. Kilani Z, Ismail R, Ghunaim S, Mohamed H, Hughes D, Brewis I, et al. Evaluation and treatment of familial globozoospermia in five brothers. Fertil Steril. 2004;82:1436-9.
172. Dirican EK, Isik A, Vicdan K, Sozen E, Suludere Z. Clinical pregnancies and livebirths achieved by intracytoplasmic injection of round headed acrosome less spermatozoa with and without oocyte activation in familial globozoospermia: case report. Asian J Androl. 2008a;10:332-6.
173. Harbuz R, Zouari R, Pierre V, Ben Khelifa M, Kharouf M, Coutton C, et al. A recurrent deletion of DPY19L2 causes infertility in man by blocking sperm head elongation and acrosome formation. Am J Hum Genet. 2011;88:351-61.
174. Koscinski I, Elinati E, Fossard C, Redin C, Muller J, Velez de la Calle J, et al. DPY19L2 deletion as a major cause of globozoospermia. Am J Hum Genet. 2011;88:344-50.
175. Perrin A, Coat C, Nguyen MH, Talagas M, Morel F, Amice J, et al. Molecular cytogenetic and genetic aspects of globozoospermia: a review. Andrologia. 2013;45:1-9.
176. Kang-Decker N, Mantchev GT, Juneja SC, McNiven MA, van Deursen JM. Lack of acrosome formation in Hrb-deficient mice. Science. 2001;294:1531-3.
177. Yao R, Ito C, Natsume Y, Sugitani Y, Yamanaka H, Kuretake S, et al. Lack of acrosome formation in mice lacking a Golgi protein, GOPC. Proc Natl Acad Sci USA. 2002;99:11211-6.
178. Xiao N, Kam C, Shen C, Jin W, Wang J, Lee KM, et al. PICK1 deficiency causes male infertility in mice by disrupting acrosome formation. J Clin Invest. 2009;119:802-12.
179. Aitken RJ, Kerr L, Bolton V, Hargreave T. Analysis of sperm function in globozoospermia: implications for the mechanism of sperm-zona interaction. Fertil Steril. 1990;54:701-7.
180. Dale B, Iaccarino M, Fortunato A, Gragnaniello G, Kyozuka K, Tosti E. A morphological and functional study of fusibility in round-headed spermatozoa in the human. Fertil Steril. 1994;61:336-40.
181. Rybouchkin AV, Vander Straeten F, Quatacker J, DeSutter P, Dhont M. Fertilization and pregnancy after assisted oocyte activation and intracytoplasmic sperm injection in a case of round-headed sperm associated with deficient oocyte activation capacity. Fertil Steril. 1997;68:1144-7.
182. Hattori H, Nakajo Y, Ito C, Toyama Y, Toshimori K, Kyono K. Birth of a healthy infant after intracytoplasmic sperm injection using pentoxifylline-activated sperm from a patient with Kartagener's syndrome. Fertil Steril. 2011;95:2431.e9-11.
183. Nodar F, DeVincentiis S, Olmedo SB, Papier S, Urrutia F, Acosta AA. Birth of twin males with normal karyotype after intracytoplasmic sperm injection with use of testicular spermatozoa from a nonmosaic patient with Klinefelter's syndrome. Fertil Steril. 1999;71:1149-52.
184. Yildirim G, Ficicioglu C, Akcin O, Attar R, Tecellioglu N, Yencilek F. Can pentoxifylline improve the sperm motion and ICSI success in the primary ciliary dyskinesia? Arch Gynecol Obstet. 2009;279:213-5.
185. Nagy ZP. Sperm centriole dysfunction and sperm immobility. Mol Cell Endocrinol. 2000;15:59-62.
186. Ortega C, Verheyen G, Raick D, Camus M, Devroey P, Tournaye H. Absolute asthenozoospermia and ICSI: what are the options? Hum Reprod Update. 2011;17:684-92.
187. Yovich JL. Pentoxifylline: actions and applications in assisted reproduction. Hum Reprod. 1993;8:1786-91.
188. Kovacic B, Vlaisavljevic V, Reljic M. Clinical use of pentoxifylline for activation of immotile testicular sperm before ICSI in patients with azoospermia. J Androl. 2006;27:45-52.
189. Terriou P, Hans E, Giorgetti C, Spach JL, Salzmann J, Urrutia V, et al. Pentoxifylline initiates motility in spontaneously immotile epididymal and testicular spermatozoa and allows normal fertilization, pregnancy, and birth after intracytoplasmic sperm injection. J Assist Reprod Genet. 2000;17:194-9.
190. Griveau JF, Lobel B, Laurent MC, Michardière L, Le Lannou D. Interest of pentoxifylline in ICSI with frozen-thawed testicular spermatozoa from patients with non-obstructive azoospermia. Reprod Biomed Online. 2006;12:14-8.
191. Tournaye H, Van der Linden M, Van den Abbeel E, Devroey P, Van Steirteghem A. Effects of pentoxifylline on in-vitro development of preimplantation mouse embryos. Hum Reprod. 1993;8:1475-80.
192. Ain R, Seshagiri PB. Micromolar concentration of pentoxifylline improves development *in vitro* of hamster 8-cell embryos: confirmation of biological viability by embryo transfer. Reprod Fertil Dev. 1997;9:697-702.
193. Ebner T, Tews G, Mayer RB, Ziehr S, Arzt W, Costamoling W Roulier R. Pharmacological stimulation of sperm motility in frozen and thawed testicular sperm using the dimethylxanthine theophylline. Fertil Steril. 2011;96:1331-6.
194. EbnerT, Shebl O, Mayer RB, Moser M, Costamoling W, Oppelt P. Healthy live birth using theophylline in a case of retrograde ejaculation and absolute asthenozoospermia. Fertil Steril. 2014;101:340-3.
195. National Toxicology Program. National Toxicology Program NTP Toxicology and Carcinogenesis Studies of Theophylline (CAS No. 58-55-9) in F344/N Rats and B6C3F1 Mice (Feed and Gavage Studies). Natl Toxicol Program Tech Rep Ser. 1998;473:1-326.
196. Soares JB, Glina S, Antunes N Jr, Wonchockier R, Galuppo AG, Mizrahi FE. Sperm tail flexibility test: a simple test for selecting viable spermatozoa for intracytoplasmic sperm injection from semen samples without motile spermatozoa. Rev Hosp Clin Fac Med Sao Paulo. 2003;58:250-3.
197. de Oliveira NM, Sanchez RV, Fiesta SR, Salgado TL, Rodriguez R, Bethencourt JCA, et al. Pregnancy with frozen-thawed and fresh testicular biopsy after motile and immotile sperm microinjection, using the mechanical touch technique to assess viability. Hum Reprod. 2004;19:262-5.
198. Nordhoff V. How to select immotile but viable spermatozoa on the day of intracytoplasmic sperm injection? An embryologists view. Andrology. 2015;3:156-62.
199. Casper RF, Meriano JS, Jarvi KA, Cowan L, Lucato ML. The hypoosmotic swelling test for selection of viable sperm for intracytoplasmic sperm injection in men with complete asthenozoospermia. Fertil Steril. 1996;65:972-6.

200. World Health Organization. WHO Laboratory Manual for the Examination and Processing of Human Semen, 5th edition. Geneva, CH: World Health Organization; 2010.
201. Stanger JD, Vo L, Yovich JL, Almahbobi G. Hypo-osmotic swelling test identifies individual spermatozoa with minimal DNA fragmentation. Reprod Biomed Online. 2010;21:474-84.
202. Bassiri F, Tavalaee M, Shiravi AH, Mansouri S, Nasr-Esfahani MH. Is there an association between HOST grades and sperm quality? Hum Reprod. 2012;27:2277-84.
203. Barros A, Sousa M, Angelopoulos T, Tesarik J. Efficient modification of intracytoplasmic sperm injection technique for cases with total lack of sperm movement. Hum Reprod. 1997a;12:1227-9.
204. Bollendorf A, Check JH, Kramer D. The majority of males with subnormal hypoosmotic test scores have normal vitality. Clin Exp Obstet Gynecol. 2012;39:25-6.
205. Sallam H, Farrag A, Agameya A, Ezzeldin F, Eid A, Sallam A. The use of a modified hypo-osmotic swelling test for the selection of viable ejaculated and testicular immotile spermatozoa in ICSI. Hum Reprod. 2001;16:272-6.
206. Hossain A, Osuamkpe C, Hossain S, Phelps JY. Spontaneously developed tail swellings (SDTS) influence the accuracy of the hypo-osmotic swelling test (HOS-test) in determining membrane integrity and viability of human spermatozoa. J Assist Reprod Genet. 2010;27:83-6.
207. Liu J, Tsai YL, Katz E, Compton G, Garcia JE, Baramki TA. High fertilization rate obtained after intracytoplasmic sperm injection with 100% nonmotile spermatozoa selected by using a simple modified hypo-osmotic swelling test. Fertil Steril. 1997;68:373-5.
208. Ved S, Montag M, Schmutzler A, Prietl G, Haidl G, van der Ven H. Pregnancy following intracytoplasmic sperm injection of immotile spermatozoa selected by the hypo-osmotic swelling-test: a case report. Andrologia. 1997;29:241-2.
209. Sallam HN, Farrag A, Agameya AF, El-Garem Y, Ezzeldin F. The use of the modified hypo-osmotic swelling test for the selection of immotile testicular spermatozoa in patients treated with ICSI: a randomized controlled study. Hum Reprod. 2005;20:3435-40.
210. Mangoli V, Mangoli R, Dandekar S, Suri K, Desai S. Selection of viable spermatozoa from testicular biopsies: a comparative study between pentoxifylline and hypoosmotic swelling test. Fertil Steril. 2011;95:631-4.
211. Geber S, Lemgruber M, Taitson PF, Valle M, Sampaio M. Birth of healthy twins after intracytoplasmic sperm injection using ejaculated immotile spermatozoa from a patient with Kartagener's syndrome. Andrologia. 2012;44(Suppl 1): 842-4.
212. Kordus RJ, Price RL, Davis JM, Whitman-Elia GF. Successful twin birth following blastocyst culture of embryos derived from the immotile ejaculated spermatozoa from a patient with primary ciliary dyskinesia: a case report. J Assist Reprod Genet. 2008;25:437-43.
213. Westlander G, Barry M, Petrucco O, Norman R. Different fertilization rates between immotile testicular spermatozoa and immotile ejaculated spermatozoa for ICSI in men with Kartagener's syndrome: case reports. Hum Reprod. 2003;18:1286-8.
214. Aktan TM, Montag M, Duman S, Gorkemli H, Rink K, Yurdakul T. Use of a laser to detect viable but immotile spermatozoa. Andrologia. 2004;36:366-9.
215. Nordhoff V, Scheuring AN, Krallmann C, Zitzmann M, Schlatt S, Kiesel L, et al. Optimising TESE-ICSI by laser-assisted selection of immotile spermatozoa and polarisation microscopy for selection of oocytes. Andrology. 2013;1: 67-74.
216. Muratori M, Tamburrino L, Marchaini S, Cambi M, Olivito B, Azzari C, et al. Investigation on the origin of sperm DNA fragmentation: role of apoptosis, immaturity and oxidative stress. Mol Med. 2015;21:109-22.
217. Lewis SE, Aitken RJ. DNA damage to spermatozoa has impacts on fertilization and pregnancy. Cell Tissue Res. 2005;322:33-41.
218. González-Marín C, Gosálvez J, Roy R. Types, causes, detection and repair of DNA fragmentation in animal and human sperm cells. Int J Mol Sci. 2012;31:14026-52.
219. Wright C, Milne S, Leeson H. Sperm DNA damage caused by oxidative stress: modifiable clinical, lifestyle and nutritional factors in male infertility. Reprod Biomed Online. 2014;28:684-703.
220. Gawecka JE, Marh J, Ortega M, Yamauchi Y, Ward MA, Ward WS. Mouse zygotes respond to severe sperm DNA damage by delaying paternal DNA replication and embryonic development. PLoS One. 2013;8:e56385.
221. Gandini L, Lombardo F, Paoli D, Caruso F, Eleuteri P, Leter G, et al. Full-term pregnancies achieved with ICSI despite high levels of sperm chromatin damage. Hum Reprod. 2004;19:1409-17.
222. Huang CC, Lin DP, Tsao HM, Cheng TC, Liu CH, Lee MS. Sperm DNA fragmentation negatively correlates with velocity and fertilisation rates but might not affect pregnancy rates. Fertil Steril. 2005;84:130-40.
223. Borini A, Tarozzi N, Bizzaro D, Bonu MA, Fava L, Flamigni C, et al. Sperm DNA fragmentation: paternal effect on early post-implantation embryo development in ART. Hum Reprod. 2006;21:2876-81.
224. Bungum M, Humaidan P, Axmon A, Spano M, Bungum L, Erenpreiss J, et al. Sperm DNA integrity assessment in prediction of assisted reproduction technology outcome. Hum Reprod 2007;22:174-9.
225. Simon L, Castillo J, Oliva R, Lewis SE. Relationships between human sperm protamines, DNA damage and assisted reproduction outcomes. Reprod Biomed Online. 2011; 23: 724-34.
226. Sakkas D. Novel technologies for selecting the best sperm for *in vitro* fertilization and intracytoplasmic sperm injection. Fertil Steril. 2013;99:1023-9.
227. PalermoGD, Neri QV, Cozzubbo T, Rosenwaks Z. Perspectives on the assessment of human sperm chromatin integrity. Fertil Steril. 2014;102:1508-17.
228. Zini A, Finelli A, Phang D, Jarvi K. Influence of semen processing technique on human sperm DNA integrity. Urology. 2000;56:1081-4.

229. Stevanato J, Bertolla RP, Barradas V, Spaine DM, Cedenho AP, Ortiz V. Semen processing by density gradient centrifugation does not improve sperm apoptotic deoxyribonucleic acid fragmentation rates. Fertil Steril. 2008;90:889-90.
230. Cayli S, Jakab A, Ovari L, Delpiano E, Celik-Ozenci C, Sakkas D, et al. Biochemical markers of sperm function: male fertility and sperm selection for ICSI. Reprod Biomed Online. 2003;7:462-8.
231. Huszar G, Ozenci CC, Cayli S, Zavaczki Z, Hansch E, Vigue L. Hyaluronic acid binding by human sperm indicates cellular maturity, viability, and unreacted acrosomal status. Fertil Steril. 2003;79:1616-24.
232. Huszar G, Jakab A, Sakkas D, Ozenci CC, Cayli S, Delpiano E, et al. Fertility testing and ICSI sperm selection by hyaluronic acid binding: clinical and genetic aspects. Reprod Biomed Online. 2007;14:650-63.
233. Parmegiani L, Cognigni GE, Bernardi S, Troilo E, Ciampaglia W, Filicori M. 'Physiologic ICSI': hyaluronic acid (HA) favors selection of spermatozoa without DNA fragmentation and with normal nucleus, resulting in improvement of embryo quality. Fertil Steril. 2010;93:598-604.
234. McDowell S, Kroon B, Ford E, Hook Y, Glujovsky D, Yazdani A. Advanced sperm selection techniques for assisted reproduction. Cochrane Database Syst Rev. 2014;10:CD010461.
235. Nasr-Esfahani MH, Razavi S, Vahdati AA, Fathi F, Tavalaee M. Evaluation of sperm selection procedure based on hyaluronic acid binding ability on ICSI outcome. J Assist Reprod Genet. 2008b;25:197-203.
236. Parmegiani L, Cognigni GE, Bernardi S, Troilo E, Taraborrelli S, Arnone A, et al. Comparison of two ready-to-use systems designed for sperm-hyaluronic acid binding selection before intracytoplasmic sperm injection: PICSI vs. Sperm Slow: a prospective, randomized trial. Fertil Steril. 2012;98:632-7.
237. Erberelli RF, Salgado RM, Pereira DHM, Wolff P. Hyaluronan-binding system for sperm selection enhances pregnancy rates in ICSI cycles associated with male factor infertility. JBRA Assit Reprod. 2017;21:02-6.
238. Said TM, Grunewald S, Paasch U, Rasch M, Agarwal A, Glander HJ. Effects of magnetic-activated cell sorting on sperm motility and cryosurvival rates. Fertil Steril. 2005;83:1442-6.
239. Grunewald S, Paasch U, Said TM, Rasch M, Agarwal A, Glander HJ. Magnetic-activated cell sorting before cryopreservation preserves mitochondrial integrity in human spermatozoa. Cell Tissue Bank. 2006;7:99-104.
240. Aziz N, Said T, Paasch U, Agarwal A. The relationship between human sperm apoptosis, morphology and the sperm deformity index. Hum Reprod. 2007;22:1413-9.
241. Lee TH, Liu CH, Shih YT, Tsao HM, Huang CC, Chen HH, et al. Magnetic-activated cell sorting for sperm preparation reduces spermatozoa with apoptotic markers and improves the acrosome reaction in couples with unexplained infertility. Hum Reprod. 2010;25:839-46.
242. Rawe VY, Boudri HU, Alvarez Sedó C, Carro M, Papier S, Nodar F. Healthy baby born after reduction of sperm DNA fragmentation using cell sorting before ICSI. Reprod Biomed Online. 2010;20:320-3.
243. Degheidy T, Abdelfattah H, Seif A, Albuz FK, Gazi S, Abbas S. Magnetic activated cell sorting: an effective method for reduction of sperm DNA fragmentation in varicocele men prior to assisted reproductive techniques. Andrologia. 2014;11:892-6.
244. Nadalini M, Tarozzi N, Di Santo M, Borini A. Annexin V magnetic-activated cell sorting versus swim-up for the selection of human sperm in ART: is the new approach better than the traditional one? J Assist Reprod Genet. 2014;31:1045-51.
245. Vendrell X, Ferrer M, García-Mengual E, Muñoz P, Triviño JC, Calatayud C, et al. Correlation between aneuploidy, apoptotic markers and DNA fragmentation in spermatozoa from normozoospermic patients. Reprod Biomed Online. 2014;28:492-502.
246. Bucar S, Goncalves A, Rocha E, Barros A, Sousa M, Sá R. DNA fragmentation in human sperm after magnetic-activated cell sorting. J Assist Reprod Genet. 2015;32:147-54.
247. Shen HM, Dai J, Chia SE, Lim A, Ong CN. Detection of apoptotic alterations in sperm in subfertile patients and their correlations with sperm quality. Hum Reprod. 2002;17:1266-73.
248. Miltenyi S, Müller W, Weichel W, Radbruch A. High gradient magnetic cell separation with MACS. Cytometry. 1990;11:231-8.
249. Paasch U, Grunewald S, Fitzl G, Glander HJ. Deterioration of plasma membrane is associated with activated caspases in human spermatozoa. J Androl. 2003;24:246-52.
250. Dirican EK, Ozgün OD, Akarsu S, Akin KO, Ercan O, Uğurlu M, et al. Clinical outcome of magnetic activated cell sorting of non-apoptotic spermatozoa before density gradient centrifugation for assisted reproduction. J Assist Reprod Genet. 2008b;25:375-81.
251. Sheikhi A, Jalali M, Gholamian M, Jafarzadeh A, Jannati S, Mousavifar N. Elimination of apoptotic spermatozoa by magnetic-activated cell sorting improves the fertilization rate of couples treated with ICSI procedure. Andrology. 2013;1:845-9.
252. Polak de Fried E, Denaday F. Single and twin ongoing pregnancies in two cases of previous ART failure after ICSI performed with sperm sorted using annexin V microbeads. Fertil Steril. 2010;94:351.e15-8.
253. Herrero MB, Delbes G, Chung JT, Son WY, Holzer H, Buckett W, et al. Case report: the use of annexin V coupled with magnetic activated cell sorting in cryopreserved spermatozoa from a male cancer survivor: healthy twin newborns after two previous ICSI failures. J Assist Reprod Genet. 2013;30:1415-9.
254. Chan PJ, Jacobson JD, Corselli JU, Patton WC. A simple zeta method for sperm selection based on membrane charge. Fertil Steril. 2006;85:481-6.
255. Focarelli R, Rosati F, Terrana B. Sialyl-glycoconjugates release during *in vitro* capacitation of human spermatozoa. J Androl. 2009;11:97-104.
256. Kheirollahi-Kouhestani M, Razavi S, Tavalaee M, Deemeh MR, Mardani M, Moshtaghian J, et al. Selection of sperm based on combined density gradient and Zeta method may improve ICSI outcome. Hum Reprod. 2009;24:2409-16.

257. Razavi SH, Nasr-Esfahani MH, Deemeh MR, Shayesteh M, Tavalaee M. Evaluation of zeta and HA-binding methods for selection of spermatozoa with normal morphology, protamine content and DNA integrity. Andrologia. 2010;42:13-9.
258. Giuliani V, Pandolfi C, Santucci R, Pelliccione F, Macerola B, Focarelli R, et al. Expression of gp20, a human sperm antigen of epididymal origin, is reduced in spermatozoa from subfertile men. Mol Reprod Dev. 2004;69:235-40.
259. Ainsworth C, Nixon B, Jansen RP, Aitken RJ. First recorded pregnancy and normal birth after ICSI using electrophoretically isolated spermatozoa. Hum Reprod. 2007;22:197-200.
260. Fleming SD, Ilad RS, Griffin AM, Wu Y, Ong KJ, Smith HC, et al. Prospective controlled trial of an electrophoretic method of sperm preparation for assisted reproduction: comparison with density gradient centrifugation. Hum Reprod. 2008;23:2646-51.
261. Boivin J, Bunting L, Koert E, Ien UC, Verhaak C. Perceived challenges of working in a fertility clinic: a qualitative analysis of work stressors and difficulties working with patients. Hum Reprod. 2017;32:403-8.
262. La Marca A, Sunkara SK. Individualization of controlled ovarian stimulation in IVF using ovarian reserve markers: from theory to practice. Hum Reprod Update. 2014;20:124-40.
263. Teixeira DM, Barbosa MA, Ferriani RA, Navarro PA, Raine-Fenning N, Nastri CO, et al. Regular (ICSI) versus ultra-high magnification (IMSI) sperm selection for assisted reproduction. Cochrane Database Syst Rev. 2013;7:CD010167.
264. Setti AS, Braga DP, Figueira RC, Iaconelli A Jr, Borges E. Intracytoplasmic morphologically selected sperm injection results in improved clinical outcomes in couples with previous ICSI failures or male factor infertility: a meta-analysis. Eur J Obstet Gynecol Reprod Biol 2014;183:96-103.

CHAPTER

16

Spermatogenesis

Nitin Lad, Neha Lad

INTRODUCTION

In the 21st century, incidence of infertility has increased significantly. One of the important causes is increased prevalence of male infertility. In last 5 decades, we have seen significant reduction in sperm count and semen volume. Hence, understanding of spermatogenesis and factors affecting spermatogenesis plays important role in managing male infertility.

Spermatogenesis is a complex phenomenon which takes place in the testis. End result of spermatogenesis is to form a mature spermatozoon which is characterized by peculiar changes like flagellum, etc. The procedure of spermatogenesis begins from puberty and continues till the end of life. Spermatogenesis is controlled by physiological as well as pathological factors.

In this chapter, we have covered various aspects of spermatogenesis.

ANATOMY OF MALE GENITAL TRACT

The *scrotum* is a sac-like organ made of skin and muscles that houses the testes (Figs. 16.1 and 16.2). It is located inferior to the penis in the pubic region. The scrotum is made up of two side-by-side pouches with a testis located in each pouch. The smooth muscles that make up the scrotum allow it to regulate the distance between the testes and the rest of the body.[1] When the testes become too

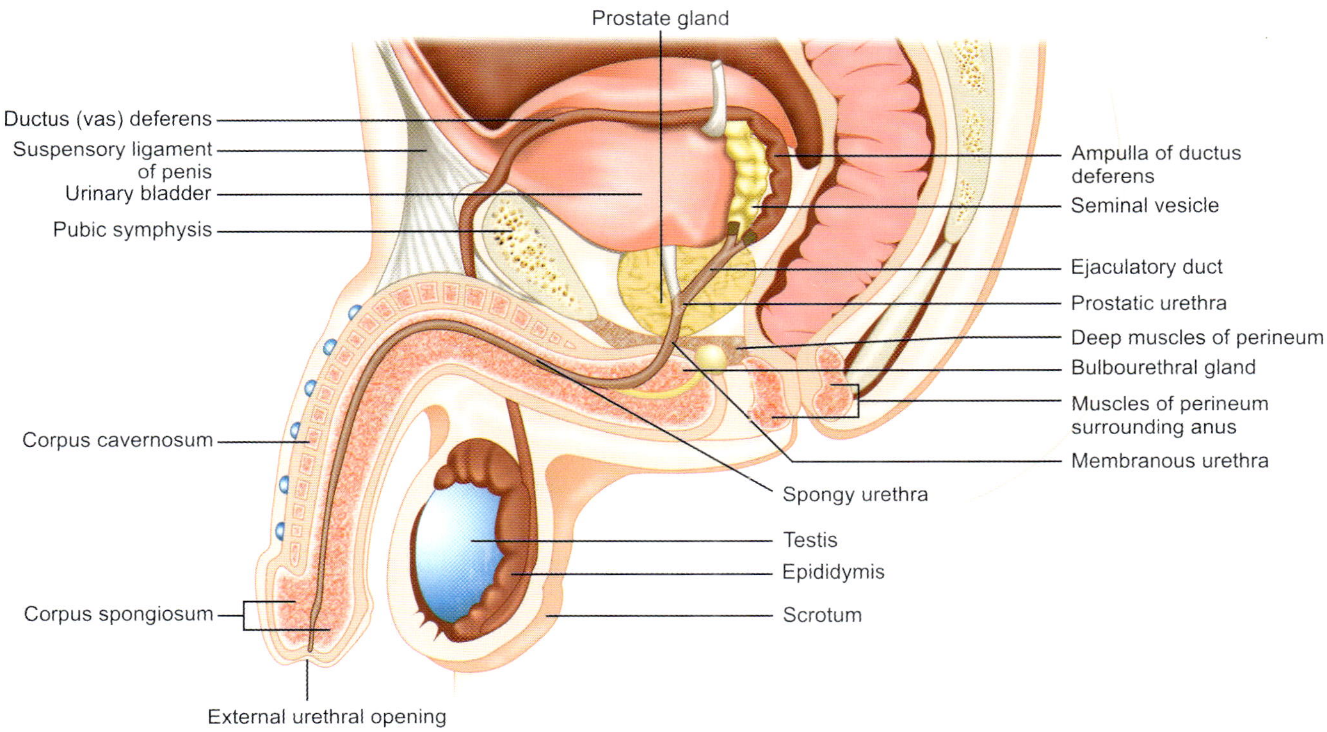

Fig. 16.1: Male reproductive tract.

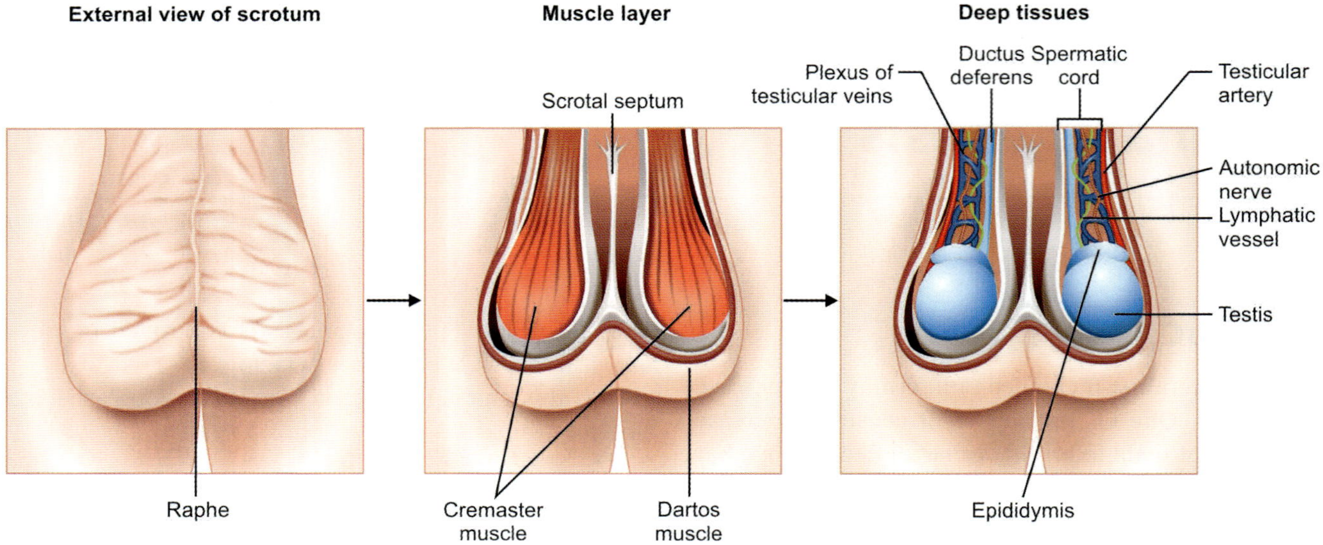

Fig. 16.2: Anterior view shows the structures of the scrotum and testes.

warm to support spermatogenesis, the scrotum relaxes to move the testes away from the body's heat. Conversely, the scrotum contracts to move the testes closer to the body's core heat when temperatures drop below the ideal range for spermatogenesis.

The two *testes*, also known as testicles, are the male gonads responsible for the production of sperm and testosterone (Figs. 16.3A and B).[2] Each testis is found inside its own pouch on one side of the scrotum and is connected to the abdomen by a spermatic cord and cremaster muscle. The cremaster muscles contract and relax along with the scrotum to regulate the temperature of the testes. The inside of the testes is divided into small compartments known as lobules. Each lobule contains a section of seminiferous tubule lined with epithelial cells. These epithelial cells contain many stem cells that divide and form sperm cells through the process of spermatogenesis. The *epididymis* is a sperm storage area that wraps around the superior and posterior edge of the testes. Sperm produced in the testes moves into the epididymis to mature before being passed on through the male reproductive organs. The length of the epididymis delays the release of the sperm and allows them time to mature.[1] The *ductus deferens*, also known as the vas deferens, is a muscular tube that carries sperm superiorly from the epididymis into the abdominal cavity to the ejaculatory duct. The ductus deferens is wider in diameter than the epididymis and uses its internal space to store mature sperm. The smooth muscles of the walls of the ductus deferens are used to move sperm toward the ejaculatory duct through peristalsis.[1] The *seminal vesicles* are a pair of lumpy exocrine glands that store and produce some of the liquid portion of semen. The liquid produced by the seminal vesicles contains proteins and mucus and has an alkaline pH to help sperm survive in the acidic environment of the vagina. The liquid also contains fructose to feed sperm cells so that they can survive long enough to fertilize the oocyte. The ductus deferens passes through the prostate and joins with the urethra at a structure known as the ejaculatory duct. The ejaculatory duct contains the ducts from the seminal vesicles as well. During ejaculation, the ejaculatory duct opens and expels sperm and the secretions from the seminal vesicles into the urethra.[1] The *prostate* is a walnut-sized exocrine gland that borders the inferior end of the urinary bladder and surrounds the urethra. The prostate produces a large portion of the fluid that makes up semen. This fluid is milky-white in color and contains enzymes, proteins, and other chemicals to support and protect sperm during ejaculation. The *Cowper's glands*, also known as the *bulbourethral glands*, are a pair of pea-sized exocrine glands located inferior to the prostate and anterior to the anus. The Cowper's glands secrete a thin alkaline fluid into the urethra that lubricates the urethra and neutralizes acid from urine remaining in the urethra after urination. This fluid enters the urethra during sexual arousal prior to ejaculation to prepare the urethra for the flow of semen. The *penis* is the male external sexual organ located superior to the scrotum and inferior to the umbilicus. The penis is roughly cylindrical in shape and contains the urethra and the external opening of the urethra. The function of the penis is to deliver

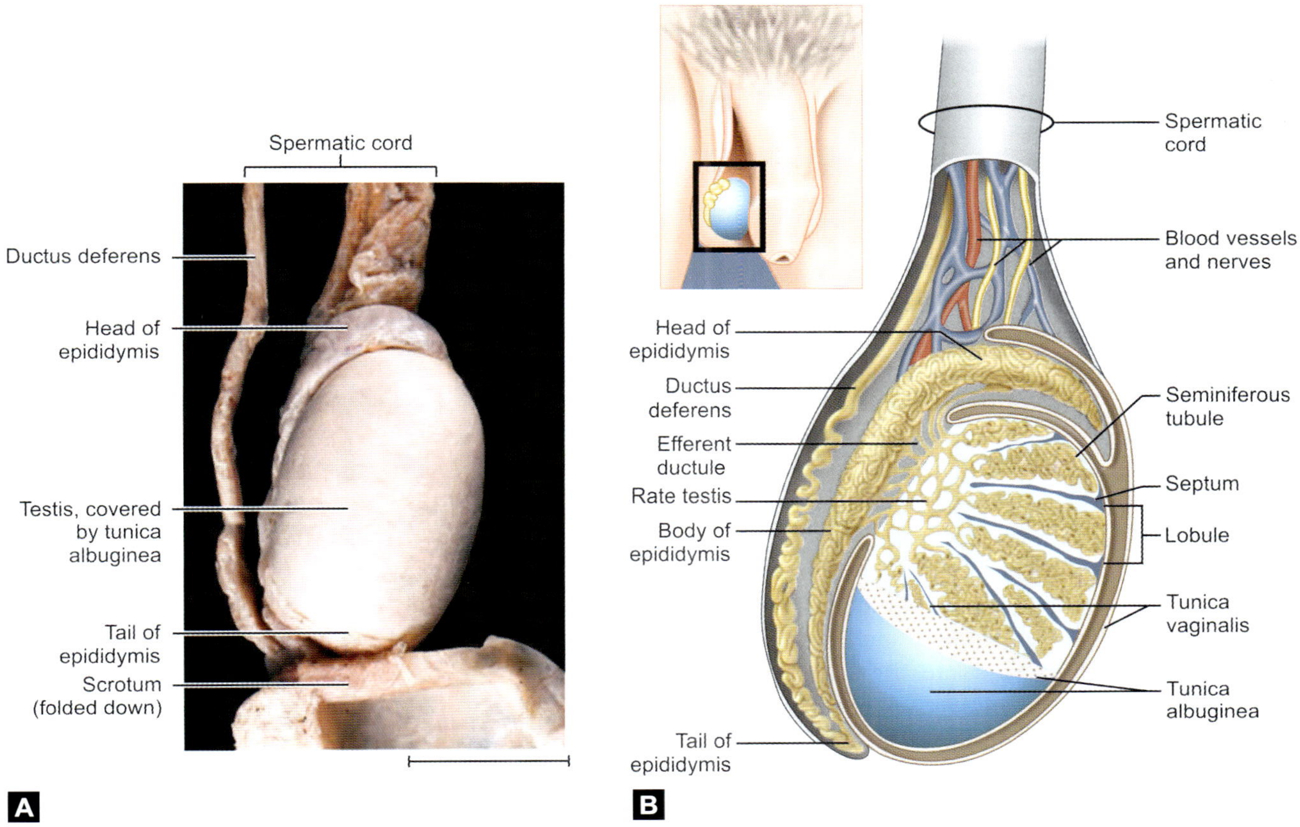

Figs. 16.3A and B: Testis and associated structures. (A) Scrotum is opened and folded downward to reveal the testis and associated organs. (B) Anatomy of the testis, epididymis, and spermatic cord.

semen into the vagina during sexual intercourse. In addition to its reproductive function, the penis also allows for the excretion of urine through the urethra to the exterior of the body. Semen is the fluid produced by males for sexual reproduction and is ejaculated out of the body during sexual intercourse. Semen contains sperm, the male reproductive gametes, along with a number of chemicals suspended in a liquid medium. The chemical composition of semen gives it a thick, sticky consistency and a slightly alkaline pH. These traits help semen to support reproduction by helping sperm to remain within the vagina after intercourse and to neutralize the acidic environment of the vagina. In healthy adult males, semen contains around 100 million sperm cells per milliliter. These sperm cells fertilize oocytes inside the female Fallopian tubes.[1]

PHYSIOLOGY

Spermatogenesis is the process of producing sperm and takes place in the testes and epididymis of adult males. Prior to puberty, there is no spermatogenesis due to the lack of hormonal triggers.[3] At puberty, spermatogenesis begins when luteinizing hormone (LH) and follicle-stimulating hormone (FSH) are produced. LH triggers the production of testosterone by the testes while FSH triggers the maturation of germ cells. Testosterone stimulates stem cells in the testes known as spermatogonium to undergo the process of developing into spermatocytes. Each diploid spermatocyte goes through the process of meiosis I and splits into two haploid secondary spermatocytes. The secondary spermatocytes go through meiosis II to form four haploid spermatid cells. The spermatid cells then go through a process known as spermiogenesis where they grow a flagellum and develop the structures of the sperm head. After spermiogenesis, the cell is finally a sperm cell, or spermatozoa. The spermatozoa are released into the epididymis where they complete their maturation and become able to move on their own.[4]

Histology

The internal male genitalia consist of the testes with the adjoining epididymis, the vas deferens, and the accessory sex glands, namely the seminal vesicles, the prostate, and the bulbourethral glands.

Testes

The testes have two functions: they produce the male gametes or spermatozoa, and they produce male sexual hormone, testosterone, which stimulates the accessory male sexual organs and causes the development of the masculine extragenital sex characteristics. The testis is surrounded by a thick capsule, the tunica albuginea, from which a conical mass of connective tissue, the mediastinum testis, projects into the testis. The tunica albuginea is covered externally by a serosa. From the mediastinum, delicate fibrous septa radiate toward the tunica albuginea and divide the parenchyma of the testis into about 300 lobuli testis, which communicate peripherally. Each lobule contains one to four convoluted seminiferous tubules (about 150–300 μm in diameter, 30–80 cm long). Interstitial tissue between the convoluted tubules is continuous with a layer of loose vascular connective tissue, the tunica vasculosa testis, which is found beneath the tunica albuginea. Each seminiferous tubule continues near the mediastinum into a straight tubule, a tubulus rectus. The straight tubules continue into the rete testis, a labyrinthine system of cavities in the mediastinum (Figs. 16.4A and B).[1]

Seminiferous Tubules

These tubules are enclosed by a thick basal lamina and surrounded by three to four layers of smooth muscle cells (or myoid cells). The insides of the tubules are lined with seminiferous epithelium, which consists of two general types of cells: spermatogenic cells and Sertoli cells (Fig. 16.5).[5]

Spermatogenic cells: Spermatogonia are the first cells of spermatogenesis. They originate in the 4th week of fetal development in the endodermal walls of the yolk sac and migrate to the primordium of the testis, where they differentiate into spermatogonia. Spermatogonia remain dormant until puberty. They are always in contact with the basal lamina of the tubule. Two types of spermatogonia can be distinguished in the human seminiferous epithelium:

Type A spermatogonia have a rounded nucleus with very fine chromatin grains and one or two nucleoli. They are stem cells, which divide to form new generations of both type A and type B spermatogonia. Type B spermatogonia have rounded nuclei with chromatin granules of variable size, which often attach to the nuclear membrane and one nucleolus. Although type B spermatogonia may divide repeatedly, they do not function as stem cells and their final mitosis always results in the formation of

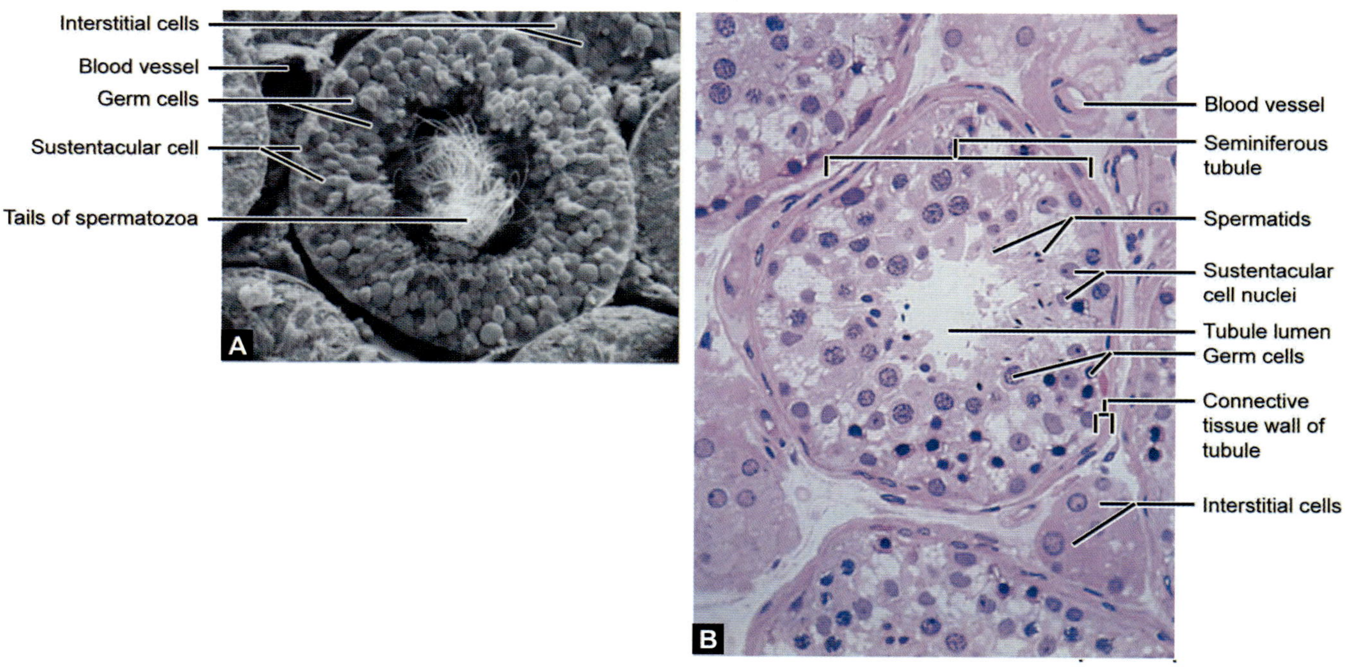

Figs. 16.4A and B: Histology of the testis. (A) Scanning electron micrograph. (B) Light micrograph.

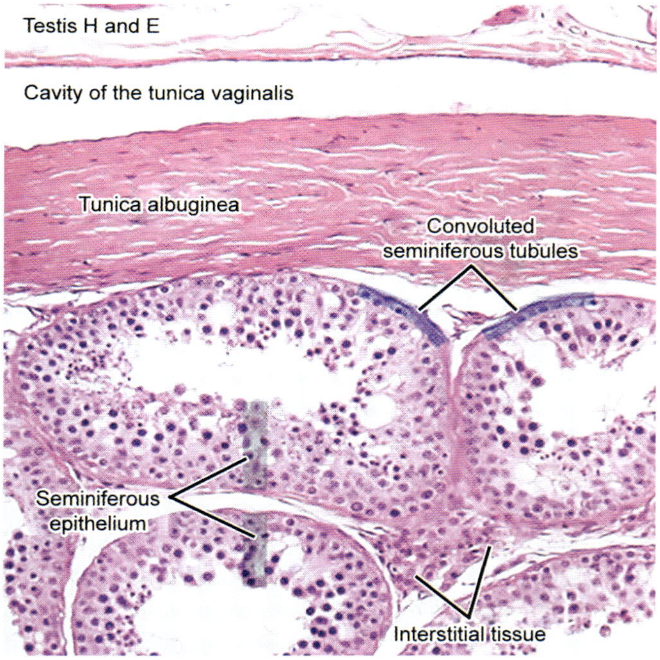

Fig. 16.5: Histology of the seminiferous tubules.

primary spermatocytes, which lie in the cell layer luminal to the spermatogonia. They appear larger than spermatogonia. They immediately enter the prophase of the first meiotic division, which is extremely prolonged (about 22 days!). A large number of primary spermatocytes are always visible in cross-sections through seminiferous tubules. Cell divisions, from the formation of primary spermatocytes and onward, to the production of the spermatocytes, are incomplete. The cells remain connected by bridges of cytoplasm. The completion of the first meiotic division results in the formation of *secondary spermatocytes*, which are smaller than primary spermatocytes. They rapidly enter and complete the second meiotic division and are, therefore, seldom seen in histological preparations. Their division results in the formation of *spermatids*, which lie in the luminal part of the seminiferous epithelium. They are small (about 10 μm in diameter) with an initially very light (often eccentric) nucleus. The chromatin condenses during the maturation of the spermatids into spermatozoa, and the nucleus becomes smaller and stains darker. The terminal phase of spermatogenesis is called spermiogenesis and consists of the differentiation of the newly formed spermatids into *spermatozoa*. The mature human spermatozoon is about 60 μm long and actively motile. It is divided into head, neck, and tail. The head (flattened, about 5 μm long and 3 μm wide) chiefly consists of the nucleus (greatly condensed chromatin!). The anterior two third of the nucleus is covered by the acrosome, which contains enzymes important in the process of fertilization. The posterior parts of the nuclear membrane form the so-called basal plate. The neck is short (about 1 μm) and attached to the basal plate. A transversely oriented centriole is located immediately behind the basal plate. The neck also contains nine segmented columns of fibrous material, which continue as the outer dense fibers into the tail. The tail is further divided into a middle piece, a principle piece, and an end piece. The axoneme begins in the middle piece. It is surrounded by nine outer dense fibers, which are not found in other cilia. In the middle piece (about 5 μm long), the axoneme and dense fibers are surrounded by a sheath of mitochondria. The middle piece is terminated by a dense ring, the annulus. The principle piece is about 45 μm long. It contains a fibrous sheath, which consists of dorsal and ventral longitudinal columns interconnected by regularly spaced circumferential hoops. Along the last part of the tail, called the end piece, the axoneme is only surrounded by a small amount of cytoplasm and the plasma membrane. It takes about 48 days from the time cells enter meiosis until morphologically mature spermatozoa are formed. Depending on the length of reproduction of spermatogonia (which is not precisely determined), it takes approximately 64 days to complete spermatogenesis.

Sertoli cells are far less numerous than the spermatogenic cells and are evenly distributed between them. Their shape is highly irregular—columnar is the best approximation. Sertoli cells extend from the basement membrane to the luminal surface of the seminiferous epithelium.[6,7] Processes of the Sertoli cells extend in between the spermatogenic cells [cell limits are, therefore, not clearly visible in the light microscope (LM)]. The nucleus of Sertoli cells is ovoid or angular, large, and lightly stained and often contains a large nucleolus. The long axis of the nucleus is oriented perpendicular to wall of the tubule. Sertoli cells provide mechanical and nutritive support for the spermatogenic cells. Sertoli cells also secrete two hormones—inhibin and activin—which provide positive and negative feedback on FSH secretion from the pituitary.

Interstitial Tissue

Leydig cells (15–20 μm), located in the interstitial tissue between the convoluted seminiferous tubules, constitute the endocrine component of the testis. They synthesize

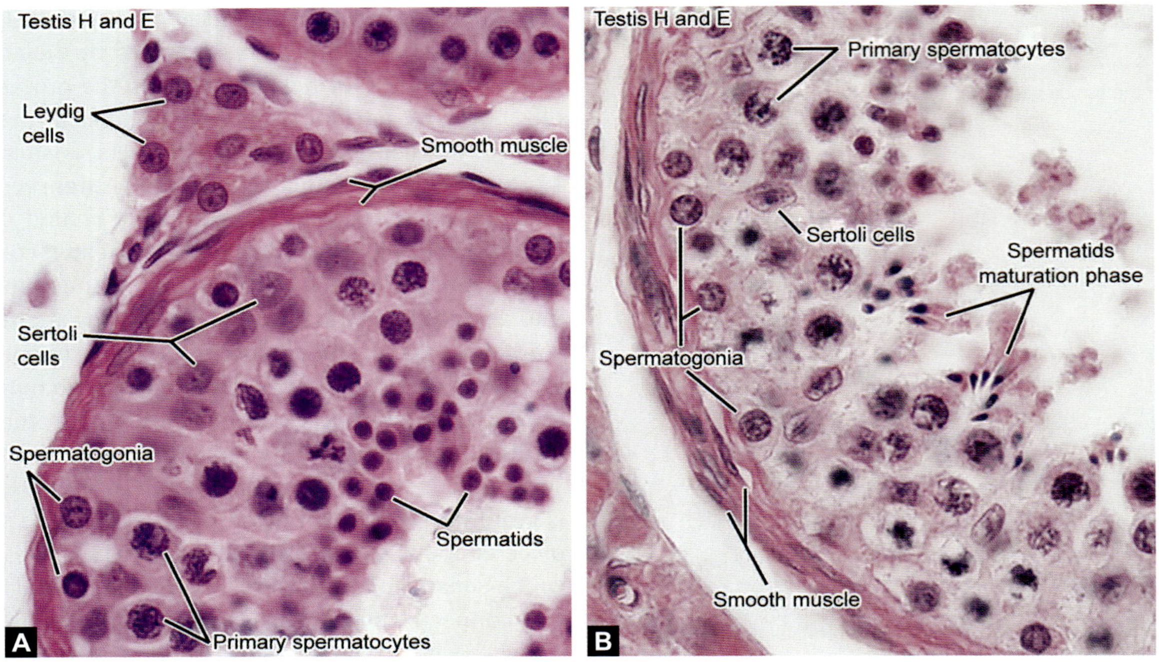

Figs. 16.6A and B: Histology of the interstitial tissue.

and secrete testosterone. Leydig cells occur in clusters, which are variable in size and richly supplied by capillaries. The cytoplasm is strongly acidophilic and finely granular. The nucleus is large, round, and often located eccentric in the cell (Figs. 16.6A and B).

Ducts of the Testis

Spermatozoa pass via the tubuli recti (low columnar epithelium) and the rete testis (flattened or cuboidal epithelium) into numerous ductuli efferentes, which are lined by a columnar epithelium, which consists of both absorptive and ciliated cells. The height of the two cells types, which form the epithelium of the ductuli efferentes is variable which gives the lumen a characteristic wavy outline. The ductuli efferentes leave the testis and open into a common duct, the ductus epididymis. Most cells of the epithelium, also called principal cells, have long stereocilia. Stereocilia are non-motile structures, which in the electron microscope (EM) resemble large microvilli. Toward the basal lamina, we see a number of small nuclei, which belong to the basal cells of the ductus epididymis. These cells regenerate the epithelium. Peristaltic contractions of smooth muscle cells surrounding the ductus epididymis move the spermatozoa toward the middle segment of the duct, which is the site of final functional maturation of the spermatozoa—now they are motile. The terminal segment of the ductus epididymis is the site of storage of the mature spermatozoa. Smooth muscle fibers of the terminal part of the ductus epididymis do not contract spontaneously. They contract during sexual stimulation concurrently with the contraction of the musculature of the duct into which it opens, the vas deferens.

Vas Deferens (Ductus Deferens)

The mucosa of the vas deferens forms low longitudinal folds. It is lined by a pseudostratified columnar epithelium. Similar to the epididymis, cells have long stereocilia. The lamina propria is unusually rich in elastic fibers. The muscularis is well developed and consists of a thick circular layer of smooth muscle between thinner inner and outer longitudinal layers. The muscularis is the structure, which makes the vas deferens palpable in the spermatic cord. The vas deferens is surrounded by an adventitia, which is slightly denser than usual (Figs. 16.7A and B).

Male Accessory Reproductive Glands

The accessory (or secondary) male sex glands consist of the seminal vesicles, the prostate, and the bulbourethral glands.

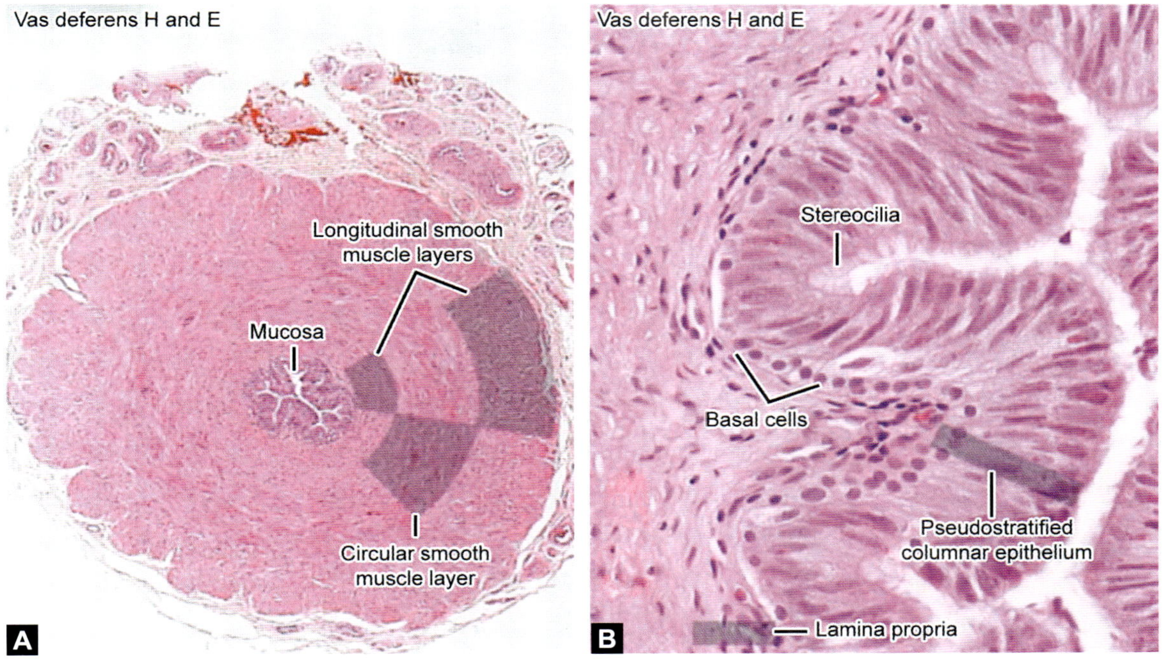

Figs. 16.7A and B: Histology of the vas deferens.

Prostate: The prostate is the largest accessory sex gland in men. It contains 30–50 tubuloalveolar glands, which empty into 15–25 independent excretory ducts. These ducts open into the urethra. The glands are embedded into a fibromuscular stroma, which mainly consists of smooth muscle separated by strands of connective tissue rich in collagenous and elastic fibers. The muscle forms a dense mass around the urethra and beneath the fairly thin capsule of the prostate. The secretory alveoli of the prostate are very irregularly shaped because of papillary projections of the mucosa into the lumen of the gland. The epithelium is cuboidal or columnar. Basal cells are again present, and the epithelium may look pseudostratified where they are found. The secretory cells are slightly acidophilic and secretory granules may be visible in the cytoplasm. Small extensions of the apical cytoplasm into the lumen of the alveoli may represent cells, which release their secretory products (secretion is apocrine/merocrine). The secretion of the prostate contains citric acid, the enzyme fibrinolysin (liquefies the semen), acid phosphatase, a number of other enzymes, and lipids. The secretion of the prostate is the first fraction of the ejaculate. The secretory ducts of the prostate are lined by a simple columnar epithelium, which changes to a transitional epithelium near the openings of the ducts into the urethra (Figs. 16.8A and B).

Seminal vesicles: The seminal vesicles develop from the vas deferens. Their histological organization resembles to some extent that of the vas deferens. All the lumina visible in sections of the seminal vesicle are in continuity in the intact organ. The mucosa shows thin, branched, anastomosing folds. The structure of the epithelium is variable appearing columnar or pseudostratified columnar. The lamina propria of the mucosa is fairly thin and loose. The muscularis consists of inner circular and outer longitudinal layers of smooth muscle. Seminal vesicles were thought to store semen—hence their name. This turned out to be wrong. They are glands, whose secretion constitutes 60–70% of the ejaculate. The secretory product of the columnar cell, which may be seen in the lumen of the seminal vesicles, is strongly acidophilic. It contains large amounts of fructose, which the spermatozoa utilize as a source of energy. Furthermore, the secretion contains prostaglandins, flavins (yellow fluorescing pigment—of use in forensic medicine to detect semen stains) and several other proteins and enzymes.

The cocktail of compounds, which is released by the seminal vesicles in addition to fructose has three main functions:

1. Formation of the sperm coagulum,
2. Regulation of sperm motility, and

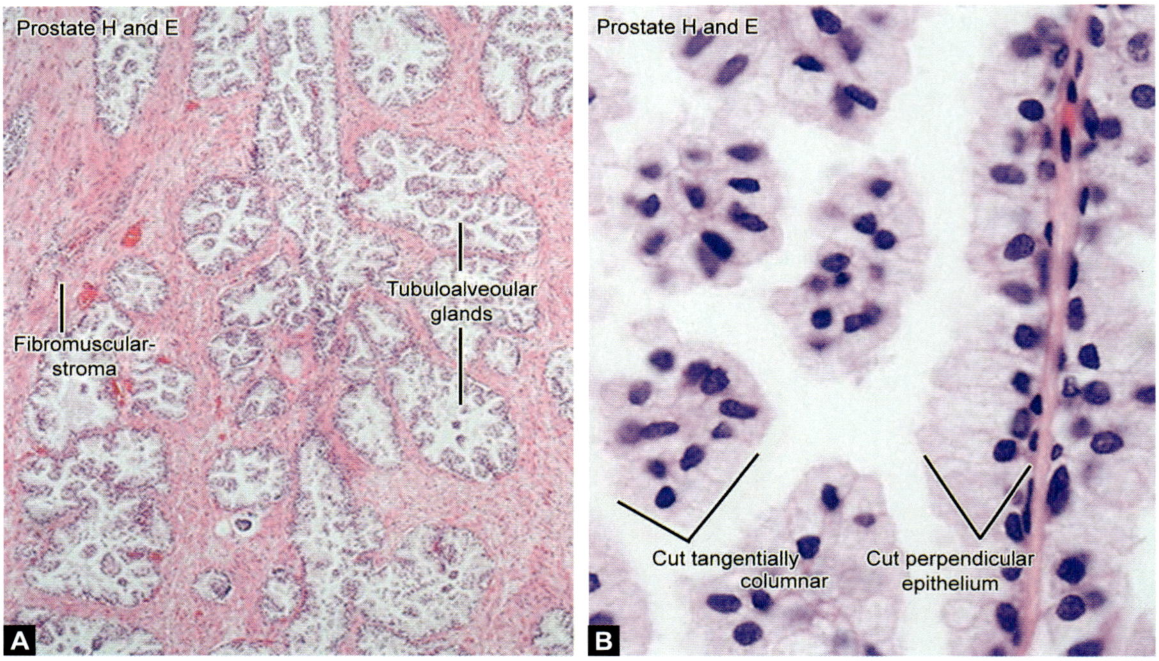

Figs. 16.8A and B: Histology of the prostate gland.

3. Suppression of immune function in the female genital tract.

The secretion of the seminal vesicles is the third fraction of the ejaculate (Figs. 16.9A and B) (the spermatozoa are released with the second fraction—the contents of the vas deferens).

STAGES OF SPERMATOGENESIS

Spermatogenesis is the sequence of developmental events by which spermatogonial stem cells give rise to functional spermatozoa. This process takes place in the seminiferous tubules of the male testis. In the mammalian testis, spermatogonia arise from primordial germ cells, which migrate into the developing testis during fetal life. Here, they become associated with the differentiating Sertoli cells, and seminiferous cords are formed. In this setting, they transform into gonocytes, which remain centrally placed, surrounded by the immature Sertoli cells. Following a period of multiplication, the gonocytes migrate to the basement membrane of the seminiferous tubule where they divide to form type A spermatogonia. Spermatogenesis can be divided into three stages:

1. Spermatogonial stage—mitotic clonal expansion
2. Meiotic stage—production of the haploid gamete
3. Spermiogenesis stage—morphological changes of spermatids into spermatozoa (Fig. 16.10)

Spermatogonial Stage

The first phase of spermatogenesis begins with the division of the spermatogonia that line the seminiferous tubule near the basement membrane. Type A spermatogonia divide to maintain the population of the stem cell pool. Some spermatogonia resulting from these mitotic divisions stay in the resting pool and do not differentiate, while the remaining type A spermatogonia proliferate and undergo several stages of division and differentiation. The number of spermatogonial cell types identified varies between species. In the human, type A pale, type A dark, and type B spermatogonial cells can be distinguished. In the rodent testis, multiple type A spermatogonia, intermediate, and type B spermatogonia have been identified (Fig. 16.11).

Meiotic Stage

The type B spermatogonia enter the preleptotene stage of the meiotic process. They are then termed primary spermatocytes (Fig. 16.12). The primary spermatocytes (ploidy = 4n) undergo the two divisions of meiosis. During the first meiotic division, each morphologic chromosome (actually two sister chromatids) aligns at the cell equator paired with its homologous partner. During this alignment, recombination between the homologous chromosomes can occur. One homologue (with both sister

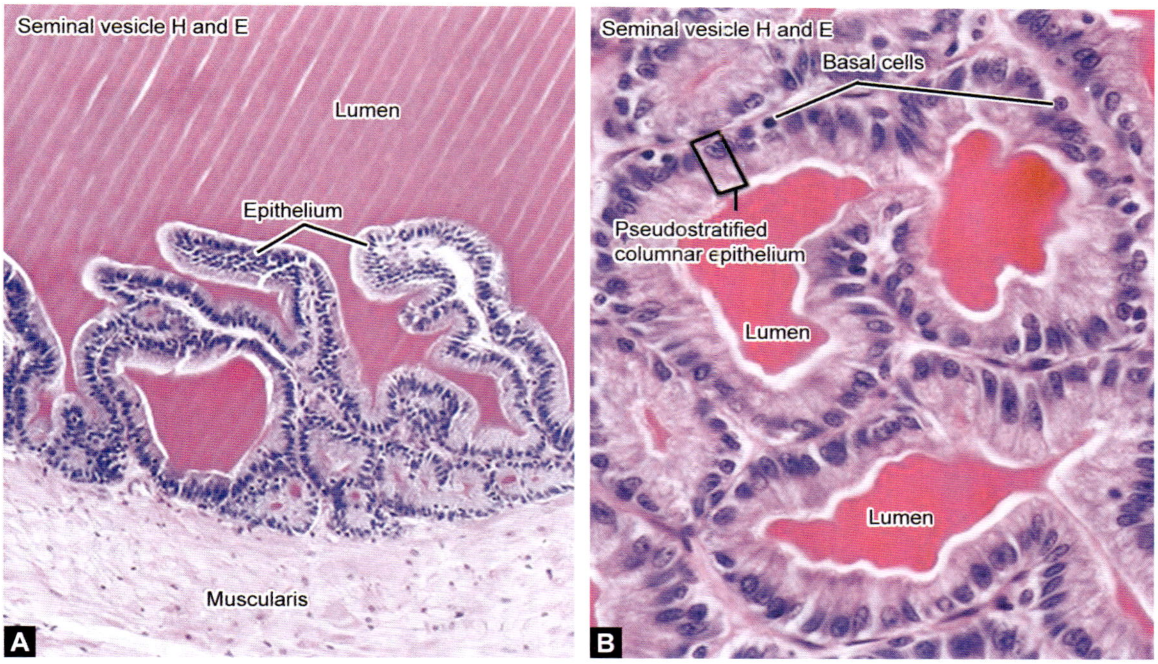

Figs. 16.9A and B: Histology of the seminal vesicle.

chromatids) is randomly selected to travel to one daughter cell, the other homologue of that chromosome goes into the other cell. No division of centromeres occurs, however, and the sister chromatids remain together. Cells passing through the prophase of the first meiotic division can be subdivided on a cytological basis into preleptotene, leptotene, zygotene, pachytene, and diplotene stage. During the second division, the centromeres do divide, as in mitosis, and one sister chromatid (now an independent chromosome) of each morphologic type is apportioned into each haploid daughter cell (ploidy = 1n). The resulting cell is termed round spermatid.

Maturation/Spermiogenesis Stage

In this stage, the round spermatid enters spermiogenesis, the third part of spermatogenesis. During this process, numerous nuclear and cytoplasmic changes occur in the spermatids, eventually leading to the formation of the spermatozoa. Restructuring of the cell includes:

- Nuclear condensation and movement of the nucleus to the periphery of the cell.
- Formation of a modified lysosome known as the acrosome, which becomes attached to the surface of the nucleus in opposition to the cell membrane.
- Flagellar formation, which includes the development of a core of microtubules, the axoneme, arises from one of the centrioles of the round spermatid. Later modifications of the axoneme lead to the formation of the tail.
- Following the completion of these events, the spermatid sheds a large part of its cytoplasm as the residual body, which is phagocytosed by the Sertoli cell. The process of spermiogenesis ends with release of the spermatozoa from the Sertoli cell. The spermatozoa are still immotile when released and must mature further during storage and transition in the epididymis (Figs. 16.13 and 16.14).[1]

Spermiation

This is the process by which mature spermatid (spermatozoa) are released into the lumen of the seminiferous tubule. After the release of the spermatozoa, the rest of the cytoplasm remains embedded in the Sertoli cells as residual bodies, which are eventually catabolized. The new released spermatozoa still have a residue of cytoplasm called the cytoplasmic droplet, attached at the point of separation. This droplet prevents forward swimming by the sperm and gets discarded during the process of maturation.[6]

Key events are the remodeling of the spermatid nucleus and cytoplasm to produce the spermatozoon, removal of Sertoli cell "ectoplasmic specialization" (ES) junctions and retraction of Sertoli cell cytoplasm, and extension of the

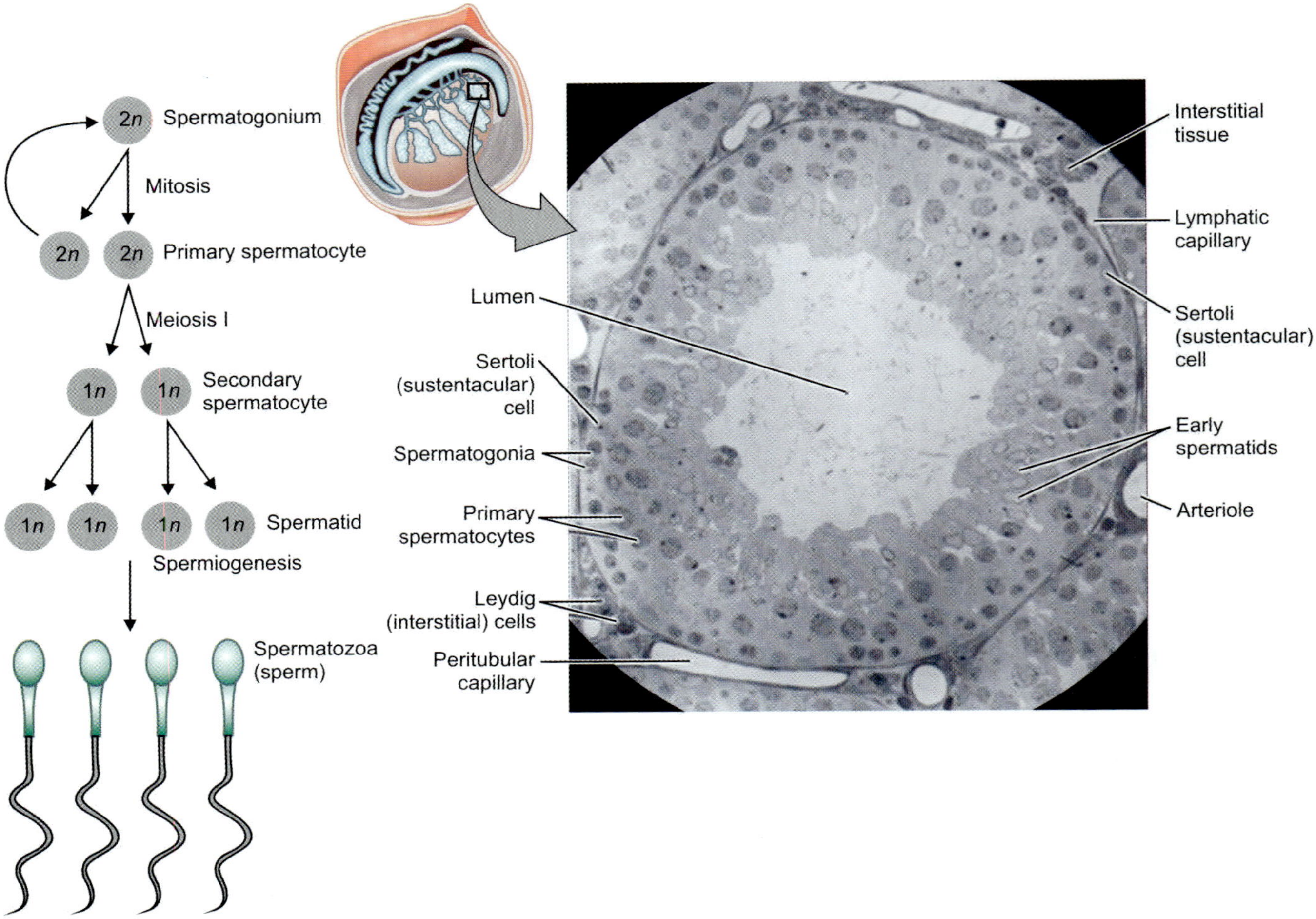

Fig. 16.10: Mammalian spermatogenesis: Spermatogenesis takes place in the seminiferous tubules of the testis. During differentiation, the germ cells, surrounded by Sertoli cells, migrate toward the lumen of the tubules, from where they are released to the epididymis. Spermatogonial stem cells at the basement membrane mitotically divide and give rise to differentiating spermatogonia.

spermatid into the lumen. Spermiation ends with release of the spermatid (now known as the spermatozoon) into the lumen and the phagocytosis of the remainder of the residual body by the Sertoli cell (Fig. 16.15).

SPERMATOGENESIS WAVES

If one closely examines serial cross-sections of a seminiferous tubule, you will discover that sperm cells differentiate in distinctive associations. Each spermatogenic association has been classified as a stage of the seminiferous epithelial cycle. A spermatogenic cycle is defined as the time it takes for the reappearance of the same stage within a given segment of the tubule. Each stage of the cycle follows in an orderly sequence along the length of the tubule. The distance between the same stage is called the spermatogenic wave. One tubule can contain numerous complete waves. Adjacent segments of the tubule evidently communicate in some unknown manner.

The number of stages within a spermatogenic cycle and the number of cycles required for the completion of spermatogenesis varies between species. Six stages have been noted in man; four 16-day cycles are needed to complete spermatogenesis (Fig. 16.16).

As in the diagram, spermatogenesis waves moves in spirals—like a corkscrew—toward the inner part of the lumen. Outside, on the edge of the tubule and at the beginning of the spiral, lie the spermatogonia; at the end of the spiral, the fully developed sperm cells are in the lumen. From the diagram, it can be seen that several differing generations can be found in a tubule cross-section. As the time goes on, the wave of spermatogenesis is shifted toward the right in order to always newly begin again.

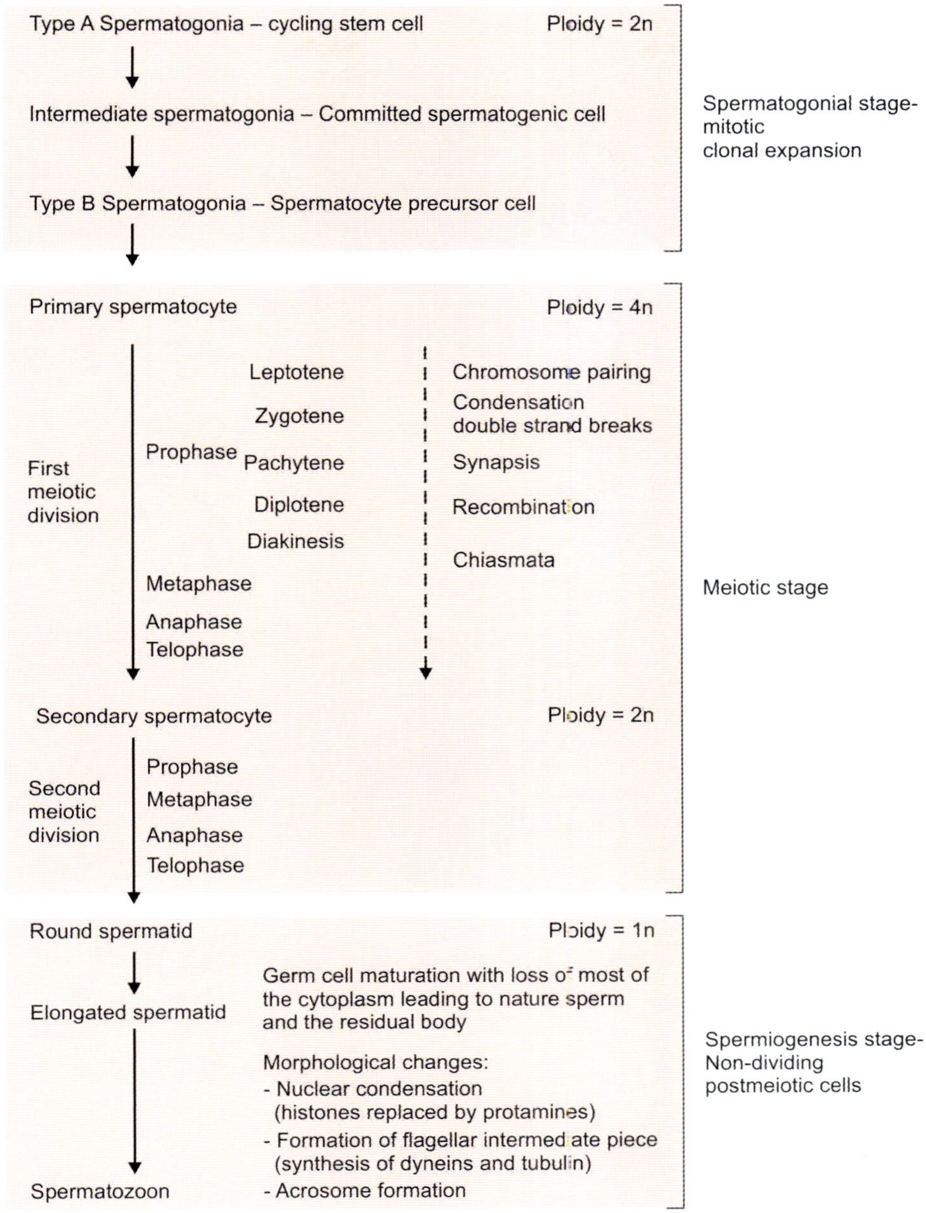

Fig. 16.11: Individual phases of spermatogenesis and their respective cell types. Spermatogenesis can be divided into three distinct phases. Shown are the specific processes and the terms for their respective cell types occurring during these stages.[7,8]

SPERM APOPTOSIS

A fundamental feature of apoptosis in the mature spermatozoon is that this process represents a default position for the cell. Indeed, it is the fate of every spermatozoon in the ejaculate to undergo an apoptotic death, apart from the few spermatozoa that achieve immortality by successfully fertilizing oocytes. For most spermatozoa, apoptosis is not induced but is a spontaneous consequence of their strenuous attempts to reach the oocyte and engage in the process of fertilization. When spermatozoa are inseminated into the female reproductive tract, they are incapable of recognizing the egg or engaging in the cascade of cellular interactions that will culminate in fertilization (Fig. 16.17).

Apoptosis is an essential part of spermatogenesis that keeps the number of proliferating germ cells in check so that their numbers are within the supportive limit of the Sertoli cells.

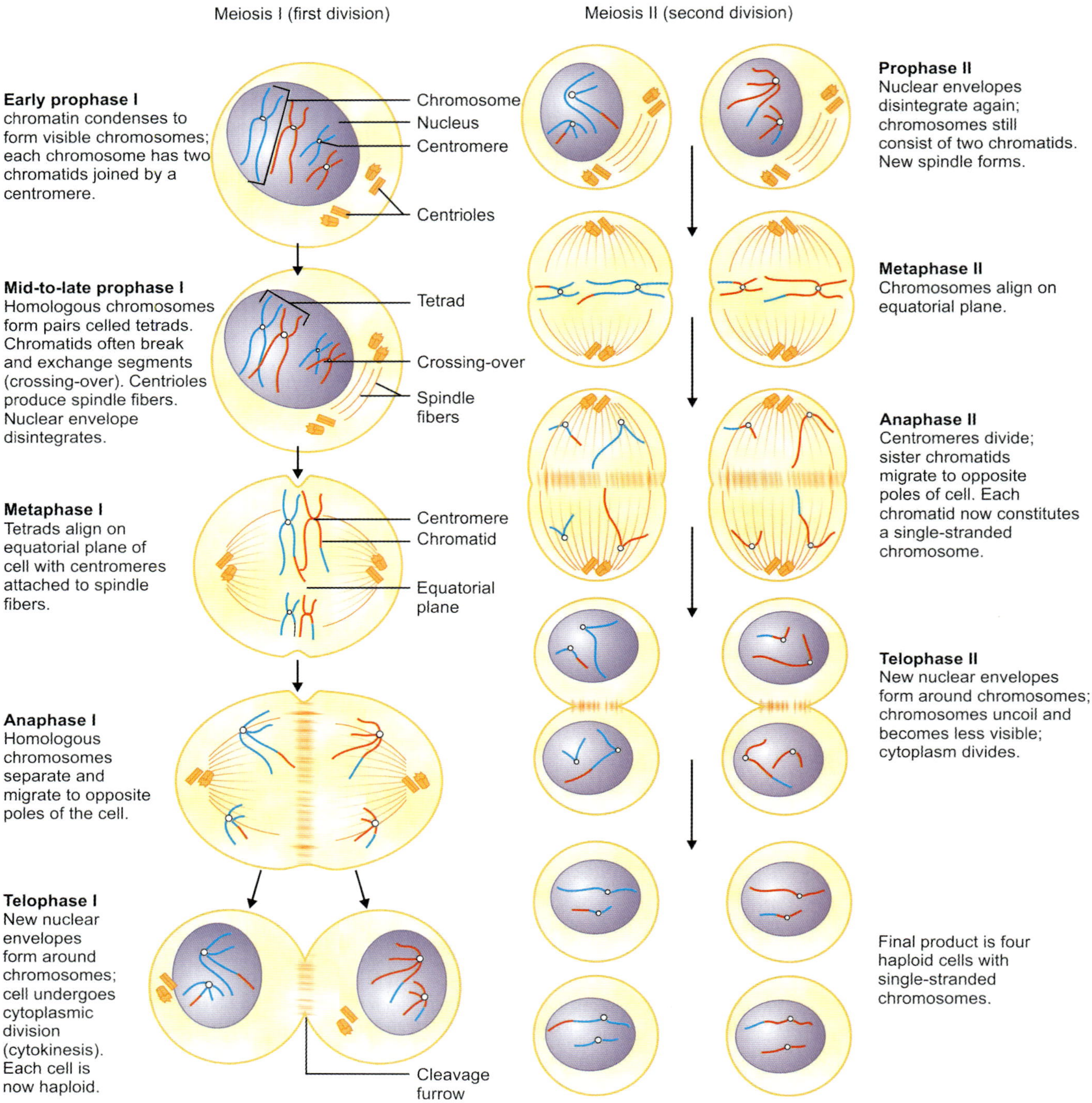

Fig. 16.12: Meiosis.[7,8]

STRUCTURE OF A MATURE SPERM

The human sperm cell is the reproductive cell in males and will only survive in warm environments; once it leaves the male body, the sperm's survival likelihood is reduced and it may die, thereby decreasing the total sperm quality (Fig. 16.18).

Human sperm cells consist of a flat, disc-shaped head 5.1 μm by 3.1 μm and a tail 50 μm long. Semen has an alkaline nature, and they do not reach full motility (hypermotility)

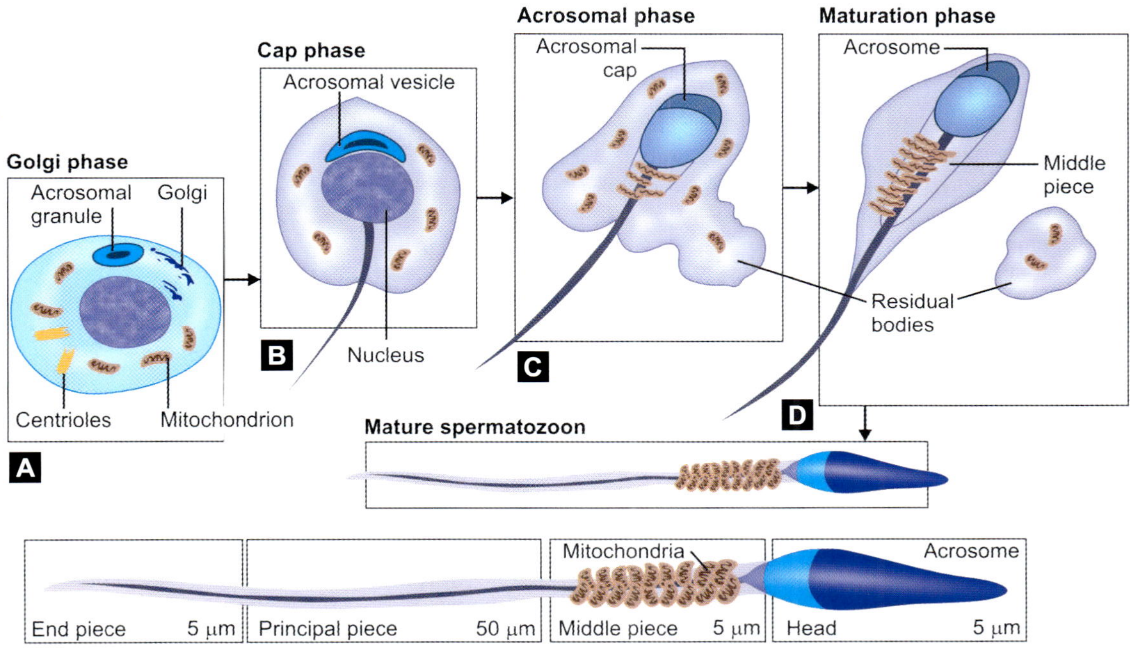

Figs. 16.13A to D: Four phases of spermiogenesis.[9] (A) Golgi phase: Acrosomic vesicle formation. (B) Cap phase: Acrosomic vesicle spreads over the nucleus of the round spermatid and the flagellum starts to form. (C) Acrosomal phase: The spermatid nucleus and cytoplasm elongates; acrosome covers the majority of the anterior nucleus. (D) Maturation phase: Mitochondria are assembled around the flagellum and the flagellum is completely formed.

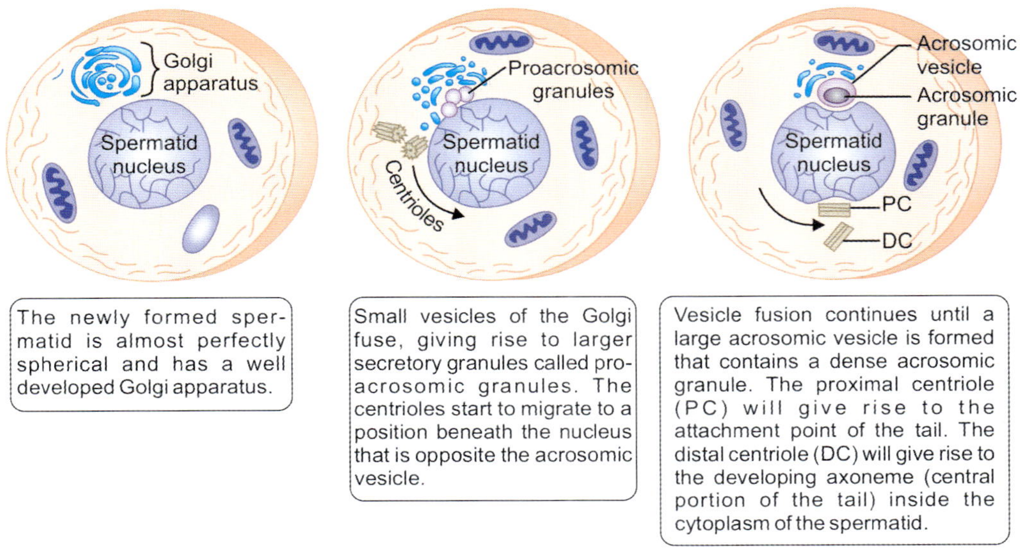

Fig. 16.14A: Golgi phase of spermatid differentiation.

until they reach the vagina where the alkaline pH is neutralized by acidic vaginal fluids. This gradual process takes 20–30 minutes. In this time, fibrinogen from the seminal vesicles forms a clot, securing and protecting the sperm. Just as they become hypermotile, fibrinolysin from the prostate dissolves the clot, allowing the sperm to progress optimally.[9,10]

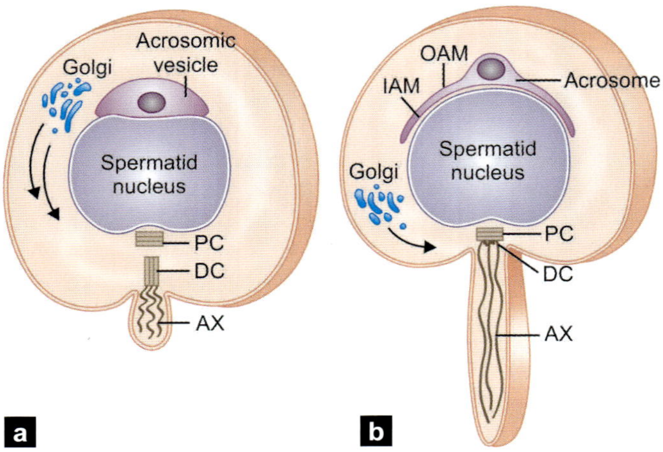

Fig. 16.14B: CAP phase. (a) The Golgi migrates toward the caudal part of the cell. The distal centriole (DC) forms the axoneme (AX) or flagellum that projects away from the nucleus toward the lumen of the seminiferous tubule. (b) The acrosomic vesicle flattens and begins to form a distinct cap consisting of an outer acrosomal membrane (OAM), an inner acrosomal membrane (IAM), and the acrosomal contents (enzymes).

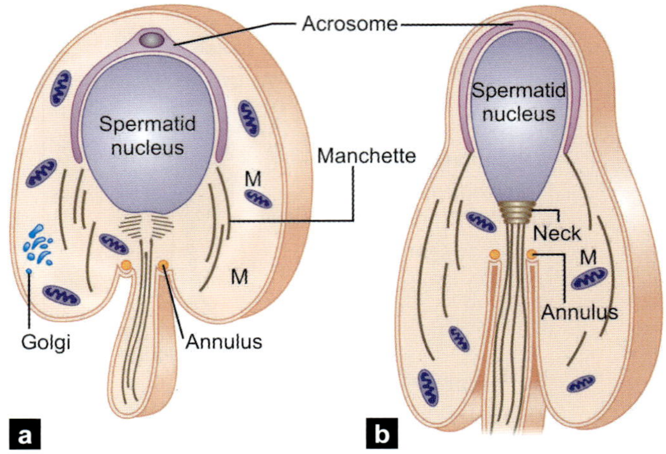

Fig. 16.14C: Acrosome phase. (a) The spermatid nucleus begins to elongate and the acrosome eventually covers the majority of the anterior nucleus. The machete forms in the region of the caudal half of the nucleus and extends down toward the developing flagellum. (b) The neck and the annulus are formed and the later will become the juncture between the middle piece and the principle piece. Notice that all components of the developing spermatids are completely surrounded by a plasma membrane. (M = Mitochondria)

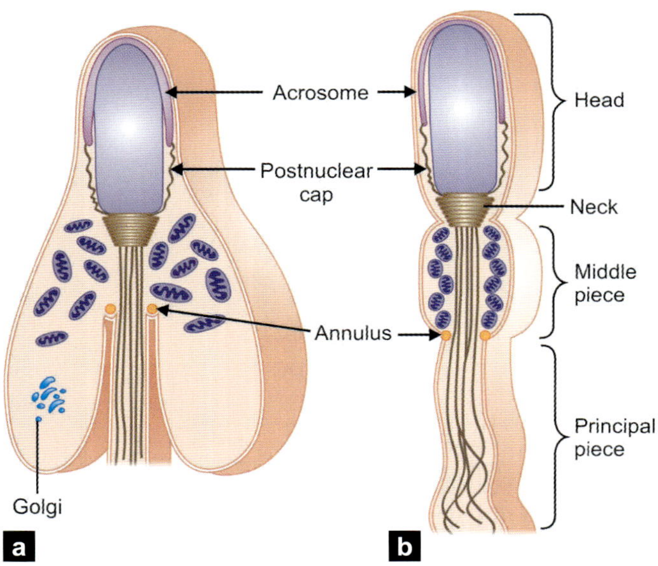

Fig. 16.14D: Maturation phases a and b. Mitochondria form a spiral assembly around the flagellum that defines the middle piece. The postnuclear cap is formed from the manchette microtubules. The annulus forms the juncture between the middle piece and the principle piece.

Peculiarities of a Mature Sperm

- Only cell which do not grow or divide
- A haploid cell
- Unique DNA chromatin condensation achieving high level of DNA stabilization using protamines
- Only human cell with motility
- Only human cell with flagellum
- Only human cell without cytoplasm
- Only human cell having an acrosome cap

Structure

Head

- Flattened ovoid structure
- Consist primarily of nucleus
- Dimension: 4–5.5 µm in length, 2.5–3.5 µm in width, 1.5 µm in height
- Length to width ratio: 1.5–1.7[11]
- Acrosome is a cap-like structure covering two-thirds of the head
- Posterior region is covered by a single membrane called the postnuclear cap
- The overlap of acrosome and postnuclear cap results in the equatorial segment (Fig. 16.19).[12]

Acrosome

- Hydrolytic enzymes: hyaluronidase, proacrosin[10,13]
- Represented by Golgi complex

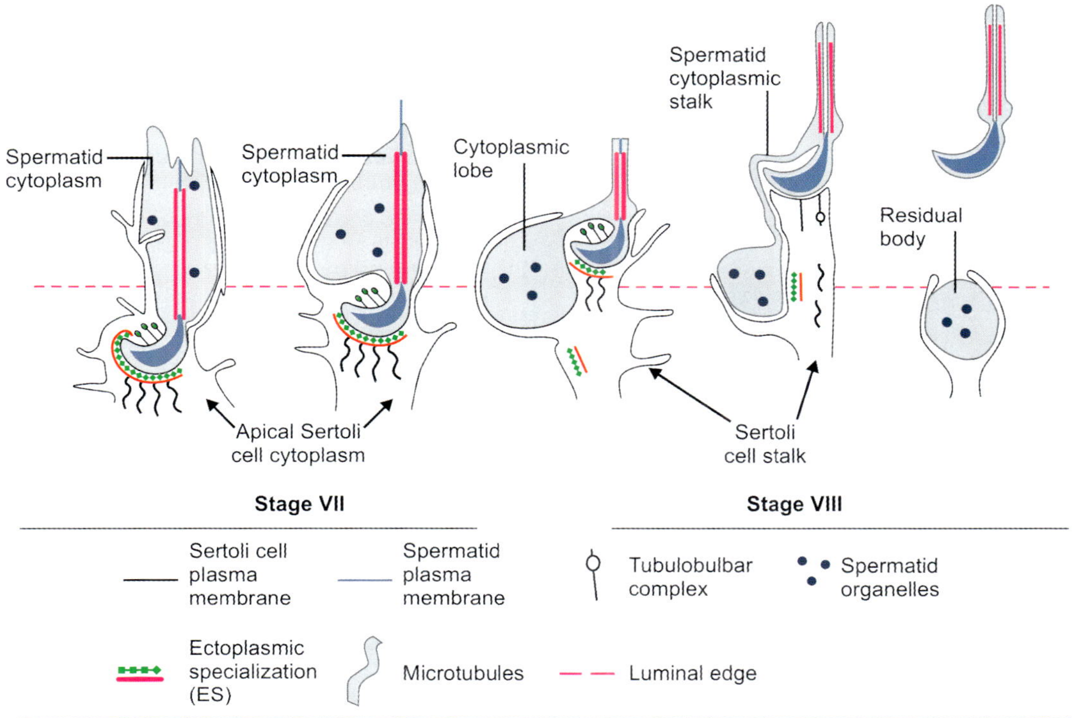

Fig. 16.15: Developmental stages of spermiogenesis.

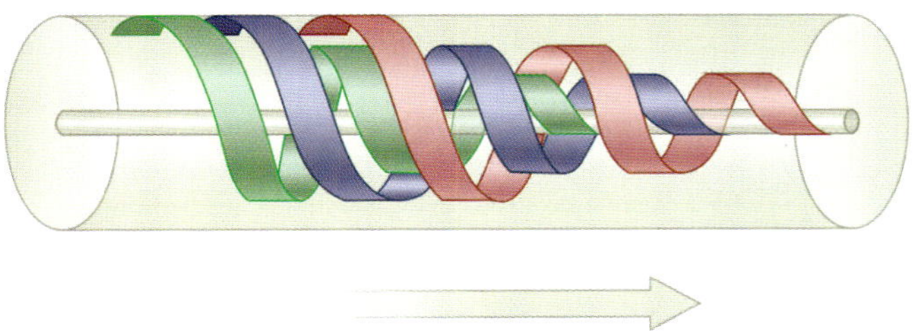

Fig. 16.16: Three waves of spermatogenesis generations.

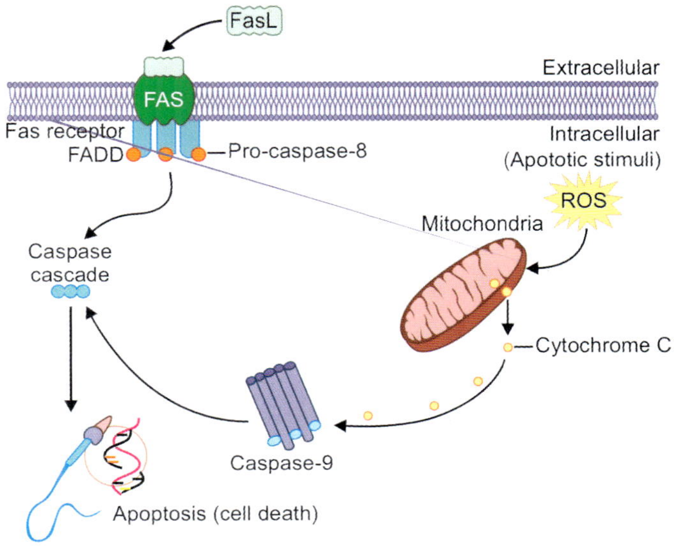

Fig. 16.17: Apoptosis in male infertility.

- It is a membrane bound vesicle
- The inner acrosomal membrane lies external to the nuclear membrane while the outer acrosomal membrane is just inside the sperm cell plasma membrane (Fig. 16.20).

Nucleus

- Comprises 65% of the head[10]
- Composed of DNA conjugated with protein
- The DNA is temporarily well protected in a semicrystalline structure stabilized by zinc.
- The chromatin is arranged like a “rope” with three intermingled strands: two DNA strands and a strand of protamines (Fig. 16.21).

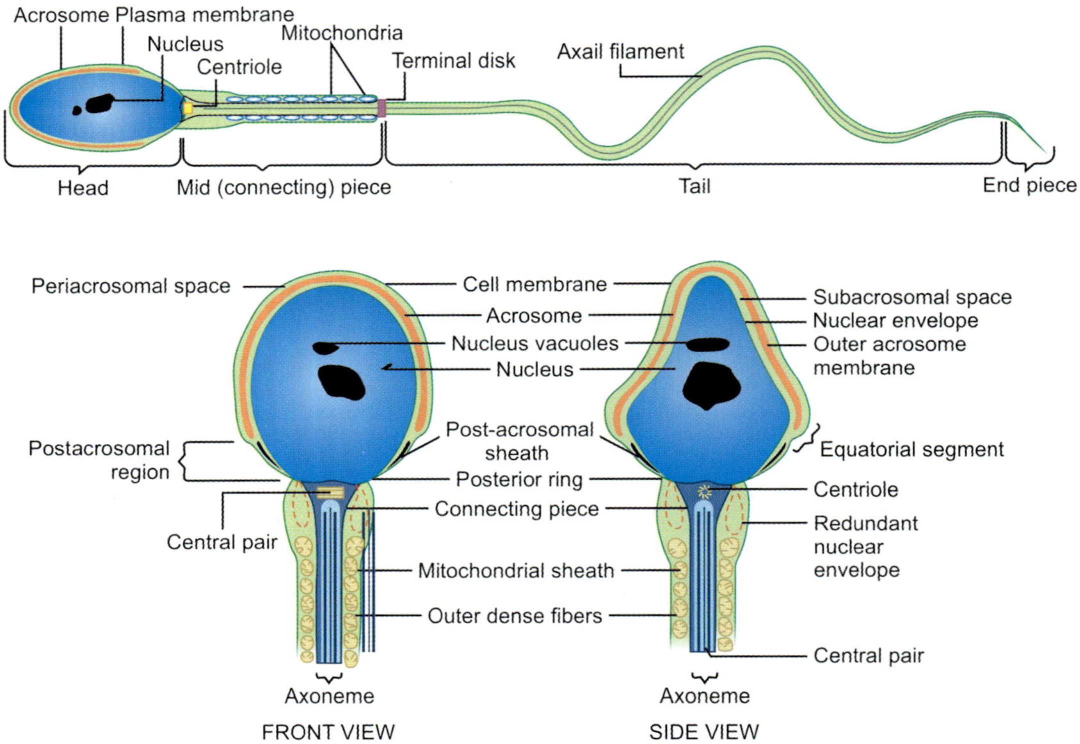

Fig. 16.18: A mature sperm.

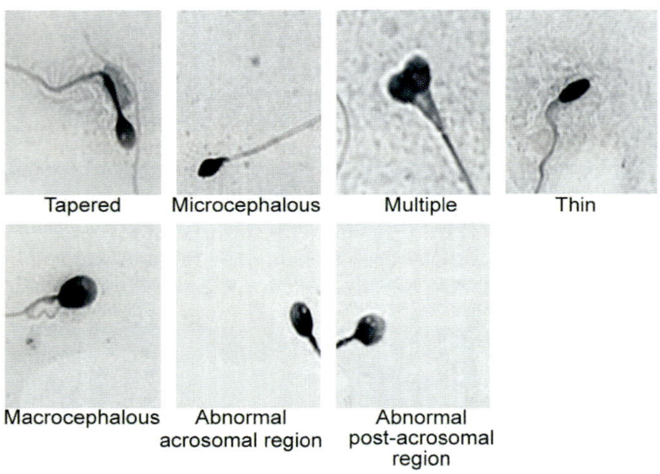

Fig. 16.19: Head defects of sperm.

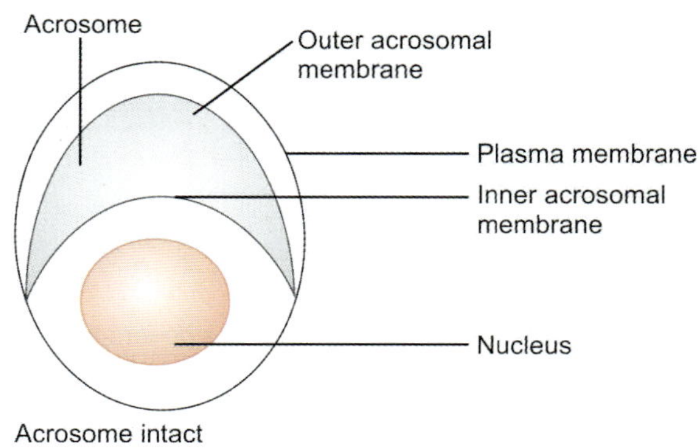

Fig. 16.20: Acrosome.

Neck

- It is small (around 1 μm). It connects the head and the middle piece.
- It contains proximal centriole and mitochondria. It provides energy for carrying device.
- It is 6–7 μm in length.
- It is quite the slender region and there are no organelles except one or two longitudinally oriented mitochondria (Fig. 16.22).

Midpiece

- Possess the cytoplasmic portion and lipid-rich mitochondrial sheath that consists of several spiral mitochondria surrounding the axial filament in a helical fashion[13]

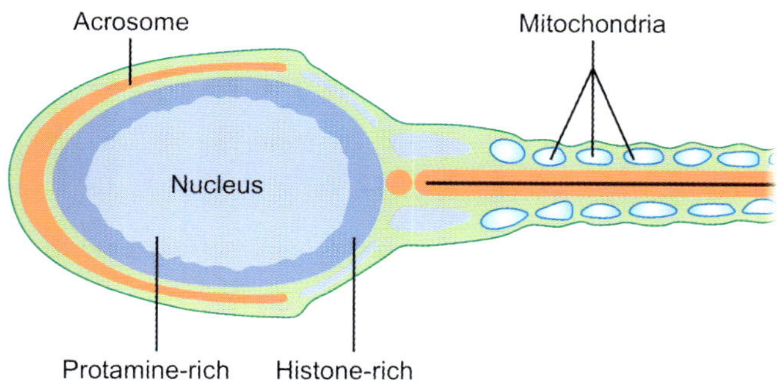

Fig. 16.21: Nucleus.

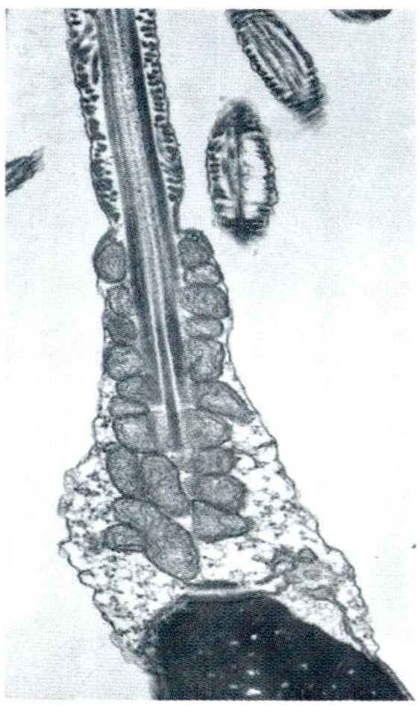

Fig. 16.23: Midpiece.

- It provides the sperm with the energy for motility (Fig. 16.23).

Sperm Flagellum

- It is based upon a unique 9 + 2 arrangement of microtubules within the sperm flagellar axoneme.[13]
- There are nine peripheral, symmetrically arranged microtubule doublets connected doublet-to-doublet by dynein arms and to the sheath of central pair of microtubules by radial spokes.
- The outer doublets, but not the central pair, are paralleled by nine outer dense fibers that provide flexible, yet firm support during flagellar movement.
- It propels by waves, which are generated in the neck region and pass distally along like a whiplash.
- Dynein is a large protein with ATPase activity.

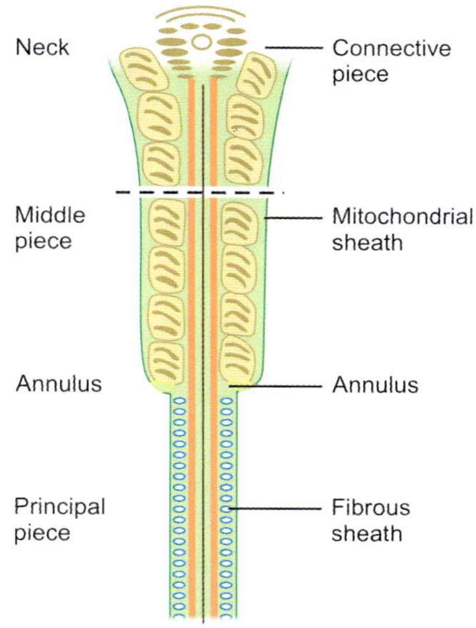

Fig. 16.22: Neck.

- Defects in the cilia and flagella of human cells are associated with some notable medical problems, a hereditary condition known as Kartagener syndrome. It is caused by problems with the dynein arms that extend between the microtubules present in the axoneme (Fig. 16.24).

Tail

- It arises at the spermatid stage.[13]
- It gives cell a straight-line movement.
- It contains the motility apparatus and is 40–55 μm long.
- The centriole differentiates into—midpiece, the main or principle piece, and endpiece.
- The mitochondria reorganize around the midpiece.

Principal piece:

- Longest part of the tail
- Provides the most of the propellant machinery
- The coarse nine fibrils of the outer ring diminish in diameter and finally disappear.

Endpiece:

- Tail terminates in the endpiece with a length of 4–10 μm and diameter of less than 1 μM.[13]
- The small diameter is due to the absence of the outer fibrous sheath and a distal fading of the microtubules (Figs. 16.25 and 16.26).

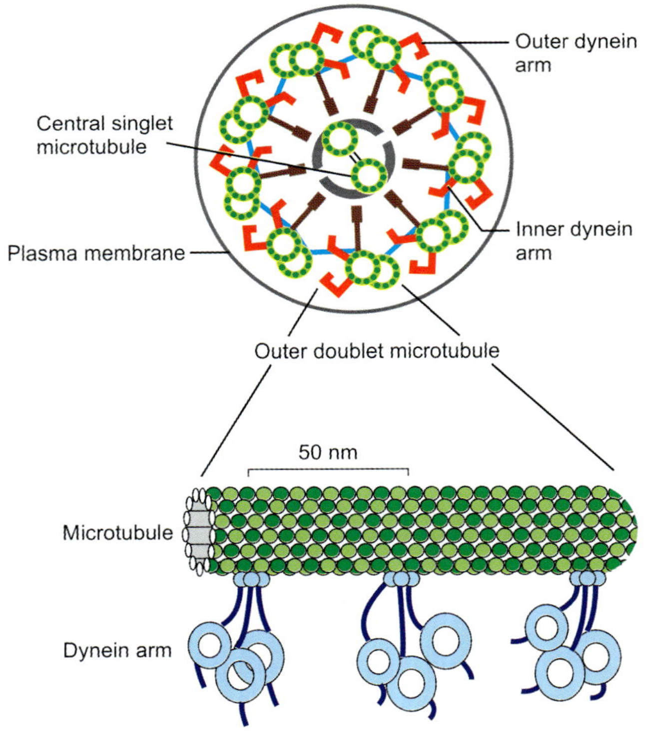

Fig. 16.24: Sperm flagellum.

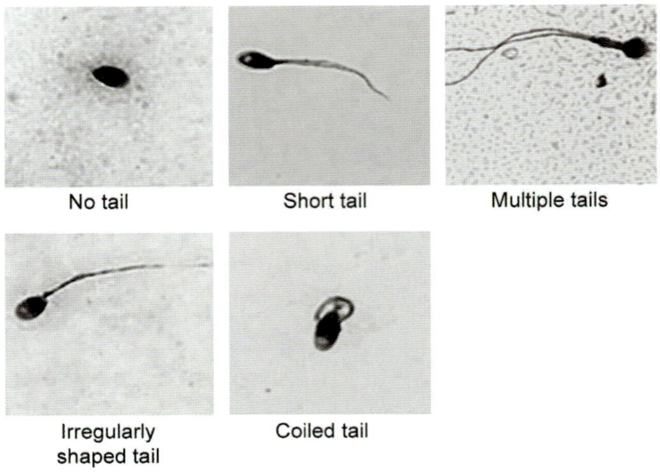

Fig. 16.25: Tail defects of spermatozoa.

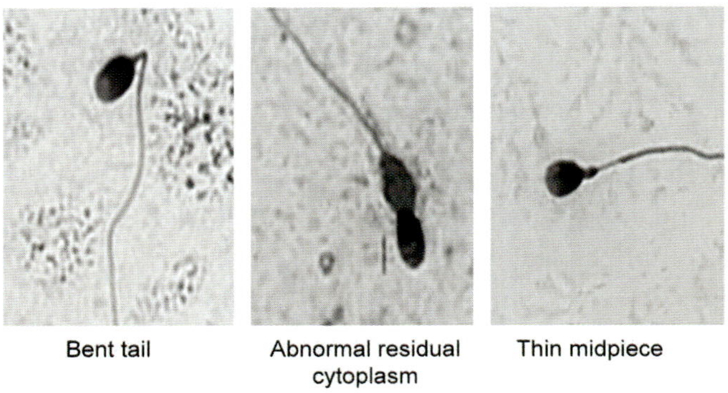

Fig. 16.26: Common sperm defects.

CHANGES IN FEMALE GENITAL TRACT

Transport of Sperm through Female Genital Tract

Vaginal Insemination

The complex process of sperm transport through the female reproductive tract begins at the time of ejaculation. During coitus, semen containing between 200 and 500 million sperm is deposited at the posterior vaginal fornix.

The optimal pH for sperm viability is between 7.0 and 8.5, and a reduction in sperm motility is seen at a pH less than 6.0. Normal vaginal pH is only 3.5–4.0, and the acidic environment of the vagina is thus toxic to sperm. However, both seminal fluid and cervical mucus present within the posterior vagina are alkaline and act as buffers. Vaginal pH rises to 7.0 within just seconds after ejaculation, and this decrease in acidity can be maintained for up to 2 hours after ejaculation.

Within about 1 minute after coitus, the ejaculate undergoes coagulation. This coagulum temporarily restricts movement of sperm out of the seminal clot, thus preventing their passage into the cervical mucus and movement up to the female reproductive tract. Over the next 20–30 minutes, however, a seminal-fluid proteolytic enzyme produced by the prostate gland gradually liquefies the clot. At this time, motile sperm may then enter the cervical mucus, leaving behind the seminal plasma. Although there are reports of motile sperm persisting within the vagina for up to 12 hours after ejaculation, motility of most vaginal sperm is diminished within about 30 minutes, and after 2 hours almost all sperm motility in the vagina has been lost.

Cervix:

Several important functions have been attributed to the cervix, and these include:

- Providing a receptive environment for sperm entry near the time of ovulation
- Preventing access of sperm, microorganisms, and particulate matter to the upper reproductive tract and thus, the peritoneal cavity

- Filtering spermatozoa and removal of seminal plasma[14]
- Preventing sperm phagocytosis by white blood cells within the female reproductive tract
- Providing a biochemical environment sufficient for sperm storage, capacitation, and migration

The structure of the human cervix facilitates performance of the these stated functions. Production of mucus is perhaps the most important function of the cervix. Cervical pH is alkaline, with a peak pH during the periovulatory period. This environment is much more hospitable to spermatozoa than the acidic pH of the vagina.

Cervical mucus: Cervical mucus is continuously secreted through exocytosis by the nonciliated epithelial cells that line the cervical canal. This biomaterial serves many important functions, including exclusion of seminal plasma, exclusion of morphologically abnormal sperm, and support of viable sperm for subsequent migration to the uterus and oviduct. The amount of mucus produced and its composition and characteristics fluctuate with circulating progesterone and estrogen levels. As estrogen levels peak at midcycle, cervical mucus is abundant in volume and thin in consistency because of increased water content. Under the influence of progesterone, water content decreases, and the mucus has a much higher viscosity.[14]

Sperm transport through the uterus: Sperm motility does not appear to be the only force directing the sperm toward the oviducts, because inert particles deposited within the uterus are transported to the Fallopian tubes. In the uterus, muscular contractions may enhance passage of sperm through the uterine cavity. A few thousand sperm swim through the uterotubal junctions to reach the Fallopian tubes (uterine tubes, oviducts) where sperm are stored in a reservoir, or at least maintained in a fertile state, by interacting with endosalpingeal (oviductal) epithelium.[15]

Fallopian tube: Sperm movement through the Fallopian tube relies on a combination of forces: intrinsic sperm motility, tubular muscular contraction, and fluid flow. Tubal fluid production is maximal at the time of ovulation, and this fluid sustains the sperm before fertilization. Tubal fluid may also facilitate both sperm capacitation and acrosomal reaction.

Although tens of millions to hundreds of millions of sperm are deposited in the vagina at the time of ejaculation, anatomic studies have shown that typically only hundreds of sperm are present in the oviduct at various postcoital time points. The tubal fluid potentiates the motility and viability of spermatozoa, thus enhancing the chances of fertilization.

Sperm Capacitation and the Acrosome Reaction

Capacitation is commonly regarded as the reversible, prefertilization activation process of sperm, which results in the spermatozoa gaining the ability to (Fig. 16.27):[16]

1. Develop hyperactivated motility
2. Bind to the zona pellucida
3. Undergo the acrosome reaction
4. Proceed eventually to fusion with the oolemma and egg fertilization

After the ejaculation, the sperm cells go through several essential physiological changes during the time in the female genital tract before they are able to penetrate the oocyte membrane. The first change in this cascade is *capacitation*. The sperm cells accomplish this, during the movement through the female genital tract, when in contact with its secretions. During capacitation the sperm cell membranes undergoes a physiological maturation process, which is seen as the precondition for the next step to follow, namely the acrosome reaction.

Capacitation is a functional maturation of a spermatozoa. The changes take place via the sperm cell membrane in which, the receptors are made available through the removal of a glycoprotein layer. The area of the acrosomal cap is also so altered thereby that the acrosome reaction becomes possible. Through the membrane alterations, the motile properties of the spermatozoon also change. *Discharging whipping movements of the tail* together with larger sideways *swinging movements of the head* take place. This type of motility is designated as hyperactivity. One can therefore say that the visible consequences of capacitation consist in hyperactivity of the spermatozoon.[16]

Capacitation occurs during transport in the female genital tract. It involves a number of changes including changes in the sperm cell membrane and signal transduction events.

Major changes occur in sperm cell membrane during capacitation:

- Changes in surface glycoproteins caused by secretions of the female genital tract
- Cholesterol is removed possibly leading to an increase fluidity of the sperm cell membrane

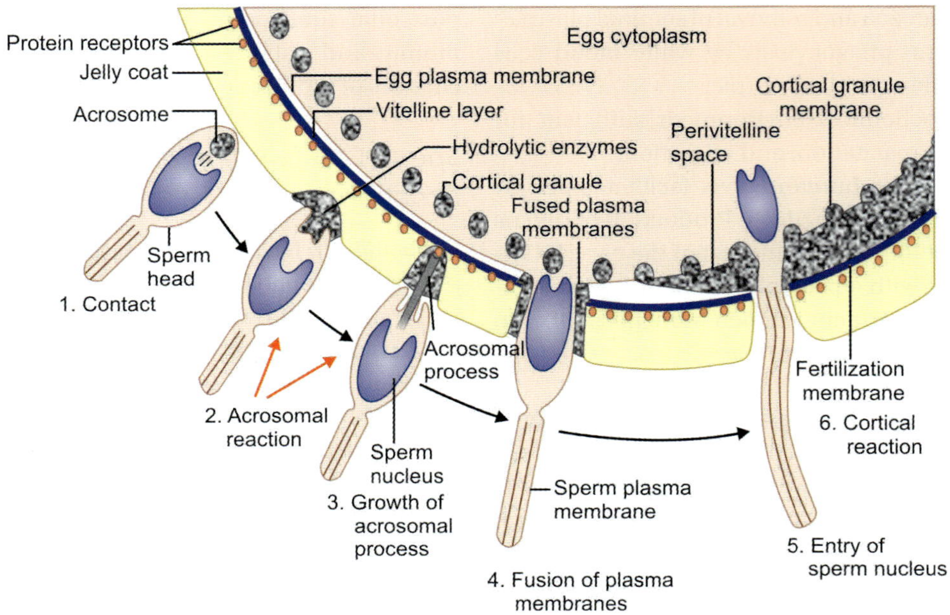

Fig. 16.27: Capacitation.

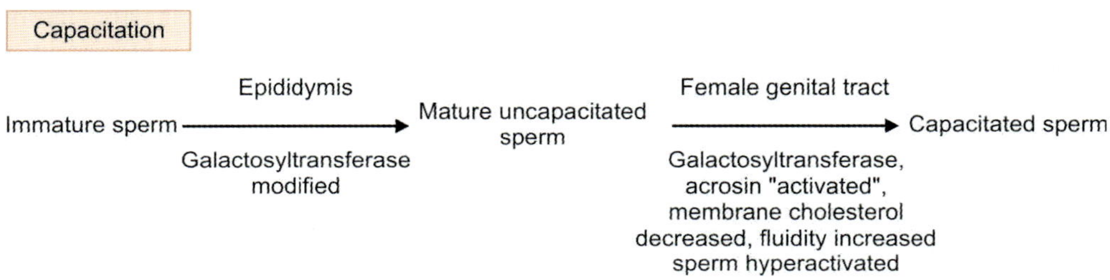

Fig. 16.28: Current model of human capacitation.

- Glycoproteins are lost which may expose the zona binding proteins
- Proteins are phosphorylated

Current model of human capacitation: This is shown in Figure 16.28.

Signal transduction events during capacitation:[17]

- Fluctuations occur in the intracellular levels of calcium ions; essential for hyperactivation
- Certain proteins are phosphorylated by tyrosine kinases under the influence of cAMP, which has been shown to be absolutely required for human sperm cell capacitation.

Effects of capacitation on sperm:

- Increased rate of metabolism
- Hyperactivation: flagellum beats more rapidly
- Changes in sperm glycoproteins allow sperm-egg binding
- Pro-Acrosin (inactive) is converted to acrosin (active)

Some Major Acrosomal Enzymes

The acrosome lies at the front end of the sperm cell just below the cell membrane. It is derived from the Golgi and, because of its content of digestive enzymes, is now considered to be a specialized lysosome-related organelle. The enzymes contained within the acrosome are designed to penetrate the egg coats during fertilization. Here is a list of those that have been characterized in humans.[16,17]

Protein digestion:

- Acid proteinase: A general protease that hydrolyzes protein at an acid pH
- Collagenase: A protease that digests collagen

- Acrosin: A special human acrosomal protease that digests zona pellucida proteins may also mediate sperm-zona pellucida binding.

Carbohydrate digestion:
- Beta-glucuronidase: An enzyme that removes beta-glucuronic acid residues from carbohydrates[16]
- Hyaluronidase: An enzyme that digests carbohydrates containing hyaluronic acid residues
- Neuraminidase: An enzyme that cleaves neuraminic (sialic) acid residues from carbohydrates

Lipid digestion:
- Phospholipase C: A lipase that hydrolyzes phosphoinositol phospholipids, in this case, in the egg membrane

Human acrosin:
- Acrosomal serine protease
- Bound to the inner surface of acrosomal membrane
- Digests pathway through the zona pellucida which is primarily made up of three proteins: ZP1, ZP2, and ZP3
- May act with other proteins to mediate the species-specific binding of sperm to the zona and hold the sperm cell in place as it digests its way through the zona.[16-18]

Cortical granules:
- The cortical granules are membrane bound vesicles that lie just below egg cell membrane.
- Many enzymes for protein and carbohydrate digestion
- Exocytosis occurs at fertilization
- Enzymes contained in the cortical granules will digest the proteins of the zona pellucida (i.e. ZP3, ZP2) to prevent more sperm binding which could lead to polyspermy.[16-18]

Acrosome Reaction

The mature human ovum possesses a number of surrounding layers that must be penetrated by the spermatozoa for normal fertilization to occur. To assist with this task, the spermatozoa has a cap-like region called the acrosome covering the anterior 80% of its head. This structure contains a number of digestive enzymes, such as hyaluronidase, corona-penetrating enzyme, and acrosin, to facilitate membrane fusion and sperm entry into the ovum.

Ultrastructurally, the acrosome reaction involves regional fusion of areas of the outer acrosomal membrane and the overlying sperm plasma membrane. These fused areas then lyse, serving as portals through which soluble contents of the acrosome can be dispersed to act on the vestments of the ovum.

The acrosome reaction is initiated as the spermatozoa arrives at the ovum. The outermost covering of the ovum, the cumulus oophorus, is degraded by hyaluronidase located on the plasma membrane of the spermatozoa. Subsequently, corona-penetrating enzyme is released to facilitate spermatozoal transit through the corona radiata. After transit through the corona radiata is completed, the sperm binds to the zona pellucida. Next, proacrosin, a zymogen within the acrosomal region, is converted to acrosin, and this facilitates breakdown of the zona pellucida glycoproteins. For this biologic process to occur, the spermatozoa plasma membrane and the outer acrosomal membrane must be removed. This, in essence, is the hallmark of the acrosomal reaction. After the spermatozoa has proceeded through the zona pellucida, the sperm head crosses the perivitelline space and attaches to the cell membrane of the ovum. Subsequently, the sperm and ovum plasma membranes fuse, the sperm enters the ovum, and fertilization follows.[17,18]

The acrosome reaction is a key component of the fertilization process, and its proper timing is essential. Initiation of the acrosome reaction seems to hinge specifically on spermatozoal binding to the zona pellucida.. The spermatozoal exposure and binding to the structural zona glycoproteins, ZP3, have been identified as the molecule that sets the events of the acrosome reaction into motion. After this binding has occurred, several changes follow:
- Influx of calcium into the spermatozoa
- Activation of the adenylate cyclase, adenosine 3',5' cyclic phosphate (cAMP), protein kinase pathway
- Activation of the guanylate cycle, cyclic guanosine monophosphate (cGMP), protein kinase pathway
- Activation of the phospholipase C, diacylglycerate, protein kinase C pathway

Together, these pathways likely share a complex regulation of the events collectively called the *acrosomal reaction*.[16-18]

Sequence of Events in Fertilization

The sperm makes its way to the surface of the egg, where the sperm cell membrane contacts with the egg cell coats. The egg is surrounded by both cellular and acellular layers. The cellular layers are stripped off so the egg is simply surrounded by the zona pellucida. The cellular layers appear to be important in activating the sperm to undergo the acrosome reaction.[16-18] The first two steps below indicate

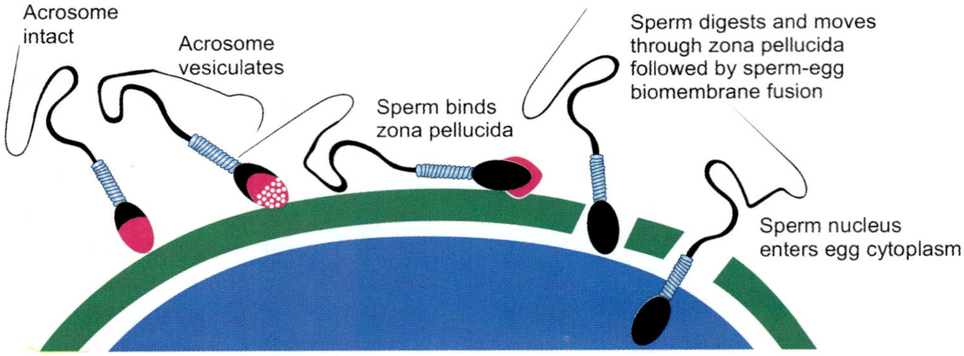

Fig. 16.29: Sequence of events in human fertilization.

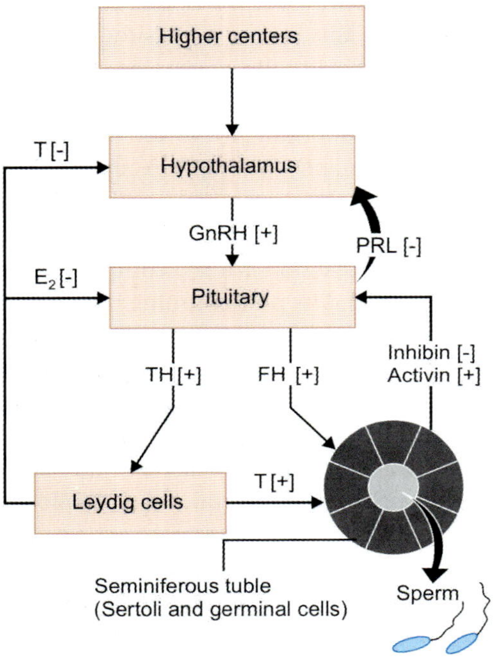

Fig. 16.30: Hypothalamic-pituitary-gonadal axis.
LH, luteinizing hormone; FSH, follicle-stimulating hormone; T, testosterone; DHT, dihydrotestosterone; E2, estradiol; GnRH, gonadotropin releasing hormone; PR, prolactin; +, positive influence; –, negative influence.

the importance of the corona radiata in the process of initiating the acrosome reaction (Fig. 16.29).

Steps in Fertilization

Passage of sperm through the corona radiata occurs as follows:

- Penetration of zona pellucida
- Fusion of plasma membranes of the sperm and oocyte
- Completion of the second meiotic division of oocyte
- Formation of female pronucleus
- Formation of male pronucleus
- Fusion of pronuclei
- Formation of a zygote

NEUROENDOCRINOLOGY OF SPERMATOGENESIS

An endocrinological cause of male infertility is uncommon (<2%); identification is important, as specific hormonal therapy is often successful (Fig. 16.30). The human testis is an organ of dual function: spermatogenesis, occurring in the seminiferous tubules, and secretion of steroid hormones (androgens) by the Leydig cells, present in the interstitial tissue. These testicular functions are intimately related, because testosterone synthesis is required not only for sperm production, but also for the development of secondary sexual characteristics and normal sexual behavior.[19] The anterior pituitary controls both these functions through the secretion of gonadotropins, LH, and FSH. In turn, the anterior pituitary is regulated by the hypothalamic secretion of gonadotropin releasing hormone (GnRH). The extrahypothalamic central nervous system then influences the hypothalamus. The hypothalamic-pituitary-gonadal axis consists of a closed-loop feedback control mechanism directed at maintaining normal reproductive function.[19]

Hypothalamus

The integrative center of the reproductive axis receives neural input from many brain centers and is the pulse generator for the cyclical secretion of pituitary and gonadal hormones. The function and anatomical association of the pituitary gland with the hypothalamus is accomplished by the hypophyseal portal microvascular system. This portal vascular system provides a direct route for the delivery of hypothalamic-releasing hormones to the anterior pituitary gland. In contrast, reverse flow through this vascular route may allow pituitary hormones direct access to the hypothalamus, e.g., men with pituitary hyperprolactinemia often have problems both with impotence and libido.[19] The excess prolactin in these individuals has direct access to, and may affect, higher brain centers.

Anterior Pituitary

Binding to high-affinity receptors on pituitary cells (gonadotrophs), GnRH influences the release of the two primary pituitary hormones (LH and FSH) that regulate testicular function. The protein component of the α-subunits are identical and similar to other pituitary hormones [thyroid-stimulating hormone (TSH) and human chorionic gonadotropin (hCG)], but biological and immunological activity are conferred by the unique β-subunit. Although both hormones are secreted in an episodic manner by the pituitary gland, the longer half-life of FSH in circulation is reflected by a more constant serum level than that of the more rapidly metabolized LH. The peak and trough pattern of blood levels of gonadotropins, particularly LH, is clinically important because a single measurement of circulating LH may be as much as 50% above or below the mean integrated hormone concentrations.[20]

Testes

The LH interacts with specific high-affinity cell surface receptors on the plasma membrane of Leydig cells. Ligand binding stimulates a membrane-bound adenylate cyclase to enhance the formation of cAMP, which binds to the regulatory subunits of protein kinase. This, in turn, causes dissociation of regulatory subunit and activation of the catalytic subunit of the enzyme. The activated Leydig cell protein kinase operates through several steps to stimulate the enzyme synthesis of testosterone synthesis. FSH targets the epithelium of the seminiferous tubule and binds to membrane receptors on the Sertoli cells. The second messenger is the cAMP, and activation of adenylate cyclase stimulates cAMP-dependent protein kinase and RNA and protein synthesis, including synthesis of the androgen-binding protein and aromatase enzyme that converts testosterone to estradiol.[20]

Feedback Control of Gonadotropins

The hypothalamic-pituitary-gonadal system is a closed-loop feedback system directed at maintaining normal reproductive function. Gonadal hormones have inhibitory effects on the secretion of LH and FSH.[19] Although testosterone—the major secretory product of the testes—is a primary inhibitor of LH secretion in men, other testes products, including estrogens and other androgens, also inhibit LH secretion. Testosterone is metabolized in peripheral tissues to the potent androgen dihydrotestosterone (DHT) or potent estrogen, estradiol.[19] Both androgens and estrogens independently appear to modulate LH secretion.[19,21] Estradiol is produced both by the testes and from peripheral conversion of androgenic precursors and is a more potent inhibitor of LH and FSH secretion. Infusions of gonadal steroids in amounts that accumulate physiological concentrations of the hormones in the blood demonstrate suppression of LH levels for testosterone and estradiol, suggesting that both hormones may have an important role in LH regulation. Gonadal sex steroids influence the frequency and/or amplitude of LH secretory pulses in men by acting at the level of the GnRH pulse generator in the hypothalamus and partly at the level of GnRH-stimulated LH secretion. The mechanism for the feedback control of FSH secretion is even more controversial than that of LH. After castration, FSH increases the indication of a negative feedback from testicular products. Like LH, both testosterone and estradiol are capable of suppressing FSH serum levels, but the influence of these two gonadal steroids in physiological function is still undefined.[22] A nonsteroidal tubular factor may also be significant in the feedback regulation of FSH. Inhibin has been isolated and characterized in follicular fluid and is produced by the Sertoli cells of the testes. Inhibin has two subunits: α and β. Two inhibin forms have been isolated—inhibin A (α and β A subunits) and inhibin B (α and β B subunits)—both of which have been shown to cause selective suppression of FSH release *in vitro*. The combination of the two β-subunits led to the formation of activins, which increase FSH secretion *in vitro*. In addition to inhibin, numerous gonadal peptides and growth factors, such as follistatin and transforming growth factor B, are also modulators of FSH secretion. Reductions in spermatogenesis are accompanied by decreased production of inhibin, and this decline in negative feedback is associated with reciprocal elevation of FSH levels. Isolated levels of FSH constitute an important and sensitive marker of the status of the germinal epithelium.[21] Even in pathological conditions with marked damage to the germinal tissue, serum FSH is not elevated to castrate levels unless Leydig cell function is also impaired. It appears that both gonadal steroids and peptides are important to maintain normal serum FSH concentrations.

Prolactin and Gonadotropins

Hyperprolactinemia is linked with disturbed reproductive function reflected by a variety of symptoms and signs of hypogonadism. LH levels are inappropriately low relative to low-serum testosterone levels, indicating that the hypothalamic-pituitary axis fails to respond to reduced testicular testosterone production.[19] Prolactin may inhibit GnRH secretion either directly or through modulation of the dopaminergic pathways. Although the pituitary responds normally to GnRH administration, the pulse frequency of LH secretion is diminished in hyperprolactinemic individuals. Bromocriptine, a dopamine agonist with prolactin-lowering activities, improves sexual function. Excessive prolactin may affect sexual functions by having a direct effect on the central nervous system and also from inhibition of androgen secretion. In individuals with elevated prolactin, libido does not return to normal as long as the prolactin levels remain elevated despite use of androgen therapy.[19]

Androgen Physiology

Androgens regulate gonadotropin secretion, initiation and maintenance of spermatogenesis, formation of male phenotype during sexual differentiation, promotion of sexual maturation at puberty, and controlling sexual drive and potency.[19,21]

Testosterone is synthesized from pregnenolone within the Leydig cells. Testosterone production in men approximates 5 mg per day and the secretion occurs in an irregular pulsatile manner. There is a diurnal pattern: the peak level is in the early morning, and the nadir is in the evening.[21] Inside androgen target cells, testosterone can be converted to DHT by 5α-reductase. Both these androgens bind to the same high-affinity-androgen receptor protein; subsequently, the hormone receptor complex is attached to acceptor sites in the nuclei to affect the biologic response. Estrogens may either be secreted directly by the testes or formed in peripheral tissues. Like other steroid hormones, androgens and estrogens initiate their effect at the cellular level by interacting with high-affinity receptor proteins and are present in the highest concentration in androgen target tissues, e.g. the accessory organs of male reproduction. In the testes, androgen receptors are present in both Sertoli cells and Leydig cells. In normal males, 2% of testosterone is free (unbound), and 44% is bound to a high-affinity sex hormone-binding globulin (SHBG), and the remainder is bound to albumin and other proteins. Free- and albumin-bound portions make up the measure known as bioavailable testosterone. It was formerly believed that the physiologic active androgen moiety was the nonprotein-bound free testosterone. Now it appears that the cellular transfer of steroid hormones is more complicated and can involve hormone dissociation from the binding proteins, such as albumin-bound testosterone, within the microcirculation of the brain and liver. SHBG has a higher affinity for testosterone than for estradiol, and changes in SHBG concentration can alter the hormonal milieu. Elevated estrogens, thyroid hormone, and healthy aging increases plasma SHBG and, therefore, decreases the free testosterone fraction. Alternatively, androgens, growth hormone, and obesity depress SHBG levels and increase the active androgen fraction.[21]

ABNORMALITIES OF SPERMATOGENESIS

Impaired Spermatogenesis

Spermatogenesis can be impaired (Table 16.1) by the following, resulting in an inadequate quantity or defective quality of sperm:[4]

- Heat
- Disorders of genitourinary system (endocrine or genetic)
- Drugs
- Toxins

Table 16.1: Causes of impaired spermatogenesis.

Condition	Examples
Endocrine disorders	Abnormalities of the hypothalamic-pituitary-gonadal axis Adrenal disorders Hyperprolactinemia Hypogonadism, sometimes related to obesity Hypothyroidism
Genetic disorders	Gonadal dysgenesis Klinefelter syndrome Microdeletions of sections of the Y chromosome (in 10–15% of men with severely impaired spermatogenesis)
GU disorders	Cryptorchidism Infections Injury Mumps orchitis Testicular atrophy Varicocele
Heat	Exposure to excessive heat within the last 3 months Fever

Causes of Impaired Spermatogenesis

Impaired Sperm Emission: Sperm emission may be impaired because of:

- Retrograde ejaculation into the bladder

  Retrograde ejaculation is often due to:
- Diabetes
- Neurologic dysfunction
- Retroperitoneal dissection (e.g. for Hodgkin lymphoma)
- Transurethral resection of the prostate

  Sperm emission can also be impaired by:
- Obstruction of the vas deferens
- Congenital absence of both vasa deferentia or epididymides, often in men with mutations of the cystic fibrosis transmembrane conductance regulator (CFTR) gene
- Absence of both seminal vesicles

FACTORS CONTROLLING SPERMATOGENESIS

Humans are constantly exposed to a range of *chemicals* and *toxins* in their *environment*, which can affect their health, including their *reproductive health*. For men, a range of environmental exposures is associated with *reduced sperm concentration* and *quality*. Men whose sperm is suboptimal in either quantity or quality are less likely to conceive, and will, on average, take longer to do so, should they manage to successfully conceive.[23]

While environmental chemicals and toxins are found in many environments, they are most commonly found at dangerous concentrations in *occupational environments*, such as chemicals used in agricultural and manufacturing sector workplaces. The environmental factors, which have evidence of an association with male infertility, include *heat*, *radiation*, *chemicals* and *trauma*.

Hormonal Control

Spermatogenesis is controlled by a complex feedback mechanism involving the *hypothalamus*, *anterior pituitary* and *testes*. *GnRH* is released by the hypothalamus in a pulsatile manner and travels through portal vessels to the anterior pituitary, where it acts of the gonadotropic cells. These cells respond to the stimulation by producing either *FSH* or *LH* depending on the pattern of GnRH secretion.

The LH and FSH travel in the bloodstream to the testes, where LH acts on the Leydig cells to stimulate them to convert steroids to *testosterone* and other androgens, which in turn contribute to the stimulation of Sertoli cells.

The FSH acts on the receptors of Sertoli cells and, in combination with testosterone, stimulates many functions, including synthesis and secretion of *estrogen*, *inhibin* and many other products, meiosis, spermatocyte maturation, and Leydig cell function.

Inhibin, testosterone, and estrogen feedback negatively on the anterior pituitary and hypothalamus to suppress secretion of gonadotropic hormones.

Genetic and Epigenetic Factors

About 10% genes in the genome are related to spermatogenesis. Genetic abnormalities account for 15–30% cases of male infertility and may lead to irreversible partial or complete spermatogenic arrest.

Other Factors that Affect Spermatogenesis

1. Primary endocrine failure involving either GnRH or gonadotropin deficiency is associated with severe disorders in spermatogenesis.
2. Dietary deficiencies (such as vitamins B, E, and A), anabolic steroids, metals (cadmium and lead), X-ray exposure, dioxin, alcohol, and infectious diseases will also adversely affect the rate of spermatogenesis.
3. Seminiferous epithelium is sensitive to elevated temperature in humans and will be adversely affected by high temperatures.

Heat Exposure

Sperm production in humans and other mammals is dependent on the temperature of the testicles. Sperm is optimally produced when the testicles are 2–4°C below body temperature.

The increased testicular temperature may affect both the quality and quantity of sperm produced.[24]

Occupational Drivers

Drivers are thought to be at greater risk of infertility because long periods of sitting can increase testicular heat, as the testicles are insulated by the thighs whilst a man is seated.[25]

Ceramic Oven Operators

The semen of the oven operators contained significantly less motile sperm (7% motile) than that of the other workers in the ceramic factory (who had 28% motile sperm).[25]

Exposure to Radiation and Toxic Substances in War Environments

Radiation and other toxic substances found in war environments negatively affect sperm quality. Compared to other body organs, the testes are very sensitive to radiation. Radiation exposure affects spermatogenesis (the production of sperm).[25]

Exposure to Pesticides, Solvents, and Other Chemicals

Men who are regularly exposed to some chemical substances are more likely to be infertile than men who are not. For example, a longitudinal study, which compared the semen samples of men with varying exposures to organophosphorus pesticides found that men with the highest exposure to these pesticides had the poorest sperm quality.[23,25]

Chemotherapy

Chemotherapy medications used to treat cancer often cause infertility and the extent to which a man's fertility is affected by chemotherapy depends on the type of chemotherapy drug used, the dose, duration of treatment, and the man's age when he is treated.[23]

Drugs that May Affect Male Fertility

1. *Testosterone*: Replacement testosterone (also called supplemental testosterone) has a strong negative effect on sperm production. When testosterone is given to a man, the hormonal signals that tell the testicles to make testosterone and to make sperm are blocked, and the man's natural testosterone production stops.
2. *Alcohol*: Light to moderate alcohol drinking does not appear to affect male fertility. Heavy alcohol drinking, however, may decrease the production of testosterone, increase the rate at which testosterone is cleared from the bloodstream, and increase a man's estrogen levels. All of this can cause a lower testosterone level, which can harm sperm production.
3. *Tobacco*: Tobacco use in general, and smoking in particular, are linked to serious health conditions. Babies in households with people who smoke are much more likely to have serious respiratory illness such as severe asthma, pneumonia, and repeated ear infection.
4. *Opiates (narcotics)*: Opiates include both prescription medications (for treating pain and addiction) and illegal street drugs. Long-term use of opiates can disrupt the signals that control testosterone production, which can cause low testosterone and decrease the quantity and quality of the sperm.[19]

Thyroid Disease and Male Fertility

Hypothyroidism may result in a decrease in the SHBG levels and a decrease in total serum testosterone (T) levels, as well as a decrease in the gonadotropins levels, specifically the LH and the FSH. In cases of prolonged prepubertal hypothyroidism due to drop in LH and FSH levels, the Leydig and Sertoli cells, respectively are less stimulated to differentiate into mature cells, negatively affecting spermatogenesis.[22]

CLINICAL MANIFESTATION

History

A detailed history of exposure to occupational and environmental toxins, excessive heat, and radiation should be elucidated. Cancer chemotherapy has a dose-dependent, potentially devastating effect on the testicular germinal epithelium and may compromise Leydig cell function. Drug history should be reviewed; anabolic steroids, cimetidine, ketoconazole, and spironolactone may affect the reproductive cycle. Exogenous androgens exert their deleterious effects on the feedback level of the pituitary and hypothalamus by inhibiting gonadotropin release. Chronic use has also been shown to inhibit gonadotropin secretion and lower testosterone levels. Additionally, alcohol, marijuana, and cocaine have been implicated as reversible gonadotoxic agents. Decreased libido and impotence are the earliest symptoms of low testosterone. Loss of libido that is associated with headaches, visual abnormalities, and galactorrhea may suggest a pituitary tumor. Anosmia may be a symptom in individuals with hypothalamic hypogonadism. Other medical problems associated with infertility include thyroid disease and liver disease.[25]

Physical Examination

When germ cell failure occurs before puberty, patients have obvious features of eunuchoidism. When failure occurs after puberty, the diagnosis is more difficult unless it is linked with adrenal failure, because the regression of secondary sexual characteristics may take years. Careful examination of the testes is essential in the physical examination. The seminiferous tubules account for approx 95% of testicular volume. The prepubertal testis measures approx 2 cm in length (2 mL volume, as assessed by Prader orchidometer) and gradually increases in size with puberty. The normal adult testis is an average of 4.6 cm long (3.6–5.5 cm range) and 2.6 cm wide (2.1–3.2 cm range) with a mean volume of 18.6 ± 4.8 mL standard deviation (SD). When the seminiferous tubules are damaged before puberty, the testes are small and firm but characteristically small and soft with postpubertal damage. Gynecomastia is a consistent feature of a feminizing state. Men with congenital hypogonadism may have related midline defects, such as anosmia, color blindness, cerebellar ataxia, hare lip, and cleft palate.[3,21,23] Hepatomegaly may be associated with problems of hormone metabolism. Proper neck examination may help rule out thyromegaly, a bruit, or nodularity linked with thyroid disease. The neurologic examination should test the visual field and reflexes.

Semen Analysis

Examination of the seminal fluid provides important information concerning the integrity of the reproductive hormonal network, spermatogenesis, and patency of the reproductive tract. A normal microscopic examination eliminates the need for any further diagnostic studies.[20]

Baseline Hormone Evaluation

The classic hormone evaluation includes a serum testosterone and serum gonadotropins (LH and FSH), an algorithm for diagnosing endocrine causes of male infertility. A low-serum testosterone with inappropriately low LH levels usually warrants the investigation of serum prolactin levels. A more recent study showed that obtaining serum FSH and testosterone only in men with sperm densities less than 10 million sperm/mL and soft testes will detect virtually all (99%) endocrine abnormalities. A single LH determination has limited prognostic accuracy (± 50%) because of the episodic nature of LH secretion and its short half-life. In contrast, serum FSH has a longer half-life, and fluctuations in serum levels are less obvious. If an abnormal LH value is obtained in a single sample, then three serum samples can be collected over a 20-minute interval and the samples pooled. Estradiol levels are measured in patients presenting with gynecomastia, testicular masses, or history compatible with excessive exogenous estrogen exposure. Testosterone secretion follows a diurnal cycle with an early morning peak around 8:00 AM followed by evening trough at 8:00 PM when the concentration falls to about 70% of the morning peak. Testosterone values should therefore be drawn in the morning. The measurement of total (bound) testosterone usually provides a correct assessment of bioavailable testosterone. Free (unbound) testosterone is a more accurate marker of bioavailable testosterone, particularly when conditions of altered SHBG concentrations exist. Elevated estrogens, thyroid hormone, and aging increase plasma SHBG and thus decrease levels of free testosterone. Alternatively, androgens, growth hormone, and obesity depress SHBG levels and increase the active androgen fraction. Measurement of the free-testosterone fraction should be made by equilibrium dialysis. Ultrafiltration or analog immunoassays are currently very unreliable.

A low-serum testosterone level is one of the best indicators of hypogonadism of hypothalamic or pituitary origin (Flowchart 16.1). Mean serum LH and FSH concentrations are significantly lower in hypogonadotropic patients than in normal men, but they can overlap with the lower limits of normal in some individuals. In patients with hypogonadotropic hypogonadism, the pituitary hormones other than LH and FSH should also be assessed (adrenocorticotropic hormone, TSH, and growth hormone) to exclude the possibility of hypopituitarism. Thyroid dysfunction is such a rare cause of infertility that routine screening is discouraged. Elevated serum FSH and LH values help to distinguish primary testicular failure (hypergonadotropic hypogonadism) from secondary testicular failure (hypogonadotropic hypogonadism). Decreases in spermatogenesis are generally accompanied by reductions in inhibin production, and this decline in negative feedback is associated with a reciprocal elevation of FSH levels. Elevated FSH is usually a reliable indicator of severe germinal epithelial damage and is usually associated with azoospermia or severe oligospermia. In azoospermic and severely oligospermic patients with normal FSH levels, primary spermatogenic defects cannot be distinguished from obstructive lesions by hormonal investigation alone. Therefore, scrotal exploration and testicular biopsy should be considered. Elevated serum FSH levels related to small atrophic testes implies severe infertility; biopsy is not warranted. Hyperprolactinemia is reported to cause oligospermia, but the diagnostic value of routine prolactin measurements is extremely low in men with semen abnormalities unless decreased libido, impotence, and evidence of hypogonadism also exist. Prolactin measurement is

Flowchart 16.1: Algorithm for the diagnosis of endocrine causes of male infertility.
*, sperm counts less than 5 × 10^6/mL.

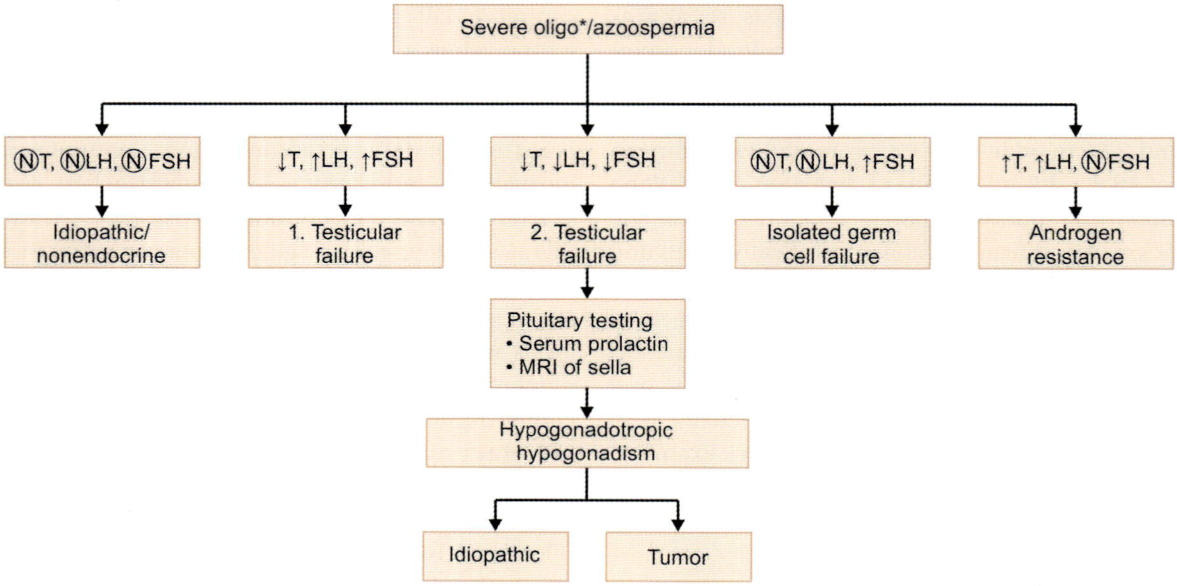

warranted in patients with low-serum testosterone without an associated increase in serum LH. Individuals with gynecomastia or suspected androgen resistance (high-serum testosterone and LH with undermasculinization) should have a serum estradiol determination. Individuals with a rapid loss of secondary sex characteristics, implying both testicular and adrenal failure, should undergo investigation of adrenal function. In men with a history of precocious puberty, congenital adrenal hyperplasia should be considered. In the common variant (21-hydroxylase deficiency), serum levels of 17-hydroxyprogesterone are elevated, as is urinary pregnanetriol. In the 11-hydroxylase deficiency, serum 11-deoxycortisol is elevated.

CONCLUSION

The blood-testis barrier provides a microenvironment for spermatogenesis to occur. The seminiferous tubules are the site of sperm production. The process of differentiation of a spermatogonium into a spermatid is known as spermatogenesis. It involves both mitotic and meiotic proliferation as well as extensive cell remodeling.

In humans, the process of spermatogenesis starts at puberty and continues throughout life. Spermatogenesis produces genetic material necessary for the replication of the species. Meiosis assures genetic diversity. Along the length of the seminiferous tubule, there are only certain cross-sections where spermatozoa are released. Sperm production is a continuous and not a pulsatile process. Spermatozoa are highly specialized cells that do not grow or divide. The spermatogenic process is maintained by different intrinsic and extrinsic influences. Spermatozoa have to undergo a series of cellular or physiological changes such as capacitation and acrosome reaction before they can fertilize. The epididymis is limited to a storage role. Nutrition, therapeutic drugs, hormones and their metabolites, increased scrotal temperature, toxic substances, or radiation can reduce or entirely inhibit spermatogenesis.

REFERENCES

1. Hess RA. Spermatogenesis, overview. In: Knobil E, Neil JD (eds). Encyclopedia of Reproduction. New York: Academic Press; 1999: pp. 539-45.
2. Middendorff R, Muller D, Mewe M, Mukhopadhyay AK, Holstein AF, Davidoff MS. The tunica albuginea of the human testis is characterized by complex contraction and relaxation activities regulated by cyclic GMP. J Clin Endocrinol Metab. 2002;87:3486-99.
3. Griffin JE, Wilson JD. Disorders of the testes and the male reproductive tract. In: Wilson JD (ed). Williams Textbook of Endocrinology, 9th ed. Philadelphia, PA: Saunders; 1998. pp. 819-75.
4. Weinbauer GF, Luetjens CM, Simoni M. Eberhard Nieschlag Physiology of Testicular Function, 2010.
5. Davidoff MS, Breuker H, Holstein AF, Seidel K. Cellular architecture of the lamina propria of human tubules. Cell Tissue Res. 1990;262:253-61.

6. Russell L. Role in spermiation. In: Russell LD, Griswold MD (eds). The Sertoli Cell. Clearwater FL: Cache River Press; 1993. pp. 269-302.
7. Russell LD, Griswold MD (eds). The Sertoli Cell. Clearwater: Cache Press; 1993.
8. Russell LD. The perils of sperm release—'let my children go.' Int J Androl. 1991;14(5):307-11.
9. Hafez ES. The human semen and fertility regulation in the male. J Reprod Med. 1976;16:91-6.
10. Menkveld R, Stander FS, Kotze TJ, Kruger TF, Van Zyl JA. The evaluation of morphological characteristics of human spermatozoa according to stricter criteria. Hum Reprod. 1990;5:586-92.
11. Katz DF, Overstreet JW, Samuels SJ, Niswander PW, Bloom TD, Lewis EL. Morphometric analysis of spermatozoa in the assessment of human male fertility. J Androl. 1986;7:203-10.
12. World Health Organization. World Health Organization laboratory manual for the examination of human semen and sperm-cervical mucus interaction.4th ed. Cambridge: Cambridge University Press; 1999.
13. Kruger TF, Menkveld R, Stander FS, Lombard CJ, Van der Merwe JP, Van Zyl JA, et al. Sperm morphologic features as a prognostic factor in vitro fertilization. Fertil Steril. 1986;46:1118-23.
14. Tredway DR, Settlage DS, Nakamura RM, Motoshima M, Umezaki CU, Mishell Jr DR. Significance of timing for the postcoital evaluation of cervical mucus. Am J Obstet Gynaecol. 1975;121:387-93.
15. Eddy EM, O'Brien DA. The spermatozoon. In: Knobill EO, NO'Nneill JD (eds). The Physiology of Reproduction. New York: Raven; 1994.
16. Mahanes MS, Oches DL, Eng LA. Cell calcium of ejaculated rabbit spermatozoa before and following in vitro capacitation. Biochem Biophys Res Commun. 1986;134: 664-70.
17. Benoff S, Hurley I, Cooper GW, Mandel FS, Hershlag A, Scholl GM, et al. Fertilization potential in vitro is correlated with head-specific mannose-ligand receptor expression, acrosome status and membrane cholesterol content. Hum Reprod. 1993;8:2155-66.
18. Ravnik SE, Zarutskie PW, Muller CH. Purification and characterization of a human follicular fluid lipid transfer protein that stimulates human sperm capacitation. Biol Reprod. 1992;47:1126-33.
19. Swerdloff RS, Wang C. Physiology of hypothalamic-pituitary function. In: Walsh PC (ed). Campbell's Urology, 7th ed. Philadelphia, PA: Saunders; 1998. p. 1239.
20. Santen RJ, Bardin CW. Episodic luteinizing hormone secretion in man: pulse analysis, clinical interpretation, physiologic mechanisms. J Clin Invest. 1973;52:2617-28.
21. Bardin CW, Paulsen CA. The testes. In: Williams RH (ed). Textbook of Endocrinology, 6th ed. Philadelphia, PA: Saunders; 1981.
22. Veldhuis JD. Male hypothalamic-pituitary-gonadal axis. In: Lipshultz LI, Howards SS (eds). Infertility in the Male, 3rd ed. St. Louis, MO: Mosby-Year Book; 1997. pp. 23-58.
23. Winters SJ. Clinical disorders of the testis. In: DeGroot LJ, Jameson JL (eds). Endocrinology, 4th ed. Philadelphia, PA: Saunders: 2001. pp. 2269-90.
24. Shapiro E, Kinsella TJ, Makuch RW, Fraass BA, Glatstein E, Rosenberg SA, et al. Effects of fractionated irradiation on endocrine aspects of testicular function. J Clin Oncol. 1985;3:1232-9.
25. Schrag SD, Dixon RL. Occupational exposures associated with male reproductive dysfunction. Ann Rev Pharmacol Toxicol. 1985;25:567-92.

CHAPTER 17

Male Reproductive Endocrinology

Satish Bharadwaj, SS Vasan

INTRODUCTION

In males, beginning of puberty is termed "adrenarche". Clinical manifestations of adrenarche in boys include testicular enlargement, development of pubic hair, release of testosterone and its effects, and onset of spermatogenesis. Adrenarche begins at an average age of 11–12 years and can last up to 17 years. Testicular enlargement is the first of the events to occur, followed by appearance and growth of pubic hair over next 2 years. Change in voice of boys occurs due to the effect of testosterone at the age of 13 years. Development of penis and scrotum to their adult size is complete by the age of 15–17 years, followed by production of sperms (spermatogenesis). Accelerated growth of the body occurs during this age, leading to the individual's adult skeletal and muscle mass by the age of 18 years. During this period of adolescence, there are also emotional changes due to the release of gonadal steroids (testosterone) that manifest in the changes in response and relationship toward parents, peers and members of the opposite sex. Violent behavior can be seen, complicated by the character and environment in which the individual is being brought up.

There could be delay in adrenarche due to dysfunction of the hypothalamic–pituitary axis, end organ failure, or unknown causes. Chronic severe illness during childhood, weight loss or malnourishment, or physical stress (including chronic strenuous exercise) can also cause delayed puberty. Other causes include pituitary or hypothalamic tumors, pituitary failure, or congenital absence of gonadotropin-releasing hormone (GnRH) expressing neurons. Sometimes, adrenarche occurs but spermatogenesis (gonadarche) may not occur due to chromosomal anomalies (Turner syndrome), exposure to high-dose chemotherapy or radiation to the pelvis in childhood, autoimmune or idiopathic causes. Boys without indication of genital growth by the age of 15 years need to be evaluated for delayed puberty.

HYPOTHALAMIC–PITUITARY–GONADAL AXIS

The hypothalamic–pituitary–gonadal pathway, shown in Figure 17.1, regulates the development of male reproductive organs and spermatogenesis, in addition to the regulation of development, reproduction, aging and many other body processes. GnRH is released from the arcuate nucleus of the hypothalamus, in a pulsatile fashion, which stimulates the pituitary gland to release several hormones called gonadotropins. Gonadotropins are glycoprotein polypeptide hormones secreted by gonadotrope cells of the anterior pituitary of vertebrates.[1] This family includes follicle-stimulating hormone (FSH), luteinizing hormone (LH), and human chorionic gonadotropin (hCG). The hypothalamic secretion of GnRH initiates spermatogenesis and testosterone production, through the action of FSH and LH on the testis. LH acts on the Leydig cells to increase

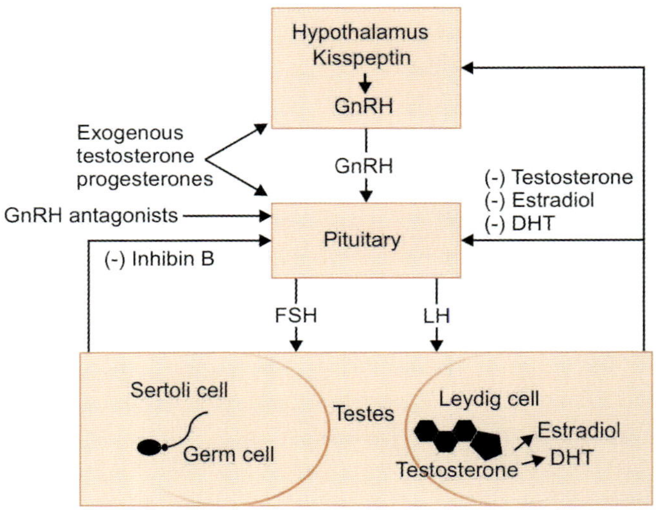

Fig. 17.1: Hypothalamus–pituitary–gonadal axis. Adapted from Manetti and Honig (2010).[4]

Table 17.1: Site of secretion, function and normal levels of reproductive hormones.

Hormone	*Site of secretion*	*Function*	*Normal levels*
Gonadotropin-releasing hormone (GnRH)	Hypothalamus	Stimulates pituitary to release LH and FSH	–
Follicle-stimulating hormone (FSH)	Anterior pituitary	Stimulates production of sperms	1–10 mIU/mL
Luteinizing hormone (LH)	Anterior pituitary	Stimulates testosterone production	1–10 mIU/mL
Testosterone	Interstitial cells of testes	Stimulates secondary sex characteristics in males; Helps stimulate spermatogenesis in the testes (with FSH)	3–10 ng/mL
Androsterone	Interstitial cells of testes	Same functions, but less effective	–
Inhibin	Sertoli cells	Negative feedback for FSH and GnRH	–
Estradiol		Negative feedback to decrease GnRH frequency	Extremely low
Dihydrotestosterone (DHT)			Extremely low

steroidogenesis, whereas FSH participates in protein synthesis and the initiation of spermatogenesis at the level of the seminiferous tubules. A brief account of the actions of FSH and LH in the testis is given below:

Luteinizing hormone stimulates the Leydig cells to produce testosterone, which has a local effect on the interstitium and seminiferous tubules leading to sperm production and maturation. This effect is manifested by very high intratesticular concentration of testosterone compared to that in the bloodstream. LH binds to Leydig cells and increases cAMP, which, in turn, increases protein secretion and the side-chain cleavage of cholesterol, as well as other likely steps, to increase steroidogenesis and the production of testosterone and other androgens. The Leydig cells, situated between the seminiferous tubules, produce the testicular steroids regulated by steroid feedback and assist in the transportation of steroids in the blood, lymph and seminiferous tubules.

Follicle-stimulating hormone exerts its effect directly on the Sertoli cells to promote spermatogenesis. Testosterone and estradiol (converted through aromatase in the testis interstitium) provide direct negative feedback to modulate GnRH, LH and FSH. Aromatase inhibition increases FSH levels suggesting that FSH regulation is more dependent on estradiol than testosterone.[2,3] FSH binds to the Sertoli cells of the seminiferous tubules, increases cAMP and protein synthesis, androgen binding in the tubules, etc. regulated by inhibin produced by the Sertoli cells. Sertoli cells, also called as "the director cells of spermatogenesis", secrete proteins that are important to spermatogenesis and comprise the blood–testis barrier. Prolactin may increase Leydig cell response to LH and/or prostate sensitivity to androgens. Steroids and other hormones may aid in the movement of sperm from the testicle by causing smooth muscle contractions. The normal values of these hormones are shown in Table 17.1.

The presence of a negative feedback control on the production of gonadotropins by the secretion of hormones produced in the Sertoli and Leydig cells has been confirmed by the rapid rise of FSH and LH after castration. Absence of hormones produced by the Sertoli and Leydig cells has a direct effect to increase the pulsatile secretion of GnRH by the hypothalamus and pituitary to increase the amplitude. Although FSH and LH are cosecreted by gonadotropic cells of the pituitary, there is a differential regulation of FSH and LH levels.

CONTROL OF LH SECRETION

Secretion of LH is controlled by the steroid hormones, testosterone, estradiol and dihydrotestosterone (DHT).[5] DHT is the most effective and nonaromatizable androgen produced by the irreversible reduction of testosterone by catalytic activity of 5α-reductase enzyme. Androgens in men act either directly by stimulation of the androgen receptor (AR), or indirectly, after aromatization, by acting at the estrogen receptor. DHT plays a role in prenatal differentiation of external genitalia being a regulatory hormone of testicular descent and development of external genitalia; it also affects skin appendages (hair follicle and sebaceous glands), maturation of spermatozoa in epididymis as well as the body composition.[6]

The mode of action of these steroid hormones to inhibit LH secretion was in question for a long time, as to whether testosterone acts directly on the AR or indirectly on the estrogen receptor, after metabolism to estradiol

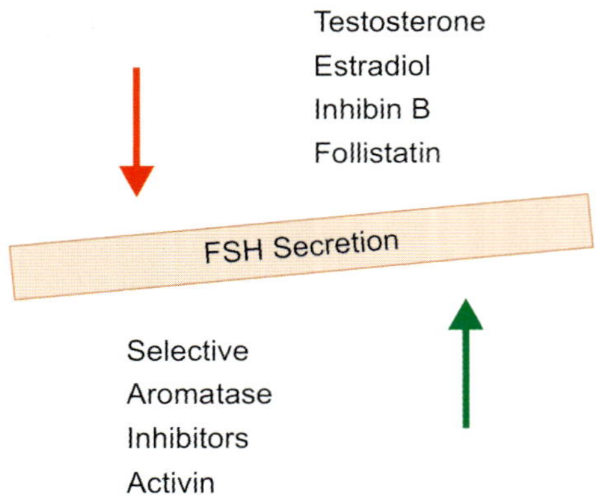

Fig. 17.2: Regulation of FSH secretion.

or DHT.[7,8] Testosterone acts at the hypothalamus level to decrease the frequency, but not amplitude of pulsatile GnRH secretion.[9] On the other hand, estradiol acts on the pituitary to bring down the amplitude of LH secretion without change in frequency. Selective aromatase inhibitor, anastrozole causes an increase in LH pulse amplitude and pulse frequency.[10] Considering all of these aspects, current understanding is that estradiol exerts a negative feedback by acting at the hypothalamus to decrease GnRH pulse frequency, and at the pituitary to decrease the responsiveness to GnRH.

CONTROL OF FSH SECRETION

Regulation of FSH secretion is brought about by several hormones as shown schematically in Figure 17.2.

Testosterone

Administration of testosterone in an amount similar or greater to its production rate can suppress FSH as well as LH in men.[5] In most cases, there was greater suppression of LH than reduction brought about by inhibin.[11] FSH, on the other hand, is totally inhibited by testosterone in primates, unlike other species. Treatment with a selective aromatase inhibitor resulted in rise in FSH and testosterone levels in men, hinting at a negative feedback control of FSH by estradiol.[10]

Inhibin

The secretion of FSH by pituitary is controlled by the protein inhibitors called "inhibin", secreted by the gonads, and follistatin, produced locally within the pituitary by the follicular-stellate cells, in addition to feedback inhibition by testosterone and estradiol.[11-13] The presence of specific regulatory hormones controlling FSH secretion had been postulated for a long time.[14] Confirmation of the existence of these glycoprotein hormones that exerts a specific negative feedback inhibition on FSH secretion at the pituitary level came in the late 1980s with the isolation of inhibin and related proteins.[15,16] Inhibin is a dimeric protein consisting of disulfide-linked α and β-subunits. Two forms of inhibin, termed A and B, which differ by the amino acid sequence of the β-subunit have been isolated. Inhibin A consists of α-βA and inhibin B consists of α-βB subunits. Inhibin is produced by the Sertoli cell, and is secreted basally across the basement membrane of the seminiferous tubule and also into the lumen.[17,18] The predominant form of inhibin secreted by the testis under FSH stimulation is inhibin B and the levels of inhibin B in males, measured by a specific ELISA, are inversely related to the levels of FSH.[19-23] There are some studies indicating the secretion of a subunit of inhibin by Leydig cells and that subunit products are released into the circulation when LH levels are high.[24-26] However, the bioactivity of inhibin produced by the Leydig cells has been controversial.[24] Testosterone-induced gonadotropin suppression also reduced circulating inhibin B and pro-alpha C levels by only 25% and 50%, respectively. Hence, it appears that secretion of inhibin B is not fully gonadotropin dependent.[27]

Activin

Dimers of the β-subunit are known as activins, have been found in follicular fluid, which stimulate pituitary FSH secretion.[28,29] Different isoforms of activin, activin A = βAβA, activin B = βBβB, activin AB = βAβB, have the capacity to stimulate FSH secretion by pituitary cells in culture. The stimulation of FSH by activin secretion is also shown by the decline in FSH levels in mice with targeted disruption of the activin type II receptor gene.[30] Activin is produced by the Sertoli cells, Leydig cells and peritubular myoid cells, but castration does not result in a decrease in circulating activin A levels.[31-34] Unfortunately, the changes after castration are not confirmed due to the lack of a suitable assay to measure activin B. Activin also stimulates spermatogonial mitosis locally within the testis.[35] Further, activin A is responsible for the stimulation of Sertoli cell mitosis during the development of the testis in both rats and mice.[36-40] Additionally, receptors for activin are present on primary spermatocytes, round spermatids and Sertoli cells.[41]

Follistatin

Follistatin is another structurally distinct protein that suppresses FSH secretion by pituitary cells, although in culture.[42] This monomeric protein binds to activin and thereby neutralizes its action of promoting FSH secretion.[43] Follistatin is produced in the Sertoli cells, spermatogonia, primary spermatocytes and round spermatids in the testis.[44,45] However, castration did not lead to a decrease in its levels in circulation suggesting that the testis does not contribute significantly to circulating levels of follistatin.[46] A rise in follistatin levels was observed in both test animals as well as the sham-operated rams indicating that it was due to the acute phase response to surgery, Further, it has been demonstrated that IL-1β could also cause an increase in follistatin levels.[47]

The principal gonadal feedback for FSH secretion is provided by inhibin, as inhibin levels in circulation decreased to undetectable levels whereas the levels of activin and follistatin did not change on castration. The studies of Plant et al. on arcuate nucleus-lesioned monkeys on a GnRH pulse regime support this fact as testosterone could prevent rise in LH, but not FSH after castration.[48] Additionally, recombinant human inhibin caused a specific fall in FSH secretion after about 6 hours following administration.[49-51] In another study, inhibin A, suppressed FSH levels into the normal range in the absence of testosterone.[52]

The role of these proteins appears to be more complex because substantial evidence shows that activin and follistatin can exert a paracrine role directly in the pituitary gland. The α- and β-subunit mRNAs are present in gonadotropes within the pituitary gland.[53] The studies of Corrigan et al. strongly suggest that these substances exert a local action on FSH secretion since the inhibition of the action of activin B by the use of a specific monoclonal antibody when added to pituitary cells in culture, caused a suppression of endogenous FSH secretion.[54] Follistatin mRNAs are also present in a number of different pituitary cell types including the folliculo-stellate cells.[53,55] This local production of follistatin also has the capacity to regulate the actions of activin.[56] Additionally, the studies of Bilizekian et al. have demonstrated that GnRH, estradiol and testosterone can modulate the local production of α, βA, βB and follistatin mRNAs within the pituitary.[57,58] Clearly, these interactions are complex and the relative importance of paracrine and endocrine actions of these glycoprotein hormones needs to be further investigated.

In a number of studies on testicular damage, the levels of circulating inhibin B is observed to be inversely related to the levels of FSH.[21,22,59] There was also a decrease in production of inhibin by Sertoli cells in parallel with the rise of FSH in a number of models of spermatogenic damage, such as cryptorchidism and intratesticular glycerol treatment.[61,62] Further, an inverse relationship between serum inhibin B levels and FSH is seen in a number of studies on normal men.[21] Hence, it appears that inhibin acts predominantly through secretion from the testis and transport via the peripheral circulation while activins and follistatin perform through paracrine actions at the level of the pituitary gland.

SPERMATOGENESIS

Spermatogenesis starts with yolk sac endoderm gives rise to primordial germ cells which give rise to type A cells. Type A stem cells form additional type A cells or differentiate into type B spermatogonia cells during early puberty. Type B cells differentiate, during late puberty and in adults, to form primary spermatocytes, secondary spermatocytes and spermatids. These events occur initially through mitosis and then reduce the chromosomes to one-half through meiosis.

Spermiogenesis transforms early spermatids into late spermatids, and further to form the "morphologically normal" sperm. The above process takes 72–74 days in the human. Sperm is released into the lumen through spermiogenesis which involves a gradual release of sperm from the Sertoli cells into the tubule lumen. Sperm transport from the testicle occurs through seminiferous tubule contractions of the myoid cells (hormone dependent), fluid buildup and pressure, and testicular capsule contractions. Epididymis is responsible for sperm maturation and motility. Usually, two-thirds of the epididymis is needed for sperm transport, to achieve normal sperm fertilization capacity. Sperms take approximately 2 weeks to get through the epididymis, and are stored near the tail portion and in the vas deferens until they are ejaculated. Carnitine and glycerol phosphocholine serve as potential markers of epididymal function. Disorders of spermatogenesis include azoospermia including Sertoli cell only syndrome, maturation arrest at a number of possible stages, and hypospermatogenesis.

Seminal vesicles and prostate glands act as accessory organs for transport and ejaculation of sperm. Seminal vesicles contribute prostaglandins and fructose and constitute up to two-thirds of the volume of ejaculate. Presence of fructose is useful to qualitatively verify the presence of the vas deferens. Prostate contributes acid phosphatase, Zn and citric acid. Chronic inflammation of the prostate may contribute to infertility.

ENDOCRINE CONTROL OF TESTICULAR FUNCTION

Apart from testosterone and estradiol, other substances have a role in this important neuroendocrine negative feedback pathway. Studies have shown that kisspeptins, a group of amino acid peptides, and kisspeptin-1 receptor (KISS1R), also known as G protein-coupled receptor (GPR54), plays a critical function in the secretion of GnRH and the negative feedback of testosterone and estradiol on the hypothalamus.[63] Studies on neuronal cell lines have shown an increase in GnRH secretion on administration of kisspeptin.[64] In addition, kisspeptin was observed to increase LH, FSH and testosterone secretion in monkeys, but prolonged treatment reduced serum LH levels.[65,66] Based on *in vivo* studies in rodents and nonhuman primates, kisspeptin has come to be recognized as critical regulator of the timing of sexual maturation, the sexual differentiation of the brain, the adult regulation of gonadotropin secretion by gonadal hormones and the control of fertility by metabolic and environmental (e.g. photoperiod) stimuli.[67,68]

Spermatogenesis is hormone dependent. Spermatogonia divide in 16-day intervals to form type B spermatogonia, which will differentiate and progress through spermatogenesis. Type B spermatogonia that differentiate will divide mitotically to form primary spermatocytes, which undergo meiosis to form secondary spermatocytes and round spermatids. The round spermatids will then undergo a process of conformational change into mature spermatids, through changes in cytoplasm and nucleus. They further develop an acrosome, flagellum and cytoplasmic organelles undergo changes to form a mature spermatozoon. The formation of a mature sperm within the testis takes about 64 days and requires high levels of testosterone.

It appears that high levels of intratesticular testosterone are required to initiate and maintain qualitative spermatogenesis. In normal sperm-producing men, intratesticular testosterone levels are 100-fold higher than in serum.[69-73] The roles of FSH and LH are not completely clear in the renewal of spermatogenesis, although FSH can initiate spermatogenesis in pubertal men. In patients with hypogonadotropic hypogonadism, FSH provides for optimized spermatogenesis in some but not all cases. A combination of FSH and high intratesticular testosterone is important for normal sperm production.[74] Suppression of gonadotropins has a direct effect on germ cell apoptosis.[75] FSH interacts in a complicated manner with testosterone and other factors to bring about spermatogenesis. Sertoli cells are activated by FSH to provide a condusive environment for the development of spermatozoa. Figure 17.3 depicts the current understanding of the role of LH, FSH and androgens on spermatogenesis.

Inhibin B is another nonsteroidal substance released by Sertoli cells after puberty and has an effect on the negative feedback of FSH secretion. However, the role of inhibin in FSH suppression and spermatogenesis is unclear, as low levels of inhibin are still present with LH-receptor mutations and chronic FSH administration.[27,65,76] Progesterone affects gonadotropins via the hypothalamic–pituitary–testis axis, as its receptors are present in these glands. However, they are also known to function directly on the testis.[77,78]

The role of DHT, a potent metabolite of testosterone, in spermatogenesis is not very clear. Reduced levels of DHT do not cause a significant drop in sperm production.[79]

Androgen receptors are found in multiple cell sites within the testes, such as immature germ cells, smooth muscle cells, myoid cells, Sertoli and Leydig cells. It has been shown that ARs in Sertoli and Lydig cells are important for spermatogenesis, but not those on germ cells and myoid cells, in specific-knockout mice.[80-84]

CONTROL OF TESTOSTERONE PRODUCTION

In men, testosterone plays a key role in the development of male reproductive tissues, such as the testis and prostate as well as promoting secondary sexual characteristics, such as increased muscle, bone mass, and the growth of body hair.[85] In addition, testosterone is essential for health and well-being as well as prevention of osteoporosis.[86,87] Testosterone is the major androgen secreted by the Leydig cells found in the intertubular spaces of the testis. These cells arise from mesenchymal precursors and studies on rat models have identified that these precursors express the platelet-derived growth factor-α but not 3β-hydroxysteroid dehydrogenase.[88] Further, they suggest that many of these precursors are situated in proximity to the external surfaces of the

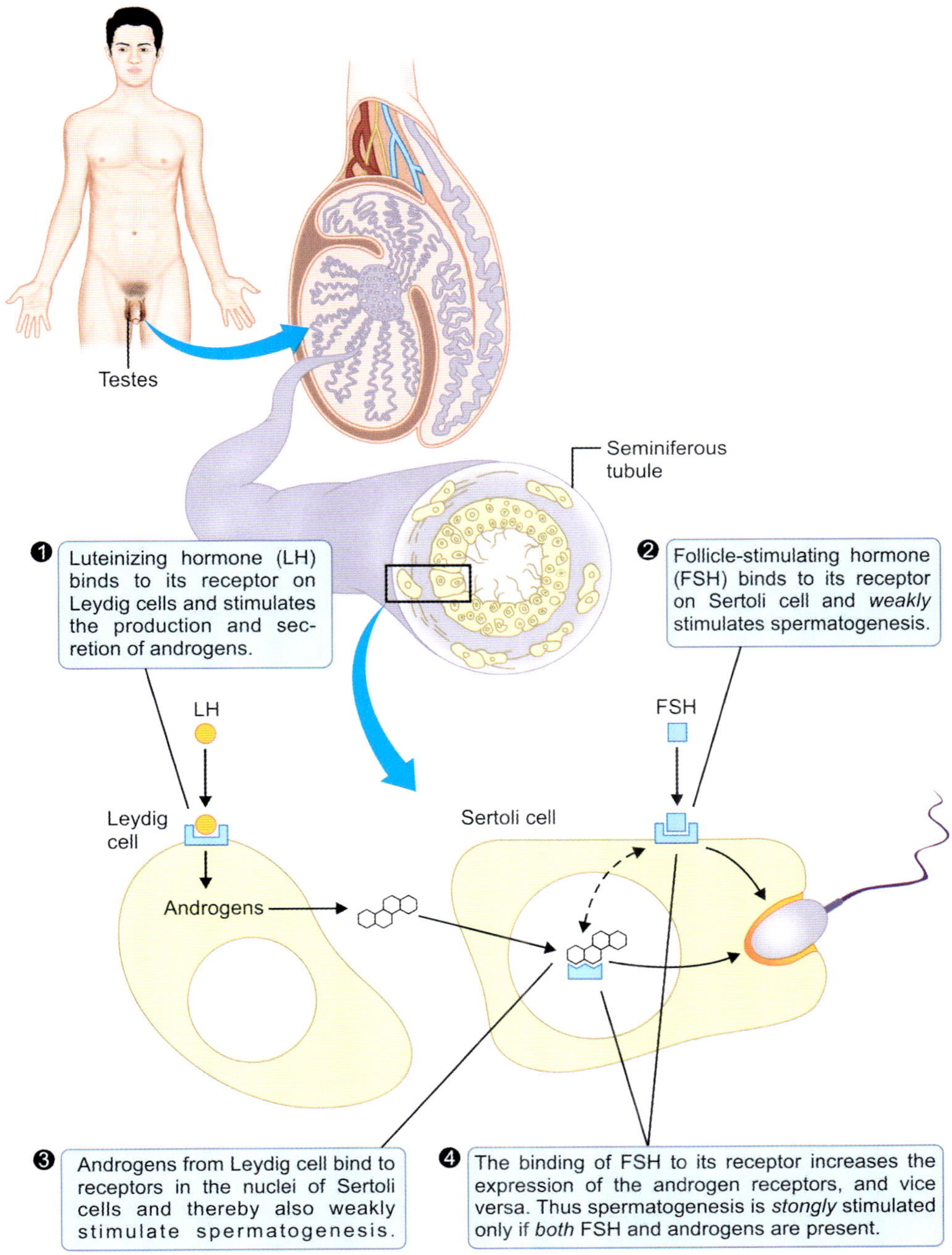

Fig. 17.3: Role of FSH, LH, and androgens in spermatogenesis. Adapted from LeVay and Baldwin (2012).[60]

seminiferous tubules. A normal male produces approximately 7 mg testosterone daily, but also produces lesser amounts of weaker androgens, such as androstenedione and dihydroepiandrosterone. In addition to testosterone, through the actions of the enzyme 5α-reductase, DHT is produced by the testis in smaller amounts. Testis also contributes approximately 25% of the total daily production of 17β-estradiol through the local action of the enzyme aromatase which converts androgenic substrates to this estrogen.[89] The remainder of the circulating estradiol is produced by the adrenal and peripheral tissue through the action of aromatase.

Cholesterol represents the major substrate for androgen production by the Leydig cells. It is derived by an uptake mechanism involving the binding of circulating low density lipoprotein to specific receptors on Leydig cells, which following internalization provides a significant source of cholesterol.[90,91] In addition, the Leydig cells are able to undertake de novo synthesis of cholesterol from acetate, and relative contributions of these two sources are partly dependent on the species and the state of stimulation of the Leydig cells. The conversion of cholesterol to testosterone involves a number of steps that are catalyzed by enzymes, predominantly belonging to cytochrome P450 family (Fig. 17.4).

The mobilization of cellular sources of cholesterol is achieved through the action of cholesterol ester hydrolase and subsequently, this is converted to pregnenolone by the enzyme cytochrome P450 cholesterol side-chain cleavage (cytochrome P450SCC).[93] The conversion of cholesterol to pregnenolone is a key step that regulates the production of androgen within the Leydig cells. Availability of cholesterol

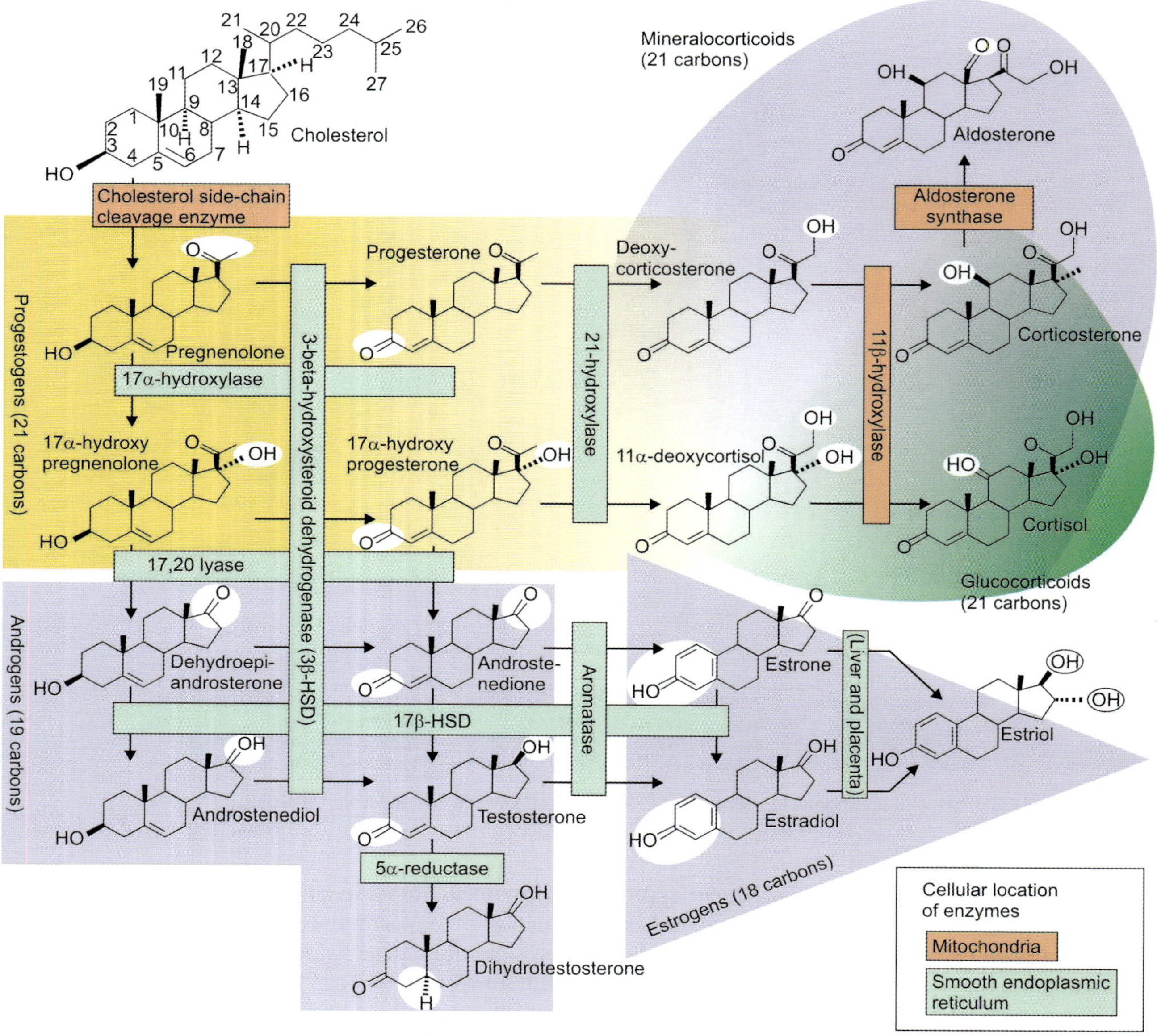

Fig. 17.4: Conversion of cholesterol to testosterone. Adapted from Häggström et al. (2014).[92]

substrate can be rate-limiting and the intracellular trafficking of cholesterol across mitochondrial membranes is dependent on the steroidogenic acute regulatory protein (STAR).[94-96] In case of congenital lipoid adrenal hyperplasia, mutations in the gene encoding STAR lead to the inability of the mitochondria in the adrenals and gonads, to convert cholesterol to pregnenolone.[97] In studies involving targeted disruption of the mouse gene encoding STAR, failure to convert cholesterol to pregnenolone, support the need for STAR protein for the conversion.[98]

Steroidogenesis Game

The purpose of this game is to explore the process of steroidogenesis, the synthesis of steroid hormones from cholesterol. This interactive website shows you how structurally similar the steroid hormones are, and how the activity of many enzymes determines which hormones can be made. If one of these enzymes is absent during development, some hormones will not be synthesized. This can lead to a variety of conditions, including some intersex conditions.

(Sara Freeman and Matt Gilbert for the "Intersex: Biology and Gender" class at Emory University. HHMI Howard Hughes Medical Institute Grant No. 52005873) Available at http://mattgilbert.net/biologygames/steroidogenesis/index.html

Pregnenolone may progress to testosterone production through two pathways. It can be converted to progesterone through the enzyme 3β-hydroxysteroid dehydrogenase (the D4 pathway) or can be hydroxylated at the 17α position by the enzyme 17α-hydroxylase to form 17α-hydroxypregnenolone (the D5 pathway). The relative importance of these two pathways varies with the species and the physiological status of the male.[99] The enzyme 17,20-lyase catalyses the conversion of 17α-hydroxypregnenolone to C19 steroid, dehydroepiandrosterone. These steps may be catalyzed by a cytochrome P450c17, microsomal enzyme encoded by a single-copy gene on chromosome 10.[100,101] The conversion of dehydroepiandrosterone to androstenediol is mediated by a microsomal enzyme 17β-hydroxysteroid dehydrogenase encoded by a single gene.[102,103]

The conversion of substrates from D5 to D4 pathway is catalyzed by the enzyme 3β-hydroxysteroid dehydrogenase.[104] In the D4 pathway, 17α-hydroxyprogesterone proceeds through the action of cytochrome P450c17 to androstenedione and testosterone. Testosterone can be converted to a DHT by the enzyme 5α-reductase[105] or can be metabolized to 17β-estradiol by the enzyme aromatase.[106]

During the production of androgen, steroid substrates such as cholesterol are transported into the mitochondrion to form pregnenolone which is transported to smooth endoplasmic reticulum for further conversion to testosterone.

Figure 17.5 shows the cells involved in the regulation of testosterone production. LH bound to specific receptors on the surface of Leydig cells also controls the production and secretion of testosterone.[108,109] The LH receptor belongs to the seven transmembrane domain, G protein-coupled receptor super family, and mutations of the receptor can lead to familial testicular resistance and male pseudohermaphroditism.[110,111] In some men, constitutively acting mutations of the LH receptor can result in precocious puberty.[112-114]

The interaction of LH with receptor on the surface of Leydig cell triggers the cyclic AMP pathway, through GTP binding proteins.[115,116] Some studies have suggested that the intracellular calcium concentration is increased by the action of LH on surface receptor, which indirectly activates phospholipases in the lipoxygenase pathway.[117] In addition, the changes in calcium can also regulate adenylate cyclase through the protein kinase C pathway. An *in vivo* injection or LH secretion induced by GnRH leads to stimulation of the side-chain cleavage enzyme and release of testosterone within 30–60 minutes of LH stimulation.[118] This acute response lasts for 24–48 hours, and is pronounced in rat and the ram, but is attenuated in men.[119] When hCG is used in place of LH, the initial stimulation is similar to LH, but a second peak of testosterone secretion is observed 48–72 hours after the initial injection.[120] This biphasic pattern has been attributed to the Leydig cells being refractory to further stimulation by either hormone[121,122] and is associated with the longer half-life of hCG compared to LH. Clinically, this suggests that a single weekly injection of hCG will suffice to maintain optimum testosterone responses in many men, rather than frequent injections of hCG.

Luteinizing hormone enhances the transcription of genes that encode a range of enzymes in the steroidogenic pathway, and continued LH stimulation results in Leydig cell hypertrophy and hyperplasia.[123-125] The episodic nature of LH stimulation in the normal male avoids prolonged periods of Leydig cell refractoriness.[126] Testosterone secretory capacity of the human testis declines with age, and so also the efficacy of the aging testis to respond to intravenous pulses of LH.[127]

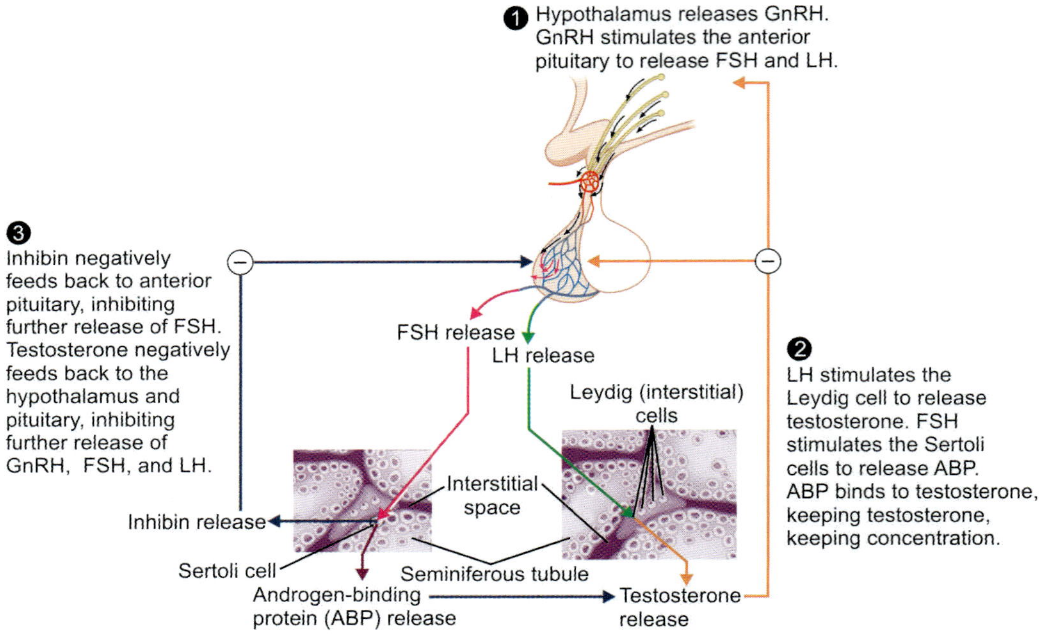

Fig. 17.5: Regulation of the production of testosterone and the cells that assist in spermatogenesis. Adapted from OpenStax (2016).[107]

The level of production of androgens and estrogens by testis also regulates the bone mass, with decreased production leading to osteoporosis. More recently, the production of osteocalcin has been shown to influence testicular function, through G protein-coupled receptors.[128-130]

CONTROL OF LEYDIG CELL FUNCTION BY SEMINIFEROUS TUBULES

Seminiferous tubules exert an influence on testosterone production in Leydig cell as confirmed by several animal studies.[131,132] Even a single episode of heat to the rodent testis has been observed to bring about changes in Leydig cell function and temporarily disrupt spermatogenesis.[133] This is further confirmed in cases like unilateral testicular damage induced by cryptorchidism or efferent duct ligation, where that Leydig cell shows an increased capacity for testosterone biosynthesis and a decrease in the number of LH receptors.[134,135] Although the molecular mechanism of such regulation is not clear at present, it has been recognized that elevated LH and low to low-normal testosterone concentrations in men indicate compromised Leydig cell function. This condition is prevalent in 15–20% of men with severe seminiferous tubule failure.

Andersson et al. have observed lower testosterone and, higher estradiol and LH concentrations in infertile men, further supporting that the state of spermatogenesis has an influence on the function of Leydig cell.[136] They have concluded that the state of spermatogenesis may reflect an extension of testicular dysgenesis to affect steroidogenesis, or alternatively, may result from intercompartment interactions in the testis. Leydig cell aggregation and malformed seminiferous tubules have been linked to impaired intratesticular testosterone levels. A decreased ano-genital distance is emerging as a marker of deficient androgen action in utero.

HORMONAL CONTROL OF SPERMATOGENESIS

A schematic diagram of the different stages of spermatogenesis and their site of occurrence are shown in Figure 17.6. The current understanding of the hormonal regulation of spermatogenesis is the result of studies over the past four decades, involving the suppression and replacement of endocrine hormones.[138-140] Modes of endocrine suppression include hypophysectomy (removal of the pituitary), suppression of pituitary gonadotropin secretion by steroid administration, and suppression of GnRH secretion by immunization or pharmacological modulation. More recently, the hpg mouse model that exhibits a major deletion within the gene encoding GnRH is used to study the role for androgens, estrogen and FSH in the initiation of

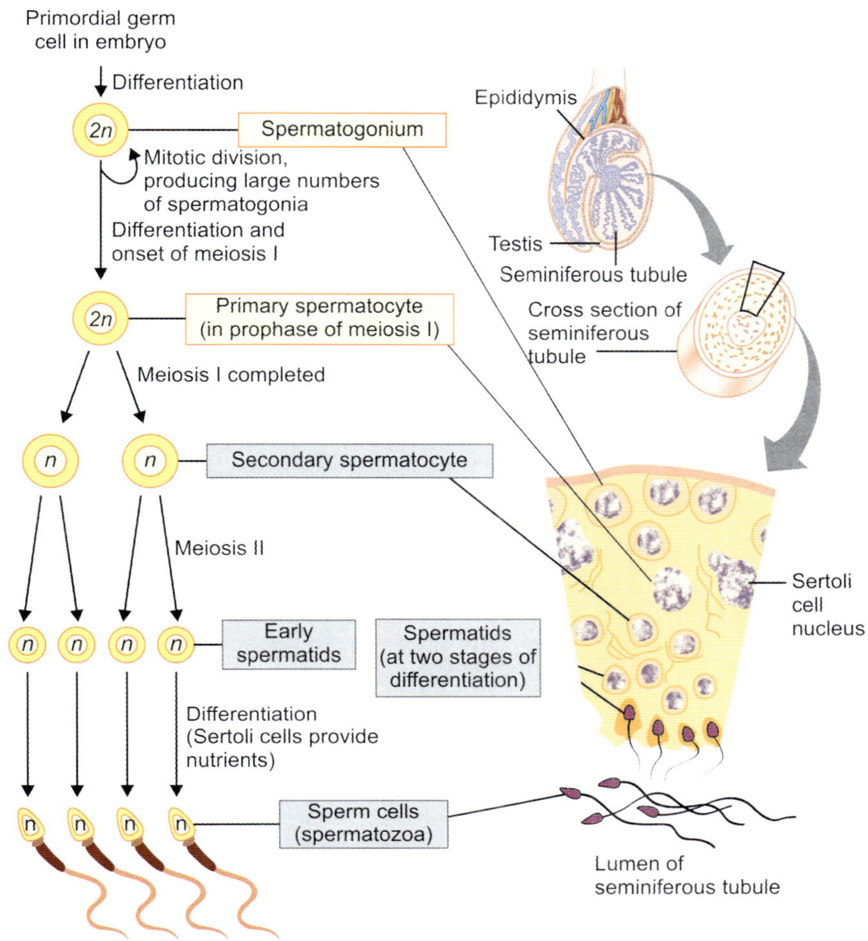

Fig. 17.6: Different stages of spermatogenesis and their site of occurrence. Adapted from Cummings.[137]

spermatogenesis.[138,141] The specific roles and sites of action of gonadotropins, androgens and estrogen have been identified using targeted genetic manipulation in mice.[138,142-144] The role of androgens, FSH and estrogen in spermatogenesis has been extensively reviewed and hence, a brief outline of their role is included here.[138,139,143,146-148]

Role of Testosterone

The primary stimulus for the initiation of spermatogenesis is the LH-induced rise in testosterone at puberty. The absolute requirement of androgen for the initiation of spermatogenesis has been demonstrated by the ability of the nonaromatizable androgen, dehydrotestosterone to initiate complete spermatogenesis in hypogonadal (hpg) mice.[149] In addition, spermatogenesis proceeds only to meiosis stage in mice lacking Sertoli cell AR expression.[150] The initiation of spermatogenesis during puberty requires a higher concentration of androgen than is required to maintain adult spermatogenesis, as observed in hpg mice studies.[151] Once initiated, androgen alone can restore or maintain adult sperm production, as seen in animal model and human studies on induced gonadotropin suppression.[138,140,143,147,152]

Concentration of testosterone in the testis is very high due to its local production. However, when testicular testosterone levels are low as in the case of pubertal testis or gonadotropin suppression, 5α-reduction of testosterone to more potent dehydrotestosterone, amplifies the androgenic signal and exerts stimulatory effects on spermatogenesis.[147] It is likely that testosterone acts directly on the ARs to maintain androgen-dependent functions, and therefore, a small amount can stimulate spermatogenesis, even in the absence of gonadotropin stimulation.[152,153]

AR is expressed in Sertoli cells, peritubular myoid cells within the testis, Leydig cells and vascular endothelial cells, whereas germ cell lack AR expression.[154-157] Recent studies in transgenic mice have revealed that androgen action on AR in each of the testicular somatic cell types is important for testicular function. In terms of androgen action on spermatogenesis, AR expression in Sertoli cells is essential as no sperm are produced in mice with targeted deletion of Sertoli cell AR expression[150] or deletion of the DNA binding domain of Sertoli cell AR.[158]

AR expression on peritubular myoid cells is also be indirectly important for normal spermatogenesis. Peritubular myoid cells support the formation of a normal and fully functional Sertoli cell population, which in turn supports germ cell development.[159] Ablation of AR from peritubular myoid cells also interferes with the normal development and function of the Leydig cell population.[160]

The autocrine action of androgen on AR on Leydig cells is required for normal steroidogenesis and hence, optimal testosteroneproduction.[80] Androgen receptor in endothelial cells of the testicular arterioles is involved in maintaining normal fluid dynamics and vasomotion in the testis.[155]

Several phases of germ cell development (Fig. 17.6) require androgen action. The progression from spermatogonia to meiotic spermatocytes can occur in the absence of androgen. However, the survival of pachytene spermatocytes during the long meiotic prophase, and entry into the final meiotic division requires action of androgen.[82,158,161] Therefore, in the absence of androgen signaling via Sertoli cells, spermatocytes cannot complete meiotic division, and haploid round spermatids are not produced. The progression of haploid spermatids through spermiogenesis (Fig. 17.7) also relies on androgens, and in the absence of androgen, spermiogenesis arrests due to defects in round spermatid survival, and in the ability of newly elongating spermatids to adhere to Sertoli cells.[83,162,163] The final release of spermatids during the process of spermiation is also sensitive to androgen and/or gonadotropin inhibition. Interestingly, the different androgen-dependent processes within germ cell development have different sensitivities and requirements for androgens.[152] The completion of meiosis requires more androgen than the completion of spermiogenesis.[149] Individual variations in the androgen sensitivities of different spermatogenic processes may explain the difficulty to establish a correlation between sperm output and testicular testosterone levels in gonadotropin-suppressed primates and humans.[27,164-166]

Many functions of Sertoli cells, such as the maintenance of tight junction function at the blood–testis barrier and the production of androgen-responsive miRNAs necessary for germ cell development are known to be androgen dependent.[168-171] The mechanisms by which Sertoli cells support each androgen-dependent phase of germ cell development need to be worked out.

Role of FSH

Figure 17.8 shows the role of FSH in spermatogenesis and formation of Sertoli cells. The specific role of FSH in initiation, restoration and maintenance of spermatogenesis has become clear after the use of transgenic mouse

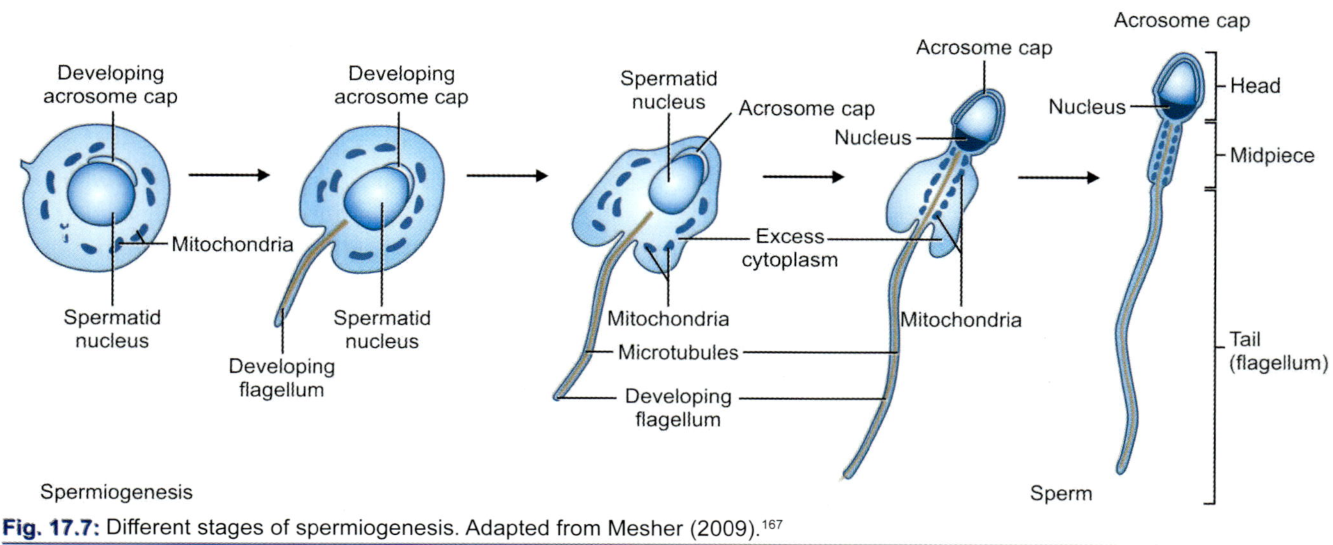

Fig. 17.7: Different stages of spermiogenesis. Adapted from Mesher (2009).[167]

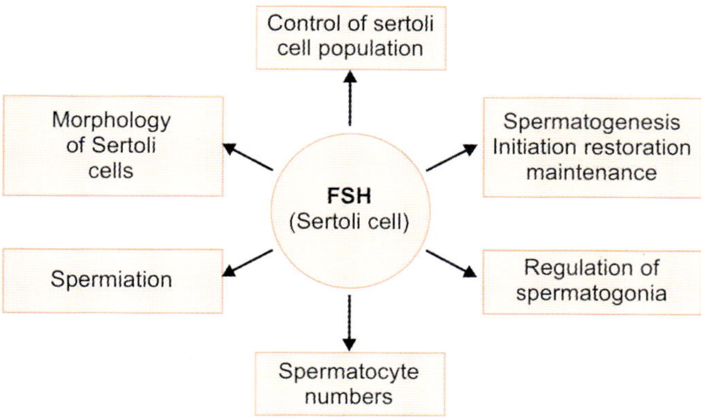

Fig. 17.8: Functions of FSH in spermatogenesis.

models.[138,142,143] Earlier, it was difficult to study action of FSH in complete absence of androgens. FSH receptors are found only on Sertoli cells and are expressed in a stage-dependent manner.[172,173] An important function of FSH is to establish a quantitatively normal adult Sertoli cell population by acting as a mitogen for postnatal Sertoli cell proliferation, as studied in mice model.[172,173] The number of Sertoli cell number determines spermatogenic output in adulthood; hence FSH has an important role in optimal sperm production.[174] Observations in transgenic mice have shown that FSH is needed for normal morphology Sertoli cells and their ability to support the maximal number of germ cells.[162,175-177]

Studies in hpg mice and primates indicate that FSH also plays an important role in the regulation of spermatogonia.[161,178-180] Number of type B spermatogonia was found to correlate more closely with circulating FSH than testicular testosterone levels in gonadotropin-suppressed monkeys and humans, indicating that these cells may be particularly supported by FSH.[73,181] FSH also exerts stimulatory effect on spermatocyte numbers, indicating a permissive effect on meiosis, as revealed by the study of hpg mice in which transgenic human FSH has been expressed.[178] On the other hand, completion of spermiogenesis is not dependent on FSH alone, although suppression of FSH leads to failure of spermiation.[182] This failure of spermiation is suspected to be due to the inability of Sertoli cell to release mature spermatids when FSH levels are very low.

Cooperation between FSH and Testosterone

It is now well established that androgen and FSH has their specific role in spermatogenesis. Several studies have also indicated the synergy between these two hormones to maximize spermatogenic output.[143,146-148] Transgenic mouse models have been used to demonstrate that androgens and FSH can have synergistic, additive and redundant effects on spermatogenesis and Sertoli cell activity.[161,178] Androgen and FSH also cooperate by supporting different aspects of germ cell development, for example, FSH stimulates spermatogonial populations and androgen stimulates spermiogenesis. FSH establishes a quantitatively normal Sertoli cell population, whereas androgen initiates and maintains sperm production. Thus, these two hormones cooperate via independent functions to enable maximal spermatogenic output.

There are many more examples of synergy between testosterone and FSH.[143,146] It has been demonstrated in many experimental settings, testosterone along with FSH has been found to support spermatogenesis at a lower dose than required individually.[147] Testosterone and FSH likely act synergistically in the control of signaling pathways and gene expression in Sertoli cells, which in turn, are important for germ cell development.[143,148] For example, under acute suppression of either androgen or FSH in rats, approximately 10% of mature spermatids failed to be released at spermiation, whereas suppression of both hormones resulted in 50% of spermatids failing tospermiate.[182] Both testosterone and FSH modulate the expression of miRNA in Sertoli cells, which likely mediate a large spectrum of proteomic changes important for Sertoli and germ cell function.[171]

Species-wise differences have been observed in the response of spermatogenesis to combined androgen and FSH suppression.[140,183,184] In humans, spermatogenesis is primarily arrested at spermatogonial development stage, but meiosis and spermiogenesis continue until all the existing spermatogonia undergo meiosis.[164,181,183]

The necessity of testosterone as well as FSH and their synergistic action to support normal spermatogenesis in men were revealed by Matsumoto et al.[185,186] They suppressed the action of gonadotropins by the administration of testosterone until spermatogenesis ceased. Then hCG was injected to stimulate Leydig cell function and to restore intratesticular testosterone concentrations, resulting in increased sperm counts but not to pretreatment levels. These observations have been attributed to the synergistic action of undetectable FSH levels with increasing intratesticular testosterone to partially restore sperm output.[186] Using the same model of halted spermatogenesis, when hFSH was injected in the presence of low intratesticular testosterone concentration, once again sperm output was partially restored.[187] In this case, a synergistic role of FSH with low testosterone is able to stimulate sperm production. These studies confirm that the combination of androgen and FSH consistently produces a better stimulatory effect on spermatogenesis than either factor alone.

Among other functions, both testosterone and FSH facilitate normal Sertoli cell morphology and function, possibly linked to the ability of Sertoli cells to support maximum number of germ cells. Both these hormones promote germ cell survival, particularly of spermatocytes and round spermatids in the midspermatogenic stage.[146,187] The fact that both these hormones can prevent germ cell apoptosis explains why either hormone can maintain germ cell development, at least in the short term, following gonadotropin suppression.[188,189]

ROLE OF ESTROGEN IN MALE REPRODUCTION

Production of estrogen in human male was demonstrated by MacDonald et al. in the year 1979.[190] The development of molecular biology, male transgenic mice lacking of functional estrogen receptors or functional aromatase enzyme, and mutations in both the human estrogen receptor-alpha and aromatase genes have facilitated comprehension of role of estrogen in men.[190-196] Currently, the presence of estrogens in the human testis is well documented and is known to exert a wide range of biological effects in men.[197-200]

The expression of aromatase enzyme, estrogen receptors, ERα and ERβ throughout both the male reproductive system and the human sperm, highlights the role of estrogens in male reproductive function.[197,201,202] Estrogens are thought to modulate sperm maturation, based on the expression of ERα and ERβ on the sperm, and are responsive to estrogens throughout their movement from the testes to the urethra.[203] However, studies on human subjects with congenital estrogen deficiency and congenital aromatase deficiency have shown a variable degree of impaired spermatogenesis.[197,202,204,205] A variable degree of germ cell arrest has been observed in cases that underwent biopsy of the testes.[195,206-208] A clear cause-effect relationship between infertility and aromatase deficiency cannot be demonstrated in these patients.[195,201] The role of estrogen in human male reproduction is far from complete. Existing data on the effects of both estrogen deficiency and excess on male reproductive function is conflicting and confusing.[198,209-211] However, the role of estrogen in controlling sperm production and quality has been recently confirmed by the association of polymorphisms of estrogen-related genes with both sperm concentration and motility, but not with sperm morphology.[212]

Regulation of Gonadotropin Feedback

The regulation of gonadotropin feedback is an important and well-documented action of estrogen in males. Till recently, testosterone was considered the key hormone for the control of gonadotropin feedback in the male. A definitive role for estrogens has recently become clear from the studies on normal men, GnRH-deficient men, and men with congenital estrogen deficiency.[206] Serum gonadotropins were found to be high in all adult patients with aromatase deficiency, in spite of serum testosterone levels being normal to high.[202] These results imply an additional regulation of circulating gonadotropins levels by estrogens in men.

Studies have demonstrated an important direct inhibitory effect of estradiol on gonadotropin secretion in normal as well as GnRH-deficient men, and indicate that the inhibitory effect is partly mediated by the conversion of testosterone to estradiol.[213,214] In line with this argument, administration of the aromatase inhibitor, letrozole to healthy adult males suppressed serum estradiol levels leading to an increase of gonadotropins. Restoration of estrogen to its normal circulating level by transdermal estrogen injections could normalize gonadotropin secretion in these males.[215] Hence, at hypothalamic as well as pituitary level, the effect of circulating estrogen seems to be more relevant than that of locally produced estrogen.[215-217] Estrogen found to act at the hypothalamic level by decreasing GnRH pulse frequency and pituitary responsiveness to GnRH.[10] All of these studies confirm the presence of a hypothalamic site of action for estrogens in men, as with women.

Current understanding about the role of estrogen, shown in Figure 17.9, is that (1) circulating estrogens are involved in gonadotropin suppression both at pituitary and hypothalamic levels and (2) its effect on the hypothalamus is independent of aromatization, but requires adequate amounts of circulating estrogens in normal healthy men, GnRH-deficient men and men with aromatase deficiency.[215-216] It is well established that androgens need to be converted to estrogens to ensure the integrity of the gonadotropin feedback mechanism in men; testosterone

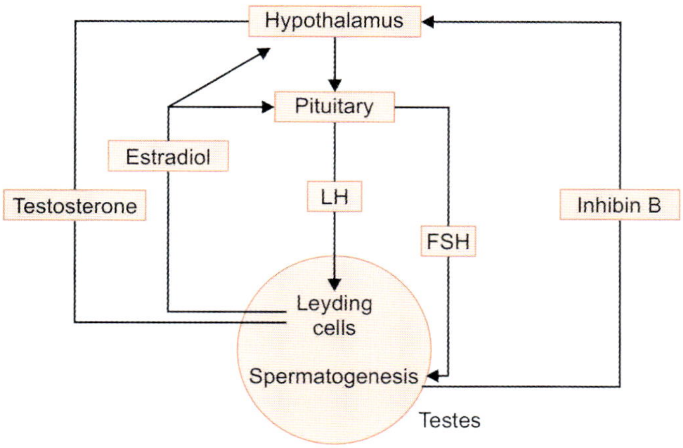

Fig. 17.9: Current understanding of the control of gonadotropin secretion. Adapted from Vincenzo et al. (2000).[200]

itself has been found to have a minor role than previously thought.

As mentioned earlier, in congenitally estrogen deficient men, gonadotropin levels were raised despite of normal to increased serum testosterone levels. The key role of estrogen is responsible for regulating circulating gonadotropins, particularly FSH, in men.[200,217,218] Accordingly, in normal men with pharmacologically induced sex steroid deprivation, estradiol but not testosterone, was able to restore normal FSH serum levels.[216] In addition, estrogens might control the responsiveness to GnRH administration.[205,217]

Estrogen affects LH secretion both at pituitary and hypothalamic levels, as shown by the reduced basal and GnRH-stimulated secretion of LH, LH pulse amplitude, and frequency, in aromatase-deficient men. In the patient with congenital aromatase deficiency diagnosed in childhood, no abnormalities were found in gonadotropin secretion and position and size of testis, unlike female newborns.[219] Lack of abnormality in childhood suggests that a role of estrogens in the hypothalamo-pituitary-testicular axis may become relevant at a later stage in life.[217] A possible role of estrogens is in the priming and maturation of hypothalamus-pituitary-gonadal axis in men.[220,221]

Role of Estrogen in Spermatogenesis

Although FSH and androgens are considered to be the principal regulators of Sertoli cell proliferation and function, and in turn, of spermatogenesis,[222] it is becoming increasingly clear that estrogens also play a role in this process.[223] The hpg mouse is an excellent animal model in which to investigate the mechanism of action of estrogens on spermatogenesis because it has arrested reproductive development without the need for surgical, endocrine, pharmacological or immunological intervention. This mouse line is infertile due to a congenital deficiency of GnRH synthesis leading to markedly reduced pituitary contents of LH and FSH and undetectable or barely measurable serum gonadotropin levels.[224,225] Consequently, the testes fail to undergo normal postnatal development and, at an adult age, hpg testicular androgen production is barely detectable.[226,227] Treatment of hpg mice with androgen alone is sufficient to induce spermatogenesis[149] and treatment with recombinant human FSH induced testicular development in hpg mice, as seen by increased proliferation of spermatogonia and increased spermatocyte numbers.[228]

In the absence of supplementary testosterone treatment, spermatogenesis was arrested at the spermatocyte stage, with little evidence of formation of round spermatids. In contrast, treatment with estradiol has shown qualitatively normal spermatogenesis.[229]

Baines et al. have observed that estradiol treatment for 10 weeks in hpg mice induced significant increases in the weight of the testes ($P < 0.001$), epididymides ($P < 0.001$) and seminal vesicles ($P < 0.001$), although lower than those in age-matched wild-type mice. Morphometric analysis confirmed that the increase in testis weight after estradiol treatment was a reflection of development of the seminiferous epithelium, resulting insignificant increases in the volume and diameter of the seminiferous tubules, although not as much as their wild-type counterparts. Round or elongating spermatids were present in all tubules examined after estradiol treatment. Estradiol treatment significantly ($P < 0.01$) increased pituitary FSH content, whereas no significant effect was observed on pituitary LH content. Consistent with the lack of increase in pituitary LH content, there was no increase in testicular testosterone content after estradiol treatment.

The studies by the same group confirm the initial observations that estradiol treatment promotes spermatogenesis in hpg mice, and provide several insights into understanding how estradiol interacts with FSH and testosterone to regulate spermatogenesis. Based on the interactions of estradiol with ERα and ERβ receptors within the pituitary gland, a model has been proposed for the role of estradiol on spermatogenesis, as depicted in Figure 17.10. The present studies confirm that estradiol treatment of male hpg mice increases FSH content,

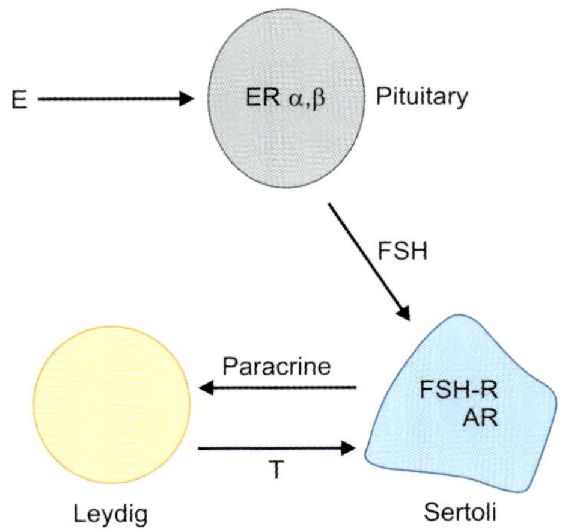

Fig. 17.10: Mode of action of estradiol on spermatogenesis. Adapted from Baines et al. (2005).[229]

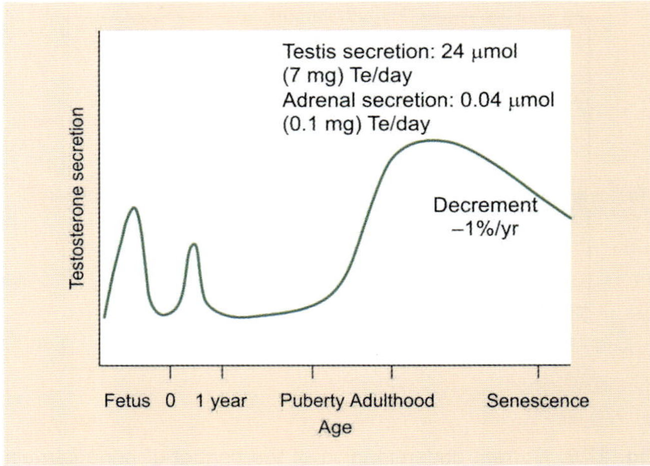

Fig. 17.11: Schematic profile of testosterone secretion over the human male lifetime. Adapted from Expert Consult (2011).[145]

but not pituitary LH content. The stimulation of FSH production is not sufficient to explain the initiation of spermatogenesis by estradiol in hpg mice. The model predicts that this increase in FSH acts upon Sertoli cells by synergizing with the low level of testosterone produced by the Leydig cells. The stimulatory actions of estradiol on the seminal vesicles and epididymides, classically considered androgen-responsive organs, are likely to be direct effects via estrogen receptors expressed in those tissues. It is likely that estradiol is important in the initial development of the male reproductive axis.

Advances in the understanding of the role of estrogens in animal and human models suggest a role for this sex steroid in the reproductive function of both sexes. The fact that both estrogen excess and estrogen deficiency influence male sexual development, testis function, the hypothalamic–pituitary–testis axis, spermatogenesis and ultimately male fertility, highlight the importance of estrogen action in male.

AGE-RELATED CHANGES IN REPRODUCTIVE HORMONES

Reduction in Testosterone Levels

There is agreement that in young men with classical hypogonadism due to known diseases of the testis, pituitary and the hypothalamus, testosterone replacement is relatively safe and has many beneficial effects in improving lean body mass, sexual function, energy, mood, and sense of well-being and reducing fat mass.[230-233] There is agreement that serum level of testosterone declines as a function of age. Several longitudinal studies have confirmed a gradual but progressive decrease in serum testosterone concentrations from age 20 to 80 (Figs. 17.11 and 17.12).[234-237] The age-related decline in men does not start at a discrete time point in age, but total testosterone concentrations decline inevitably after reaching a peak in the second and third decade. The rate of age-related decline is greater in older men with chronic illness and adiposity than in healthy, nonobese older men.[238-240] Epidemiological studies of older men have reported associations between low testosterone levels and health outcomes, although these associations are weak. For instance, in a number of epidemiologic studies, low bioavailable testosterone levels were associated with low appendicular skeletal muscle mass.[241-244] Low bioavailable testosterone levels also have been associated with decreased strength of upper as well as lower extremity muscles and decreased performance in self-reported as well as performance-based measures of physical function.[242,245] Aging of humans is also associated with a decline in cognitive function, such as verbal memory, visual memory, spatial ability, and executive function, are associated with the age-related decline in testosterone.[246-251]

Decline in testosterone levels has an influence on the bone metabolism, affecting both osteoblast and osteoclast activity, as shown in Figure 17.13. Several epidemiologic studies of older men have found that bioavailable testosterone and estradiol levels but not total testosterone levels, are associated with bone mineral density. In the MrOS study, the odds of osteoporosis in men with a total testosterone less than 200 ng/dL were 3.7-fold higher than in men with

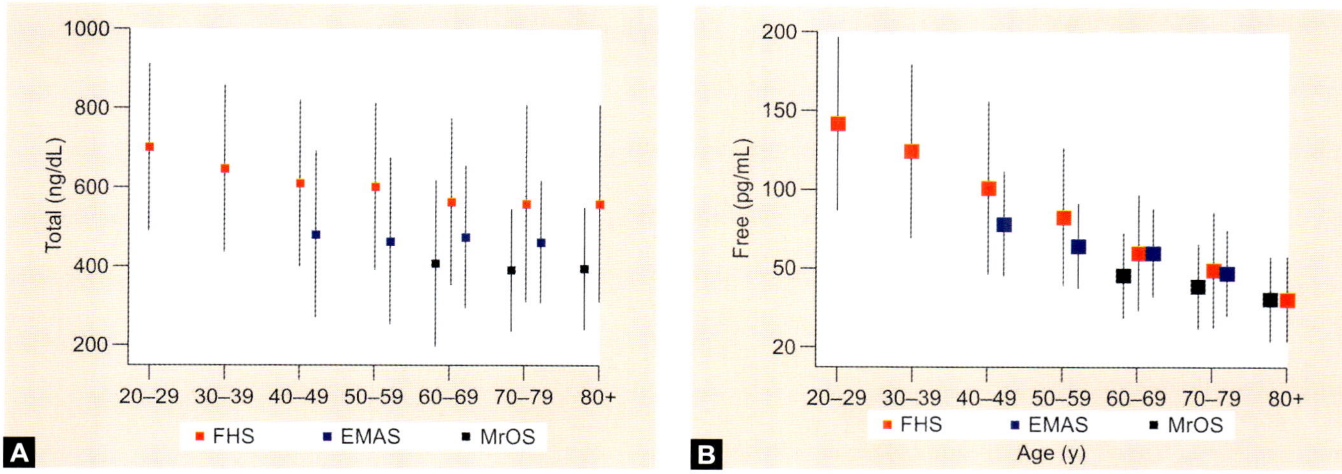

Figs. 17.12A and B: Decline in testosterone concentration by decades of age, observed in the Framingham heart study (FHS), the European male aging study (EMAS) and the study of osteoporotic fractures in men (MrOS). Mean ± SD are shown. Reproduced with permission from Bhasin et al. (2010).[230]

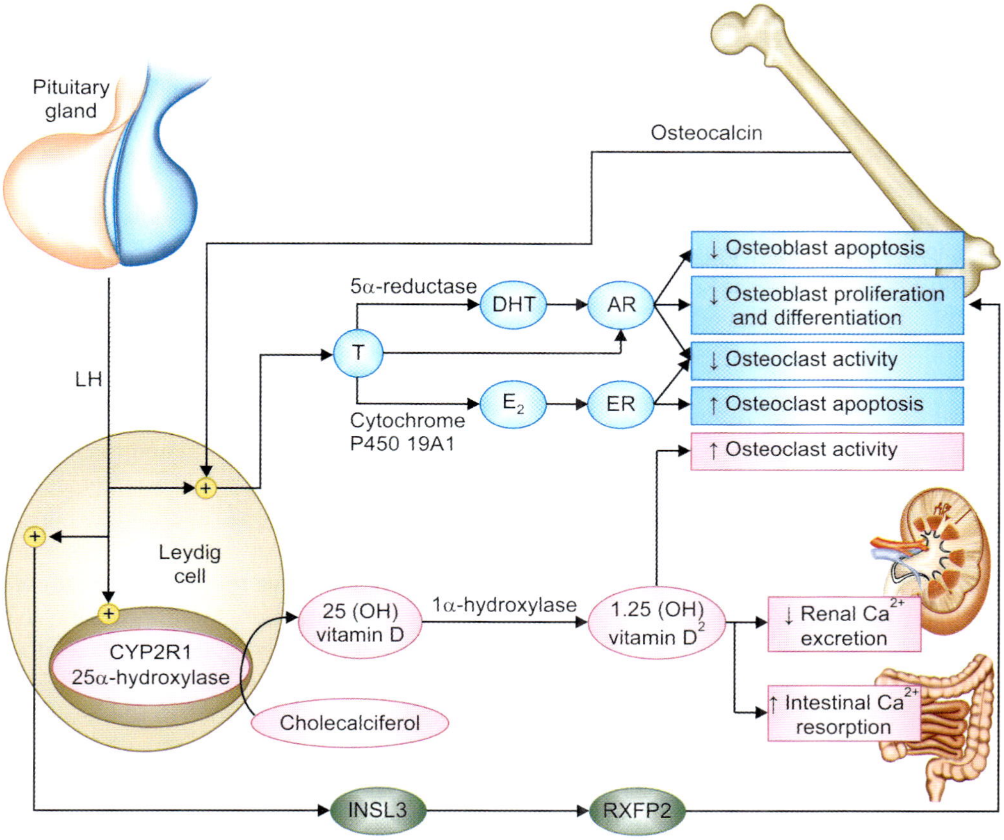

Fig. 17.13: Testosterone influences bone mineral density. Adapted from Ferlin et al. (2013).[254]

normal testosterone level.[252] Free testosterone level has been found to be a predictor of osteoporotic bone fractures.[253]

The association of testosterone levels with sexual dysfunction has been inconsistent across studies because of the heterogeneity of instruments used to define sexual dysfunction, varying quality of instruments used to assess sexual function, problems of testosterone assay quality, and failure to distinguish among various categories of sexual dysfunction.[246,247,255,256] In general, serum total and bioavailable testosterone levels were not significantly different between men who reported erectile dysfunction and those who did not.[247,256]

Circulating testosterone concentrations are dependent on testosterone production and clearance rates. The age-related decline in serum testosterone concentrations is primarily a consequence of decreased production rates in older men[257-260] and lower plasma clearance rates in older men than in younger men.[240,261] Testosterone production in older men is reduced due to abnormalities at many levels of the hypothalamic–pituitary–testicular axis.[257,258,262,263] Testicular testosterone secretion in healthy, young men is characterized by a diurnal rhythm with higher concentrations in the morning and lower levels in later afternoon. Many studies have revealed that the diurnal rhythm of testosterone secretion is dampened in older men.[264,265] Testosterone response to LH and hCG is also decreased in older men.[257,258,262]

There are potential benefits of supplementation in older men with low testosterone levels, to raise it to minnormal levels. Supplementation is expected to improve physical function and mobility, some domains of sexual and cognitive functions, energy and sense of wellbeing, bone health and overall quality of life. However, the effects of testosterone supplementation on health-related outcomes in older men have not been studied. A number of randomized trials have demonstrated improvements in surrogate markers, such as lean and fat mass; however, there are very few long-term, placebo-controlled, randomized trials that are adequately powered to detect clinically meaningful changes in health outcomes, such as fracture rates, physical function, disability, progression to dementia, etc. Long-term data on the effects of testosterone supplementation on the risk of prostate disease and cardiovascular events are also lacking.

A review of studies examining fertility at different ages demonstrated significant age-related differences in fertility rates men, including lower pregnancy rates, increased time to pregnancy, and subfecundity in men older than 50 years.[266-270] A literature review found no significant change in sperm concentration with aging, when comparing men under the age of 30 with those greater than 50 years.[271] However, in general, semen volume, sperm motility, and the number of morphologically normal sperm decrease with advancing age (Table 17.2).

Table 17.2: Comparison of semen quality and fertility in men with aging[271]

Parameter	*Age comparison*	*Change*
Semen volume	30 vs. 50 years	3–22% decrease
Sperm concentration	Varying	None
Abnormal sperm morphology	30 vs. 50 years	4–18% increase
Time to pregnancy	<30–35 vs. >30–50 years	5–20% increase
Pregnancy rates	<30 vs. >50 years	23–38% decrease
Subfecundity	Varying	11–250% increase

Gonadotropin Secretion and Regulation

There are significant variations in the circulating LH and FSH concentrations in individual older men. Therefore, both hypogonadotropic and hypergonadotropic hypogonadism are known in older men.[240,272] Serum LH and FSH concentrations have been found to be raised in older men than in young men.[235,236] Serum LH and FSH levels show an age-related increase in longitudinal studies, although no simple relationship has been observed between serum LH concentrations and age-related decline in circulating testosterone levels. Studies of Urban et al. and Zwart et al. on LH responsiveness to GnRH to have opposite trends; the former have observed a diminished response in older men, while the latter have reported an increased response.[273,274] This has been attributed to the changes in GnRH secretion and alterations in gonadal steroid feedback and feedforward relationships. Both of the feedback and feed-forward mechanisms are operative in older men, in contrast with younger men.[263,275] Studies on synchronization of LH and testosterone secretion have revealed that there is greater variability in LH pulse frequency, amplitude, and secretory mass in older men, in comparison to younger men, leading to the disruption of the synchrony.[275,276]

REFERENCES

1. Parhar IS. Gonadotropin-Releasing Hormone: Molecules and Receptors. Amsterdam: Elsevier; 2002. ISBN 0-444-50979-8.
2. Hayes FJ, DeCruz S, Seminara SB, Boepple PA, Crowley Jr WF. Differential regulation of gonadotropin secretion by testosterone in the human male: absence of a negative feedback effect of testosterone on follicle-stimulating hormone. J Clin Endocrinol Metab. 2001;86:53-8.
3. Schnorr JA, Bray MJ, Veldhuis JD. Aromatization mediates testosterone's short term feedback restraint of 24-hour endogenously driven and acute endogenous gonadotropin releasing hormone stimulated luteinizing hormone and follicle stimulating hormone secretion in young men. J Clin Endocrinol Metab. 2001;86:2600-6.
4. Manetti GJ, Honig SC. Update on male hormonal contraception: is the vasectomy in jeopardy? Intl J Impotence Res. 2010;22:159-70.
5. Sherins RJ, Loriaux DL. Studies of the role of sex steroids in the feedback control of FSH concentrations in men. J Clin Endocrinol Metab. 1973;36:886-93.
6. Aumueller G, Eicheler W, Renneberg H, Adermann K, Vilja P, Forssmann WG. Immunocytochemical evidence for differential subcellular localization of 5 alpha-reductase isoenzymes in human tissues. Acta Anat. 1996;156:241-52.
7. Naftolin F, Ryan KJ, Petro Z. Aromatization of androstenedione by the diencephalon. J Clin Endocrinol Metab. 1971;33:368-70.
8. Santen RJ. Is aromatization of testosterone to estradiol required for inhibition of luteinizing hormone secretion in men? J Clin Invest. 1975;56:1555-63.
9. Santen RJ, Bardin CW. Episodic luteinizing hormone secretion in man. Pulse analysis, clinical interpretation, physiologic mechanisms. J Clin Invest. 1973;52:2617-28.
10. Hayes FJ, Seminara SB, Decruz S, Boepple PA, Crowley WF, Jr. Aromatase inhibition in the human male reveals a hypothalamic site of estrogen feedback. J Clin Endocrinol Metab. 2000;85:3027-35.
11. Decker MH, Loriaux DL, Cutler GB, Jr. A seminiferous tubular factor is not obligatory for regulation of plasma follicle stimulating hormone in the rat. Endocrinology. 1981;108:1035-9.
12. Phillips DJ, de Kretser DM. Follistatin: a multifunctional regulatory protein. Front Neuroendocrinol. 1998;19:287-322.
13. O'Donnell L, Stanton P, de Kretser DM. Endocrinology of the male reproductive system.In: De Groot LJ, Chrousos G, Dungan K, Feingold KR, Grossman A, Hershman JM, Koch C, Korbonits M, McLachlan R, New M, Purnell J, Rebar R, Singer F, Vinik A (Eds). Endotext [Internet]. South Dartmouth, MA: MDText.com, Inc.; 2000. Available from: http://www.ncbi.nlm.nih.gov/books/NBK279031/ [Updated 8 Jan 2013].
14. McCullagh DR. Dual endocrine activity of the testes. Science. 1932;76:19-20.
15. de Kretser DM, Robertson DM. The isolation and physiology of inhibin and related proteins. Biol Reprod. 1989;40:33-47.
16. McNeilly AS1, Tsonis CG, Baird DT. Inhibin. Hum Reprod. 1988;3(1):45-9.
17. Le Gac F, de Kretser DM. Inhibin production by Sertoli cell cultures. Mol Cell Endocrinol. 1982;28:487-98.
18. Steinberger A, Steinberger E. Secretion of an FSH-inhibiting factor by cultured Sertoli cells. Endocrinology. 1976;99:918-21.
19. Klaij IA, Timmerman MA, Blok LJ, Grootegoed JA, de Jong FH. Regulation of inhibin beta B-subunit mRNA expression in rat Sertoli cells: consequences for the production of bioactive and immunoreactive inhibin. Mol Cell Endocrinol. 1992;85:237-46.
20. Sharpe RM, Turner KJ, McKinnell C, Groome NP, Atanassova N, Millar MR, et al. Inhibin B levels in plasma of the male rat from birth to adulthood: effect of experimental manipulation of Sertoli cell number. J Androl. 1999;20:94-101.
21. Anawalt BD, Bebb RA, Matsumoto AM, Groome NP, Illingworth PJ, McNeilly AS, et al. Serum inhibin B levels reflect Sertoli cell function in normal men and men with testicular dysfunction. J Clin Endocrinol Metab. 1996;81:3341-5.
22. Anderson RA, Wallace EM, Groome NP, Bellis AJ, Wu FC. Physiological relationships between inhibin B, follicle stimulating hormone secretion and spermatogenesis in normal men and response to gonadotrophin suppression by exogenous testosterone. Hum Reprod. 1997;12:746-51.
23. Krummen LA, Toppari J, Kim WH, Morelos BS, Ahmad N, Swerdloff RS, et al. Regulation of testicular inhibin subunit messenger ribonucleic acid levels *in vivo*: effects of hypophysectomy and selective follicle-stimulating hormone replacement. Endocrinology. 1989;125:1630-7.
24. Risbridger GP, Clements J, Robertson DM, Drummond AE, Muir J, Burger HG, et al. Immuno- and bioactive inhibin and inhibin alpha-subunit expression in rat Leydig cell cultures. Mol Cell Endocrinol. 1989;66:119-22.
25. McLachlan RI, Matsumoto AM, Burger HG, de Kretser DM, Bremner WJ. Relative roles of follicle-stimulating hormone and luteinizing hormone in the control of inhibin secretion in normal men. J Clin Invest. 1988;82:880-4.
26. Tena-Sempere M, Kero J, Rannikko A, Yan W, Huhtaniemi I. The pattern of inhibin/activin alpha- and betaB subunit messenger ribonucleic acid expression in rat testis after selective Leydig cell destruction by ethylene dimethane sulfonate. Endocrinology. 1999;140:5761-70.
27. Matthiesson KL, Robertson DM, Burger HG, McLachlan RI. Response of serum inhibin B and pro-alphaC levels to gonadotrophic stimulation in normal men before and after steroidal contraceptive treatment. Hum Reprod. 2003;18:734-43.
28. Ling N, Ying SY, Ueno N, Shimasaki S, Esch F, Hotta M, et al. Pituitary FSH is released by a heterodimer of the beta-subunits from the two forms of inhibin. Nature. 1986;321:779-82.
29. Vale W, Rivier J, Vaughan J, McClintock R, Corrigan A, Woo W, et al. Purification and characterization of an FSH releasing protein from porcine ovarian follicular fluid. Nature. 1986;321:776-9.
30. Matzuk MM, Kumar TR, Bradley A. Different phenotypes for mice deficient in either activins or activin receptor type II. Nature. 1995;374:356-60.

31. de Winter JP, Vanderstichele HM, Verhoeven G, Timmerman MA, Wesseling JG, de Jong FH. Peritubular myoid cells from immature rat testes secrete activin-A and express activin receptor type II *in vitro*. Endocrinology. 1994;135: 759-67.
32. de Winter JP, Vanderstichele HM, Timmerman MA, Blok LJ, Themmen AP, de Jong FH. Activin is produced by rat Sertoli cells *in vitro* and can act as an autocrine regulator of Sertoli cell function. Endocrinology. 1993;132:975-82.
33. Lee W, Mason AJ, Schwall R, Szonyi E, Mather JP. Secretion of activin by interstitial cells in the testis. Science. 1989;243:396-8.
34. McFarlane JR, Foulds LM, Pisciotta A, Robertson DM, de Kretser DM. Measurement of activin in biological fluids by radioimmunoassay, utilizing dissociating agents to remove the interference of follistatin. Eur J Endocrinol. 1996;134:481-9.
35. Mather JP, Attie KM, Woodruff TK, Rice GC, Phillips DM. Activin stimulates spermatogonial proliferation in germ-Sertoli cell cocultures from immature rat testis. Endocrinology. 1990;127:3206-14.
36. Boitani C, Stefanini M, Fragale A, Morena AR. Activin stimulates Sertoli cell proliferation in a defined period of rat testis development. Endocrinology. 1995;136:5438-44.
37. Meehan T, Schlatt S, O'Bryan MK, de Kretser DM, Loveland KL. Regulation of germ cell and Sertoli cell development by activin, follistatin, and FSH. Dev Biol. 2000;220:225-37.
38. Archambeault DR, Yao HH. Activin A, a product of fetal Leydig cells, is a unique paracrine regulator of Sertoli cell proliferation and fetal testis cord expansion. Proc Natl Acad Sci U S A. 2010;107:10526-31.
39. Buzzard JJ, Farnworth PG, De Kretser DM, O'Connor AE, Wreford NG, Morrison JR. Proliferative phase sertoli cells display a developmentally regulated response to activin *in vitro*. Endocrinology. 2003;144:474-83.
40. Mendis SH, Meachem SJ, Sarraj MA, Loveland KL. Activin A balances Sertoli and germ cell proliferation in the fetal mouse testis. Biol Reprod. 2011;84:379-91.
41. de Winter JP, Themmen AP, Hoogerbrugge JW, Klaij IA, Grootegoed JA, de Jong FH. Activin receptor mRNA expression in rat testicular cell types. Mol Cell Endocrinol. 1992;83:R1-8.
42. Robertson DM, Klein R, de Vos FL, McLachlan RI, Wettenhall RE, Hearn MT, et al. The isolation of polypeptides with FSH suppressing activity from bovine follicular fluid which are structurally different to inhibin. Biochem Biophys Res Commun. 1987;149:744-9.
43. Nakamura T, Takio K, Eto Y, Shibai H, Titani K, Sugino H. Activin-binding protein from rat ovary is follistatin. Science. 1990;247:836-8.
44. Meinhardt A, O'Bryan MK, McFarlane JR, Loveland KL, Mallidis C, Foulds LM, et al. Localization of follistatin in the rat testis. J Reprod Fertil. 1998;112:233-41.
45. Michel U, Albiston A, Findlay JK. Rat follistatin: gonadal and extragonadal expression and evidence for alternative splicing. Biochem Biophys Res Commun. 1990;173:401-7.
46. Tilbrook AJ, de Kretser DM, Dunshea FR, Klein R, Robertson DM, Clarke IJ, et al. The testis is not the major source of circulating follistatin in the ram. J Endocrinol. 1996;149: 55-63.
47. Phillips DJ, Hedger MP, McFarlane JR, Klein R, Clarke IJ, Tilbrook AJ, et al. Follistatin concentrations in male sheep increase following sham castration/castration or injection of interleukin-1 beta. J Endocrinol. 1996;151:119-24.
48. Dubey AK, Zeleznik AJ, Plant TM. In the rhesus monkey (Macaca mulatta), the negative feedback regulation of follicle-stimulating hormone secretion by an action of testicular hormone directly at the level of the anterior pituitary gland cannot be accounted for by either testosterone or estradiol. Endocrinology. 1987;121:2229-37.
49. Ramaswamy S, Pohl CR, McNeilly AS, Winters SJ, Plant TM. The time course of follicle-stimulating hormone suppression by recombinant human inhibin A in the adult male rhesus monkey (Macaca mulatta). Endocrinology. 1998;139:3409-15.
50. Robertson DM, Prisk M, McMaster JW, Irby DC, Findlay JK, de Kretser DM. Serum FSH-suppressing activity of human recombinant inhibin A in male and female rats. J Reprod Fertil. 1991;91:321-8.
51. Tilbrook AJ, de Kretser DM, Clarke IJ. Human recombinant inhibin A and testosterone act directly at the pituitary to suppress plasma concentrations of FSH in castrated rams. J Endocrinol. 1993;138:181-9.
52. Tilbrook AJ, De Kretser DM, Clarke IJ. Human recombinant inhibin A suppresses plasma follicle-stimulating hormone to intact levels but has no effect on luteinizing hormone in castrated rams. Biol Reprod. 1993;49:779-88.
53. Roberts V, Meunier H, Vaughan J, Rivier J, Rivier C, Vale W, et al. Production and regulation of inhibin subunits in pituitary gonadotropes. Endocrinology. 1989;124:552-4.
54. Corrigan AZ, Bilezikjian LM, Carroll RS, Bald LN, Schmelzer CH, Fendly BM, et al. Evidence for an autocrine role of activin B within rat anterior pituitary cultures. Endocrinology. 1991;128:1682-4.
55. Gospodarowicz D, Lau K. Pituitary follicular cells secrete both vascular endothelial growth factor and follistatin. Biochem Biophys Res Commun. 1989;165:292-8.
56. Kogawa K, Nakamura T, Sugino K, Takio K, Titani K, Sugino H. Activin-binding protein is present in pituitary. Endocrinology. 1991;128:1434-40.
57. Bilezikjian LM, Corrigan AZ, Blount AL, Vale WW. Pituitary follistatin and inhibin subunit messenger ribonucleic acid levels are differentially regulated by local and hormonal factors. Endocrinology. 1996;137:4277-84.
58. Bilezikjian LM, Vaughan JM, Vale WW. Characterization and the regulation of inhibin/activin subunit proteins of cultured rat anterior pituitary cells. Endocrinology. 1993;133:2545-53.
59. Jensen TK, Andersson AM, Hjollund NH, Scheike T, Kolstad H, Giwercman A, et al. Inhibin B as a serum marker of spermatogenesis: correlation to differences in sperm concentration and follicle-stimulating hormone levels. A study of 349 Danish men. J Clin Endocrinol Metab. 1997;82:4059-63.

60. LeVay S, Baldwin J. Human sexuality. 4th edition. Sunderland, MA: Sinauer Associates, Inc; 2012.
61. Gonzales GF, Risbridger GP, de Krester DM. *In vivo* and *in vitro* production of inhibin by cryptorchid testes from adult rats. Endocrinology. 1989;124:1661-8.
62. Weinbauer GF, Bartlett JM, Fingscheidt U, Tsonis CG, de Kretser DM, Nieschlag E. Evidence for a major role of inhibin in the feedback control of FSH in the male rat. J Reprod Fertil. 1989;85:355-62.
63. George JT, Seminara SB. Kisspeptin and the hypothalamic control of reproduction: lessons from the human. Endocrinology. 2012;153(11):5130-6.
64. Novaira HJ, Ng Y, Wolfe A, Radovick S. Kisspeptin increases GnRH mRNA expression and secretion in GnRH secreting neuronal cell lines. Mol Cell Endocrinol. 2009;311:126-34.
65. Page ST, Amory JK, Bremner WJ. Advances in male contraception. Endocr Rev. 2008;29:465-93.
66. Seminara SB, Dipietro MJ, Ramaswamy S, Crowley Jr WF, Plant TM. Continuous human metastin 45-54 infusion desensitizes G protein-coupled receptor 54-induced gonadotropin-releasing hormone release monitored indirectly in the juvenile male Rhesus monkey (Macaca mulatta): A finding with therapeutic implications. Endocrinology. 2006;147:2122-6.
67. Oakley AE, Clifton DK, Steiner RA. Kisspeptin signaling in the brain. Endocr Rev. 2009;30:713-43.
68. Roa J, Navarro VM, Tena-Sempere M. Kisspeptins in reproductive biology: consensus knowledge and recent developments. Biol Reprod. 2011;85:650-60.
69. Coviello AD, Bremner WJ, Matsumoto AM, Herbst KL, Amory JK, Anawalt BD, et al. Intratesticular testosterone concentrations comparable with serum levels are not sufficient to maintain normal sperm production in men receiving a hormonal contraceptive regimen. J Androl. 2004;25:931-8.
70. Coviello AD, Matsumoto AM, Bremner WJ, Herbst KL, Amory JK, Anawalt BD, et al. Low-dose human chorionic gonadotropin maintains intratesticular testosterone in normal men with testosterone-induced gonadotropin suppression. J Clin Endocrinol Metab. 2005;90:2595-602.
71. Heller CG, Rowley MJ, Heller GV. Clomiphene citrate: a correlation of its effect on sperm concentration and morphology, total gonadotropins, ICSH, estrogen and testosterone excretion, and testicular cytology in normal men. J Clin Endocrinol Metab. 1969;29:638-49.
72. Huhtaniemi I, Nikula H, Rannikko S. Pituitary-testicular function of prostatic cancer patients during treatment with a gonadotropin-releasing hormone agonist analog. I. Circulating hormone levels. J Androl. 1987;8:355-62.
73. McLachlan RI, O'Donnell L, Stanton PG, Balourdos G, Frydenberg M, de Kretser DM, et al. Effects of testosterone plus medroxyprogesterone acetate on semen quality, reproductive hormones, and germ cell populations in normal young men. J Clin Endocrinol Metab. 2002;87:546-56.
74. Simoni M, Weinbauer GF, Gromoll J, Nieschlag E. Role of FSH in male gonadal function. Ann Endocrinol (Paris). 1999;60:102-6.
75. Ruwanpura SM, McLachlan RI, Matthiesson KL, Meachem SJ. Gonadotrophins regulate germ cell survival, not proliferation, in normal adult men. Hum Reprod. 2008;23:403-11.
76. Soriano-Guillen L, Mitchell V, Carel JC, Barbet P, Roger M, Lahlou N. Activating mutations in the luteinizing hormone receptor gene: a human model of non-follicle-stimulating hormone-dependent inhibin production and germ cell maturation. J Clin Endocrinol Metab. 2006;91:3041-7.
77. McLachlan RI, Robertson DM, Pruysers E, Ugoni A, Matsumoto AM, Anawalt BD, et al. Relationship between serum gonadotropins and spermatogenic suppression in men undergoing steroidal contraceptive treatment. J Clin Endocrinol Metab. 2004;89:142-9.
78. Shah C, Modi D, Sachdeva G, Gadkar S, Puri C. Coexistence of intracellular and membrane-bound progesterone receptors in human testis. J Clin Endocrinol Metab. 2005;90:474-83.
79. Amory JK, Wang C, Swerdloff RS, Anawalt BD, Matsumoto AM, Bremner WJ, et al. The effect of 5-alpha-reductase inhibition with dutasteride and finasteride on semen parameters and serum hormones in healthy men. J Clin Endocrinol Metab. 2007;92:1659-65.
80. Tsai MY, Yeh SD, Wang RS, Yeh S, Zhang C, Lin HY, et al. Differential effects of spermatogenesis and fertility in mice lacking androgen receptor in individual testis cells. Proc Natl Acad Sci U S A. 2006;103:18975-80.
81. Chang C, Chen YT, Yeh SD, Xu Q, Wang RS, Guillou F, et al. Infertility with defective spermatogenesis and hypotestosteronemia in male mice lacking the androgen receptor in Sertoli cells. Proc Natl Acad Sci U S A. 2004;101:6876-81.
82. De Gendt K, Swinnen JV, Saunders PT, Schoonjans L, Dewerchin M, Devos A, et al. A Sertoli cell-selective knockout of the androgen receptor causes spermatogenic arrest in meiosis. Proc Natl Acad Sci U S A. 2004;101:1327-32.
83. Holdcraft RW, Braun RE. Androgen receptor function is required in Sertoli cells for the terminal differentiation of haploid spermatids. Development. 2004;131:459-67.
84. Zhang C, Yeh S, Chen YT, Wu CC, Chuang KH, Lin HY, et al. Oligozoospermia with normal fertility in male mice lacking the androgen receptor in testis peritubular myoid cells. Proc Natl Acad Sci U S A. 2006;103:17718-23.
85. Mooradian AD, Morley JE, Korenman SG. Biological actions of androgens. Endocr Rev. 1987;8(1):1-28.
86. Bassil N, Alkaade S, Morley JE. The benefits and risks of testosterone replacement therapy: a review. Ther Clin Risk Manage. 2009;5(3):427-48.
87. Tuck SP, Francis RM. Testosterone, bone and osteoporosis. Front Horm Res. 2009;37:123-32.
88. Stanley E, Lin CY, Jin S, Liu J, Sottas CM, Ge R, et al. Identification, proliferation, and differentiation of adult leydig stem cells. Endocrinology. 2012;153(10):5002-10.
89. Baird DT, Galbraith A, Fraser IS, Newsam JE. The concentration of oestrone and oestradiol-17 in spermatic venous blood in man. J Endocrinol. 1973;57:285-8.
90. Chen YD, Kraemer FB, Reaven GM. Identification of specific high density lipoprotein-binding sites in rat testis and

regulation of binding by human chorionic gonadotropin. J Biol Chem. 1980;255:9162-7.
91. Freeman DA, Ascoli M. The low-density lipoprotein pathway of cultured Leydig tumor cells. Utilization of low density lipoprotein-derived cholesterol for steroidogenesis. Biochim Biophys Acta. 1983;754:72-81.
92. Häggström M, Richfield D. Diagram of the pathways of human steroidogenesis. Wikiversity Journal of Medicine. 2014;1(1):1-5.
93. Chung BC, Matteson KJ, Voutilainen R, Mohandas TK, Miller WL. Human cholesterol side-chain cleavage enzyme, P450scc: cDNA cloning, assignment of the gene to chromosome 15, and expression in the placenta. Proc Natl Acad Sci U S A. 1986;83:8962-6.
94. Clark BJ, Wells J, King SR, Stocco DM. The purification, cloning, and expression of a novel luteinizing hormone induced mitochondrial protein in MA-10 mouse Leydig tumor cells. Characterization of the steroidogenic acute regulatory protein (StAR). J Biol Chem. 1994;269:28314-22.
95. Pollack SE, Furth EE, Kallen CB, Arakane F, Kiriakidou M, Kozarsky KF, et al. Localization of the steroidogenic acute regulatory protein in human tissues. J Clin Endocrinol Metab. 1997;82:4243-51.
96. Stocco DM, Clark BJ. Regulation of the acute production of steroids in steroidogenic cells. Endocr Rev. 1996;17:221-44.
97. Lin D, Sugawara T, Strauss JF, 3rd, Clark BJ, Stocco DM, Saenger P, et al. Role of steroidogenic acute regulatory protein in adrenal and gonadal steroidogenesis. Science. 1995;267:1828-31.
98. Caron KM, Soo SC, Wetsel WC, Stocco DM, Clark BJ, Parker KL. Targeted disruption of the mouse gene encoding steroidogenic acute regulatory protein provides insights into congenital lipoid adrenal hyperplasia. Proc Natl Acad Sci U S A. 1997;94:11540-45.
99. Weusten JJ, Smals AG, Hofman JA, Kloppenborg PW, Benraad TJ. Early time sequence in pregnenolone metabolism to testosterone in homogenates of human and rat testis. Endocrinology. 1987;120:1909-13.
100. Chung BC, Picado-Leonard J, Haniu M, Bienkowski M, Hall PF, Shively JE, et al. Cytochrome P450c17 (steroid 17 alpha-hydroxylase/17,20 lyase): Cloning of human adrenal and testis cDNAs indicates the same gene is expressed in both tissues. Proc Natl Acad Sci U S A. 1987;84:407-11.
101. Matteson KJ, Picado-Leonard J, Chung BC, Mohandas TK, Miller WL. Assignment of the gene for adrenal P450c17 (steroid 17 alpha-hydroxylase/17,20 lyase) to human chromosome 10. J Clin Endocrinol Metab. 1986;63:789-91.
102. Inano H, Ishii-Ohba H, Sugimoto Y, Ohta Y, Morikawa T, Yoshida M, et al. Purification and properties of enzymes related to steroid hormone synthesis. Ann N Y Acad Sci. 1990;595:17-25.
103. Luu-The V, Labrie C, Simard J, Lachance Y, Zhao HF, Couet J, et al. Structure of two in tandem human 17 beta-hydroxysteroid dehydrogenase genes. Mol Endocrinol. 1990;4:268-75.
104. Lorence MC, Corbin CJ, Kamimura N, Mahendroo MS, Mason JI. Structural analysis of the gene encoding human 3 beta-hydroxysteroid dehydrogenase/delta 5-4 isomerase. Mol Endocrinol. 1990;4:1850-5.
105. Andersson S, Russell DW. Structural and biochemical properties of cloned and expressed human and rat steroid 5 alpha-reductases. Proc Natl Acad Sci U S A. 1990;87: 3640-4.
106. Chen SA, Besman MJ, Sparkes RS, Zollman S, Klisak I, Mohandas T, et al. Human aromatase: cDNA cloning, Southern blot analysis, and assignment of the gene to chromosome 15. DNA. 1988;7(1):27-38.
107. OpenStax. (2016). Anatomy and physiology of the male reproductive system. [online] OpenStax CNX. Available from http://cnx.org/contents/370d6d11-8e11-4b2b-8fa4-a70c14b0554b@6 [Accessed February 2016].
108. De Kretser DM, Catt KJ, Paulsen CA. Studies on the *in vitro* testicular binding of iodinated luteinizing hormone in rats. Endocrinology. 1971;88:332-7.
109. Loosfelt H, Misrahi M, Atger M, Salesse R, Vu Hai-Luu Thi MT, Jolivet A, et al. Cloning and sequencing of porcine LH-hCG receptor cDNA: variants lacking transmembrane domain. Science. 1989;245:525-8.
110. Latronico AC, Chai Y, Arnhold IJ, Liu X, Mendonca BB, Segaloff DL. A homozygous microdeletion in helix 7 of the luteinizing hormone receptor associated with familial testicular and ovarian resistance is due to both decreased cell surface expression and impaired effector activation by the cell surface receptor. Mol Endocrinol. 1998;12:442-50.
111. Simoni M, Gromoll J, Nieschlag E. Molecular pathophysiology and clinical manifestations of gonadotropin receptor defects. Steroids. 1998;63:288-93.
112. Gromoll J, Partsch CJ, Simoni M, Nordhoff V, Sippell WG, Nieschlag E, et al. A mutation in the first transmembrane domain of the lutropin receptor causes male precocious puberty. J Clin Endocrinol Metab. 1998;83:476-80.
113. Muller J, Gondos B, Kosugi S, Mori T, Shenker A. Severe testotoxicosis phenotype associated with Asp578-->Tyr mutation of the lutrophin/choriogonadotrophin receptor gene. J Med Genet. 1998;35:340-1.
114. Stavrou SS, Zhu YS, Cai LQ, Katz MD, Herrera C, Defillo-Ricart M, et al. A novel mutation of the human luteinizing hormone receptor in 46XY and 46XX sisters. J Clin Endocrinol Metab. 1998;83:2091-8.
115. Dufau ML. Endocrine regulation and communicating functions of the Leydig cell. Annu Rev Physiol. 1988;50:483-508.
116. Dufau ML, Tsuruhara T, Horner KA, Podesta E, Catt KJ. Intermediate role of adenosine 3':5'-cyclic monophosphate and protein kinase during gonadotropin-induced steroidogenesis in testicular interstitial cells. Proc Natl Acad Sci U S A. 1977;74:3419-23.
117. Cooke BA. Is cyclic AMP an obligatory second messenger for luteinizing hormone? Mol Cell Endocrinol. 1990;69:C11-15.
118. Payne AH, Hardy MP, Russell LD. The Leydig Cell. Illinois: Cache River Press; 1996. pp. 1-802.
119. Hodgson YM, de Kretser DM. Serum Testosterone response to single injection of hCG ovine-LH and LHRH in male rats. Int J Androl. 1982;5:81-91.

120. Padron RS, Wischusen J, Hudson B, Burger HG, de Kretser DM. Prolonged biphasic response of plasma testosterone to single intramuscular injections of human chorionic gonadotropin. J Clin Endocrinol Metab. 1980;50:1100-4.
121. Cigorraga SB, Sorrell S, Bator J, Catt KJ, Dufau ML. Estrogen dependence of a gonadotropin-induced steroidogenic lesion in rat testicular Leydig cells. J Clin Invest. 1980;65:699-705.
122. Sharpe RM. hCG-induced decrease in availability of rat testis receptors. Nature. 1976;264:644-6.
123. Christensen A. Leydig cells. In: Hamilton DW, Greep RO (Eds), Handbook of Physiology, Section 7, Endocrinology, Vol. 5 (Male Reproductive System). Washington, D.C.:American Physiological Society; 1975. pp. 57-94.
124. Hodgson YM, de Kretser DM. Acute responses of Leydig cells to hCG: evidence for early hypertrophy of Leydig cells. Mol Cell Endocrinol. 1984;35:75-82.
125. Waterman MR, Simpson ER. Regulation of steroid hydroxylase gene expression is multifactorial in nature. Recent Prog Horm Res. 1989;45:533-63; discussion 563-6.
126. Wu FC, Irby DC, Clarke IJ, Cummins JT, de Kretser DM. Effects of gonadotropin-releasing hormone pulse frequency modulation on luteinizing hormone, follicle-stimulating hormone and testosterone secretion in hypothalamo/pituitary-disconnected rams. Biol Reprod. 1987:37:501-10.
127. Veldhuis JD, Liu PY, Keenan DM, Takahashi PY. Older men exhibit reduced efficacy of and heightened potency downregulation by intravenous pulses of recombinant human LH: a study in 92 healthy men. Am J Physiol Endocrinol Metab. 2012;302:E117-22.
128. Oury F, Sumara G, Sumara O, Ferron M, Chang H, Smith CE, et al. Endocrine regulation of male fertility by the skeleton. Cell. 2011;144:796-809.
129. Karsenty G. The mutual dependence between bone and gonads. J Endocrinol. 2012;213:107-14.
130. Karsenty G, Oury F. Biology without walls: the novel endocrinology of bone. Annu Rev Physiol. 2012;74:87-105.
131. de Kretser DM. Germ cell-Sertoli cell interactions. Reprod Fertil Dev. 1990;2:225-35.
132. Aoki A, Fawcett DW. Is there a local feedback from the seminiferous tubules affecting activity of the Leydig cells? Biol Reprod. 1978:19:144-58.
133. Jegou B, Laws AO, de Kretser DM. Changes in testicular function induced by short-term exposure of the rat testis to heat: further evidence for interaction of germ cells, Sertoli cells and Leydig cells. Int J Androl. 1984;7:244-57.
134. Risbridger GP, Kerr JB, de Kretser DM. Evaluation of Leydig cell function and gonadotropin binding in unilateral and bilateral cryptorchidism; evidence for local control of Leydig cell function by the seminiferous tubule. Biol Reprod. 1981;24:534-40.
135. Risbridger GP, Kerr JB, Peake RA, de Kretser DM. An assessment of Leydig cell function after bilateral or unilateral efferent duct ligation: further evidence for local control of Leydig cell function. Endocrinology. 1981;109:1234-41.
136. Andersson AM, Jorgensen N, Frydelund-Larsen L, Rajpert-De Meyts E, Skakkebaek NE. Impaired Leydig cell function in infertile men: a study of 357 idiopathic infertile men and 318 proven fertile controls. J Clin Endocrinol Metab. 2004;89:3161-7.
137. Cummings, B. Pearson Education Inc., Available from http://images.slideplayer.com/25/7878850/slides/slide_16.jpg
138. Handelsman DJ. Hormonal regulation of spermatogenesis: insights from constructing genetic models. Reprod Fertil Dev. 2011;23:507-19.
139. Zirkin BR. Spermatogenesis: its regulation by testosterone and FSH. Semin Cell Dev Biol. 1998;9:417-21.
140. McLachlan RI, O'Donnell L, Meachem SJ, Stanton PG, de Kretser DM, Pratis K, et al. Identification of specific sites of hormonal regulation in spermatogenesis in rats, monkeys, and man. Recent Prog Horm Res. 2002;57:149-79.
141. Mason AJ, Hayflick JS, Zoeller RT, Young WS, 3rd, Phillips HS, Nikolics K, et al. A deletion truncating the gonadotropin-releasing hormone gene is responsible for hypogonadism in the hpg mouse. Science. 1986;234:1366-71.
142. Allan CM, Handelsman DJ. Transgenic models for exploring gonadotropin biology in the male. Endocrine. 2005;26:235-9.
143. O'Shaughnessy PJ, Morris ID, Huhtaniemi I, Baker PJ, Abel MH. Role of androgen and gonadotrophins in the development and function of the Sertoli cells and Leydig cells: data from mutant and genetically modified mice. Mol Cell Endocrinol. 2009;306:2-8.
144. Wang RS, Yeh S, Tzeng CR, Chang C. Androgen receptor roles in spermatogenesis and fertility: lessons from testicular cell-specific androgen receptor knockout mice. Endocr Rev. 2009;30:119-32.
145. Testicular Steroidogenesis. (2011). Expert Consult. Available from http://www.hapmd.com/home/hapmdcom/public_html/wp-content/uploads/2009/03/sub/articulos-e-imagenes/20110501_testicular_steroidogenesis.pdf.
146. Ruwanpura SM, McLachlan RI, Meachem SJ. Hormonal regulation of male germ cell development. J Endocrinol. 2010;205:117-31.
147. O'Donnell L, Meachem SJ, Stanton PG, McLachlan RI. Endocrine regulation of spermato-genesis. In: Neill JD (Ed). Knobil and Neill's Physiology of Reproduction, 3rd edition. San Diego, CA: Elsevier; 2006. pp. 1017-69.
148. Walker WH, Cheng J. FSH and testosterone signaling in Sertoli cells. Reproduction. 2005;130:15-28.
149. Singh J, O'Neill C, Handelsman DJ. Induction of spermatogenesis by androgens in gonadotropin-deficient (hpg) mice. Endocrinology. 1995;136:5311-21.
150. De Gendt K, Swinnen JV, Saunders PT, Schoonjans L, Dewerchin M, Devos A, et al. A Sertoli cell-selective knockout of the androgen receptor causes spermatogenic arrest in meiosis. Proc Natl Acad Sci U S A. 2004;101:1327-32.
151. Handelsman DJ, Spaliviero JA, Simpson JM, Allan CM, Singh J. Spermatogenesis without gonadotropins: maintenance has a lower testosterone threshold than initiation. Endocrinology. 1999;140:3938-46.
152. O'Donnell L, McLachlan RI. The role of testosterone in spermatogenesis. In: Nieschlag E, Behre HM, Nieschlag S (Eds). Testosterone: Action, Deficiency, Substitution, 4th

edition. New York, USA: Cambridge University Press; 2012. pp. 123-153.
153. Grino PB, Griffin JE, Wilson JD. Testosterone at high concentrations interacts with the human androgen receptor similarly to dihydrotestosterone. Endocrinology. 1990;126:1165-72.
154. Bremner WJ, Millar MR, Sharpe RM, Saunders PT. Immunohistochemical localization of androgen receptors in the rat testis: evidence for stage-dependent expression and regulation by androgens. Endocrinology. 1994;135:1227-34.
155. Van Roijen JH, Van Assen S, Van Der Kwast TH, De Rooij DG, Boersma WJ, Vreeburg JT, et al. Androgen receptor immunoexpression in the testes of subfertile men. J Androl 1995; 16:510-6.
156. Welsh M, Sharpe RM, Moffat L, Atanassova N, Saunders PT, Kilter S, et al. Androgen action via testicular arteriole smooth muscle cells is important for Leydig cell function, vasomotion and testicular fluid dynamics. PLoS One. 2010;5:e13632.
157. Johnston DS, Russell LD, Friel PJ, Griswold MD. Murine germ cells do not require functional androgen receptors to complete spermatogenesis following spermatogonial stem cell transplantation. Endocrinology. 2001;142:2405-8.
158. Lim P, Robson M, Spaliviero J, McTavish KJ, Jimenez M, Zajac JD, et al. Sertoli cell androgen receptor DNA binding domain is essential for the completion of spermatogenesis. Endocrinology. 2009;150:4755-65.
159. Welsh M, Saunders PT, Atanassova N, Sharpe RM, Smith LB. Androgen action via testicular peritubular myoid cells is essential for male fertility. FASEB J. 2009;23:4218-30.
160. Welsh M, Moffat L, Belling K, de Franca LR, Segatelli TM, Saunders PT, et al. Androgen receptor signalling in peritubular myoid cells is essential for normal differentiation and function of adult Leydig cells. Int J Androl. 2012;35:25-40.
161. Abel MH, Baker PJ, Charlton HM, Monteiro A, Verhoeven G, De Gendt K, et al. Spermatogenesis and Sertoli cell activity in mice lacking Sertoli cell receptors for follicle-stimulating hormone and androgen. Endocrinology. 2008;149:3279-85.
162. O'Donnell L, McLachlan RI, Wreford NG, de Kretser DM, Robertson DM. Testosterone withdrawal promotes stage-specific detachment of round spermatids from the rat seminiferous epithelium. Biol Reprod. 1996;55:895-901.
163. O'Donnell L, Pratis K, Stanton PG, Robertson DM, McLachlan RI. Testosterone-dependent restoration of spermatogenesis in adult rats is impaired by a 5alpha-reductase inhibitor. J Androl. 1999;20:109-17.
164. Zhengwei Y, Wreford NG, Royce P, de Kretser DM, McLachlan RI. Stereological evaluation of human spermatogenesis after suppression by testosterone treatment: heterogeneous pattern of spermatogenic impairment. J Clin Endocrinol Metab. 1998;83:1284-91.
165. Weinbauer GF, Schlatt S, Walter V, Nieschlag E. Testosterone-induced inhibition of spermatogenesis is more closely related to suppression of FSH than to testicular androgen levels in the cynomolgus monkey model (Macaca fascicularis). J Endocrinol. 2001;168:25-38.
166. Narula A, Gu YQ, O'Donnell L, Stanton PG, Robertson DM, McLachlan RI, et al. Variability in sperm suppression during testosterone administration to adult monkeys is related to follicle stimulating hormone suppression and not to intratesticular androgens. J Clin Endocrinol Metab. 2002;87:3399-406.
167. Mesher AL. (2009). Junqueira's Basic Histology: Text and Atlas, 12th edition. The McGraw-Hill Companies Inc. Available from http://www.accessmedicine.com
168. Meng J, Holdcraft RW, Shima JE, Griswold MD, Braun RE. Androgens regulate the permeability of the blood testis barrier. Proc Natl Acad Sci U S A. 2005;102:16696-700.
169. McCabe MJ, Allan CM, Foo CF, Nicholls PK, McTavish KJ, Stanton PG. Androgen initiates sertoli cell tight junction formation in the hypogonadal (hpg) mouse. Biol Reprod. 2012;87:38.
170. Willems A, Batlouni SR, Esnal A, Swinnen JV, Saunders PT, Sharpe RM, et al. Selective ablation of the androgen receptor in mouse Sertoli cells affects Sertoli cell maturation, barrier formation and cytoskeletal development. PLoS One. 2010;5:e14168.
171. Nicholls PK, Harrison CA, Walton KL, McLachlan RI, O'Donnell L, Stanton PG. Hormonal regulation of Sertoli cell micro-RNAs at spermiation. Endocrinology. 2011;152: 1670-83.
172. Heckert L, Griswold MD. Expression of the FSH receptor in the testis. Recent Prog Horm Res. 1993;48:61-77.
173. Rannikko A, Penttila TL, Zhang FP, Toppari J, Parvinen M, Huhtaniemi I. Stage-specific expression of the FSH receptor gene in the prepubertal and adult rat seminiferous epithelium. J Endocrinol. 1996;151:29-35.
174. Petersen C, Soder O. The Sertoli cell--a hormonal target and 'super' nurse for germ cells that determines testicular size. Horm Res. 2006;66:153-61.
175. Allan CM, Garcia A, Spaliviero J, Zhang FP, Jimenez M, Huhtaniemi I, et al. Complete Sertoli cell proliferation induced by follicle-stimulating hormone (FSH) independently of luteinizing hormone activity: evidence from genetic models of isolated FSH action. Endocrinology. 2004;145:1587-93.
176. Grover A, Sairam MR, Smith CE, Hermo L. Structural and functional modifications of Sertoli cells in the testis of adult follicle-stimulating hormone receptor knockout mice. Biol Reprod. 2004;71:117-29.
177. Wreford NG, Rajendra Kumar T, Matzuk MM, de Kretser DM. Analysis of the testicular phenotype of the follicle-stimulating hormone beta-subunit knockout and the activin type II receptor knockout mice by stereological analysis. Endocrinology. 2001;142:2916-20.
178. Haywood M, Spaliviero J, Jimemez M, King NJ, Handelsman DJ, Allan CM. Sertoli and germ cell development in hypogonadal (hpg) mice expressing transgenic follicle-stimulating hormone alone or in combination with testosterone. Endocrinology. 2003;144:509-17.
179. Weinbauer GF, Behre HM, Fingscheidt U, Nieschlag E. Human follicle-stimulating hormone exerts a stimulatory effect on spermatogenesis, testicular size, and serum inhibin levels in the gonadotropin-releasing hormone antagonist

treated nonhuman primate (Macaca fascicularis). Endocrinology. 1991;129:1831-9.
180. Marshall GR, Zorub DS, Plant TM. Follicle-stimulating hormone amplifies the population of differentiated spermatogonia in the hypophysectomized testosterone-replaced adult rhesus monkey (Macaca mulatta). Endocrinology. 1995;136:3504-11.
181. O'Donnell L, Narula A, Balourdos G, Gu YQ, Wreford NG, Robertson DM, et al. Impairment of spermatogonial development and spermiation after testosterone-induced gonadotropin suppression in adult monkeys (Macaca fascicularis). J Clin Endocrinol Metab. 2001;86:1814-22.
182. Saito K, O'Donnell L, McLachlan RI, Robertson DM. Spermiation failure is a major contributor to early spermatogenic suppression caused by hormone withdrawal in adult rats. Endocrinology. 2000;141:2779-85.
183. McLachlan RI, O'Donnell L, Meachem SJ, Stanton PG, de K, Pratis K, et al. Hormonal regulation of spermatogenesis in primates and man: insights for development of the male hormonal contraceptive. J Androl. 2002;23:149-62.
184. Meachem SJ, Wreford NG, Stanton PG, Robertson DM, McLachlan RI. Follicle-stimulating hormone is required for the initial phase of spermatogenic restoration in adult rats following gonadotropin suppression. J Androl. 1998;19:725-35.
185. Matsumoto AM, Karpas AE, Paulsen CA, Bremner WJ. Reinitiation of sperm production in gonadotropin suppressed normal men by administration of follicle-stimulating hormone. J Clin Invest. 1983;72:1005-15.
186. Matsumoto AM, Paulsen CA, Bremner WJ. Stimulation of sperm production by human luteinizing hormone in gonadotropin-suppressed normal men. J Clin Endocrinol Metab. 1984;59:882-7.
187. Bremner WJ, Matsumoto AM, Sussman AM, Paulsen CA. Follicle-stimulating hormone and human spermatogenesis. J Clin Invest. 1981;68:1044-52.
188. El Shennawy A, Gates RJ, Russell LD. Hormonal regulation of spermatogenesis in the hypophysectomized rat: cell viability after hormonal replacement in adults after intermediate periods of hypophysectomy. J Androl. 1998;19:320-34; discussion 341-42.
189. Matthiesson KL, McLachlan RI, O'Donnell L, Frydenberg M, Robertson DM, Stanton PG, et al. The relative roles of follicle-stimulating hormone and luteinizing hormone in maintaining spermatogonial maturation and spermiation in normal men. J Clin Endocrinol Metab. 2006;91:3962-9.
190. MacDonald PC, Madden JD, Brenner PF, Wilson JD, Siiteri PK. Origin of estrogen in normal men and in women with testicular feminization. J Clin Endocrinol Metab. 1979;49:905-16.
191. Couse JF, Lindzey J, Grandien K, Gustafsson JA, Korach KS Tissue distribution and quantitative analysis of estrogen receptor-α (ERα) and estrogen receptor-β (ERβ) messenger ribonucleic acid in the wild-type and ERα-knock-out mouse. Endocrinology. 1997;138:4613-21.
192. Simpson ER, Mahendroo MS, Means GD, Kilgore MW, Hinshelwood MM, Graham-Lorence S, Amarneh B, et al. Aromatase cytochrome P450, the enzyme responsible for estrogen biosynthesis. Endocr Rev. 1994;15: 342-55.
193. Couse JF, Korach KS. Estrogen receptor null mice: what have we learned and where will they lead us? Endocrine Rev 1999;20:358-417.
194. Smith EP, Boyd J, Frank GR, Takahashi H, Cohen RM, Specker B, et al. Estrogen resistance caused by a mutation in the estrogen-receptor gene in a man. N Engl J Med. 1994;331:1056-61.
195. Carani C, Qin K, Simoni M, Faustini-Fustini M, Serpente S, Boyd J. Effect of testosterone and estradiol in a man with aromatase deficiency. N Engl J Med. 1997;337:91-5.
196. Morishima A, Grumbach MM, Simpson ER, Fisher C, Qin K. Aromatase deficiency in male and female sibling caused by a novel mutation and the physiological role of estrogens. J Clin Endocrinol Metab. 1995;80:3689-99.
197. Carreau S, Bouraima-lelong H, Delalande C. Role of estrogen in spermatogenesis. Front Bioscence. 2012;1:1-11.
198. Sharpe RM. The roles of oestrogen in the male. Trends Endocrinol Metab. 1998;9:371-7.
199. Deroo BJ, Korach KS. Estrogen receptors and human disease. J. Clin Invest. 2006;116:561-70.
200. Vincenzo R, Bruno M, Chiara D, Lucia Z, Santi D, Cesare C. Estrogens and male reproduction. In: De Groot LJ, De Groot LJ, Chrousos G, Dungan K, Feingold KR, Grossman A, Hershman JM, Koch C, Korbonits M, McLachlan R, New M, Purnell J, Rebar R, Singer F, Vinik A (Eds). Endotext [Internet]. South Dartmouth, MA: MDText.com, Inc; 2000. Available from: http://www.ncbi.nlm.nih.gov/books/NBK278933/ [Updated 6 Feb 2013]
201. Rochira V, Granata ARM, Madeo B, Zirilli L, Rossi G, Carani C. Estrogens in males: what have we learned in the last 10 years? Asian J Androl. 2005;7:3-20.
202. Rochira V, Carani C. Aromatase deficiency in men: a clinical perspective. Nature Reviews. 2009;5:559-68.
203. Luconi M, Muratori M, Forti G, Baldi E. Identification and characterization of a novel functional estrogen receptor on human sperm membrane which interferes with progesterone effects. J Clin Endocr Metab. 1999;84:1670-8.
204. Zirilli L, Rochira V, Diazzi C, Caffagni G, Carani C. Human models of aromatase deficiency. J Steroid Biochem Molec Biol. 2008;109:212-8.
205. Rochira V, Balestrieri A, Madeo B, Spaggiari A, Carani C. Congenital estrogen deficiency in men: a new syndrome with different phenotypes; clinical and therapeutic implications in men. Mol Cell Endocrinol. 2002;193:19-28.
206. Faustini-Fustini M, Rochira V, Carani C. Oestrogen deficiency in men: where are we today? Eur J Endocrinol. 1999;140:111-29.
207. Bouillon R, Bex M, Vanderschueren D, Boonen S. Estrogens are essential for male pubertal periosteal bone expansion. J Clin Endocrinol Metab. 2004;89:6025-9.
208. Maffei L, Murata Y, Rochira V, Tubert G, Aranda C, Vasquez M, et al. Dysmetabolis syndrome in a man with a novel mutation of the aromatase gene: effects of testosterone,

alendronate, and estradiol treatment. J Clin Endocrinol Metab. 2004;89:61-70.
209. Sharpe RM, Skakkebaek NE. Are oestrogens involved in falling sperm counts and disorders of the male reproductive tract? Lancet. 1993;341:1392-5.
210. Toppari J, Larsen JC, Christiansen P, Giwercman A, Grandjean P, Guillette Jr LJ, et al. Male reproductive health and environmental xenoestrogens. Environ Health Persp. 1996;104:741-803.
211. Pflieger-Bruss S, Schuppe HC, Schill WB. The male reproductive system and its susceptibility to endocrine disrupting chemicals. Andrologia. 2004;36:337-45.
212. Lee IW, Kuo PH, Su MT, Kuan LC, Hsu CC, Kuo PL. Quantitative trait analysis suggests polymorphisms of estrogen-related genes regulate human sperm concentrations and motility. Hum Reprod. 2011;26:1585-96.
213. Finkelstein JS, O'Dea L StL, Whitcomb RW, Crowley WF. Sex steroid control of gonadotropin secretion in the human male. II. Effect of estradiol administration in normal and gonadotropin-releasing hormone-deficient men. J Clin Endocrinol Metab. 1991;73:621-8.
214. Finkelstein JS, Whitcomb RW, O'Dea LS, Longcope C, Schoenfeld DA, Crowley WF Jr. Sex steroid control of gonadotropin secretion in the human male. I. Effect of testosterone administration in normal and gonadotropin-releasing hormone-deficient men. J Clin Endocrinol Metab. 1991a;73:609-20.
215. Raven G, de Jong FH, Kaufman JM, de Ronde W. In men, peripheral estradiol levels directly reflect the action of estrogens at the hypothalamopituitary level to inhibit gonadotropin secretion. J Clin Endocrinol Metab. 2006;91:3324-8.
216. Pitteloud N, Dwyer AA, DeCruz S, Lee H, Boepple PA, Crowley WF Jr, et al. Inhibition of luteinizing hormone secretion by testosterone in men requires aromatization for its pituitary but not its hypothalamic effects: evidence from the tandem study of normal and gonadotropin-releasing hormone-deficient men. J Clin Endocrinol Metab. 2008;93:784-791.
217. Rochira V, Zirilli L, Genazzani AD, Balestrieri A, Aranda C, Fabre B, et al. Hypothalamic-pituitary-gonadal axis in two men with aromatase deficiency: evidence that circulating estrogens are required at the hypothalamic level for the integrity of gonadotropin negative feedback. Eur J Endocrinol. 2006;155:513-22.
218. Rochira V, Balestrieri A, Madeo B, Baraldi E, Faustini-Fustini M, Granata AR, et al. Congenital estrogen deficiency: in search of the estrogen role in human male reproduction. Mol Cell Endocrinol. 2001;178:107-15.
219. Deladoëy J, Flück C, Bex M, Yoshimura N, Harada N, Mullis PE. Aromatase deficiency caused by a novel P450arom gene mutation: impact of absent estrogen production on serum gonadotropin concentration in a boy. J Clin Endocrinol Metab. 1999;84:4050-4.
220. Herrman BL, Saller B, Janssen OE, Gocke P, Bockish A, Sperling H, et al. Impact of estrogen replacement therapy in a male with congenital aromatase deficiency caused by a novel mutation in the CYP19 gene. J Clin Endocrinol Metab 2002;87:5476-84.
221. Carani C, Granata AR, Rochira V, Caffagni G, Aranda C, Antunez P, et al. Sex steroid and sexual desire in a man with a novel mutation of aromatase gene and hypogonadism. Psychoneuroendocrinol. 2005;30:413-7.
222. Sharpe RM, McKinnell C, Kivlin C, Fisher JS. Proliferation and functional maturation of Sertoli cells, and their relevance to disorders of testis function in adulthood. Reproduction. 2003;125:769-784.
223. O'Donnelll L, Robertson KM, Jones ME, Simpson ER. Estrogen and spermatogenesis. Endocr Rev. 2001;22:289-318.
224. Cattanach BM, Iddon CA, Charlton HM, Chiappa SA, Fink G. Gonadotropin releasing hormone deficiency in a mutant mouse with hypogonadism. Nature. 1977;269:338-40.
225. Charlton HM, Halpin DMG, Iddon C, Rosie R, Levy G, McDowell IFW, et al., The effects of daily administration of single and multiple injections of gonadotropin releasing hormone on pituitary and gonadal function in the hypogonadal (hpg) mouse. Endocrinology. 1983;113:535-43.
226. Sheffield JW, O'Shaughnessy PJ. Effect of injection of gonadotropin-releasing hormone on testicular steroidogenesis in the hypogonadal (hpg) mouse. J Reprod Fert. 1989;86:609-17.
227. Scott IS, Charlton HM, Cox BS, Grocock CA, Sheffield JW, O'Shaughnessy PJ. Effect of LH injections on testicular steroidogenesis, cholesterol P450scc mRNA content and Leydig cell morphology in hypogonadal mice. J Endocrinol. 1990;125:131-8.
228. Singh J, Handelsman DJ. The effects of recombinant FSH on testosterone-induced spermatogenesis in gonadotrophin-deficient (hpg) mice. J Androl. 1996;17:382-92.
229. Baines H, Nwagwu MO, Furneaux EC, Stewart J, Kerr JB, Mayhew TM, et al. Estrogenic induction of spermatogenesis in the hypogonadal (hpg) mouse: role of androgens. Reproduction. 2005;130:643-54.
230. Bhasin S, Cunningham GR, Hayes FJ, Matsumoto AM, Snyder PJ, Swerdloff RS, et al. Testosterone therapy in adult men with androgen deficiency syndromes: an endocrine society clinical practice guideline. J Clin Endocrinol Metab. 2010;95:2536-44.
231. AACE Guidelines for evaluation and treatment of hypogonadism in adult male patients - 2002 update. Endocrine Practice. 2002;8:439-56.
232. Bhasin S, Fisher CE. (2003). Male Hypogonadism. In: PIER [online database]. Philadelphia: American College of Physicians. Available from http://pier.acponline.org/physicians/diseases/d169.
233. Wang C, Nieschlag E, Swerdloff R, Behre HM, Hellstrom WJ, Gooren LJ, et al. Investigation, treatment, and monitoring of late-onset hypogonadism in males: ISA, ISSAM, EAU, EAA, and ASA recommendations. J Androl. 2009;30:1-9.
234. Harman SM, Metter EJ, Tobin JD, Pearson J, Blackman MR; Baltimore Longitudinal Study of Aging. Longitudinal effects of aging on serum total and free testosterone levels in healthy

men. Baltimore Longitudinal Study of Aging. J Clin Endocrinol Metab. 2001;86:724-31.
235. Feldman HA, Longcope C, Derby CA, Johannes CB, Araujo AB, Coviello AD, et al. Age trends in the level of serum testosterone and other hormones in middle-aged men: longitudinal results from the Massachusetts male aging study. J Clin Endocrinol Metab. 2002;87(2):589-98.
236. Morley JE, Kaiser FE, Perry HM 3rd, Patrick P, Morley PM, Stauber PM, et al. Longitudinal changes in testosterone, luteinizing hormone, and follicle stimulating hormone in healthy older men. Metabolism. 1997;46:410-3.
237. Zmuda JM, Cauley JA, Kriska A, Glynn NW, Gutai JP, Kuller LH. Longitudinal relation between endogenous testosterone and cardiovascular disease risk factors in middle-aged men. A 13-year follow-up of former Multiple Risk Factor Intervention Trial participants. Am J Epidemiol. 1997;146:609-17.
238. Gray A, Feldman HA, McKinlay JB, Longcope C. Age, disease, and changing sex hormone levels in middle-aged men: results of the Massachusetts Male Aging Study. J Clin Endocrinol Metab. 1991;73:1016-25.
239. Mohr BA, Bhasin S, Link CL, O'Donnell AB, McKinlay JB. The effect of changes in adiposity on testosterone levels in older men: longitudinal results from the Massachusetts Male Aging Study. Eur J Endocrinol. 2006;155(3):443-52.
240. Wu FC, Tajar A, Pye SR, Silman AJ, Finn JD, O'Neill TW, et al. Hypothalamic-pituitary-testicular axis disruptions in older men are differentially linked to age and modifiable risk factors: the European Male Aging Study. J Clin Endocrinol Metab. 2008;93:2737-45.
241. Bhasin S, Tenover JS. Age-associated sarcopenia-issues in the use of testosterone as an anabolic agent in older men. J Clin Endocrinol Metab. 1997;82:165960.
242. Perry HM 3rd, Miller DK, Patrick P, Morley JE. Testosterone and leptin in older African-American men: relationship to age, strength, function, and season. Metabolism. 2000;49:1085-91.
243. Baumgartner RN, Koehler KM, Gallagher D, Romero L, Heymsfield SB, Ross RR, et al. Epidemiology of sarcopenia among the elderly in New Mexico [published erratum appears in Am J Epidemiol 1999;149(12):1161]. Am J Epidemiol. 1998;147:755-63.
244. Baumgartner RN, Waters DL, Gallagher D, Morley JE, Garry PJ. Predictors of skeletal muscle mass in elderly men and women. Mech Ageing Dev. 1999;107:123-36.
245. Melton LJ, 3rd, Khosla S, Riggs BL. Epidemiology of sarcopenia. Mayo Clin Proc. 2000;75 Suppl:S10-2; discussion S12-3.
246. Zitzmann M, Faber S, Nieschlag E. Association of specific symptoms and metabolic risks with serum testosterone in older men. J Clin Endocrinol Metab. 2006;91(11): 4335-43.
247. Kaiser FE, Viosca SP, Morley JE, Mooradian AD, Davis SS, Korenman SG. Impotence and aging: clinical and hormonal factors. J Am Geriatr Soc. 1988;36:511-9.
248. O'Connor DB, Lee DM, Corona G, Forti G, Tajar A, O'Neill TW, et al., European Male Ageing Study Group. The relationships between sex hormones and sexual function in middle-aged and older European men. J Clin Endocrinol Metab. 2011;96(10):E1577-87.
249. Liu-Ambrose T, Pang MY, Eng JJ. Executive function is independently associated with performances of balance and mobility in community-dwelling older adults after mild stroke: implications for falls prevention. Cerebrovasc Dis. 2007;23(2-3):203-10.
250. Janowsky JS, Oviatt SK, Orwoll ES. Testosterone influences spatial cognition in older men. Behav Neurosci. 1994;108(2):325-32.
251. Shute VJ PJ, Hubert L, Reynolds RW. The relationship between androgen levels and human spatial abilities. Bull Psychonomic Soc. 1983;21:465-8.
252. Fink HA, Ewing SK, Ensrud KE, Barrett-Connor E, Taylor BC, Cauley JA, et al. Association of testosterone and estradiol deficiency with osteoporosis and rapid bone loss in older men. J Clin Endocrinol Metab. 2006;91(10):3908-15.
253. Mellstrom D, Johnell O, Ljunggren O, Eriksson AL, Lorentzon M, Mallmin H, et al. Free testosterone is an independent predictor of BMD and prevalent fractures in elderly men: MrOS Sweden. J Bone Miner Res. 2006;21(4):529-35.
254. Ferlin A, Selice R, Carraro U, Foresta C. Testicular function and bone metabolism beyond testosterone. Nat Rev Endocrinol. 2013;9:548-54.
255. Travison TG, Morley JE, Araujo AB, O'Donnell AB, McKinlay JB. The relationship between libido and testosterone levels in aging men. J Clin Endocrinol Metab. 2006;91(7): 2509-13.
256. Korenman SG, Morley JE, Mooradian AD, Davis SS, Kaiser FE, Silver AJ, et al. Secondary hypogonadism in older men: its relation to impotence. J Clin Endocrinol Metab. 1990;71:963-9.
257. Harman SM, Tsitouras PD, Costa PT, Blackman MR. Reproductive hormones in aging men. II. Basal pituitary gonadotropins and gonadotropin responses to luteinizing hormone-releasing hormone. J Clin Endocrinol Metab. 1982;54:547-51.
258. Murono EP, Nankin HR, Lin T, Osterman J. The aging Leydig cell: VI. Response of testosterone precursors to gonadotropin in men. Acta Endocrinologica. (Copenhagen) 1982;100:455-61.
259. Nieschlag E, Lammer U, Freischem CW, Langer K, Wickings EJ. Reproductive function in young fathers and grandfathers. J Clin Endocrinol Metab. 1982;51:675-81.
260. Bhasin S, Pencina M, Jasuja GK, Travison TG, Coviello A, Orwoll E, et al. Reference ranges for testosterone in men generated using liquid chromatography tandem mass spectrometry in a community-based sample of healthy non-obese young men in the Framingham Heart Study and applied to three geographically distinct cohorts. J Clin Endocrinol Metab. 2011;96:2430-9.
261. Sartorius G, Spasevska S, Idan A, Turner L, Forbes E, Zamojska A, et al., Serum testosterone, dihydrotestosterone and estradiol concentrations in older men self-reporting very good health: the healthy man study. Clin Endocrinol (Oxford). 2012;77(5):755-63.

262. Harman SM, Tsitouras PD. Reproductive hormones in aging men I. Measurement of sex steroids, basal luteinizing hormone and Leydig cell response to human chorionic gonadotropin. J Clin Endocrinol Metab. 1980;51:35-41.
263. Bhasin S, Huang G, Travison TG, Shehzad B. Age-Related Changes in the Male Reproductive Axis.In: De Groot LJ, De Groot LJ, Chrousos G, Dungan K, Feingold KR, Grossman A, Hershman JM, Koch C, Korbonits M, McLachlan R, New M, Purnell J, Rebar R, Singer F, Vinik A (Eds). Endotext [Internet]. South Dartmouth, MA: MDText.com, Inc.; 2002. Available from: http://www.ncbi.nlm.nih.gov/books/NBK278998/ [Updated 14 Feb 2014].
264. Bremner WJ, Prinz PN. A loss of circadian rhythmicity in blood testosterone levels with aging in normal men. J Clin Endocrinol Metab. 1983;56:1278-81.
265. Zumoff B, Strain GW, Kream J, O'Connor J, Rosenfeld RS, Levin J, et al. Age variation of the 24 hour mean plasma concentration of androgens, estrogens, and gonadotropins in normal adult men. J Clin Endocrinol Metab. 1982;54:534-8.
266. Plas E, Berger P, Hermann M, Pfluger H. Effects of aging on male fertility? Exp Gerontol. 2000;35:543-51.
267. Rolf C, Nieschlag E. Reproductive functions, fertility and genetic risks of ageing men. Exp Clin Endocrinol Diabetes. 2001;109:68-74.
268. Sloter ED, Marchetti F, Eskenazi B, Weldon RH, Nath J, Cabreros D, et al. Frequency of human sperm carrying structural aberrations of chromosome 1 increases with advancing age. Fertil Steril. 2007;87:1077-86.
269. Wiener-Megnazi Z, Auslender R, Dirnfeld M. Advanced paternal age and reproductive outcome. Asian J Andrology. 2012;14:69-79.
270. Hellstrom WJ, Overstreet JW, Sikka SC, Denne J, Ahuja S, Hoover AM, et al., Semen and sperm reference ranges for men 45 years of age and older. J Androl. 2006;27(3):421-8.
271. Kidd SA, Eskenazi B, Wyrobek AJ. Effects of male age on semen quality and fertility: a review of the literature. Fertil Steril. 2001;75:237-48.
272. Tajar A, Huhtaniemi IT, O'Neill TW, Finn JD, Pye SR, Lee DM. et al. Characteristics of androgen deficiency in late-onset hypogonadism: results from the European Male Aging Study (EMAS). J Clin Endocrinol Metab. 2012;97:1508-16.
273. Urban RJ, Veldhuis JD, Blizzard RM, Dufau ML. Attenuated release of biologically active luteinizing hormone in healthy aging men. J Clin Invest. 1988;81(4):1020-9.
274. Zwart AD, Urban RJ, Odell WD, Veldhuis JD. Contrasts in the gonadotropin-releasing hormone dose-response relationships for luteinizing hormone, follicle-stimulating hormone and alpha-subunit release in young versus older men: appraisal with high-specificity immunoradiometric assay and deconvolution analysis. Eur J Endocrinol. 1996;135:399-406.
275. Pincus SM, Mulligan T, Iranmanesh A, Gheorghiu S, Godschalk M, Veldhuis JD. Older males secrete luteinizing hormone and testosterone more irregularly, and jointly more asynchronously, than younger males. Proc Natl Acad Sci U S A. 1996;93(24):14100-5.
276. Keenan DM, Veldhuis JD. Disruption of the hypothalamic luteinizing hormone pulsing mechanism in aging men. Am J Physiol Regul Integr Comp Physiol. 2001;281(6): R1917-924.

CHAPTER

18 Male Endocrine Disorders

Satish Bharadwaj, SS Vasan

INTRODUCTION

Male sexual development and hormonal function depend on a complex feedback circuit involving the hypothalamus-pituitary-gonadal (HPG) axis modulated by the central nervous system. Male sexual dysfunction can be a consequence of malfunctions of the HPG axis, neurovascular disorders, drugs, or other disorders. The hypothalamus produces gonadotropin-releasing hormone (GnRH), in a pulsatile fashion every 60–120 minute. GnRH acts on the anterior pituitary gland which releases corresponding pulses of luteinizing hormone (LH) and follicle-stimulating hormone (FSH). LH acts on the Leydig cells which produce testosterone while FSH stimulates the Sertoli cells to induce spermatogenesis. Hypogonadotropic hypogonadism (HH) develops when the GnRH pulses do not occur with the proper amplitude, frequency and diurnal variation.

The Leydig cells of the testes produce 5–10 mg of testosterone daily, in response to LH secretion. Testosterone is synthesized from cholesterol through several intermediates, such as dehydroepiandrosterone (DHEA) and androstenedione. Circulating testosterone is mostly protein-bound, about 40% bound to sex hormone-binding globulin (SHBG) and 58% loosely bound to albumin. Thus, only about 2% of circulating testosterone is bio-available in its free form. Testosterone undergoes conversion to estradiol and dihydrotestosterone (DHT). Testosterone, DHT and estradiol provide negative feedback on the hypothalamic-pituitary axis. In males, estradiol is the main inhibitor of LH production, whereas both estradiol and inhibin B, produced by Sertoli cells of the testes, inhibit production of FSH.

SEXUAL DIFFERENTIATION AND PUBERTY

In the embryo, the presence of a Y chromosome triggers the development and growth of the testes. Testes begin secreting testosterone and a Müllerian duct inhibitor by about 7th week of gestation. Testosterone virilizes the wolffian duct to develop into the epididymis, vas deferens, and seminal vesicles. DHT promotes development of the external genitals. Testosterone levels peak in the 2nd trimester and fall to almost zero by birth, but its production rises briefly during the first 6 months of life, after which testosterone levels remain low until puberty. LH and FSH are elevated at birth, but fall to low levels within a few months, and remain low or undetectable until puberty. Through an unknown mechanism, blood levels of the adrenal androgens DHEA and DHEA sulfate begin to increase several years before puberty. Their conversion to testosterone in small amounts initiates pubic and axillary hair growth (adrenarche). Figure 18.1 shows the changes occurring at puberty and their mean time frames.[1]

TESTICULAR ENDOCRINE DISORDERS

Hypogonadism is defined as testosterone deficiency that may result from a disorder of the testes (primary hypogonadism) or of the hypothalamic-pituitary axis (secondary hypogonadism). Additionally, a number of congenital enzyme deficiencies cause varying degrees of target organ androgen resistance. Table 18.1 lists different kinds of hypogonadism observed along with their etiologies.[2]

Congenital Hypothalamic Diseases

Kallmann syndrome (KS) is a rare genetic disorder that affects both men and women. The condition is characterized by a failure to commence or complete puberty and

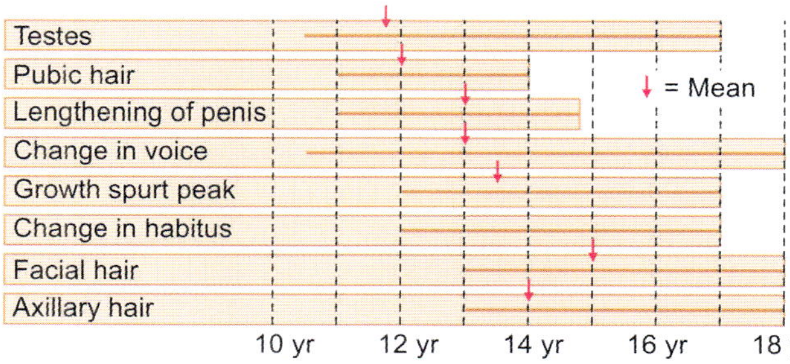

Fig. 18.1: Changes occurring at puberty. Bars indicate normal ranges. Adapted from Ref. 1.

Table 18.1: Causes of hypogonadism.*

Type	*Congenital causes*	*Acquired causes*
Primary (testicular)	Klinefelter syndrome	
	Anorchia (bilateral)	Chemotherapy
	Cryptorchidism	Radiation therapy
	Myotonic dystropy	Testicular infection (e.g., mumps, echovirus, flavivirus)
	Enzymatic defects in testosterone synthesis	High doses of antiandrogen drugs (e.g., cimetidine, spironolactone, ketoconazole, flutamide, cyproterone)
	Leydig cell aplasia	
	Noonan syndrome	
Secondary (hypothalamic–pituitary)		Any acute systemic illness
	Idiopathic, hypogonadotropic, hypogonadism	Hypopituitarism (tumor, infarction, infiltrative disease, infection, trauma, irradiation)
	Kallmann syndrome	Hyperprolactinemia
	Prader–Willi syndrome	Iron overload (hemochromatosis)
	Dandy–Walker malformation	Certain drugs (e.g., estrogens, psychoactive drugs, metoclopramide, opioids, leuprolide, goserelin, triptorelin, newer androgen biosynthesis inhibitors for prostate cancer)
	Isolated LH deficiency	Cushing syndrome
		Cirrhosis
		Morbid obesity
		Idiopathic
Mixed		Aging
		Alcoholism
		Systemic disease (e.g., uremia, liver failure, AIDS, sickle cell disease)
		Drugs (ethanol, corticosteroids)

*Adapted from Ref. 4.

is accompanied by very low levels of the sex-related hormones, specifically testosterone in males.[3] It is estimated that approximately 1 in every 10,000 males has Kallmann syndrome. It is typically inherited by one of the two parents, although there are some reported cases that have no family history of the condition. The most commonly inherited form is the "X-linked form", which is the result of a mutation in the KAL1 gene located on the X chromosome. The KAL1 gene plays a crucial role in the proper development of the olfactory system and this is why most KS patients experience partial or total anosmia (lack of sense of smell). Other inherited form of KS result from a mutated KAL2 gene on chromosome 8, and mutation of KAL3 gene.[3,4]

Symptoms of KS include failure to go through or complete puberty, partial or total lack of smell, infertility and poorly defined secondary sex characteristics. Rarely, the symptoms may include osteroporosis, having only one kidney, mental retardation and obesity.[5] Inability to smell is usually a positive sign for KS, as it is the only disease associated with a partial or total lack of smell, and is confirmed by the "smell" test which is quick, easy and noninvasive. Physical examination to check for small genitals or undescended testes, and blood tests to measure the levels of LH, FSH, and testosterone are performed for diagnosis of KS.

Treatment for KS is to increase the levels of hormones, usually by testosterone injections. Cryptorchidism and microphallus, very common in patients with KS, are treated by surgery and testosterone replacement, respectively. A recent study has also showed that human chorionic gonadotropin (hCG) injections are effective in treating the condition in adolescents and adults.[6] Other treatments for microphallus include dihydrotestosterone therapy.[7]

Kisspeptin is a protein that regulates the release of GnRH from the hypothalamus, which in turn regulates the release of LH and to a lesser extent, FSH from the anterior pituitary gland. Kisspeptin and its associated receptor ligand GPR54 are known to be involved in the regulation of puberty. Studies have shown that Kisspeptin could be used in the diagnosis and treatment of conditions such as Kallmann syndrome and congenital HH in certain cases.[8,9] At present, there are some limitations to the potential therapeutic role of Kisspeptin in cases of Kallmann syndrome and congenital HH. Studies have shown that GnRH release, and hence LH and FSH response does decrease over time with continuous Kisspeptin administration and there have to be sufficient GnRH releasing neurones present in the hypothalamus in order for the Kisspeptin to be effective. Further research on Kallmann syndrome and other clinical conditions linked to the dysregulation of the HPG axis is necessary to develop Kisspeptin as a therapeutic agent for HH.

In the prepubertal male, differentiating between Kallmann's syndrome and delayed sexual maturation may be very difficult. A family history of Kallmann's syndrome or the presence of somatic midline defects or anosmia may help in the prepubertal diagnosis. As the first sign of puberty is testicular growth, a patient who has testes greater than 2 cm^3 is experiencing delayed puberty rather than HH. Delayed pubertal males, respond to clomiphene citrate with a rise in serum LH levels, but not patients with Kallmann's syndrome. Patients of Kallmann's syndrome have an absent or blunted rise in gonadotropins following GnRH administration; however, repeated GnRH injections may prime the pituitary resulting in rise of LH and FSH. Unfortunately, this pattern of response is also found in prepubertal boys. However, doses of 5,000 IU of hCG induces larger rises in testosterone levels in these boys than KS patients.

Androgen replacement with testosterone or hCG is adequate treatment for the teenager and usually results in virilization. Gonadotropin therapy is required for the initiation of spermatogenesis. Given as hCG (2,000 IU IM three times per week) initiates spermatogenesis in most patients, but only 20% of patients complete spermatogenesis with hCG therapy alone. FSH is required in most patients for the completion of spermatogenesis, and is commonly given after 6 months of hCG therapy, in the form of human menopausal gonadotropin (hMG). Stimulation of the testes with FSH and LH results in testicular growth, although the final testis volume may remain below normal. Oligospermia (sperm count <10 million/mL) are common although motility parameters are usually quite good. In contrast to patients with idiopathic oligospermia who are often infertile with these sperm densities, many patients with HH are able to conceive despite these low sperm densities.

In addition to KS, there are several other congenital hypothalamic hypogonadal syndromes which differ in their presentation. The *Prader-Willi syndrome* consists of obesity, hypotonic musculature, mental retardation, small hands and feet, short stature, micropenis and hypogonadism. This syndrome may be associated with abnormalities of chromosome 15. Patients demonstrate an LH and FSH deficiency because of a lack of GnRH. Treatment is identical to that for KS. A similar situation is observed in *Laurence-Moon Bardet-Biedl syndrome* which consists of HH, retinitis pigmentosa and polydactyly.

Acquired Hypothalamic Diseases

Pituitary function may be impaired in case of pituitary surgery, infarction, tumors, radiation or infectious diseases. Patients with prepubertal onset of pituitary disease are usually diagnosed prior to a fertility evaluation as a result of growth retardation or adrenal or thyroid deficiency. Infertility, impotence, visual field abnormalities and severe headaches may be presenting symptoms in the adult male with pituitary dysfunction. Normal male secondary sexual characteristics are usually present unless adrenal insufficiency also exists. Small, soft testes may be demonstrated on physical examination, in contrast to small testes that are firm to palpation in cases of primary testicular failure with tubular and peritubular sclerosis. Plasma testosterone levels are low and gonadotropin levels are low to normal. Therefore, a normal LH value associated with a low serum testosterone level is abnormal and indicates need for further evaluation of other pituitary hormones and endocrine functions.[10]

Fertile Eunuch Syndrome

Isolated LH deficiency occurs rarely in patients with normal FSH levels. These men demonstrate a variably eunuchoid habitus, large testes and small volume ejaculates containing few spermatozoa. Plasma testosterone and LH levels are low, but FSH levels are in the normal range. Testicular biopsy specimens demonstrate maturation of the germinal epithelium with Leydig cell hypoplasia because of insufficient LH stimulation. A rise in serum testosterone following hCG therapy supports normal Leydig cell function in these patients. Sufficient intratesticular testosterone is produced for spermatogenesis, but inadequate peripheral androgen levels lead to poor virilization.[11]

Isolated FSH Deficiency

This is a rare disorder in which patients have adequate virilization, normal LH- and testosterone levels, and normal-sized testes. Due to a lack of FSH, oligospermia or azoospermia is present. Administration of hMG improves spermatogenesis, but a more specific treatment may be given in the form of pure FSH.[12]

Hyperprolactinemia

Hyperprolactinemia is known to interfere with reproductive functions lowering serum testosterone levels resulting in classic symptoms of hypogonadism. The mechanisms by which hyperprolactinemia induces testosterone deficiency are complex. Serum LH levels are suppressed or inappropriately low, indicating that the hypothalamic-pituitary axis fails to respond to reduced testicular testosterone production. Prolactin inhibits GnRH secretion. Prompt and dramatic improvement in sexual function occurs in many hyperprolactinemic men treated with bromocriptine (dopamine agonist with PRL-lowering activity). There is evidence to suggest that hyperprolactinemia may impair sexual function in men, both by direct effect on the CNS and by inhibition of androgen secretion. The direct CNS effect is supported by clinical data demonstrating that androgen replacement therapy did not improve libido to normal as long as PRL levels remained elevated. Finally, it must be recognized that some patients with prolactinomas will have HH produced by the mass lesion itself.[13]

Primary Testicular Disorders

Sex-determining Region Y (SRY) and Azoospermic Factor (AZF) Genes

The sex-determining region Y gene is found on the short (p) arm of the Y chromosome at position 11.3 (Yp11.3). It provides instructions for making a protein called the sex-determining region Y protein. The SRY protein produced from this gene acts as a transcription factor, initiating the processes that cause a fetus to develop male gonads (testes) and prevent the development of female reproductive structures (uterus and fallopian tubes). The SRY protein is also called the testis-determining factor (TDF). Changes occurring in the SRY gene are responsible for various disorders of sex development.[14,15]

An abnormal exchange of genetic material between chromosomes (translocation) resulting in the 46, XX testicular disorder of sex development, occurs as a random event during the formation of sperm cells in the affected person's father. The SRY gene is misplaced in this disorder, almost always onto an X chromosome. A fetus with an X chromosome that carries the SRY gene will develop male characteristics despite not having a Y chromosome.[16]

Mutations in the SRY gene cause Swyer syndrome, also known as complete or pure 46, XY gonadal dysgenesis. SRY gene mutations may lead to absence of the SRY protein or result in the production of a nonfunctioning protein. A fetus carrying such mutation will not develop testes but will develop a uterus and fallopian tubes, despite having a typically male karyotype.[17] Partial gonadal dysgenesis can also occur in a small number of individuals having SRY gene mutations that impair but not eliminate the function of the SRY protein. Affected individuals acquire two X chromosomes with one carrying a misplaced copy of the SRY gene that leads to development of ambiguous genitalia (ovotesticular disorder of sex development) or other abnormalities of the reproductive organs.

An AZF gene has been found to be localized to the long arm of the Y chromosome. This locus is subdivided into a, b and c, of which AZFc contains the gene DAZ which is deleted in case of azoospermia. Men with complete deletions of the entire AZFa region uniformly show a Sertoli cell only pattern. The AZFa region contains a gene DBY, a transcriptional regulator that appears to be critical for the completion of spermatogenesis. No patient with AZFb deletion has shown completely developed spermatozoa present on testicular biopsy. Approximately 6% of infertile men are found to have chromosomal abnormalities, with the incidence increasing as the sperm count decreases.[18] The highest incidence is found in azoospermic patients, with up to 21% of cases demonstrating abnormalities of the karyotype. The majority of these cases are associated with Klinefelter's syndrome or XXY syndrome.

Klinefelter's Syndrome

The presence of an extra X chromosome is the genetic hallmark of Klinefelter's syndrome. This is due to nondysjunction of the meiotic chromosomes of the gametes from either parent. Hypogonadism, with the classic triad of small, firm testes, gynecomastia, and elevated urinary gonadotropins, has an incidence of 1 of every 600 male births, but clinically may not be identifiable until puberty. Although secondary sexual characteristics begin developing at the appropriate time, the completion of puberty is usually delayed with features of eunuchoidism, gynecomastia, and impotence. Virilization may be complete in some patients and the diagnosis for them delayed until adulthood, at which point the patient may present with infertility (azoospermia) with associated gynecomastia and small, firm testes. Mental retardation and various psychiatric disturbances may also occur. Testicular biopsy reveals seminiferous tubular sclerosis and an occasional Sertoli cells or spermatozoa. Owing to the absence of normal seminiferous tubules, Leydig cells may appear hyperplastic. Plasma FSH levels are usually markedly elevated as a result of the severe seminiferous tubular injury, whereas LH levels may be elevated or normal. Total plasma testosterone levels are decreased in 60% of patients and normal in 40%. The physiologically active free testosterone concentrations are usually decreased. In addition, plasma estradiol levels are usually increased, stimulating increased levels of testosterone-binding globulin and resulting in a decreased testosterone to estrogen ratio resulting in gynecomastia. The diagnosis may be made with a chromatin-positive buccal smear, indicating the presence of an extra X chromosome. Karyotypes usually demonstrate 47 XXY or, less commonly, a mosaic pattern 46 XY/47 XXY. Less severe abnormalities are present in patients with the mosaic form of Klinefelter's syndrome, and occasional patients are fertile.[19]

XYY Syndrome

This karyotype occurs in 0.1–0.4% of newborn infants, and has been linked to aggressive and criminal behavior. Not all investigators agree that this behavior is secondary to the karyotype, but feel it may be secondary to tall stature, which may predispose individuals to this behavior. Patients are characteristically tall, whereas semen analyses typically reveal severe oligospermia or azoospermia. Testicular biopsy specimens reveal patterns of maturation arrest to complete germinal aplasia as well as occasional cases demonstrating seminiferous tubular sclerosis. Plasma gonadotropins and testosterone levels are most often within the normal range in these patients. However, elevations of plasma FSH levels may be found in association with more severe patterns of testicular dysfunction.[20]

XX Disorder

Patients with the XX male syndrome (sex reversal syndrome) have findings similar to those of Klinefelter's syndrome. These patients demonstrate small, firm testes, frequent gynecomastia, small to normal-sized penises, and azoospermia. Testicular biopsy may demonstrate seminiferous tubule sclerosis, resulting in elevated gonadotropins and decreased testosterone levels. In contrast to Klinefelter's syndrome, these individuals have average heights to shorter than normal heights, no mental deficiency, and hypospadias. Although karyotypes are 46 XX, molecular biologic mapping has suggested that portions of the Y chromosome including the testis-determining gene SRY are present in some but not all of these individuals. Because none of the AZF region is present, it is unlikely that sperm could be recovered from testicular tissue.[21]

Noonan's Syndrome

The appearance of these patients is similar to that of Turner's syndrome (XO), having short stature, hypertelorism, webbed neck, low-set ears, cubitus valgus, ptosis, and cardiovascular abnormalities. Chromosomal analysis reveals a 46 XY karyotype. A gene on chromosome 12 has been linked to this defect. Cryptorchidism and testicular atrophy results in elevations of gonadotropins. Androgens may be given to complete virilization, but these patients remain infertile.

Androgen Insensitivity Syndrome

Androgens act by binding to androgen receptors that travel to the cell nucleus and interact with the nuclear matrix, stimulating messenger RNA synthesis. Abnormalities in this process result in androgen-resistant syndromes. Karyotypically, these patients are 46 XY males, with phenotypes ranging from pseudohermaphroditism to a normal male phenotype with infertility. Owing to a defect in testosterone action, these patients are found to have elevated serum levels of LH and testosterone.

Bilateral Anorchia (Vanishing Testis Syndrome)

Vanishing testis syndrome is bilateral anorchia found in genetic XY males with nonpalpable testes. Patients have prepubertal male phenotypes, suggesting that testicular tissue capable of secreting androgens must have been present at one time in utero. It is theoretical that the testes may have been lost in utero, secondary to vascular injury or testicular torsion. Low plasma testosterone and elevated gonadotropin levels are present in these males. Virilization may be induced with testosterone administration, but the infertility is not treatable.[22]

Cryptorchidism

Cryptorchidism is present in about 3% of full term boys. By the age of 1 year, approximately 1% of boys demonstrate undescended testes and approximately 0.8% of adult males have undescended testes. After 1 year of age, the undescended testis is unlikely to descend. Two thirds of cases are unilateral, whereas one third of cases are bilateral. Sperm concentrations below 12–20 million/mL are found in 50% of patients with bilateral cryptorchidism, and in 25% of patients with unilateral cryptorchidism. Testicular biopsy of the cryptorchid testis reveals decreased numbers of Leydig cells. Until the first 6 months of life, the number of germ cells in the cryptorchid testis is within the normal range. By about 2 years of age, 38% of unilateral and bilaterally cryptorchid testes will have lost their germ cells. The descended testis, in cases of unilateral cryptorchidism, also may demonstrate abnormalities with low numbers of germ cells. The higher the cryptorchid testis, the more severe is the testicular dysfunction. Absence of germ cells is found in 20–40% of inguinal or prescrotal testes, in contrast to 90% of intra-abdominal testes. Both mechanical and hormonal etiologic factors have been suggested to explain the mechanism of cryptorchidism. Increasing evidence points to a defect in the hypothalamic–pituitary–gonadal axis in these patients.[23] Histologic changes in cryptorchid testis within the first year of life have supported therapy directed toward correction of cryptorchidism by 12 months of age. Retrospective studies report reasonably high fertility rates in patients with surgically corrected unilateral cryptorchidism.[24]

Sertoli Cell-only Syndrome

Although the etiology of *Sertoli cell-only* syndrome is unknown, patients usually present with bilaterally small testes and azoospermia. Phenotypically, these patients have normal secondary characteristics. Seminiferous tubules are lined by Sertoli cells with a complete absence of germ cells. The testes of patients with *Sertoli cell-only* syndrome are reasonably normal in consistency. Plasma FSH levels are often elevated, but not in all patients. Plasma testosterone and LH levels are normal.[25]

Myotonic Dystrophy

Myotonia is a condition of delayed muscle relaxation after contraction. These patients also demonstrate premature frontal baldness, posterior subcapsular cataracts and cardiac conduction defects. Testicular atrophy may develop in up to 80% of patients. Testicular damage usually occurs in adulthood; Leydig cells typically are uninvolved, with biopsy specimens demonstrating severe tubular sclerosis. Serum FSH is elevated with severe tubular atrophy. Disease is transmitted as an autosomal dominant trait with variable penetrance. There is no therapy for the testicular dysfunction in these patients.[26]

Influence of Exogenous Hormones

Androgen Excess

Production of LH and FSH is inhibited by negative feedback from estrogens and androgens at both the hypothalamus and pituitary levels. Androgen excess, from exogenous sources or by endogenous production, may induce a hypogonadal state such as a metabolic abnormality or an androgen-producing tumor. Congenital adrenal hyperplasia is the most common cause of endogenous androgen excess. A congenital deficiency of 21-hydroxylase is the most common cause of the five enzyme defects responsible for this syndrome. A deficiency of 21-hydroxylase results in a decrease in cortisone synthesis, which leads to increased pituitary production of adrenocorticotropic hormone (ACTH). Elevated levels of ACTH result in hyperstimulation of the adrenal gland and in increased production of adrenal androgens.[27] Excess androgens feedback to the pituitary, inhibiting the production and secretion of gonadotropins and leading to hypogonadism. Short stature and precocious puberty develop in these patients. As a result of androgen stimulation, premature enlargement of the penis may occur; however, because of a lack of gonadotropin stimulation, the testes remain underdeveloped. Basal plasma 17-hydroxyprogesterone levels are often elevated 50–200 times above normal levels. In addition, elevated urinary 17-ketosteroid and pregnanetriol levels may occur. Glucocorticoid therapy results in a reduction of ACTH levels, which induces a decrease in peripheral testosterone, thus stimulating endogenous gonadotropin secretion. HH has also been identified after the use of anabolic steroids by athletes. This condition is usually reversible after medications are discontinued, but permanent suppression of gonadotropin may occur.

Estrogen Excess

Pituitary gonadotropin secretion is suppressed by peripheral estrogens. A state of secondary testicular failure may be induced by estrogen-secreting tumors in the adrenal cortex or in the testis. Testicular Sertoli cell tumors or interstitial cell tumors may produce estrogen. Excess peripheral estrogens may also result from hepatic dysfunction. Peripheral adipose tissue converts androgen into estrogen. Elevated estrogen levels have been identified in morbidly obese patients. Impotence, gynecomastia and testicular atrophy may result from estrogen excess. Hormonal studies demonstrate low levels of FSH, LH, and testosterone in the presence of elevated estrogens. Treatment is directed at the underlying condition.[28]

Prolactin Excess

Impotence and infertility have been associated with hyperprolactinemia. In patients with pituitary adenomas, prolactin levels are elevated and gonadotropins and testosterone levels are depressed. The majority of patients with hyperprolactinemia, however, demonstrate mild elevations and investigations reveal no evidence of pituitary tumors. These patients are classified as having idiopathic hyperprolactinemia which may be caused by microadenomas that are too small to be detected by current imaging techniques. Hypoglycemia, hyperaminoacidemia and dopaminergic antagonists and agonists, as well as other neurotransmitters, stimulate prolactin release. Pathologic stimuli include chronic renal failure, cirrhosis, intercostal nerve stimulation, and pituitary and hypothalamic tumors. Gynecomastia and galactorrhea are uncommon findings in men. Although most women present with microadenomas, most men presenting with prolactinomas have macroadenomas (≥1.0 cm). Patients who have persistent elevation of prolactin should undergo a CT scan or a MRI study of the head. Bromocriptine, cabergoline, surgery and radiation therapy have been used for the treatment of macroadenomas. Bromocriptine therapy alone is usually successful for the treatment of microadenomas.[29]

Gonadotoxic Agents

Many physical and chemical agents are known to injure the germinal epithelium. Seminiferous epithelium consists of rapidly dividing cells and is susceptible to agents that interfere with cell division. In addition, since spermatogenesis is an androgen dependent process, drugs that interfere with androgen production or action also adversely affect fertility.[30]

Chemotherapy

Spermatogenesis is adversely affected by most chemotherapeutic agents. Cells that are most actively dividing are the most susceptible to chemotherapeutic agents, and consist of spermatogonia and spermatocytes up to the preleptotene stage. Nondividing spermatids and mature spermatozoa are relatively less susceptible. Repopulation of the seminiferous tubules occurs as long as some spermatogonial stem cells remain. These cells divide slowly, eventually resulting in a resumption of spermatogenesis. The specific combination of drugs used for therapy, the dose administered, and the age of the patient at the time of treatment are all determinants of the specific effect on the gonads. Studies of large groups of patients who survived cancers in childhood have demonstrated that fertility rates of patients treated with alkylating agents were 60% lower than in nontreated controls.[31] As single drugs, alkylating agents and procarbazine seem to result in the greatest amount of testicular damage. The use of multidrug chemotherapeutic regimens has made it difficult to determine which specific agents are responsible for specific defects. A resumption of spermatogenesis occurs in 50–60% of testis cancer patients treated with combination chemotherapy, such as cisplatin, vinblastine and bleomycin. During chemotherapy, most patients demonstrate elevations of serum FSH levels that correlate with azoospermia and then levels decline if and when spermatogenesis resumes.[32]

Radiation

Germinal epithelium has a high rate of cell division, making it very radiosensitive. Spermatids are more resistant to radiation than spermatogonia or spermatocytes. Leydig cells are reasonably radio-resistant; and testosterone levels usually remain normal after radiation exposure. Serum FSH levels may increase and revert to normal after the return of spermatogenesis. Azoospermia results from dosages greater than 65 cGy. At dosages lower than 100 cGy, recovery takes approximately 12 months. Following dosages of 200–300 cGy, recovery may take 30 months; at dosages of 400–600 cGy, more than 5 years may be required for spermatogenesis to return. Semen quality will usually return to baseline within 2 years of radiation therapy for seminoma, however, approximately 25% may become permanently infertile. After radiation therapy, most patients are advised to avoid conception for 2 years, although pregnancies after treatment have revealed no evidence of an increase in the prevalence of congenital anomalies.[33]

Systemic Illnesses

Uremia is associated with decreased libido, impotence, gynecomastia and defects in spermatogenesis, secondary to decreased plasma testosterone levels and elevated gonadotropins. These abnormalities persist even in patients undergoing chronic hemodialysis. The elevated gonadotropin levels and subnormal responses of the testes to hCG administration suggest an impairment of testosterone production. An improvement in spermatogenesis and testicular function occurs following renal transplantation.[34] Testicular failure is also common in patients with cirrhosis of the liver also resulting in impotence, gynecomastia, and testicular atrophy. Patients with sickle cell disease may demonstrate delayed secondary characteristics, small testicles, and oligospermia.[35]

Postpubertal mumps results in orchitis in approximately 30% of patients with bilateral involvement in 10–30% of cases. Permanent testicular atrophy may develop within several months to several years following infection. An intense interstitial edema and mononuclear infiltration is noted pathologically. This may result in hypergonadotropic hypogonadism and gynecomastia. This entity has become uncommon since the advent of the mumps vaccine. Syphilis may affect both the testis and epididymis, resulting in diffuse interstitial inflammation with endarteritis and gumma formation.[36]

Lifestyle-related Factors

Lifestyle-related factors may have a significant impact on male reproductive parameters. It is well known that the length of the period of abstinence affects sperm concentration and total sperm counts[37] and that cigarette smoking,[38] alcohol consumption[39,40] and dietary habits[41] also play a role. Lifestyle-related habits are known to be subject to geographic as well as time related variation, and if associated with male reproductive function, may at least partly explain some of the observed epidemiological trends.

Alcohol

Moderate alcohol intake does not seem to affect the fertility potential of a male,[42] but chronic and excessive alcohol intake is known to affect reproductive parameters.[39,40] Both the testes and the liver are directly affected by ethanol. Testicular atrophy is commonly found in chronic alcoholics. Free testosterone levels are often decreased, whereas total testosterone levels may be within the normal range, secondary to elevated levels of testosterone–estradiol-binding globulin. Testicular specimens demonstrate peritubular fibrosis and a reduction in the number of germ cells. Patients may demonstrate impotence, gynecomastia, and feminization. Gonadotropin levels may be increased.[43] Acute consumption of alcohol in nonalcoholics also demonstrates a fall in testosterone levels.

Smoking

Recent data show that cigarette smoking has an antiandrogenic effect, leading to a 30% reduction in sperm count and 10% decrease in seminal volume.[44] Maternal smoking during pregnancy is also shown to hamper spermatogenesis in the sons,[45] a finding which has been confirmed by several other studies.[46,47] Additionally, a recent report indicated 30% lower sperm numbers in sons of men smoking during pregnancy even after adjustment for the smoking habits of the mother.[48] This effect was more pronounced than that when the mother alone was smoking, it could indicate some preconception damage to spermatozoa mediated through genetic or epigenetic mechanisms. In the Nordic countries, the pattern of increased smoking among females mirrors the rise in the incidence of testicular cancer, but so far, no association between maternal smoking during pregnancy and the risk of TGCC among their sons has been disclosed.

Pain Killers and Recreational Drugs

It has been shown by an epidemiological study of 47,000 Scandinavian women and their live born sons that intake of mild analgesics, such as acetaminophen, was associated with congenital cryptorchidism in boys.[49,50] Later animal studies have shown that the effect also applies to malformations in animals and that these drugs inhibit testosterone synthesis in rodents.[51,52] *In vitro* studies on human testicular tissue have shown significantly reduced steroidogenesis in the presence of analgesics.[53] Taken together, these compounds act like endocrine disruptors, which may be of concern, since more than 50% of pregnant women in Europe and the USA use weak analgesics frequently.

Endocrine-disrupting Factors

On the basis of a rapid increase observed in testicular germ-cell cancer (TGCC) as well as in congenital genital anomalies in boys, it seems reasonable to propose that environmental, rather than genetic factors have a greater role in the increase of these disorders. Many of these compounds have the capability to interfere with hormone synthesis or hormone receptors. Animal models have convincingly shown the adverse effects of these compounds on the male reproductive system. It has been debated for decades as to whether these compounds are truly causing genital malformations or TGCC in humans, with one exception diethylstilbestrol (DES). Millions of women in the USA and Europe used this estrogenic compound from 1940s to 1971 to prevent abortions and pregnancy complications. DES was banned in 1971 after it was shown to be associated with uncommon vaginal cancer (vaginal clear cell adenocarcinoma) in in utero exposed girls.[54] In exposed boys, increased risk of cryptorchidism, epididymal cysts, and testicular infection was shown,[55] whereas studies on increased risk of TGCC have been inconclusive. An increased risk was suggested in a report in 1983, but this was not confirmed for 20 years, until a study on women taking DES at an early stage of pregnancy, the most critical developmental window for the fetus.[56,57] In a multigenerational study on 529 families, an increased risk of hypospadias in grandsons of women prescribed DES during pregnancy was observed, but no other abnormalities were found.[58]

A number of environmental chemical exposures have been shown to promote epigenetic transgenerational inheritance of cryptochidism and the transgenerational epigenetic changes may be used as biomarkers of exposure and disease.[58] None of the human studies have investigated transgenerational (four generations) effects of DEHP (di-2-ethylhexyl phthalate). Animal models have been used to study the toxicological effects of DEHP. DEHP has been shown to produce reproduction toxicity in newborn rats.[59]

There a few studies regarding the effects of exposure to estrogenic or antiandrogenic compounds effects in the general population. The INUENDO study, an EU financed project, was conducted between 2002 and 2006 to identify and characterize the impact of dietary, persistent organic pollutants (POP) on fertility in European populations, and to provide epidemiologic evidence on possible health impacts of environmental exposure to xenobiotics which have a hormone-like action.[60] The study populations ranged from Greenland Inuit, with the highest body burdens of POP in the world, to Swedish fishermen from the polluted east coast as well as from the west coast, to Ukrainians, who are mostly exposed by use of pesticides, and to a Polish population, as a low exposure group. The POP exposure was negatively correlated to sperm motility and sperm DNA integrity, but, no association with fecundity or sperm concentrations was found, despite the fact that some of the subjects included in the study presented with extremely high POP levels in serum.[61] From the same cohorts, a negative association between serum levels of perfluorooctane sulfonate and sperm morphology has been found recently.[62]

Exposure to phthalates, another type of compounds belonging to the family of endocrine disrupters, has also been reported to be associated with the deterioration of classical sperm parameters and sperm DNA integrity.[63,64] Anogenital distance (AGD), a marker of prenatal androgen exposure in newborn boys, was found to be negatively correlated to the levels of phthalates in the serum of the mothers.[65] In adult men, the same parameter was found to be negatively associated with signs of testicular dysfunction, hypogonadism and nonobstructive azoospermia.[66,67]

GYNECOMASTIA

Abnormal development of breast glandular tissue in males is called gynecomastia. In some cases, there is only an increase breast fat, but not that of breast glandular tissue. Such a condition is called pseudogynecomastia, which must be ruled out in genuine cases of gynecomastia.[68] Some enlargement of male breast tissue occurs normally during infancy and puberty. Enlargement is temporary, tender, bilateral and is distributed uniformly under the areola, and is known as physiologic gynecomastia, which resolves in 6 months to 2 years. Similar enlargement also occurs in old age due to the proliferation of stroma, not of breast ducts. Diminished effect of androgen due to decreased production, blockade and androgen receptor defects, and/or increased effect of estrogen caused by a rise in estrogen production and release of bound estrogen from sex hormone-binding globulin (SHBG) appears to be responsible for gynecomastia.[69] In adults, the common causes of gynecomastia are persistent pubertal gynecomastia and use of drugs, otherwise, it is idiopathic gynecomastia where the cause is unknown. Some causes and findings of gynecomastia and corresponding diagnostic approaches are shown in Table 18.2.

Use of drugs is another major cause of gynecomastia. A variety of drugs, listed in Table 18.3 have been shown to be associated with the disorder. However, not all drugs that have been associated have been shown to cause gynecomastia through challenge–rechallenge testing.

Table 18.2: Causes of gynecomastia.*

Causes	*Suggestive findings*	*Diagnostic approach*
Chronic kidney disease (CKD)	History of chronic kidney disease	Serum electrolytes, BUN, and creatinine, urinalysis, possibly urine culture and urinary levels of Na, K, and creatinine
Cirrhosis	Liver disease, alcohol use ascites, spider angiomas, dilated abdominal veins	Routine laboratory testing, sometimes liver biopsy
Drugs	History of use	Trial of stopping the drug
Feminizing adrenocortical tumor	Palpable mass, testicular atrophy	Imaging (MRI or CT)
Hyperthyroidism	Tremor, heat intolerance, diarrhea, tachycardia, weight loss, goiter, exophthalmos	Thyroid function tests
Hypogonadism	*Prepubertal onset:* Underdeveloped secondary sexual characteristics *Postpubertal onset:* Decreased libido, erectile dysfunction, mood changes, decreased muscle and increased fat mass, osteopenia, testicular atrophy, mild cognitive changes	Serum FSH, LH, and testosterone levels
Paraneoplastic ectopic production of hCG	Possibly signs of primary tumor or symptoms and signs of hypogonadism	Evaluation for suspected primary tumor
Testicular tumors	Testicular mass, possibly symptoms and signs of hypogonadism	Ultrasonography
Feeding after undernutrition	Muscle and fat wasting, hair loss, skin changes, frequent infections, fatigue, signs of vitamin deficiencies (e.g., osteopenia)	Clinical evaluation, selective laboratory testing
Idiopathic gynecomastia	No abnormal findings other than gynecomastia, no symptoms, no apparent cause	Repeat clinical evaluation in 6 months, possibly serum testosterone level

*Adapted from Ref. 68.

Table 18.3: Common drug causes of gynecomastia.*

Category	*Drugs*
Inhibitors of androgen synthesis/ activity	Cyproterone (an antiandrogen), dutasteride and finasteride (5α-reductase inhibitors), goserelin, histrelin, leuprolide, and triptorelin (LH–RH agonists), flutamide, bicalutamide, enzalutamide and nilutamide (antiandrogens used to treat prostate cancer)
Antimicrobials	Efavirenz, ethionamide, isoniazid, ketoconazole, metronidazole
Antineoplastic drugs	Alkylating drugs, imatinib, methotrexate, vinca alkaloids
Cardiovascular drugs	ACE inhibitors (e.g., captopril, enalapril), amiodarone, Ca channel blockers (e.g., nifedipine, diltiazem), methyldopa, reserpine, spironolactone
CNS-acting drugs	Diazepam, haloperidol, methadone, phenothiazines, tricyclic antidepressants
Antiulcer drugs	Cimetidine, ranitidine, omeprazole
Hormones	Androgens, anabolic steroids, estrogens, human growth hormone
Recreational drugs	Amphetamines, ethanol, heroin, marijuana
OTC herbal drugs	Lavender oil, tea tree oils
Other drugs	Auranofin, diethylpropion, domperidone, metoclopramide, phenytoin, penicillamine, sulindac, theophylline

*Adapted from Ref. 68.

Evaluation and Treatment

The first and foremost aspect of evaluation is to examine patient's medical history for duration of symptoms, presence of secondary sexual characteristics, puberty and presence of symptoms, such as decreased libido, erectile dysfunction, pain in the breast area and nipple discharge. Medical history should also look for disorders that can cause gynecomastia and include a history of all prescribed and OTC drugs. Complete physical examination should include vital signs, skin and general appearance, the neck for possible goiter, the abdomen for ascites, venous distention and suspected adrenal masses, assessment of the penis, pubic hair, auxiliary hair and the testes for masses or atrophy. The breasts are examined while patients are recumbent with their hands behind the head. Using thumb and forefinger together from opposite sides of the nipple until they meet, the examiner should look for possible nipple discharge. Lumps are assessed and characterized in terms of location, consistency, fixation to underlying tissues, and skin changes. The axilla is examined for lymph node involvement in men who have breast lumps. With pseudogynecomastia, there is no resistance between the thumb and forefinger, whereas in the case of gynecomastia, a rim of tissue more than 0.5 cm in diameter surrounds the nipple symmetrically and is similar in consistency to the nipple itself. Symptoms are evaluated for presence of underlying systemic conditions like chronic kidney disease (CKD), cirrhosis, undernutrition, hypogonadism and hyperthyroidism. While weight loss and fragile, discolored skin indicate CKD, undernutrition and cirrhosis; tachycardia, tremor, goiter, exophthalmos along with weight loss indicate hyperthyroidism. Hypogonadism is suspected in case of underdeveloped secondary sexual characteristics (prepuberty) and testicular atrophy (postpuberty). Hypogonadism is common with aging. If other findings suggest hypogonadism, therefore, in adults without a drug or evident pathologic cause, measurement of serum levels of LH, FSH, testosterone, estradiol and hCG are recommended, once in 6 months. Findings of particular concern are presence of localized or eccentric breast swelling, particularly with nipple discharge, fixation to the skin, or hard consistency suggesting breast cancer, although uncommon in males. Presence of testicular mass may suggest testicular (Leydig cell) tumor.[69]

Specific treatment is not required in most cases as gynecomastia usually remits spontaneously. If a drug, except for anabolic steroids is the cause for gynecomastia, symptoms usually disappear once the use of drugs is stopped. Treatment for underlying diseases like CKD, cirrhosis, hyperthyroidism, etc. is provided if that is the major cause. Tamoxifen is indicated in men and adolescents when pain and tenderness in breast are particularly troublesome, and in cases of prostate cancer patients treated with anti-androgen therapy. Surgical removal of excess breast tissue by suction lipectomy alone or with cosmetic surgery may be recommended if appearance is unacceptable.[69]

TESTICULAR CANCER

Testicular germ cell tumors are derived from carcinoma in situ (CIS) germ cells, which are arrested and transformed fetal gonocytes that failed to mature to spermatogonia. There has been a significant increase in the incidence of testicular germ cell cancer (TGCC), among Caucasians, which to date is 23 times higher than 30–40 years ago.[70] The TGCC is the most common form of testicular malignancy, mainly appearing among males aged 25–40 years. The risk of TGCC has been shown to be strongly linked to the birth year.[71] Environmental or Lifestyle-related factors are especially important in the etiology and pathogenesis of this malignancy, and possible affect prenatally.[72]

Testicular germ cell tumors may occur in any age, but more than 90% of the cases are seen in young adult men, with the peak prevalence in the age range of 25–40 years. Unusually, incidence rate of testicular cancer has a small peak in the postnatal period and a major peak in the young adult age, starting at puberty. This hints at a plausible relationship between gonadal hormone activity and invasive transformation of germ cells, as these are periods of activation of gonadal hormones. Certain groups, such as individuals with developmental abnormalities of the gonads and sex differentiation have an increased risk of developing germ cell neoplasia. Among them, individuals with the so-called mixed gonadal dysgenesis and the 45,X/46,XY karyotype are at particular risk of harboring carcinoma in situ (CIS) or gonadoblastoma and developing testicular germ cell tumor in adolescence.[73-74] Several developmental abnormalities, like cryptorchidism,[75,76] Down syndrome,[77] low birth weight and unspecific perinatal factors, e.g., premature birth, birth order, high levels of maternal estrogens or bleeding during pregnancy, high maternal age and neonatal jaundice[78-80] have been linked to TGCC. This association of testicular cancer with poor testicular function, cryptorchidism, hypospadias

Flowchart 18.1: Etiology and pathogenesis of disorders grouped within testicular dysgenesis syndrome. Adapted from Ref. 85.

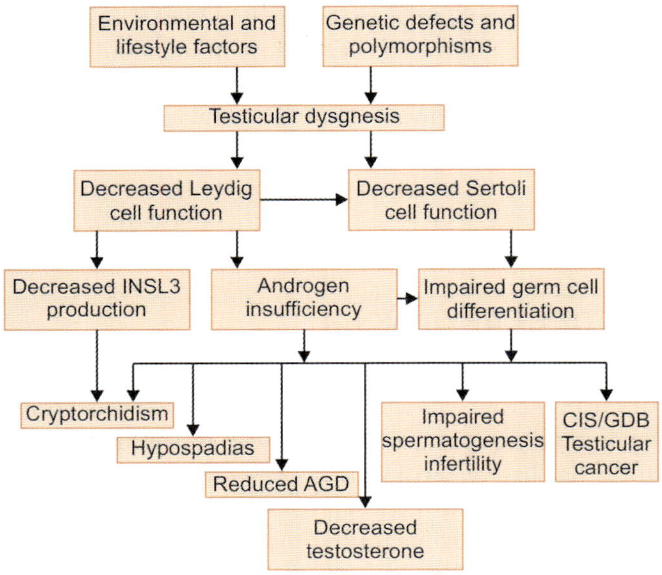

and abnormal testicular differentiation has led to the concept of testicular dysgenesis syndrome (TDS) suggesting that poor gonadal development and testicular neoplasia are etiologically linked. Among the several variations of TDS, testicular cancer is the rarest but also one of the most severe symptoms.[81] Flowchart 18.1 shows the concept of TDS schematically. Testicular dysgeneic features, such as undifferentiated tubules with immature Sertoli cells or hyaline bodies, are also seen in association with testicular cancer, thereby supporting the TDS hypothesis.[82,83] However, this concept cannot be generalized to all genital malformations and infertility cases, but needs to be applied with caution to poor development of the testis in fetal stage.[84] Poor development of the genitals may be a consequence of disturbed functions of testicular somatic cells (Leydig and Sertoli cells) caused by inherited genetic mutations/polymorphisms or environmental/lifestyle factors acting during early development. This, in turn, affects hormonal homeostasis and causes impaired germ cell differentiation. Depending on the severity of the impairment, multiple outcomes or phenotypes may occur, ranging from reduced AGD, genital malformations to testicular cancer. Among these, the most severe forms of TDS like gonadoblastoma or CIS are rarely seen. The most common and mildest is impaired spermatogenesis.

The prevalence of testicular cancer has been observed to be high in the well-developed countries such as Western Europe and the Scandinavian countries.[70] The high incidence rate of testicular cancer in developed countries suggests a possible adverse influence of environmental or Lifestyle-related factors. In recent decades, a great number of potent natural and synthetic hormones and hormone antagonists have been identified in environment. Observations in wildlife and experiments in laboratory animals exposed to the synthetic hormones and a broad range of "endocrine disrupters" suggest that these substances can cause a disturbance of hormonal milieu of the developing gonad and disturb differentiation of early germ cells.[81,86,87] The problem may even be more complicated due to possible mixtures of possible contaminating factors present in food, packaging, cosmetics and other products of daily life. In fact, a high serum levels of some POP is found in mothers of men with testicular cancer,[88] and a greater burden of p,p′-DDE (a DDT metabolite) has been found in serum of testicular cancer patients.[89-92]

Leydig Cell Hyperplasia and Tumors

Leydig cell tumors account for 1–3% of testicular neoplasms and occur in all age groups.[93-95] About 20% of the cases are found before the age of 10 years, most often between 5 and 10 years of age. The breakdown of hypothalamo-pituitary-testicular axis leading to an excessive stimulation of Leydig cells by LH has been found to play a central role in the development of Leydig cell hyperplasia.[96] There are other possible molecular pathways that remain largely unknown. Activating mutations of the LH receptor and G proteins have been detected in some cases.[97-100]

Among the symptoms of Leydig cell hyperplasia, precocious puberty is almost always the presenting symptom in these cases. Pubertal development, indicated by the growth of penis, pubic hair, accelerated skeletal and muscle growth, advancement of bone age, skin changes (acne, comedos, hair greasing) and adult type odor of sweat, are all seen as the tumors produce androgens, mainly testosterone. This secretion of testosterone being gonadotropin independent, and therefore LH and FSH remain low in spite of external signs of puberty.

Sertoli Cell Tumors

Most testicular tumors are large cell calcifying Sertoli cell tumors that are multifocal and bilateral and appear usually during the second decade of life.[101-103] Sertoli cell tumors are frequently found in association with two distinct multiple neoplasm syndromes, Carney complex and Peutz–Jeghers syndrome. When the Sertoli cell tumors cannot be classified to any of the above mentioned histopathological groups, they are referred to as Sertoli cell tumors, not otherwise specified (NOS).[104] Large-cell calcifying Sertoli cell tumors are usually not hormonally active, although elevated levels of serum inhibin B or testosterone have been reported, but other tumors of Carney complex, including Leydig cell tumors, can cause endocrine manifestations.[105,106]

Endocrine Aspects

Relative imbalance of androgen signaling (excess or deficiency) causes the most pronounced secondary endocrine symptoms associated with testicular tumors. Testosterone is produced by tumors, such as Leydig cell tumors, or by normal Leydig cells stimulated by large amounts of hCG from some germ cell tumors. In addition, aromatization of androgens leads to a relative excess of estrogens, which causes impairment of spermatogenesis and gynecomastia.[107]

Testicular dysfunction in young adult patients with testicular cancer, who usually are in their best reproductive age, is a serious clinical problem. Patients with testicular tumors have poor spermatogenesis and decreased fertility, even before the overt tumor has developed[84,108,109] and before cytotoxic treatment.[110] Features include oligozoospermia, elevated LH levels, and a variable degree of testicular dysgenesis or atrophy in the biopsy. In some cases it is further complicated by the presence of CIS. Examination of a contralateral biopsy in a patient with a unilateral tumor may show a similar picture with at least 5% risk of presence of CIS cells.[82] Testicular function is further disturbed by treatment of neoplasm. In recent years there is growing concern about adverse endocrinological sequelae of testicular irradiation and chemotherapy.[111] Refinement of the dosage must be considered in each patient individually, to eradicate the neoplasm with least possible damage to the endocrine function. The eradication of CIS or a tumor by irradiation in bilateral cancer cases also invariably destroys all germ cells leading to sterility. This underlines the importance of semen cryopreservation before treatment which will allow assisted reproduction treatment, if needed.[112-114] If the patient has a very severe oligozoospermia or cryptozoospermia, testicular sperm extraction (TESE) at the time of orchidectomy (oncoTESE) may be attempted in specialized centers.[115] The TESE and subsequent intracytoplasmic sperm injection (ICSI) may be also an option for fertility treatment in some cases of postchemotherapy azoospermia.[116] All the patients treated for testicular cancer, require careful assessment of their reproductive hormones and spermatogenic capacity by an endocrinologist or andrologist with respect to their future fertility, sexual potency, possible need for androgen replacement therapy and general wellbeing.

Diagnosis and Management

Surgical testicular biopsy is currently the only sure diagnostic procedure for testicular cancer. Examination for CIS by immunohistochemistry can be recommended in the leftover material after TESE in fertility clinics.[117] The histological examination of the biopsy should be aided by immunohistochemical staining for one of the known CIS marker proteins, such as placenta-like alkaline phosphatase (PLAP).[118-120]

Poor spermatogenesis is a good indication that the patient may be at risk of harboring CIS.[121-125] In addition, it has been known for a long time that CIS cells may be occasionally found in semen and immunocytochemical detection of CIS cells in semen has also been described.[126-128] An improved automated double staining based assay has been recently developed, although further improvement of sensitivity is needed.[129] Semen analysis is a noninvasive approach which may, in the future, eliminate the need for the contralateral biopsy.

Scrotal ultrasonography has become increasingly popular for assessment of the testicles and should be performed routinely, if testicular malignancy is suspected. Testicles afflicted with CIS have frequently an irregular echo pattern that may be associated with the presence of testicular microliths or hyaline bodies.[130,131]

A majority of primary and metastatic germ cell tumors secrete protein products that can be detected in circulating blood. These biochemical serum tumor markers are very helpful in diagnosis and monitoring of testicular cancer.[132] Some of the most important markers in clinical practice are hCG and AFP, very sensitive markers for nonseminomas, which in many cases have a more malignant clinical course than seminoma.[132] Choriocarcinoma which resembles gestational trophoblast, produces large quantities of hCG and yolk sac tumor, which is similar in morphology to the embryonic yolk sac, secretes alpha-fetoprotein (AFP).[133] Lactate dehydrogenase (LDH) may be secreted by both nonseminoma and seminoma.[134]

Sertoli cell tumors can be treated by orchiectomy, which has the highest assured success rate, consists of removal of a testis with CIS or localized tumor when the second testis is not affected. In cases where radiographically detected retroperitoneal involvement is observed, retroperitoneal lymphadenectomy is indicated.[105]

Low-dose radiotherapy is another good alternative to orchiectomy in cases where CIS is present in the contralateral testis, so the patient can be spared a total castration and lifelong androgen replacement therapy. The efficacy of radiotherapy with doses as low as 16 Gy has been demonstrated, but more studies are needed to confirm the best regimen.[135,136]

Chemotherapy has also been used to treat testicular cancer, but not with much success, as incomplete cure or relapse of CIS has been reported.[137,138] In some cases of extragonadal germ cell tumors treated with chemotherapy, testicular CIS progressed to metachronous overt testicular tumors.[139]

Surveillance is potentially hazardous since CIS may progress to invasive cancer at any time. However, if the patient desires to defer treatment temporarily for the purpose of paternity, surveillance with ultrasound monitoring may be considered after careful informed discussion of risks with the patient. In all cases of desired fatherhood, and in all cases of very young men, semen analysis and cryopreservation of semen samples, if viable spermatozoa are detected, is an appropriate option.

REFERENCES

1. Shenot PJ. Male Reproductive Endocrinology, Genitourinary Disorders. Merck Manuals, Professional Edition.
2. Irvin H, Hirsch M. Male Hypogonadism. Merck Manuals, Professional Edition 2015.
3. Pitteloud N, Quinton R, Pearce S, Raivio T, Acierno J, Dwyer A, et al. Digenic mutations account for variable phenotypes in idiopathic hypogonadotropic hypogonadism. J Clin Invest. 2007;117(2):457-63.
4. MacColl G, Bouloux P, Quinton R. Kallmann syndrome: adhesion, afferents, and anosmia. Neuron. 2002;34(5):675-8.
5. Valdes-Socin H. Reproduction, smell, and neurodevelopmental disorders: genetic defects in different hypogonadotropic hypogonadal syndromes. Front Endocrinol. 2014;5:109.
6. Kim S-O, Ryu KH, Hwang IS, Jung SI, Oh KJ, Park K. Penile growth in response to human chorionic gonadotropin (hcg) treatment in patients with idiopathic hypogonadotrophic hypogonadism. Chonnam Med J. 2011;47(1):39-42.
7. Choi SK, Han SW, Kim DH, de Lignieres B. Transdermal dihydrotestosterone therapy and its effects on patients with microphallus. J Urol. 1993;150(2 Pt. 2):657-60.
8. George JT, Seminara SB. Kisspeptin and the hypothalamic control of reproduction: lessons from the human. Endocrinology. 2012;153(11):5130-6.
9. Skorupskaite K, George JT, Anderson RA. The kisspeptin-GnRH pathway in human reproductive health and disease. Hum Reprod Update. 2014;20(4):485-500.
10. Carmichael JD, Braunstein GD. Diseases of hypothalamic origin. In: Pfaff DW, Arnold AP, Fahrbach SE, Etgen AM, Rubin RT (Eds). Hormones, Brain and Behavior. Los Angeles, CA: Academic Press; 2009. pp. 3005-48.
11. Smals AG, Kloppenborg PW, van Haelst UJ, Lequin R, Benraad TJ. Fertile eunuch syndrome vs. classic hypogonadotrophic hypogonadism. Acta Endocrinol (Copenh). 1978;87(2):389-99.
12. Mantovani G1, Borgato S, Beck-Peccoz P, Romoli R, Borretta G, Persani L. Isolated follicle-stimulating hormone (FSH) deficiency in a young man with normal virilization who did not have mutations in the FSHbeta gene. Fertil Steril. 2003;79(2):434-6.
13. Torre DL, Falorni A. Pharmacological causes of hyperprolactinemia. Therapeutics and Clin Risk Manage. 2007;3(5):929-51.
14. Fan W, Wang B, He S, Zhang T, Tin C, Chen Y, et al. A novel Missense Mutation 224G>T (R75M) in SRY Coding Region Interferes with Nuclear Import and Results in 46 XY Complete Gonadal Dysgenesis. PLoS One. 2016;11(12):e0168484.
15. Peng D, Zhang YS, Zhang XY, Hu C, Miu MH, Miu RZ. An infertile 45 X male with a SRY-bearing chromosome 13: a clinical case report and literature review. J Assist Reprod Genet. 2015;32(1):107-9.
16. Wu QY, Li N, Li WW, Li TF, Zhang C, Cui YX, et al. Clinical, molecular and cytogenetic analysis of 46, XX testicular disorder of sex development with SRY-positive. BMC Urol. 2014;14:70.
17. Mutlu GY, Kırmızıbekmez H, Aydın H, Çetiner H, Moralıoğlu S, Celayir AC. Pure gonadal dysgenesis (Swyer syndrome) due to microdeletion in the SRY gene: a case report. J Pediatr Endocrinol Metab. 2015;28(1-2):207-10.
18. Esteves SC, Miyaoka R, Agarwal A. An update on the clinical assessment of the infertile male. Clinics. 2011;66(4): 691-700.
19. Lanfranco F, Kamischke A, Zitzmann M, Nieschlag E. Klinefelter's syndrome. The Lancet. 2004;364(9430): 273-83.
20. Robinson DO, Jacobs PA. The origin of the extra Y chromosome in males with a 47,XYY karyotype. Hum Mol Genet. 1999;8(12):2205-9.
21. Délot EC, Vilain EJ. Nonsyndromic 46,XX Testicular Disorders of Sex Development. 2003 Oct 30. In: Pagon RA, Adam MP, Ardinger HH, Wallace SE, Amemiya A, Bean LJH, Bird TD, Ledbetter N, Mefford HC, Smith RJH, Stephens K (Eds). GeneReviews® [Internet]. Seattle (WA): University of Washington, Seattle; 1993-2016.
22. Pirgon Ö, Dündar BN. Vanishing testes: a literature review. J Clin Res Pediatric Endocrinol. 2012;4(3):116-20. doi: 10.4274/Jcrpe.728. PubMed PMID: 22985611; PubMed Central PMCID: PMCPMC3459158.

23. Abacı A, Çatlı G, Anık A, Böber E. Epidemiology, classification and management of undescended testes: does medication have value in its treatment? J Clin Res Pediatric Endocrinol. 2013;5(2):65-72. doi: 10.4274/Jcrpe.883. PubMed PMID: 23748056; PubMed Central PMCID: PMCPMC3701924.
24. Fawzy F, Hussein A, Eid MM, El Kashash AM, Salem HK. Cryptorchidism and fertility. Clin Med Insights Reprod Health. 2015;9:39-43. doi: 10.4137/CMRH.S25056. PubMed PMID: 26740750; PubMed Central PMCID: PMCPMC4689328.
25. Silber SJ, Van Steirteghem AC, Devroey P. Editorial: sertoli cell only revisited. Hum Reprod. 1995;10(5):1031-2. PubMed PMID: 7657732.
26. Bird TD. Myotonic dystrophy type 1. In: Pagon RA, Adam MP, Ardinger HH, Wallace SE, Amemiya A, Bean LJH, Bird TD, Ledbetter N, Mefford HC, Smith RJH, Stephens K (Eds). GeneReviews® [Internet]. Seattle (WA): University of Washington, Seattle; 1993-2016. 1999 Sep 17.
27. Voutilainen R, Jääskeläinen J. Premature adrenarche: etiology, clinical findings, and consequences. J Steroid Biochem Mol Biol. 2015;145:226-36. doi: 10.1016/j.jsbmb.2014.06.004. PubMed PMID: 24923732.
28. Rochira V, Granata AR, Madeo B, Zirilli L, Rossi G, Carani C. Estrogens in males: what have we learned in the last 10 years? Asian J Androl. 2005;7(1):3-20. doi: 10.1111/j.1745-7262.2005.00018.x. PubMed PMID: 15685347.
29. Serri O, Chik CL, Ur E, Ezzat S. Diagnosis and management of hyperprolactinemia. CMAJ. 2003;169:575-81. PubMed PMID: 12975226; PubMed Central PMCID: PMCPMC191295.
30. Pasqualotto FF, Lucon AM, Sobreiro BP, Pasqualotto EB, Arap S. Effects of medical therapy, alcohol, smoking, and endocrine disruptors on male infertility. Rev Hosp Clin Fac Med Sao Paulo. 2004;59(6):375-82. doi: /S0041-87812004000600011. PubMed PMID: 15654492.
31. Byrne J, Mulvihill JJ, Myers MH, Connelly RR, Naughton MD, Krauss MR, et al. Effects of treatment on fertility in long-term survivors of childhood or adolescent cancer. N Engl J Med. 1987;317:1315-21. doi: 10.1056/NEJM198711193172104. PubMed PMID: 3683460.
32. Berthelsen JG. Sperm counts and serum follicle-stimulating hormone levels before and after radiotherapy and chemotherapy in men with testicular germ cell cancer. Fertil Steril. 1984;41(2):281-6. PubMed PMID: 6199233.
33. Winther J, Boice J, Frederiksen K, Bautz A, Mulvihill J, Stovall M, et al. Radiotherapy for childhood cancer and risk for congenital malformations in offspring: a population-based cohort study. Clin Genet. 2009;75:50-6. doi: 10.1111/j.1399-0004.2008.01109.x. PubMed PMID: 19021636; PubMed Central PMCID: PMCPMC2697125.
34. Handelsman DJ. Hypothalamic-pituitary gonadal dysfunction in renal failure, dialysis and renal transplantation. Endocr Rev. 1985;6(2):151-82. PubMed PMID: 3891321.
35. Smith-Whitley K. Reproductive issues in sickle cell disease. Blood. 2014;124(24):3538-43. doi: 10.1182/blood-2014-07-577619. PubMed PMID: 25472967.
36. Mackenzie H, Mahmalji W, Raza A. The gumma and the gonad: syphilitic orchitis, a rare presentation of testicular swelling. Int J STD AIDS. 2011;22:531-3. doi: 10.1258/ijsa.2009.009442. PubMed PMID: 21890556.
37. Richthoff J, Rylander L, Hagmar L, Malm J, Giwercman A. Higher sperm counts in Southern Sweden compared with Denmark. Hum Reprod. 2002;17(9):2468-73. PubMed PMID: 12202443.
38. Jensen TK, Henriksen TB, Hjollund NH, Scheike T, Kolstad H, Giwercman A, et al. Adult and prenatal exposures to tobacco smoke as risk indicators of fertility among 430 Danish couples. Amer J Epidemiol. 1998;148(10):9927. PubMed PMID: 9829871.
39. Jensen TK, Hjollund NH, Henriksen TB, Scheike T, Kolstad H, Giwercman A, et al. Does moderate alcohol consumption affect fertility? Follow up study among couples planning first pregnancy. BMJ. 1998;317(7157):505-10. PubMed PMID: 9712595; PubMed Central PMCID: PMCPMC28642.
40. Ramlau-Hansen CH, Toft G, Jensen MS, Strandberg-Larsen K, Hansen ML, Olsen J. Maternal alcohol consumption during pregnancy and semen quality in the male offspring: two decades of followup. Hum Reprod. 2010;25(9):2340-5. doi: 10.1093/humrep/deq140. PubMed PMID: 20587536.
41. Jensen TK, Giwercman A, Carlsen E, Scheike T, Skakkebaek NE. Semen quality among members of organic food associations in Zealand, Denmark. Lancet. 1996;347(9018):1844. PubMed PMID: 8667966.
42. Dunphy BC, Barratt CL, Cooke ID. Male alcohol consumption and fecundity in couples attending an infertility clinic. Andrologia. 1991;23(3):219-21. PubMed PMID: 1741485.
43. Pajarinen JT, Karhunen PJ. Spermatogenic arrest and 'Sertoli cell-only' syndrome—common alcohol-induced disorders of the human testis. Int J Androl. 1994;17:292-9.
44. Richthoff J, Elzanaty S, Rylander L, Hagmar L, Giwercman A. Association between tobacco exposure and reproductive parameters in adolescent males. Int J Androl. 2008;31(1):319. doi: 10.1111/j.1365-2605.2007.00752.x. PubMed PMID: 17376217.
45. Storgaard L, Bonde JP, Ernst E, Spano M, Andersen CY, Frydenberg M, et al. Does smoking during pregnancy affect sons' sperm counts? Epidemiology. 2003;14(3):27886. PubMed PMID: 12859027.
46. Jensen TK, Jorgensen N, Punab M, Haugen TB, Suominen J, Zilaitiene B, et al. Association of in utero exposure to maternal smoking with reduced semen quality and testis size in adulthood: a cross-sectional study of 1,770 young men from the general population in five European countries. Amer J Epidemiol. 2004;159(1):4958. PubMed PMID: 14693659.
47. Ravnborg TL, Jensen TK, Andersson AM, Toppari J, Skakkebaek NE, Jorgensen N. Prenatal and adult exposures to smoking are associated with adverse effects on reproductive hormones, semen quality, final height and body mass index. Hum Reprod. 2011;26(5):1000-11. doi: 10.1093/humrep/der011. PubMed PMID: 21335416.
48. Axelsson J, Rylander L, Rignell-Hydbom A, Silfver KA, Stenqvist A, Giwercman A. The impact of paternal and maternal smoking on semen quality of adolescent men. PLoS one. 2013;8(6):e66766. doi: 10.1371/journal.pone.0066766.

PubMed PMID: 23840528; PubMed Central PMCID: PMCPMC3694111.

49. Jensen MS, Henriksen TB, Rebordosa C, Thulstrup AM, Toft G, Sorensen HT, et al. Analgesics during pregnancy and cryptorchidism: additional analyses. Epidemiology. 2011;22(4):610-2. doi: 10.1097/EDE.0b013e3181f20bed. PubMed PMID: 20805751.
50. Jensen MS, Rebordosa C, Thulstrup AM, Toft G, Sorensen HT, Bonde JP, et al. Maternal use of acetaminophen, ibuprofen, and acetylsalicylic acid during pregnancy and risk of cryptorchidism. Epidemiology. 2010;21(6): 779-85. doi: 10.1097/EDE.0b013e31821eca69. PubMed PMID: 21642784.
51. Kristensen DM, Hass U, Lesne L, Lottrup G, Jacobsen PR, Desdoits-Lethimonier C, et al. Intrauterine exposure to mild analgesics is a risk factor for development of male reproductive disorders in human and rat. Hum Reprod. 2011;26(1):235-44. doi: 10.1093/humrep/deq323. PubMed PMID: 21059752.
52. Kristensen DM, Lesne L, Le Fol V, Desdoits-Lethimonier C, Dejucq-Rainsford N, Leffers H, et al. Paracetamol (acetaminophen), aspirin (acetylsalicylic acid) and indomethacin are anti-androgenic in the rat foetal testis. Int J Androl. 2012;35(3):377-84.
53. Albert O, Desdoits-Lethimonier C, Lesne L, Legrand A, Guille F, Bensalah K, et al. Paracetamol, aspirin and indomethacin display endocrine disrupting properties in the adult human testis *in vitro*. Hum Reprod. 2013;28(7):189-208.
54. Herbst AL, Ulfelder H, Poskanzer DC. Adeno-carcinoma of the vagina. Association of maternal stilbestrol therapy with tumor appearance in young women. New Engl J Med. 1971;284(15):878-81.
55. Strohsnitter WC, Noller KL, Hoover RN, Robboy SJ, Palmer JR, Titus-Ernstoff L, et al. Cancer risk in men exposed in utero to diethylstilbestrol. J Natl Cancer Inst. 2001;93(7): 545-51.
56. Depue RH, Pike MC, Henderson BE. Estrogen exposure during gestation and risk of testicular cancer. J Natl Cancer Inst. 1983;71(6):1151-5.
57. Kalfa N, Paris F, Soyer-Gobillard MO, Daures JP, Sultan C. Prevalence of hypospadias in grandsons of women exposed to diethylstilbestrol during pregnancy: a multigenerational national cohort study. Fertil Steril. 2011;95(8):2574-7.
58. Skinner MK, Manikkam M, Guerrero-Bosagna C. Epigenetic transgenerational actions of environmental factors in disease etiology. Trends Endocrinol Metabol. 2010;21(4): 214-22.
59. Wu S, Zhu J, Li Y, Lin T, Gan L, Yuan X, et al. Dynamic epigenetic changes involved in testicular toxicity induced by di2-(ethylhexyl) phthalate in mice. Basic Clin Pharmacol Toxicol 2010;106(2):118-223.
60. Jönsson BA, Rylander L, Lindh C, Rignell-Hydbom A, Giwercman A, Toft G, et al. Inter-population variations in concentrations, determinants of and correlations between 2,2',4,4',5,5'-hexachlorobiphenyl (CB-153) and 1,1-dichloro-2,2-bis (p-chlorophenyl)-ethylene (p,p'-DDE): a cross-sectional study of 3161 men and women from Inuit and European populations. Environmental Health. 2005;4:27. http://www.inuendo.dk
61. Toft G, Rignell-Hydbom A, Tyrkiel E, Shvets M, Giwercman A, Lindh CH, et al. Semen quality and exposure to persistent organo-chlorine pollutants. Epidemiology. 2006;17(4): 450-8.
62. Toft G, Jonsson BA, Lindh CH, Giwercman A, Spano M, Heederik D, et al. Exposure to perfluorinated compounds and human semen quality in Arctic and European populations. Hum Reprod. 2012;27(8):2532-40.
63. Hauser R, Meeker JD, Singh NP, Silva MJ, Ryan L, Duty S, et al. DNA damage in human sperm is related to urinary levels of phthalate monoester and oxidative metabolites. Hum Reprod. 2007;22(3):688-95.
64. Pant N, Shukla M, Kumar Patel D, Shukla Y, Mathur N, Kumar Gupta Y, et al. Correlation of phthalate exposures with semen quality. Toxicol Appl Pharmacol. 2008;231(1):112-6.
65. Swan SH, Main KM, Liu F, Stewart SL, Kruse RL, Calafat AM, et al. Decrease in anogenital distance among male infants with prenatal phthalate exposure. Environ Health Perspect. 2005;113(8):1056-61.
66. Eisenberg ML, Jensen TK, Walters RC, Skakkebaek NE, Lipshultz LI. The relationship between anogenital distance and reproductive hormone levels in adult men. J Urol. 2012;187(2):594-8. doi: 10.1016/j.juro.2011.10.041. PubMed PMID: 22177168.
67. Eisenberg ML, Shy M, Walters RC, Lipshultz LI. The relationship between anogenital distance and azoospermia in adult men. Int J Androl. 2012;35(5):726-30. doi: 10.1111/j.1365-2605.2012.01275.x. PubMed PMID: 22519659.
68. Irvin H. Hirsch M, Thomas Jefferson University. Gynecomastia. MERCK MANUALS, Professional Version. 2016.
69. Johnson RE, Murad MH. Gynecomastia: pathophysiology, evaluation, and management. Mayo Clinic Proc, 2009;84(11):1010-1015.
70. Rosen A, Jayram G, Drazer M, Eggener SE. Global trends in testicular cancer incidence and mortality. Eur Urol. 2011;60(2):349.
71. Ekbom A, Akre O. Increasing incidence of testicular cancer birth cohort effects. APMIS: Acta Pathologica, Microbiologica, et Immunologica Scandinavica. 1998;106(1): 225-9; discussion 9-31.
72. Giwercman A, Giwercman YL. Epidemiology of male reproductive disorders. In: De Groot LJ, Chrousos G, Dungan K, Feingold KR, Grossman A, Hershman JM, Koch C, Korbonits M, McLachlan R, New M, Purnell J, Rebar R, Singer F, Vinik A (Eds). Endotext [Internet]. South Dartmouth, MA: MDText.com, Inc.; 2000.
73. Müller J, Skakkebaek NE, Ritzén M, Ploen L, Petersen KE. Carcinoma in situ of the testis in children with 45,X/46,XY gonadal dysgenesis. J Pediatr. 1985;106:431-6.
74. Cools M, Wolffenbuttel KP, Drop SL, Oosterhuis JW, Looijenga LH. Gonadal development and tumor formation at the crossroads of male and female sex determination. Sex Dev. 2011;5:167-80.

75. Dieckmann KP, Pichlmeier U. Clinical epidemiology of testicular germ cell tumors. World J Urol. 2004;22(1):2-14. doi: 10.1007/s00345-004-0398-8. PubMed PMID: 15034740.
76. Giwercman A, Grindsted J, Hansen B, Jensen OM, Skakkebaek NE. Testicular cancer risk in boys with maldescended testis: a cohort study. J Urol. 1987;138(5):1214-6. PubMed PMID: 2889833.
77. Dieckmann KP, Rube C, Henke RP. Association of Down's syndrome and testicular cancer. J Urol. 1997;157:1701-4.
78. Cook MB, Akre O, Forman D, Madigan MP, Richiardi L, McGlynn KA. A systematic review and meta-analysis of perinatal variables in relation to the risk of testicular cancer—experiences of the son. Int J Epidemiol. 2010;39(6):1605-18. doi: 10.1093/ije/dyq120. PubMed PMID: 20660640; PubMed Central PMCID: PMCPMC2992627.
79. Swerdlow AJ, Huttly SR, Smith PG. Prenatal and familial associations of testicular cancer. Br J Cancer. 1987;55:571-7.
80. Weir HK, Marrett LD, Kreiger N, Darlington GA, Sugar L. Prenatal and perinatal exposures and risk of testicular germ cell cancer. Int J Cancer. 2000;87:438-43.
81. Skakkebaek NE, Rajpert-De Meyts E, Main KM. Testicular dysgenesis syndrome: an increasingly common developmental disorder with environmental aspects. Hum Reprod. 2001;16:972-8.
82. Hoei-Hansen CE, Holm M, Rajpert-De Meyts E, Skakkebaek NE. Histological evidence of testicular dysgenesis in contralateral biopsies of 218 patients with testicular germ cell cancer. J Pathol. 2003;200:370-4.
83. Skakkebæk NE, Rajpert-De Meyts E, Jørgensen N, Main KM, Leffers H, Andersson AM, et al. Testicular cancer trends as "whistle blowers" of testicular developmental problems in populations. Int J Androl. 2007;30:198-205.
84. Jørgensen N, Rajpert-De Meyts E, Main KM, Skakkebæk NE. Testicular dysgenesis syndrome comprises some but not all cases of hypospadias and impaired spermatogenesis. Int J Androl. 2010;33:298-303.
85. Rajpert-De Meyts E, Skakkebaek NE, Toppari J. Testicular Cancer Pathogenesis, Diagnosis and Endocrine Aspects. In De Groot LJ, Chrousos G, Dungan K, Feingold KR, Grossman A, Hershman JM, Koch C, Korbonits M, McLachlan R, New M, Purnell J, Rebar R, Singer F, Vinik A (Eds). Endotext [Internet]. South Dartmouth (MA): MDText.com, Inc.; 2000.
86. Sharpe RM, Skakkebaek NE. Testicular dysgenesis syndrome: mechanistic insights and potential new downstream effects. Fertil Steril. 2008;89(2 Suppl):e33-8. doi: 10.1016/j.fertnstert.2007.12.026. PubMed PMID: 18308057.
87. Toppari J, Larsen JC, Christiansen P, Giwercman A, Grandjean P Guillette LJ, et al. Male reproductive health and environmental xenoestrogens. Environ Health Perspect. 1996;104(Suppl 4):741-803.
88. Hardell L, Bavel B, Lindstrom G, Eriksson M, Carlberg M. In utero exposure to persistent organic pollutants in relation to testicular cancer risk. Int J Androl. 2006;29(1):228-34. doi: 10.1111/j.1365-2605.2005.00622.x. PubMed PMID: 16371110.
89. Cook MB, Trabert B, McGlynn KA. Organochlorine compounds and testicular dysgenesis syndrome: human data. Int J Androl. 2011;34(4 Pt 2):e68-84; discussion e-5. doi: 10.1111/j.1365-2605.2011.01171.x. PubMed PMID: 21668838; PubMed Central PMCID: PMCPMC3145030.
90. Del-Mazo J, Brieno-Enriquez MA, Garcia-Lopez J, Lopez-Fernandez LA, De-Felici M. Endocrine disruptors, gene deregulation and male germ cell tumors. Int J Dev Biol. 2013;57(2-4):225-39. doi: 10.1387/ijdb.130042jd. PubMed PMID: 23784834.
91. Giannandrea F, Paoli D, Figa-Talamanca I, Lombardo F, Lenzi A, Gandini L. Effect of endogenous and exogenous hormones on testicular cancer: the epidemiological evidence. Int J Dev Biol. 2013;57(2-4):255-63. doi: 10.1387/ijdb.130015fg. PubMed PMID: 23784836.
92. McGlynn KA, Quraishi SM, Graubard BI, Weber JP, Rubertone MV, Erickson RL. Persistent organochlorine pesticides and risk of testicular germ cell tumors. J Natl Cancer Inst. 2008;100(9):663-71. doi: 10.1093/jnci/djn101. PubMed PMID: 18445826.
93. Bertram KA, Bratloff B, Hodges GF, Davidson H. Treatment of malignant Leydig cell tumor. Cancer. 1991;68(10):2324-9. PubMed PMID: 1913469.
94. Dilworth JP, Farrow GM, Oesterling JE. Nongerm cell tumors of the testis. Urology. 1991;37:399-417.
95. Rich MA, Keating MA. Leydig cell tumors and tumors associated with congenital adrenal hyperplasia. Urol Clin North Am. 2000;27:519-28.
96. Holm M, Rajpert-De Meyts E, Andersson AM, Skakkebaek NE. Leydig cell micronodules are a common finding in testicular biopsies from men with impaired spermatogenesis and are associated with decreased testosterone/LH ratio. J Pathol. 2003;199(3):378-86. doi: 10.1002/path.1309. PubMed PMID: 12579540.
97. Fragoso MC, Latronico AC, Carvalho FM, Zerbini MC, Marcondes JA, Araujo LM, et al. Activating mutation of the stimulatory G protein (gsp) as a putative cause of ovarian and testicular human stromal Leydig cell tumors. J Clin Endocrinol Metab. 1998;83(6):2074-8. doi: 10.1210/jcem.83.6.4847. PubMed PMID: 9626141.
98. Iiri T, Herzmark P, Nakamoto JM, van Dop C, Bourne HR. Rapid GDP release from Gs alpha in patients with gain and loss of endocrine function. Nature. 1994;371(6493):164-8. doi: 10.1038/371164a0. PubMed PMID: 8072545.
99. Liu G, Duranteau L, Carel JC, Monroe J, Doyle DA, Shenker A. Leydig cell tumors caused by an activating mutation of the gene encoding the luteinizing hormone receptor. N Engl J Med. 1999;341:173-6.
100. Shenker A, Laue L, Kosugi S, Merendino JJ, Jr., Minegishi T, Cutler GB, Jr. A constitutively activating mutation of the luteinizing hormone receptor in familial male precocious puberty. Nature. 1993;365(6447):652-4. doi: 10.1038/365652a0. PubMed PMID: 7692306.
101. Kratzer SS, Ulbright TM, Talerman A, Srigley JR, Roth LM, Wahle GR, et al. Large cell calcifying Sertoli cell tumor of the testis: contrasting features of six malignant and six benign tumors and a review of the literature. Am J Surg Pathol. 1997;21(11):1271-80. PubMed PMID: 9351565.
102. Proppe KH, Scully RE. Large cell calcifying Sertoli cell tumor of the testis. Am J Clin Pathol. 1980;74:607-19.

103. Washecka R, Dresner MI, Honda SA. Testicular tumors in Carney's complex. J Urol. 2002;167:1299-302.
104. Thomas M. Ulbright MBA, Robert H. Young. Atlas of Tumor Pathology: Tumors of the Testis, Adnexa, Spermatic Cord, and Scrotum 1999. International Journal of Andrology. 2000;23(4):254. doi: 10.1046/j.1365-2605.2000.00231.x.
105. Giglio M, Medica M, De Rose AF, Germinale F, Ravetti JL, Carmignani G. Testicular sertoli cell tumours and relative sub-types. Analysis of clinical and prognostic features. Urol Int. 2003;70(3):205-10. doi: 68770. PubMed PMID: 12660458.
106. Toppari, J, Kaipia A, Kaleva M, Laato M, de Kretser DM, Krummen LA, et al. Inhibin gene expression in a large cell calcifying Sertoli cell tumour and serum inhibin and activin levels. APMIS. 1998;106:101-13.
107. Morrish DW, Venner PM, Siy O, Barron G, Bhardwaj D, Outhet D. Mechanisms of endocrine dysfunction in patients with testicular cancer. J Natl Cancer Inst. 1990;82(5):412-8. PubMed PMID: 2304089.
108. Petersen PM, Giwercman A, Hansen SW, Berthelsen JG, Daugaard G, Rorth M, et al. Impaired testicular function in patients with carcinoma-in-situ of the testis. J Clin Oncol. 1999;17(1):173-9. doi: 10.1200/JCO.1999.17.1.173. PubMed PMID: 10458231.
109. Petersen PM, Skakkebaek NE, Giwercman A. Gonadal function in men with testicular cancer: biological and clinical aspects. APMIS. 1998;106(1):24-34; discussion -6. PubMed PMID: 9524559.
110. van Casteren NJ, Boellaard WP, Romijn JC, Dohle GR. Gonadal dysfunction in male cancer patients before cytotoxic treatment. Int J Androl. 2010;33(1):73-9. doi: 10.1111/j.1365-2605.2009.00956.x. PubMed PMID: 19538481.
111. Haugnes HS, Bosl GJ, Boer H, Gietema JA, Brydoy M, Oldenburg J, et al. Long-term and late effects of germ cell testicular cancer treatment and implications for follow-up. J Clin Oncol. 2012;30(30):3752-63. doi: 10.1200/JCO.2012.43.4431. PubMed PMID: 23008318.
112. Brydoy M, Fossa SD, Klepp O, Bremnes RM, Wist EA, Bjoro T, et al. Sperm counts and endocrinological markers of spermatogenesis in long-term survivors of testicular cancer. Br J Cancer. 2012;107(11):1833-9. doi: 10.1038/bjc.2012.471. PubMed PMID: 23169336; PubMed Central PMCID: PMCPMC3504949.
113. Rives N, Perdrix A, Hennebicq S, Saias-Magnan J, Melin MC, Berthaut I, et al. The semen quality of 1158 men with testicular cancer at the time of cryopreservation: results of the French National CECOS Network. J Androl. 2012;33(6):1394-401. doi: 10.2164/jandrol.112.016592. PubMed PMID: 22837112.
114. Schmidt KL, Carlsen E, Andersen AN. Fertility treatment in male cancer survivors. Int J Androl. 2007;30(4):413-8; discussion 8-9. doi: 10.1111/j.1365-2605.2007.00761.x. PubMed PMID: 17573855.
115. Schrader M, Muller M, Sofikitis N, Straub B, Krause H, Miller K. "Onco-tese": testicular sperm extraction in azoospermic cancer patients before chemotherapy-new guidelines? Urology. 2003;61(2):421-5. PubMed PMID: 12597960.
116. Hsiao W, Stahl PJ, Osterberg EC, Nejat E, Palermo GD, Rosenwaks Z, et al. Successful treatment of postchemotherapy azoospermia with microsurgical testicular sperm extraction: the Weill Cornell experience. J Clin Oncol. 2011;29(12):1607-11. doi: 10.1200/JCO.2010.33.7808. PubMed PMID: 21402606.
117. Hessel M, Ramos L, Hulsbergen AF, D'Hauwers KW, Braat DD, Hulsbergen-van de Kaa CA. A novel cell-processing method 'AgarCytos' in conjunction with OCT3/4 and PLAP to detect intratubular germ cell neoplasia in non-obstructive azoospermia using remnants of testicular sperm extraction specimens. Hum Reprod. 2013;28(10):2608-20. doi: 10.1093/humrep/det311. PubMed PMID: 23900208.
118. Dieckmann KP, Kulejewski M, Heinemann V, Loy V. Testicular biopsy for early cancer detection--objectives, technique and controversies. Int J Androl. 2011;34(4 Pt 2):e7-13. doi: 10.1111/j.1365-2605.2011.01152.x. PubMed PMID: 21615417.
119. McLachlan RI, Rajpert-De Meyts E, Hoei-Hansen CE, de Kretser DM, Skakkebaek NE. Histological evaluation of the human testis--approaches to optimizing the clinical value of the assessment: mini review. Hum Reprod. 2007;22(1):2-16. doi: 10.1093/humrep/del279. PubMed PMID: 16887924.
120. Oosterhuis JW, Stoop H, Dohle G, Boellaard W, van Casteren N, Wolffenbuttel K, et al. A pathologist's view on the testis biopsy. Int J Androl. 2011;34(4 Pt 2):e14-9; discussion e20. doi: 10.1111/j.1365-2605.2011.01204.x. PubMed PMID: 21790650.
121. Harland SJ, Cook PA, Fossa SD, Horwich A, Mead GM, Parkinson MC, et al. Intratubular germ cell neoplasia of the contralateral testis in testicular cancer: defining a high risk group. J Urol. 1998;160(4):1353-7. PubMed PMID: 9751353.
122. Jacobsen R, Bostofte E, Engholm G, Hansen J, Olsen JH, Skakkebaek NE, et al. Risk of testicular cancer in men with abnormal semen characteristics: cohort study. BMJ. 2000;321(7264):789-92. PubMed PMID: 11009515; PubMed Central PMCID: PMCPMC27489.
123. Petersen PM, Skakkebaek NE, Vistisen K, Rorth M, Giwercman A. Semen quality and reproductive hormones before orchiectomy in men with testicular cancer. J Clin Oncol. 1999;17(3):941-7. doi: 10.1200/JCO.1999.17.3.941. PubMed PMID: 10071288.
124. Rud CN, Daugaard G, Rajpert-De Meyts E, Skakkebaek NE, Petersen JH, Jorgensen N. Sperm concentration, testicular volume and age predict risk of carcinoma in situ in contralateral testis of men with testicular germ cell cancer. J Urol. 2013;190(6):2074-80. doi: 10.1016/j.juro.2013.06.023. PubMed PMID: 23770148.
125. Skakkebaek NE. Carcinoma in situ of the testis: frequency and relationship to invasive germ cell tumours in infertile men. Histopathology. 1978;2(3):157-70. PubMed PMID: 27442.
126. Giwercman A, Marks A, Skakkebaek NE. Carcinoma-in-situ germ-cells exfoliated from seminiferous epithelium into seminal fluid. Lancet. 1988;1(8584):530. PubMed PMID: 2893940.
127. Hoei-Hansen CE, Carlsen E, Jorgensen N, Leffers H, Skakkebaek NE, Rajpert-De Meyts E. Towards a non-invasive method for early detection of testicular neoplasia in semen samples by identification of fetal germ cell-specific markers. Hum Reprod. 2007;22(1):167-73. doi: 10.1093/humrep/del320. PubMed PMID: 16920726.

128. van Casteren NJ, Stoop H, Dohle GR, de Wit R, Oosterhuis JW, Looijenga LH. Noninvasive detection of testicular carcinoma in situ in semen using OCT3/4. Eur Urol. 2008;54(1):153-8. doi: 10.1016/j.eururo.2007.10.042. PubMed PMID: 17996359.
129. Almstrup K, Lippert M, Mogensen HO, Nielsen JE, Hansen JD, Daugaard G, et al. Screening of subfertile men for testicular carcinoma in situ by an automated image analysis-based cytological test of the ejaculate. Int J Androl. 2011;34(4 Pt 2):e21-30; discussion e-1. doi: 10.1111/j.1365-2605.2011.01192.x. PubMed PMID: 21696398.
130. Holm M, Hoei-Hansen CE, Rajpert-De Meyts E, Skakkebaek NE. Increased risk of carcinoma in situ in patients with testicular germ cell cancer with ultrasonic microlithiasis in the contralateral testicle. J Urol. 2003;170(4 Pt 1):1163-7. doi: 10.1097/01.ju.0000087820.94991.21. PubMed PMID: 14501716.
131. Holm M, Lenz S, De Meyts ER, Skakkebaek NE. Microcalcifications and carcinoma in situ of the testis. BJU Int. 2001;87(2):144-9. PubMed PMID: 11167632.
132. Ehrlich Y, Beck SD, Foster RS, Bihrle R, Einhorn LH. Serum tumor markers in testicular cancer. Urol Oncol. 2013;31(1):17-23. doi: 10.1016/j.urolonc.2010.04.007. PubMed PMID: 20822927.
133. A GDP. Synthesis of serum albumin, prealbumin, alphafetoprotein, alpha 1-antitrypsin and transferrin by the human yolk sac. Popline. 1970;228(5275):995-7.
134. von Eyben FE, de Graaff WE, Marrink J, Blaabjerg O, Sleijfer DT, Koops HS, et al. Serum lactate dehydrogenase isoenzyme 1 activity in patients with testicular germ cell tumors correlates with the total number of copies of the short arm of chromosome 12 in the tumor. Mol Gen Genet. 1992;235(1):140-6. PubMed PMID: 1435725.
135. Bang AK, Petersen JH, Petersen PM, Andersson AM, Daugaard G, Jorgensen N. Testosterone production is better preserved after 16 than 20 Gray irradiation treatment against testicular carcinoma in situ cells. Int J Radiat Oncol Biol Phys. 2009;75(3):672-6. doi: 10.1016/j.ijrobp.2008.11.057. PubMed PMID: 19250763.
136. Giwercman A, von der Maase H, Berthelsen JG, Rorth M, Bertelsen A, Skakkebaek NE. Localized irradiation of testes with carcinoma in situ: effects on Leydig cell function and eradication of malignant germ cells in 20 patients. J Clin Endocrinol Metab. 1991;73(3):596-603. doi: 10.1210/jcem-73-3-596. PubMed PMID: 1908483.
137. Christensen TB, Daugaard G, Geertsen PF, von der Maase H. Effect of chemotherapy on carcinoma in situ of the testis. Ann Oncol. 1998;9(6):657-60. PubMed PMID: 9681081.
138. Kleinschmidt K, Dieckmann KP, Georgiew A, Loy V, Weissbach L. Chemotherapy is of limited efficacy in the control of contralateral testicular intraepithelial neoplasia in patients with testicular germ cell cancer. Oncology. 2009;77(1):33-9. doi: 10.1159/000218202. PubMed PMID: 19440001.
139. Fossa SD, Aass N, Heilo A, Daugaard G, N ES, Stenwig AE, et al. Testicular carcinoma in situ in patients with extragonadal germ-cell tumours: the clinical role of pretreatment biopsy. Ann Oncol. 2003;14(9):1412-8. PubMed PMID: 12954581.

CHAPTER

19

Semen Analysis

Natachandra Chimote

INTRODUCTION

Semen analysis is considered to be a diagnostic cornerstone when evaluating male fertility. In its most basic element, it reports the functioning of the testicular machinery for sperm production and the fluid volume contributed by the accessory glands. The production and packaging from spermatogonia to spermatozoa in the testes is critically important because without that functional process there are no cells and no fertility.

In a perfect world, every laboratory performing semen analyses would follow the same methodology and, where applicable, adhere to criteria for making quantitative measurements. For the past several decades, the World Health Organization (WHO) laboratory manual for the examination of human sperm and sperm-cervical mucus interaction[1-4] has been the primary reference for methods of semen analysis. The premise for the manual was to provide a "cookbook" of standardized procedures for infertility studies and for assessing the effects of contraceptives and toxicants on spermatogenesis; with a goal being to afford a more direct comparison of data between either clinical or research laboratories.

The recently published WHO 2010 laboratory manual[5] presents, for the first time, statistically derived 5th centile lower reference limits derived from semen analysis studies from around the world. Important to acknowledge is that these values are not to be viewed as cutoffs but rather as probabilities or likelihoods.

Semen is a mixture of concentrated suspension of spermatozoa, which are stored in epididymis and fluid secretions from various accessory sex glands such as epididymis, ampulla, seminal vesicles, prostate and bulbourethric glands. It is ejaculated as several spurts or boluses. The fluid secretions from seminal vesicles and prostate glands constitute about 90% of semen volume. The vitality, motility and morphology characteristics of spermatozoa and the composition of seminal fluid mainly are determinant factors for sperm function.

In the laboratory setting, semen is collected in a container for analysis. Semen comprises the entire volume of seminal fluids in which spermatozoa are trapped in a coagulum formed by proteins of seminal vesicle fluid. This is subsequently liquefied by the action of prostatic proteases, during this time its osmolality rises.[6,7]

The results of laboratory measurements of semen quality depend on:

- The first two to three spurts of ejaculate mainly contains sperm-rich prostatic fluid, whereas spurts subsequently followed are usually seminal vesicular fluid.[6] Hence, the spilling out of first spurt can adversely influence the result of semen analysis as compared to last spurt spillage.
- Sperm concentration is not a direct measure of testicular sperm output as functioning of accessory sex glands influences it. As the age grows, both the volume and total sperm output decrease.[8]
- Abstinence or the time since last ejaculation also has an impact on semen quality. In the absence of ejaculation, spermatozoa accumulate in the epididymis, then overflow into the urethra and are flushed out in urine.[7,9] Sperm vitality and chromatin remain same even though abstinence length is increased[9,10] unless epididymal function is disturbed.[11]
- Some spermatozoa still remain in epididymis from the time of previous ejaculation as epididymis does not empty completely in one ejaculate.[12] This influences the range of age and quality of spermatozoa in the ejaculate.[13] The extent of this influence is difficult to ascertain and it is rarely taken into account.
- The testicular size amounts to spermatogenic activity. It also influences sperm morphology.[14] Therefore, testicular size influences sperm production.[15-17]

These variables and uncontrollable events actually influence the intraindividual variations in semen composition.[18,19]

Therefore, it is impossible to characterize a man's semen quality from evaluation of a single semen sample.

Hence, it is wise to examine at least 2–3 semen samples to establish a baseline data while evaluating male factor.

Most importantly, semen analysis provides essential information on the clinical status of an individual. All aspects of semen collection and analysis must be done by properly standardized procedures if the results are to provide valid and useful information.

SEMEN ANALYSIS

Sample Collection for Analysis/Diagnosis

- Although it has been suggested that ejaculates produced by masturbation and collected into containers in a room near the laboratory can be of lower quality than those recovered from nonspermicidal condoms used during intercourse at home[20]; it is still preferred that sample should be collected in a private room near laboratory to avoid fluctuations in temperature.
- When collection of semen sample is done at home, spoken as well as clear written instructions should be given to man regarding collection and transportation. Similarly, while using condom to collect semen, only special nontoxic condoms designed for semen collection should be used. Ordinary latex condoms must not be used. Coitus interruptus is not a reliable means of semen collection as the first portion of ejaculate that contains highest number of spermatozoa may be lost.
- Ejaculated in wide mouthed nontoxic glass or plastic sterile clean container.
- Abstinence: 2–7 days.
- Clear/written instructions should be provided about collection of semen sample (a complete collection of sample, no spillage). The male should report any loss of any fraction of the sample. If first bolus of semen is lost while collecting sample, a second sample should be collected again after 2–7 days abstinence.
- ID and recording: Name of patient, code number, period of abstinence, date and timing of collection, completeness of sample, any difficulties in producing sample and interval between collection and start of semen analysis.
- Throughout the process, care must be taken that he specimen container, pipettes, tips used for mixing must be sterile.
- Semen samples may contain dangerous infectious agents such as HIV, hepatitis viruses, or herpes simplex virus, which therefore should be handled as a biohazard.
- Container should then be placed on stage warmer maintained at 37°C.

Between 30 and 60 minutes:

- Assessing liquefaction and appearance of the semen
- Measuring semen volume.
- Measuring semen pH (if required)
- Preparing a wet preparation for assessing microscopic appearance, sperm motility and the dilution required for assessing sperm number.
- Assessing sperm vitality (if the percentage of motile cells is low).
- Making semen smears for assessing sperm morphology.
- Making semen dilutions for assessing sperm concentration.
- Assessing sperm number.
- Performing the mixed antiglobulin reaction (MAR) test (if required).
- Assessing peroxidase-positive cells (if round cells are present).
- Preparing spermatozoa for the immunobead test (if required).
- Centrifuging semen (if biochemical markers are to be assayed).

Within 3 hours:

- Sending samples to the microbiology laboratory (if required).

After 4 hours:

- Fixing, staining and assessing smears for sperm morphology.
- Later on the same day (or on a subsequent day if samples are frozen).
- Assaying accessory gland markers (if required).
- Performing the indirect immunobead test (if required).

Initial Macroscopic Examination

Soon after liquefaction (during 30 minutes), semen analysis should begin.

Liquefaction

Initially, the semen ejaculate in the container is a semisolid coagulated lump or mass. After a few minutes, it starts to liquefy, becomes thinner and more homogenous. After 15 minutes, it becomes almost watery. Within 30 minutes, it becomes more and more homogenous indicating liquefaction is complete. In very rare cases, it takes 60 minutes or more time. Normally liquefied semen samples may contain jelly-like granules, which are of no significance. The presence of mucus strands, however, may interfere with semen analysis. Continuous gentle mixing at room temperature should be done during liquefaction to avail a homogenous whole semen sample.

In case of delayed liquefaction, mechanical mixing or enzymatic digestion may be necessary.

- Some samples can be induced to liquefy by the addition of an equal volume of physiological medium (e.g., Dulbecco's phosphate-buffered saline) followed by repeated pipetting.
- Inhomogeneity can be reduced by repeated (6–10 times) gentle passage through a blunt gauge 18 (internal diameter 0.84 mm) or gauge 19 (internal diameter 0.69 mm) needle attached to a syringe.
- Digestion by bromelain, a broad-specificity proteolytic enzyme may help to promote liquefaction.

Semen Viscosity

Viscosity measures the seminal fluids' resistance to flowing. It can be estimated by gently aspirating it into a wide-bore (approximately 1.5 mm diameter) plastic disposable pipette, allowing the semen to drop by gravity and observing the length of any thread. A normal sample leaves the pipette in small discrete drops. If viscosity is abnormal (Fig. 19.1), the drop will form a thread more than 2 cm long. Viscous samples can be treated by a viscosity treatment system containing a premeasured vial of chymotrypsin (5 mg/vial). The sample can be swirled and left in the incubator for another 10–15 minutes till viscosity is completely broken down and the sample is suitable for analysis.

High viscosity can interfere with determination of sperm motility, sperm concentration, detection of antibody-coated spermatozoa and measurement of biochemical markers.

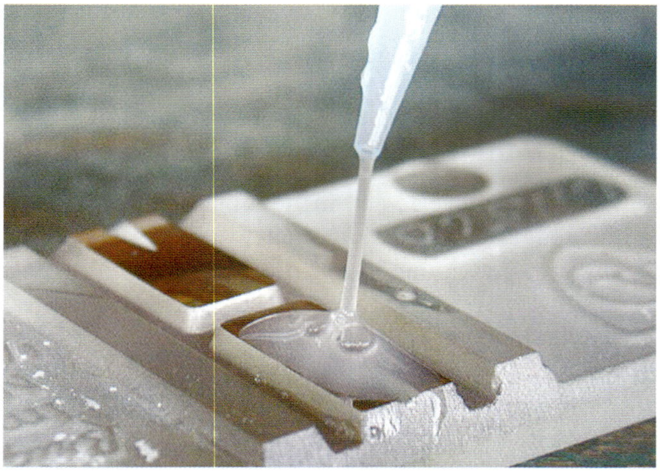

Fig. 19.1: Extremely viscous seminal fluid.

Appearance

A normal liquefied semen sample has a homogeneous, gray-opalescent appearance. It may appear less opaque if the sperm concentration is very low; the color may also be different, i.e. red-brown when red blood cells are present (hemospermia), or yellow in a man with jaundice or taking certain vitamins or drugs.

Semen Volume

Precise measurement of volume is essential in any evaluation of semen because it allows the total number of spermatozoa and nonsperm cells in the ejaculate to be calculated. The volume can be measured directly.

- Collect the sample directly into a modified graduated glass measuring cylinder with a wide mouth.
- Read the volume directly from the graduations (0.1 mL accuracy).

The lower reference limit for semen volume is 1.5 mL [5th centile, 95% confidence interval (CI) 1.4–1.7].

Low semen volume is characteristic of obstruction of the ejaculatory duct or congenital bilateral absence of the vas deferens (CBAVD),[21-24] a condition in which the seminal vesicles are also poorly developed.

For clinical purpose, semen volume is differentiated into three categories to facilitate interpretation and diagnosis:

- Aspermia: No semen produced after orgasm.
- Hypospermia: Less than 0.5 mL of semen ejaculated (partial or retrograde flow of sperm, accessory glands impairment).
- Hyperspermia: More than 6 mL of semen ejaculated (long period of sexual abstinence or overproduction of fluids from the accessory glands).

Low semen volume can also be the result of collection problems (loss of a fraction of the ejaculate), partial retrograde ejaculation or androgen deficiency.

High semen volume may reflect active exudation in cases of active inflammation of the accessory organs.

pH

The pH of semen reflects the balance between the pH values of the different accessory gland secretions, mainly the alkaline seminal vesicular secretion and the acidic prostatic secretion. The pH should be measured after liquefaction at a uniform time, preferably after 30 minutes.

For normal samples, pH paper in the range 6.0–10.0 should be used.

- Mix the semen sample well to be homogenous.
- Spread a drop of semen evenly onto the pH paper.
- Wait for the color of the impregnated zone to become uniform (<30 seconds).
- Compare the color with the calibration strip to read the pH.

The consensus value of 7.2 is considered as a lower threshold value for pH.

If the pH is less than 7.0 in a semen sample with low volume and low sperm numbers, there may be ejaculatory duct obstruction or congenital bilateral absence of the vas deferens,[21-24] a condition in which seminal vesicles are also poorly developed. pH increases with time, as natural buffering decreases, so high pH values may provide little clinically useful information.

Initial Microscopic Investigation

All examinations of unstained preparations of fresh semen sample should be carried out preferably under phase-contrast microscope. An initial microscopic examination of the sample involves scanning the preparation at a total magnification of ×100 (i.e. a combination of a ×10 objective lens with a ×10 ocular lens).

This provides an overview of the sample, to reveal:

- Mucus strand formation;
- Sperm aggregation or agglutination;
- The presence of cells other than spermatozoa, e.g., epithelial cells, "round cells" (leukocytes and immature germ cells) and isolated sperm heads or tails.

The preparation should then be observed at ×200 or ×400 total magnification (i.e. a combination of a ×20 or a ×40 objective with a ×10 ocular). This permits

- Assessment of sperm motility;
- Determination of the dilution required for accurate assessment of sperm number.

If the sample is not well mixed, analysis of two separate aliquots may show marked differences in sperm motility, vitality, concentration and morphology. Before removing an aliquot of semen for assessment, mix the sample well in the original container, but not so vigorously that air bubbles are created!

Wet Preparation

The volume of semen and the dimensions of the coverslip must be standardized, so that the analyses are carried out on a preparation of fixed depth of about 20 μm, which allows the spermatozoa to swim freely:

- Place a standard volume of semen10 μL, onto a clean glass slide.
- Cover it with a coverslip, e.g., 22 mm × 22 mm for 10 μL, to provide a chamber approximately 20 μm deep. The weight of the coverslip spreads the sample.
- Take care to avoid the formation and trapping of air bubbles between the coverslip and the slide.
- Assess the freshly made wet preparation as soon as the contents are no longer drifting.

A chamber depth of less than 20 μm constrains the rotational movement of spermatozoa.[25,26] If the chamber is too deep, it will be difficult to assess spermatozoa as they move in and out of focus. If the number of spermatozoa per visual field varies considerably, the sample is not homogeneous. In such cases, the semen sample should be mixed again thoroughly and a new slide prepared as above.

Lack of homogeneity may also result from abnormal consistency, abnormal liquefaction and aggregation of spermatozoa or sperm agglutination.

Aggregation of Spermatozoa

The adherence either of immotile spermatozoa to each other or of motile spermatozoa to mucus strands, nonsperm cells or debris is considered to be nonspecific aggregation and should be recorded as such (Fig. 19.2).

Agglutination of Spermatozoa

Agglutination specifically refers to motile spermatozoa sticking to each other, head-to-head, tail-to-tail or in a mixed way. The motility is often vigorous with a frantic shaking motion, but sometimes the spermatozoa are so agglutinated that their motion is limited. Any motile spermatozoa that stick to each other by their heads, tails or midpieces should be noted.

The major type of agglutination (Fig. 19.3) reflecting the degree (grades 1–4) and the site of attachment (grades A–E) should be recorded.[27]

- Grade 1: isolated: <10 spermatozoa per agglutinate, many free spermatozoa;
- Grade 2: moderate: 10–50 spermatozoa per agglutinate, free spermatozoa;
- Grade 3: large: agglutinates of >50 spermatozoa, some spermatozoa still free;
- Grade 4: gross: all spermatozoa agglutinated and agglutinates interconnected.

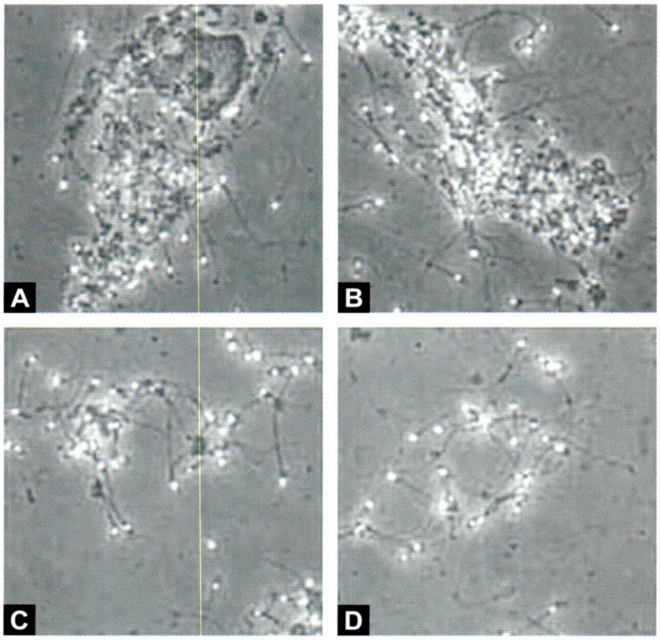

Figs. 19.2A to D: Views of spermatozoa aggregated with an epithelial cell (A), debris (B) or spermatozoa (C and D).
Micrographs courtesy of C Brazil.
WHO Laboratory manual for the examination and processing of Human Semen (Ed. V; 2010), page 19, Standard Procedures, fig. 2.2.

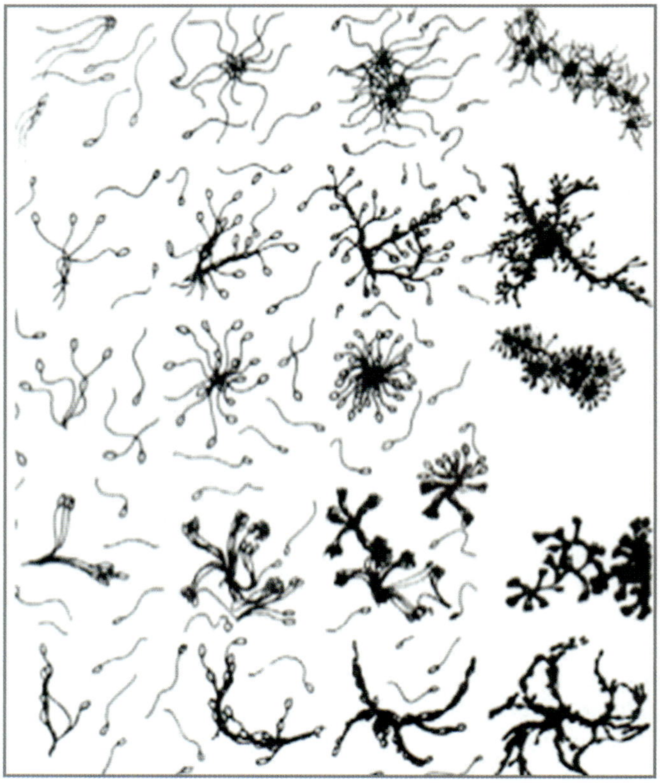

Fig. 19.3: Degree of agglutination.
WHO Laboratory Manual for the examination and processing of Human Semen (Ed. V; 2010), page 20, fig. 2.3.

Motile spermatozoa stuck to cells or debris or immotile spermatozoa stuck to each other (aggregation) should not be scored as agglutination.

The presence of agglutination is not sufficient evidence to deduce an immunological cause of infertility, but is suggestive of the presence of antisperm antibodies; further testing is required. Severe agglutination can affect the assessment of sperm motility and concentration.

Sperm Motility

It is the ratio of the number of motile sperm to the total number of sperm in a given volume and is expressed as a percentage. Several scoring systems exist for sperm motility assessments, but a simple grading system is recommended. This provides an assessment of motility without requiring ultramodern equipment.

The extent of progressive sperm motility is related to pregnancy rates.[28-30] It should be assessed soon after liquefaction in grades to avoid deleterious effects of dehydration, pH and changes in temperature on motility. Approximately 200 spermatozoa should be examined for different grades of motility at ×200 or ×400 magnification of phase-contrast microscope in the wet preparation. The procedure may be performed at room temperature or at 37°C with a heated microscope stage, prewarmed slides and coverslips. Assess progressive motility first, then nonprogressive motility and immotility.

- Progressive motility (PR): spermatozoa moving actively, either linearly or in a large circle, regardless of speed. Rapid progressive motility, i.e. more than 25 μm/s at 37°C or 5 head lengths/half a tail length.
- Nonprogressive motility (NP): all other patterns of motility with an absence of progression, e.g., swimming in small circles, the flagellar force hardly displacing the head or when only a flagellar beat can be observed. Slow and sluggish progressive motility.
- Nonprogressive motility: less than 5 μm/s.
- Immotility (IM): no movement. Assess only intact spermatozoa (defined as having a head and a tail), since only intact spermatozoa are counted for sperm concentration. Do not count motile pinheads. Report the average percentage for each motility grade to the nearest whole number.

- An eyepiece reticle makes it easier to count motile and immotile spermatozoa.
- Systematic selection of fields for assessment of sperm motility, at least 5 mm from the edges of the coverslip.

The lower reference limit for total motility (PR + NP) is 40% (5th centile, 95% CI 38–42). The lower reference limit for progressive motility (PR) is 32% (5th centile, 95% CI 31–34).

Computer-assisted Semen Analysis (CASA)

Manual semen analysis lacks the ability to measure the kinematics of sperm motion. CASA due to its potential benefits has been given more attention for analyzing sperm motility, i.e., sperm head and flaggelar kinematics. Some of these motion characteristics have been shown to be related to IVF outcome. This important kinematics are

- *Curvilinear velocity* (VCL) is the measure of the rate of travel of the centroid of the sperm head over a given time period. This is calculated from the sum of the straight lines joining the sequential positions of the sperm along the sperm's track. Values are reported as µm/s.
- *Average path velocity* (VAP) is the velocity along the average path of the spermatozoon. It is reported as µm/s.
- *Straight-line velocity* (VSL) is the linear or progressive velocity of the cell. It is also the straight-line distance between the first and the last centroid position for a given period of time. It is reported as µm/s.
- *Linearity*: Linearity of the forward progression (LIN) is the ratio of VSL to VSL and is expressed as percentage. A value of 100% represents cells swimming a perfect straight line.
- *Amplitude of lateral head displacement* (ALH) of the sperm head is calculated from the amplitude of its lateral deviation about the cells axis of progression or average path. It is reported as µm.

A man is considered to be asthenozoospermic if the spermatozoa in his ejaculate show less than 40% forward progressive movement within 60 minutes of ejaculation and necrozoospermic if all sperms are immotile.

Sperm Vitality

The membrane integrity of spermatozoa is determined by vitality test. Though carried out routinely in all the semen samples, it is of utmost importance when the progressive motility of sperm is less than 40%. This test can provide a check on the motility evaluation, since the percentage of dead cells should not exceed (within sampling error) the percentage of immotile spermatozoa. The percentage of viable cells normally exceeds that of motile cells.

The percentage of live spermatozoa is assessed by identifying those with an intact cell membrane, from dye exclusion or by hypotonic swelling. The dye exclusion method is based on the principle that damaged plasma membranes, such as those found in nonvital (dead) cells, and allow entry of membrane-impairment stains. The hypo-osmotic swelling test presumes that only cells with intact membranes (live cells) will swell in hypotonic solutions.

It is clinically important to know whether immotile spermatozoa are alive or dead. Vitality results should be assessed in conjunction with motility results from the same semen sample. The presence of a large proportion of vital but immotile cells may be indicative of structural defects in the flagellum[31]; a high percentage of immotile and nonviable cells (necrozoospermia) may indicate epididymal pathology.[11,32]

Vitality Test Using Eosin–Nigrosin

This one-step staining technique uses nigrosin to increase the contrast between the background and the sperm heads, which makes them easier to discern. It also permits slides to be stored for re-evaluation and quality control purposes.[6]

Preparing the reagents:

- Eosin Y: dissolve 0.67 g of eosin Y (color index 45380) and 0.9 g of sodium chloride (NaCl) in 100 mL of purified water with gentle heating.
- Eosin–nigrosin: add 10 g of nigrosin (color index 50420) to the 100 mL of eosin Y solution.
- Boil the suspension, and then allow to cool to room temperature.
- Filter through filter paper (e.g., 90 g/m^2) to remove coarse and gelatinous precipitates and store in a sealed dark-glass bottle.

Procedure:

- Mix the semen sample well.
- Remove a 50-Pl aliquot of semen and mix with an equal volume of eosin–nigrosin suspension, e.g., in a porcelain spot plate well or test-tube, and wait for 30 seconds.
- Remix the semen sample before removing a replicate aliquot and mixing with eosin–nigrosin and treating as in step 2 above.
- For each suspension make a smear on a glass slide and allow it to dry in air.

- Examine immediately after drying, or later after mounting with a permanent nonaqueous mounting medium.
- Examine each slide with brightfield optics at ×1,000 magnification and oil immersion.
- Tally the number of stained (dead) or unstained (vital) cells with the aid of a laboratory counter.
- Evaluate 200 spermatozoa in each replicate, in order to achieve an acceptably low sampling error.
- Calculate the average and difference of the two percentages of vital cells from the replicate slides.
- Report the average percentage of vital spermatozoa to the nearest whole number.

The lower reference limit for vitality (membrane-intact spermatozoa) is 58% (5th centile, 95% CI 55–63).

Vitality Test Using Hypo-osmotic Swelling

The hypo-osmotic swelling (HOS) test may be used to assess vitality[33] (Fig. 19.4). This is useful when staining of spermatozoa must be avoided, e.g., when choosing spermatozoa for ICSI. Spermatozoa with intact membranes swell within 5 minutes in hypo-osmotic medium and all flagellar shapes are stabilized by 30 minutes.[34]

Thus, use

- 30 minutes incubation for routine diagnostics, but
- 5 minutes incubation when spermatozoa are to be processed for therapeutic use.

Preparing the reagents:

- Swelling solution for diagnostic purposes: dissolve 0.735 g of sodium citrate dihydrate and 1.351 g of D-fructose in 100 mL of purified water. Freeze 1-mL aliquots of this solution at –20°C.
- For therapeutic use: dilute the medium to be used 1 + 1 (1:2) with sterile, purified water.

Procedure:

- Thaw the frozen swelling solution and mix well before use.
- Warm 1 mL of swelling solution or 1 mL of 1 + 1 (1:2) diluted medium in a closed microcentrifuge tube at 37°C for 5 minutes.
- Mix the semen sample well.
- Remove a 100-Pl aliquot of semen and add to the swelling solution. Mix gently by drawing it in and out of the pipette.
- Incubate at 37°C for exactly 5 minutes or 30 minutes (see above), then transfer a 10-Pl aliquot to a clean slide and cover with a 22 mm × 22 mm coverslip.
- Remix the semen sample, remove a replicate aliquot, mix with swelling solution, incubate and prepare a replicate slide, as above.
- Examine each slide with phase-contrast optics at ×200 or ×400 magnification.
- Tally the number of unswollen (dead) and swollen (vital) cells with the aid of a laboratory counter.

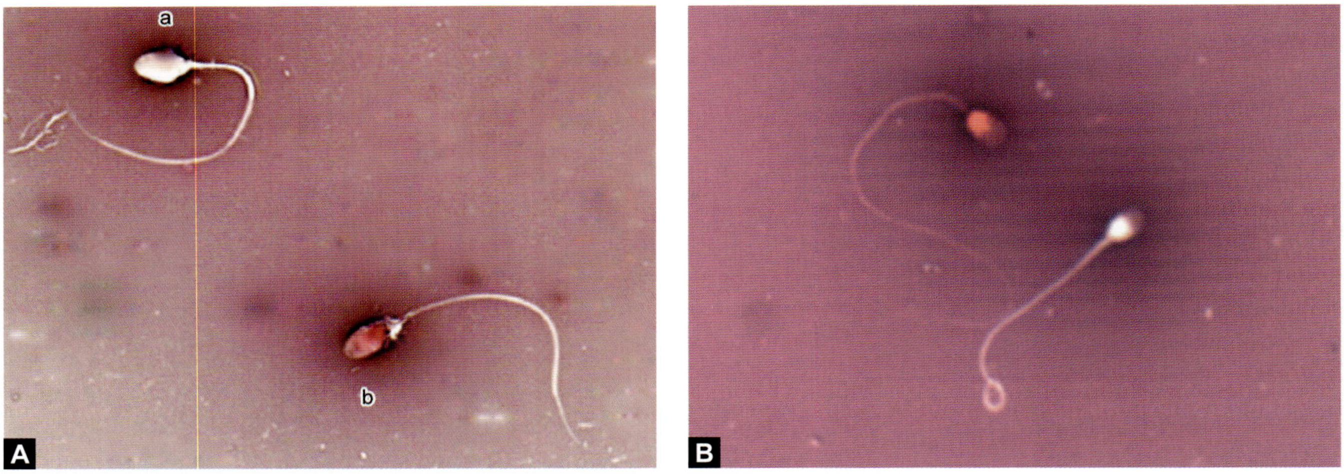

Fig. 19.4: Vitality test: (A) Unstained (white) alive spermatozoa, (B) Stained (red) dead spermatozoa.
(A) Mohammad Ali Khalili; Iman Halvaei; Ali Nabi Urology Journal: Vol. 11:2; 1467, 2014; (B) http://fertilitysolutions.com/controls/aqc107.htm.

- Evaluate 200 spermatozoa in each replicate, to achieve an acceptably low sampling error.
- Report the average percentage of vital spermatozoa to the nearest whole number.

Scoring:

- Swollen spermatozoa are identified by changes in the shape of the cell, as indicated by coiling of the tail.
- Live cells are distinguished by evidence of swelling of the sperm tail; score all forms of swollen tails as live spermatozoa.

Cells that swell under hypo-osmotic conditions (those with a coiled tail) are alive whereas those with straight tails are dead

Lower reference limit: HOS test values approximate those of the eosin test.[35] The lower reference limit for vitality (membrane-intact spermatozoa) is 58% (5th centile, 95% CI 55–63). The total number of membrane-intact spermatozoa in the ejaculate is of biological significance. This is obtained by multiplying the total number of spermatozoa in the ejaculate by the percentage of membrane-intact cells.

Sperm Count

The total number of spermatozoa per ejaculate and the sperm concentration are related to both time to pregnancy[36] and pregnancy rates and are predictors of conception.[29,37]

The number of spermatozoa in the ejaculate is calculated from the concentration of spermatozoa, which is measured during semen evaluation. For normal ejaculates, when the male tract is unobstructed and the abstinence time short, the total number of spermatozoa in the ejaculate is correlated with testicular volume[16,17] and thus is a measure of the capability of the testes to produce spermatozoa[38] and the patency of the male tract. The concentration of spermatozoa in the semen, while related to fertilization and pregnancy rates, is influenced by the volume of the secretions from the seminal vesicles and prostate[39]) and is not a specific measure of testicular function.

The terms "total sperm number" and "sperm concentration" are not synonymous. Sperm concentration refers to the number of spermatozoa per unit volume of semen and is a function of the number of spermatozoa emitted and the volume of fluid diluting them. Total sperm number refers to the total number of spermatozoa in the entire ejaculate and is obtained by multiplying the sperm concentration by the semen volume.

Sperm Concentration

Determining accurate sperm concentration (million/mL of ejaculate), and total sperm count (million sperm per ejaculate) is important. The most accurate method of determining sperm concentration is volumetric dilution and hemocytometry. Gently mixing the semen sample using a positive displacement pipette before the volume is withdrawn is essential for an accurate determination of sperm concentration.

Types of Counting Chamber

The use of 100-Pm-deep hemacytometer chambers is recommended (Figs. 19.5 and 19.6). Other deep hemacytometer chambers may be used, but they will have different volumes and grid patterns and will require different factors for calculation. Disposable chambers are available for determining sperm concentration,[40-42] but they may produce different results from those of the improved Neubauer hemacytometer (Fig. 19.7). Shallow chambers that fill by capillary action may not have a uniform distribution of spermatozoa because of streaming.[43,44] It may be possible to correct for this[43] but it is not advised.[45] For accurate assessment of low sperm concentrations, large-volume counting chambers may be necessary.

Hemacytometer

A fixed volume of liquefied semen aliquot is used and fixed sperm are counted in a Neubauer hemacytometer

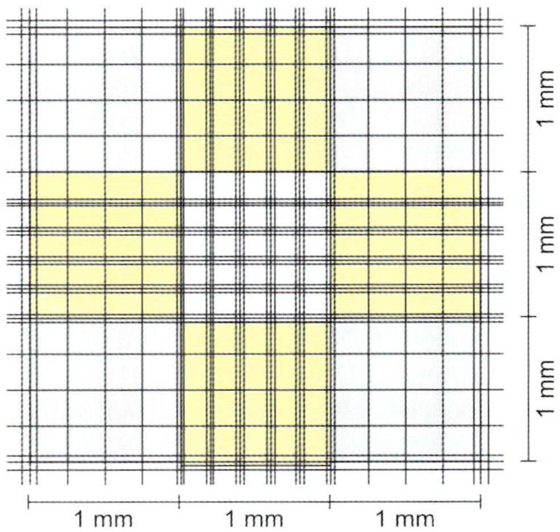

Fig. 19.5: Standard hemacytometer chamber. http/ www. Neubauer improved schema.gif

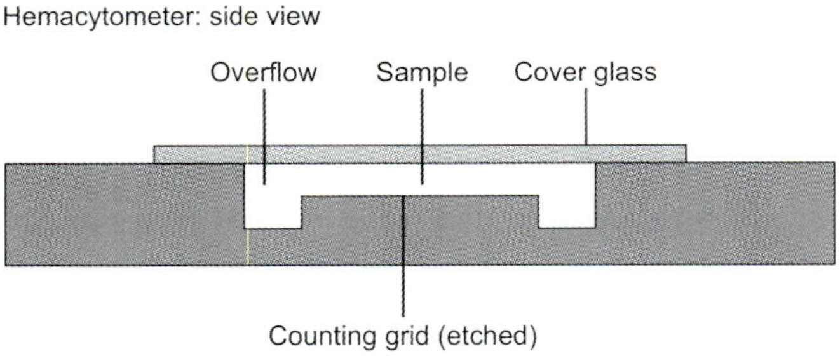

Fig. 19.6: Profile view of hemocyto meter
http://www.microbehunter.com/wp/wp-content/uploads/2010/06/counting_chamber6.jpg.

chamber. Dilution of 1:19 is usually employed. Dilutions may be made in small clean, glass or plastic vials. Extreme care must be taken while making dilutions and preparing the hemacytometer. Figure 19.6 shows the microscopic view of hemacytometer.

Semen or sperm suspension (SS) is diluted with sperm-counting (SC) diluent (sodium acid carbonate-formaldehyde solution) and counted according to the procedure indicated in the WHO laboratory manual (2010).

Reagents:
- The diluent consists of 50 g sodium bicarbonate
- 10 mL of 35% of formaldehyde solution, and 0.25 g trypan blue dissolved in reagent water up to 1 L.

Procedure:
- Filter the solution through Whatman no. 1 paper into a clean bottle and store it at 4°C.
- Add 50 μL liquefied semen to 950 diluent. Use a positive displacement pipette to ensure accurate handling of the viscous semen.
- These dilutions can be stored for 4 weeks at 4°C.
- Place the hemacytometer cover slip over the chamber.
- Vortex the diluent for 10 seconds. Transfer 10 μL to each chamber.
- Leave the hemacytometer in a humid chamber for 10–15 minutes for the spermatozoa to settle down on to the counting grid.
- Count the spermatozoa using ×20 objective phase-contrast optics. The central square of the grid in an improved Neubauer chamber contains 25 large squares, each containing 16 small squares. The number of squares counted depends on the number of spermatozoa seen in the first large square as follows (Fig. 19.8):
- <10 spermatozoa in the first large square-count the whole grid of 25 large squares;

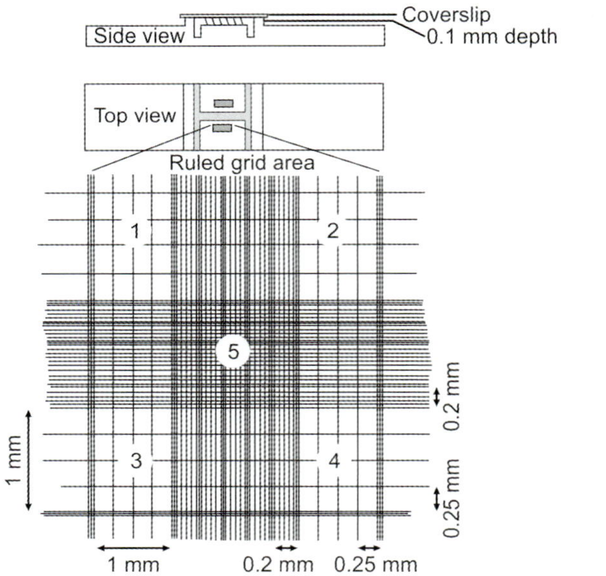

Fig. 19.7: Improved neubauer hemacytometer.
http://homepages.gac.edu/~cellab/chpts/chpt1/figure8.html

- 10–40 spermatozoa per square—count only 10 large squares (two vertical and two horizontal rows);
- >40 spermatozoa per square - count spermatozoa in five large squares (the four corners and the central one).

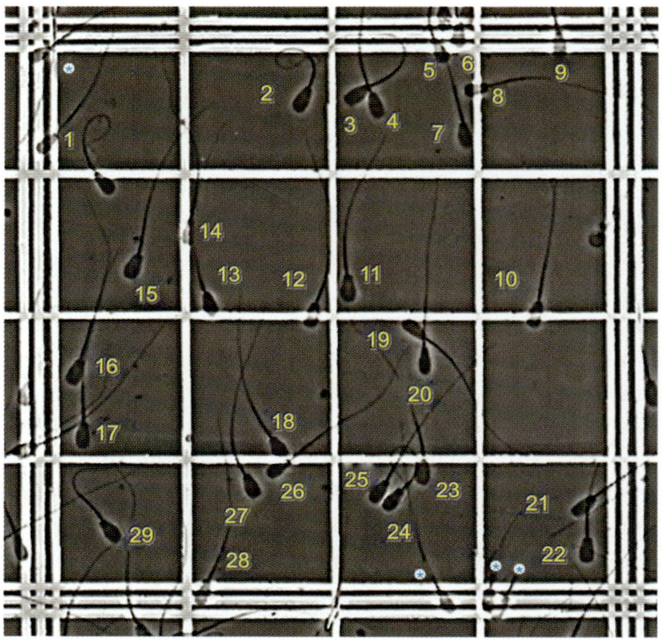

Fig. 19.8: Determining concentration of sperm.
http://www.ansci.wisc.edu/jjp1/ansci_repro/lab/procedures/hemacytometer/hemacytometer20use.html.

Results:

- Counts of two hemacytometer chambers should be within 5% of their average. If not, discard, remix sample and prepare another sample to be loaded on the hemacytometer, i.e. (higher value – lower value) must be < (sum of values /20) for the counts to be acceptable.
- Sperm concentration (10^6/mL) = total number of spermatozoa/appropriate correction factor
- Total sperm count = sperm concentration × ejaculate volume.

Samples with low numbers of spermatozoa (<2/field, 400×) should be centrifuged, a small aliquot of supernatant discarded, and the sample mixed and counted again after correcting for the volume of the supernatant that was removed. The sample in which no spermatozoa are seen must be centrifuged and examined for the presence of spermatozoa in the pellet.

Cell-VU

The Cell-VU sperm-counting method involves the use of a dual-chamber glass slide and two pieces of 0.5-mm thick coverslip containing a laser-etched grid on the reverse side. The grid area is 1 mm × 1 mm and is divided into 100 smaller squares, each of which is 0.1 mm × 0.1 mm. The chamber has a reported depth of 20 µm. Semen or SS sample is vortexed prior to sperm counting according to the manufacturer's instructions. Briefly, a 4 µL volume of semen or SS is loaded into the left and right chambers and the number of sperm counted based on those sperm which touched the upper and left sides instead of the lower and right sides of each square of a counting chamber. To ensure consistent counting, a minimum of 200 sperm is counted in each chamber.

Makler Chamber

The Makler chamber is designed specifically for the determination of sperm concentration and motility in undiluted semen. It has a reported depth of 0.01 mm. The grid area in the center of the coverslip is 1 mm × 1 mm and is divided into 100 smaller squares, each of which is 0.1 mm × 0.1 mm. A 5 µL volume of semen or SS is loaded into the chamber and the number of sperm counted as indicated above for the cell-VU method (Fig. 19.9).

The lower reference limit for sperm concentration is 15 × 10^6 spermatozoa per mL (5th centile, 95% CI 12–16 × 10^6).

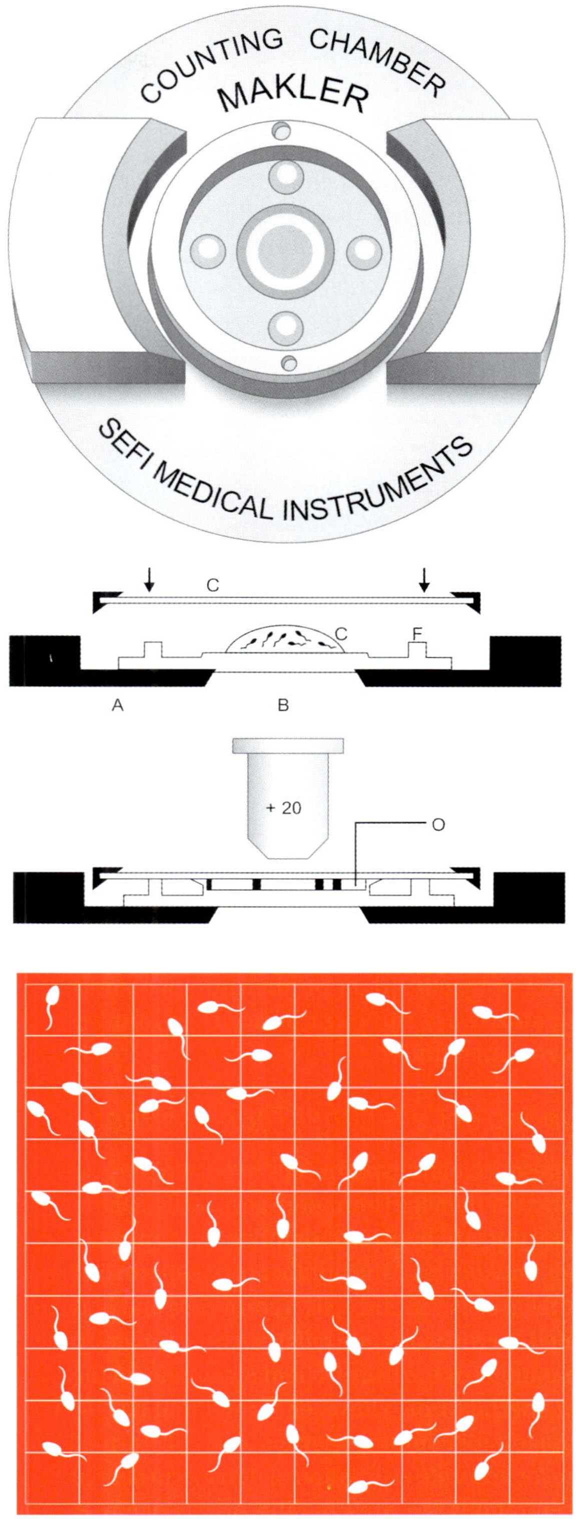

Fig. 19.9: Makler chamber for sperm count. http://www.galaxyivf.com/Equ_Mackler_Sperm_Counting_Chambers.php.

Calculation of the total number of spermatozoa in the ejaculate: It is recommended to calculate and report the total number of spermatozoa per ejaculate, as this parameter provides a measure of the capability of the testes to produce spermatozoa and the patency of the male tract. This is obtained by multiplying the sperm concentration by the volume of the whole ejaculate.

The lower reference limit for total sperm number is 39×10^6 spermatozoa per ejaculate (5th centile, 95% CI $33–46 \times 10^6$).

Low Sperm Numbers: Cryptozoospermia and Suspected Azoospermia

If no spermatozoa are observed in the replicate wet preparations, azoospermia can be suspected. Although it has been suggested that the definition should change,[46,47] azoospermia remains a description of the ejaculate rather than a statement of its origin or a basis for diagnosis and therapy. It is generally accepted that the term azoospermia can only be used if no spermatozoa are found in the sediment of a centrifuged sample.[48]

However, it should be borne in mind that

- whether or not spermatozoa are found in the pellet depends on the centrifugation time and speed[49,50] and on how much of the pellet is examined;
- centrifugation at 3,000 g for 15 minutes does not pellet all spermatozoa from a sample[51]; and
- after centrifugation, motility can be lost[52] and concentration will be underestimated.[53]

The way these samples are handled depends on whether subjective data on the presence and motility of spermatozoa are sufficient or accurate numbers of spermatozoa are required.

Counting of Cells Other Than Spermatozoa

The presence of nonsperm cells in semen may be indicative of testicular damage (immature germ cells), pathology of the efferent ducts (ciliary tufts) or inflammation of the accessory glands (leukocytes). The number of nonsperm cells in semen (epithelial cells, "round cells" (germ cells and leukocytes) or isolated sperm heads and tails) can be estimated in fixed wet preparations by the use of a hemacytometer in the same way as for spermatozoa. However, semen that has been diluted adequately for counting spermatozoa will normally be more dilute for accurate estimation of nonsperm cells, unless high concentrations are present. The prevalence of round cells relative to spermatozoa can be assessed from slides. Alternatively, their concentration can be assessed during the estimation of peroxidase-positive cells.

Sperm Morphology

Determination of sperm morphology comprises the following steps:

- Preparing a smear of semen on a slide.
- Air-drying, fixing and staining the slide.
- Mounting the slide with a coverslip if the slide is to be kept for a long time.
- Assessing approximately 200 spermatozoa per replicate for the percentage of normal forms or of normal and abnormal forms.
- Comparing replicate values to see if they are acceptably close: if so, proceeding with calculations; if not, re-reading the slides.

Semen Smearing Methods for Sperm Morphology

- "Feathering" method for undiluted semen. The semen drop spreads along the back edge of the angled slide and is pulled forward over the slide to form the smear.
- Pipette method for washed samples. A drop of the SS is spread over the surface of the slide by pushing the horizontal pipette.

Staining Methods

Once the semen smears have been air-dried, they should be fixed and stained to highlight details of the spermatozoa. The use of the Papanicolaou, Shorr or Diff-Quik stain is recommended.

With all three stains in brightfield optics, the head is stained pale blue in the acrosomal region and dark blue in the post-acrosomal region. The midpiece may show some red staining and the tail is stained blue or reddish. Excess residual cytoplasm, usually located behind the head and around the midpiece, is stained pink or red (Papanicolaou stain) or reddish-orange (Shorr stain).

Papanicolaou stain: It is the most widely used staining method. It is recommended by the WHO (2010) laboratory manual because it gives a good staining to spermatozoa and other cells as it distinguishes basophilic cell components and acidophilic cell components. It allows a comprehensive examination of nuclear chromatin pattern.

Reagents:

- Fixative: A freshly prepared solution of equal parts of analytical grade absolute ethanol and diethyl ether;
- Graded ethanol (50%, 70%, 80%, 95%, and 99.5% v/v).

Staining Solutions:

- Hematoxylin: Orange G6 and EA-50 are commercially available.
- Acid ethanol: Prepared by mixing 300 mL of 95% (v/v) ethanol and 2.0 mL concentrated hydrochloric acid (36% HCL) in 100 mL reagent water.
- Scott's solution: Prepare by dissolving 3.5 g $NaHCO_3$ and 20.0 g $MgSO_4 \cdot 7H_2O$ in reagent water to a total volume of 1,000 mL

Procedure:

Prepare the air-dried smear and fix as explained above. Proceed with staining according to the sequence.

- Graded ethanol (80%, 70%, 50%): 10 dips each
- Running water: 12–15 dips
- Hematoxylin: 3 minutes
- Running water: 3–5 dips
- Acid ethanol: 2 dips
- Scott's solution: 4 minutes
- Distilled water: 1 dip
- Graded ethanol (50%, 70%, 80%, 90%): 10 dips
- Orange G6: 2 minutes
- Ethanol 95%: 10 dips
- EA-50: 5 minutes
- Ethanol 95% (3 jars): 5 dips
- Ethanol 99.5%: 2 minutes
- Xylene (3 staining jars): 1 minute

With this stain, the head stains pale blue in the acrosomal region and dark blue in the post-acrosomal region. The midpiece may show some red staining. The tail is stained bluish or reddish and the cytoplasmic droplets stain green.

Examining the Stained Preparation

With stained preparations, a ×100 oil-immersion bright-field objective and at least a ×10 eyepiece should be used. Clearer images are obtained when a fluid of similar refractive index (RI) to those of cells (approximately 1.5) and glass (1.50–1.58) is placed between the lens and the unmounted section or glass coverslip. This is usually immersion oil (RI 1.52).

Classification of Normal Sperm Morphology

The method recommended is a simple normal/abnormal classification, with optional tallying of the location of abnormalities in abnormal spermatozoa.

Spermatozoa consist of a head, neck, middle piece (midpiece), principal piece and endpiece (Fig 19.10). As the endpiece is difficult to see with a light microscope, the cell can be considered to comprise a head (and neck) and tail (midpiece and principal piece). For a spermatozoon to be considered normal, both its head and tail must be normal. All borderline forms should be considered abnormal (Fig. 19.11).

- The head should be smooth, regularly contoured and generally oval in shape. There should be a well-defined acrosomal region comprising 40–70% of the head area.[54] The acrosomal region should contain no large vacuoles, and not more than two small vacuoles, which should not occupy more than 20% of the sperm head. The postacrosomal region should not contain any vacuoles.
- The midpiece should be slender, regular and about the same length as the sperm head. The major axis of the midpiece should be aligned with the major axis of the sperm head. Residual cytoplasm is considered an anomaly only when in excess, i.e. when it exceeds one third of the sperm head size.[55]
- The principal piece should have a uniform caliber along its length, be thinner than the midpiece, and be approximately 45 μm long (about 10 times the head length). It may be looped back on itself, provided there is no sharp angle indicative of a flagellar break (Fig. 19.11).

Classification of Abnormal Sperm Morphology

Human semen samples contain spermatozoa with different kinds of malformations. Defective spermatogenesis and some epididymal pathologies are commonly associated with an increased percentage of spermatozoa with abnormal shapes. The morphological defects are usually mixed. Abnormal spermatozoa generally have a lower fertilizing potential, depending on the types of anomalies, and may also have abnormal DNA. Morphological defects have been associated with increased DNA fragmentation,[56] an increased incidence of structural chromosomal aberrations,[57] immature chromatin[58] and aneuploidy.[59,60] Emphasis is therefore given to the form of the head, although the sperm tail (midpiece and principal piece) is also considered.

The following categories of defects should be noted:

- Head defects: large or small, tapered, pyriform, round, amorphous, vacuolated (more than two vacuoles or >20% of the head area occupied by unstained vacuolar areas), vacuoles in the post-acrosomal region, small or large acrosomal areas (<40% or >70% of the head area), double heads, or any combination of these (Fig 19.12).

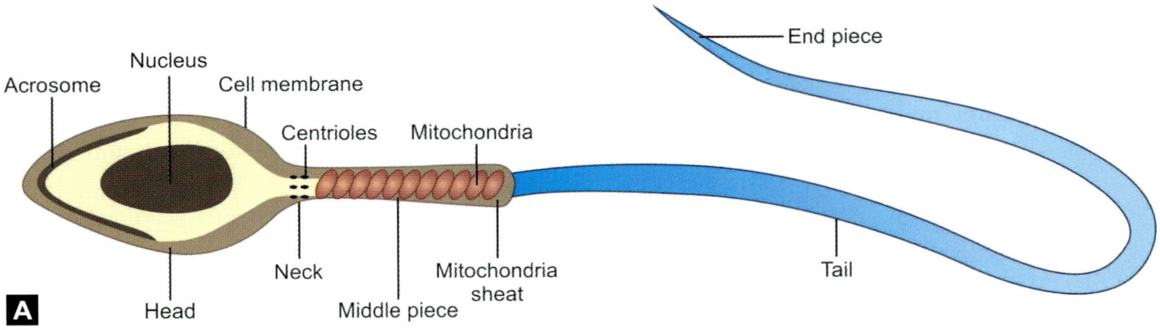

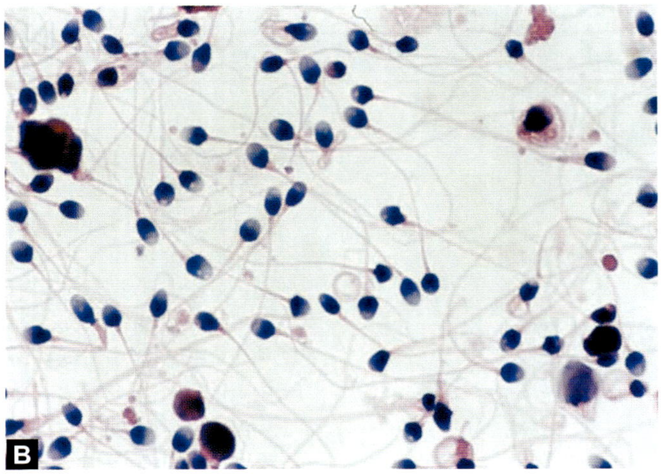

Figs. 19.10: (A) Sperm Components (B) Sperm components. Papanicolaou staining combines a nuclear stain, Harris Hematoxylin with two cytoplasmic stains, OG6 and EA50 Papanicolaou solutions. It allows carrying out the morphological study of spermatozoa (spermocytogram). (A) http://www.jetanin.com/vn/service/archive_detail/23. (B) http://www.scielo.cl/scielo.php?script=sci_arttext&pid=S0717-95022012000400045

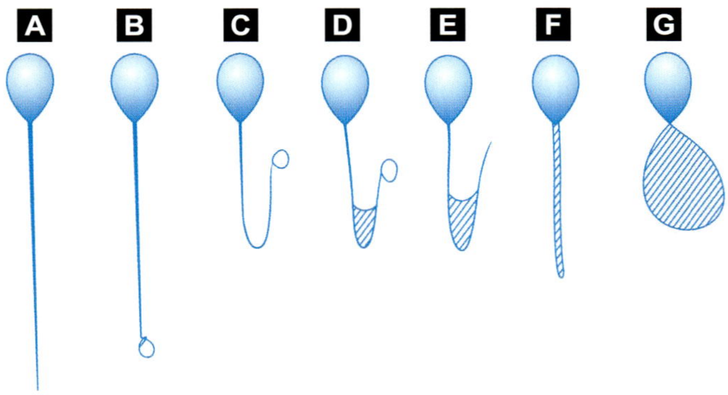

Figs. 19.11A to G: Schematic representation of typical morphological changes in human spermatozoa subjected to hypo-osmotic stress. (A) No change. (B to G) Various types of tail changes. Swelling in tail is indicated by the gray area.
Reproduced from Jayendran RE, Vander ven HH, Perez Pelaez, M, Crabo BG, Zeneveld LJD (1984), Journal of Reproduction & Fertility 70:219-228 @ Society for Reproduction & Fertility (1984) [From WHO Manual ed. V 2010, page 32].

- Neck and midpiece defects: asymmetrical insertion of the midpiece into the head, thick or irregular, sharply bent, abnormally thin or any combination of these (Fig 19.12).
- Principal piece defects: short, multiple, broken, smooth hairpin bends, sharply angulated bends, of irregular width, coiled or any combination of these (Fig 19.12).
- Excess residual cytoplasm (ERC): this is associated with abnormal spermatozoa produced from a defective spermatogenic process. Spermatozoa characterized by large amounts of irregular stained cytoplasm, one third or more of the sperm head size, often associated with defective midpieces[55] are abnormal. This abnormal excess cytoplasm should not be called a cytoplasmic droplet[61] (Fig 19.12).

Assess only intact spermatozoa, defined as having a head and a tail, since only intact spermatozoa are counted for sperm concentration. Do not count immature germ (round) cells.

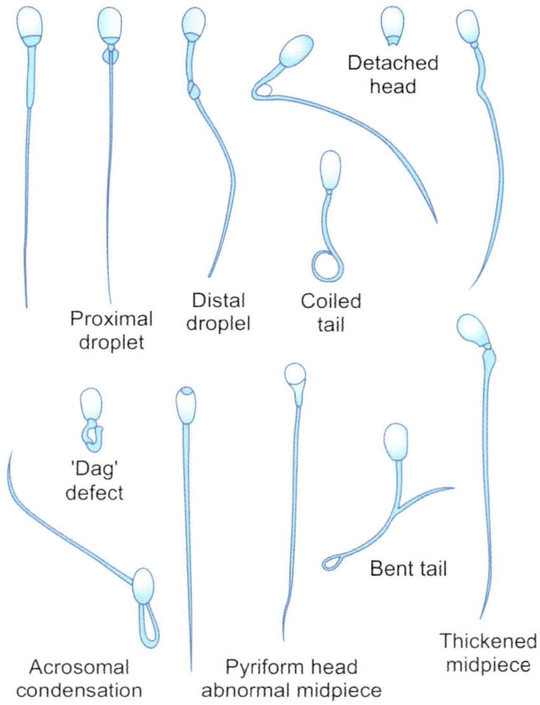

Figs. 19.12: Morphology of human sperm using diff-quick stain. Reproduced from Liu et al. (2003) European Society for Human Reproduction & Embryology and Menkveld & Kruger (1990) as mentioned in WHO Manual (Ed. V, 2010), Page 58.

The lower reference limit for normal forms is 4% (5th centile, 95% CI 3.0–4.0).

Standardized Classification of Normal and Abnormal Human Sperm Morphology

Morphologically normal spermatozoa are defined as in the 5th WHO manual (World Health Organization, 2010) except that all borderline aspects are considered normal; tapered head: increased major axis length and normal minor axis length; thin head: normal major axis length and decreased minor axis length; microcephalic: decreased major and minor axes lengths; macrocephalic: increased major and minor axes lengths; multiple heads: more than one head per sperm cell; abnormal post-acrosomal region: any type of outline and/or size and/or texture abnormality of the posterior part of the head; abnormal acrosomal region: any type of outline and/or size and/or texture abnormality of the anterior part of the head; abnormal (or excess) residual cytoplasm (or abnormal cytoplasmic remnant): residual cytoplasmic area. 30% of the head area, in any part of the sperm cell; thin midpiece: midpiece diameter, smaller than the principal piece diameter for 40% of the whole midpiece length; bent/misaligned tail: may include neck anomalies, misalignment of the head major axis and midpiece axis or an acute angle (≤120°) between the head major axis and midpiece axis or an acute angle (≤120°) between the midpiece and the principal piece axes ; no tail: isolated head, no tail observed; short tail: a tail length (midpiece + principal piece) no more than five times the major axis length of the head; irregularly shaped tail: irregular or changing caliber along the tail; coiled tail: completely or partially coiled tail, with the coil close to or around the head (flat coiling or coiling at the extremity of the tail reminiscent of hypo-osmotic coiling aspects should not be included in this category); multiple tails: more than one tail per sperm cell. Many of the spermatozoa presented more than one type of abnormality. The classification method encompasses all the abnormalities.

Do not assess overlapping spermatozoa and those lying with the head on edge; these cannot be analyzed adequately. They should not be present in a good smear, but may occur when debris and a large amount of particulate material are present (such as in viscous semen). These samples should be washed and the slides examined before staining.

The total number of morphologically normal spermatozoa in the ejaculate is of biological significance. This is obtained by multiplying the total number of spermatozoa in the ejaculate by the percentage of normal forms.

Pinheads (free tails) are not counted as head defects, since they possess no chromatin or head structure anterior to the basal plate. Because free tails (pinheads) and free heads are not counted as spermatozoa (defined as having a head and tail), they are not considered to be sperm abnormalities.

Assessment of Leukocytes in Semen

Leukocytes, predominantly polymorphonuclear leukocytes (PMN, neutrophils), are present in most human ejaculates.[62,63] They can sometimes be differentiated from spermatids and spermatocytes in a semen smear stained with the Papanicolaou procedure. Differentiation is based on differences in staining coloration, and on nuclear size and shape[63] (Fig 19.13). Polymorphonuclear leukocytes can easily be confused morphologically with multinucleated spermatids, but stain a bluish color, in contrast to the more pinkish color of spermatids.[63] Nuclear size may also help identification: monocyte nuclei exhibit a wide variation

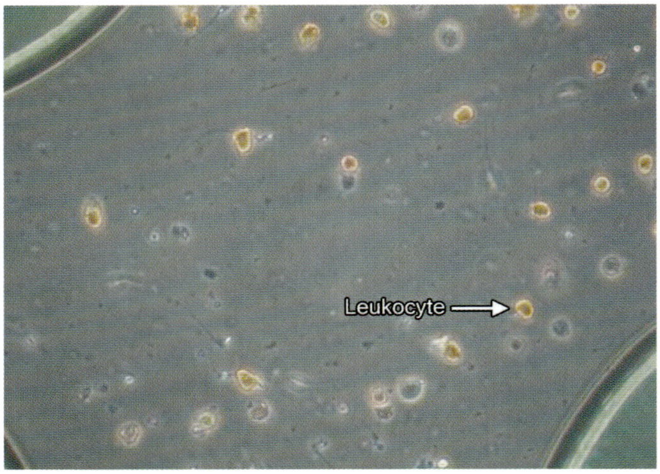

Fig. 19.13: Various defects in spermatozoa (morphology). http://www.tupbebek-genetik.com/en/laboratory-procedures/andrology-laboratory/

in size, from approximately 7 µm for lymphocytes to over 15 µm for macrophages. These sizes are only guidelines, since degeneration and division affect the size of the nucleus.

There are several other techniques for quantifying the leukocyte population in semen. As peroxidase-positive granulocytes are the predominant form of leukocytes in semen, routine assay of peroxidase activity is useful as an initial screening technique.[63,64]

Leukocytes can be further differentiated with more time-consuming and expensive immunocytochemical assays against common leukocyte and sperm antigens.[65,66]

Staining Cellular Peroxidase Using Ortho-toluidine

This test is quick and inexpensive, and is a useful initial screening for granulocytes.

Reagents:

1. Phosphate buffer, 67 mmol/L, pH 6.0: dissolve 9.47 g of sodium hydrogen phosphate (Na_2HPO_4) in 1,000 mL of purified water and 9.08 g of potassium dihydrogen phosphate (KH_2PO_4) in 1,000 mL of purified water. Add one solution to the other (approximately 12 mL of Na_2HPO_4 solution to 88 mL of KH_2PO_4 solution) until the pH is 6.0.
2. Saturated ammonium chloride (NH_4Cl) solution: add 250 g of NH_4Cl to 1,000 mL of purified water.
3. Disodium ethylenediamine tetra-acetic acid (Na 2EDTA) 148 mmol/L: dissolve 50 g/L in phosphate buffer (pH 6.0) prepared in step 1.
4. Substrate: dissolve 2.5 mg of o-toluidine in 10 mL of 0.9% (9 g/L) saline.
5. Hydrogen peroxide (H_2O_2) 30% (v/v): as purchased
6. Working solution: to 9 mL o-toluidine substrate, add 1 mL of saturated NH_4Cl solution, 1 mL of 148 mmol/L Na_2EDTA, and 10 µL of 30% (v/v) H_2O_2 and mix well. This solution can be used up to 24 hours after preparation.

Procedure:

1. Mix the semen sample well.
2. Remove a 0.1-mL aliquot of semen and mix with 0.9 mL of working solution (1 + 9 (1:10) dilution).
3. Vortex the SS gently for 10 seconds and incubate at room temperature for 20–30 minutes. Alternatively, shake continuously with a tube-rocking system.
4. Remix the semen sample before removing a replicate aliquot and mixing with working solution as above.

Assessing peroxidase-positive cell number in the hemacytometer chambers:

1. After 20–30 minutes, mix the SSs again and fill each side of a hemacytometer with one of the replicate preparations.
2. Store the hemacytometer horizontally for at least 4 minutes at room temperature in a humid chamber (e.g., on water-saturated filter paper in a covered Petri dish) to prevent drying out and to allow the cells to settle.
3. Examine the chamber with phase-contrast optics at ×200 or ×400 magnification.
4. Count at least 200 peroxidase-positive cells in each replicate, in order to achieve an acceptably low sampling error. Peroxidase-positive cells are stained brown, while peroxidase-negative cells are unstained.
5. Examine one chamber, grid by grid, and continue counting until at least 200 peroxidase-positive cells have been observed and a complete grid has been examined. Counting must be done by complete grids; do not stop in the middle of a grid.
6. Make a note of the number of grids assessed to reach at least 200 peroxidase-positive cells. The same number of grids will be counted from the other chamber of the hemacytometer.
7. Tally the number of peroxidase-positive cells and grids with the aid of a laboratory counter.

8. Switch to the second chamber of the hemacytometer and perform the replicate count on the same number of grids as the first replicate, even if this yields fewer than 200 peroxidase-positive cells.
9. Calculate the sum and difference of the two numbers of peroxidase-positive cells.
10. Report the average concentration of peroxidase-positive cells to two significant figures.
11. Calculate the total number of peroxidase-positive cells per ejaculate

This procedure can be used to calculate round cell concentration when the total number of round cells counted (peroxidase-positive and -negative) is used for N in the calculation. The absence of peroxidase-positive cells from the aliquot examined does not necessarily mean that they are absent from the rest of the sample.

Excessive numbers of leukocytes in the ejaculate (leukocytospermia, pyospermia) may be associated with infection and poor sperm quality. Leukocyte-dependent damage to spermatozoa depends on the total leukocyte number in the ejaculate and the number of leukocytes relative to the number of spermatozoa. Leukocytes can impair sperm motility and DNA integrity through an oxidative attack. However, whether the level of leukocytic infiltration observed is damaging depends on factors that are impossible to infer from a semen sample, such as the reason for, timing and anatomical location of the infiltration, as well as the nature of the leukocytes involved and whether they are in an activated state.[62,67,68]

There is currently no reference range for peroxidase-positive cells in semen from fertile men. Pending additional evidence, WHO (2010) manual retains the consensus value of 1.0×10^6 peroxidase-positive cells per mL as a threshold value. The total number of peroxidase-positive cells in the ejaculate may reflect the severity of an inflammatory condition.[69] This is obtained by multiplying the concentration of peroxidase-positive cells by the volume of the whole ejaculate.

Assessment of immature germ cells in semen: Germ cells include round spermatids and spermatocytes, but rarely spermatogonia. They can be detected in stained semen smears, but may be difficult to distinguish from inflammatory cells when the cells are degenerating.

Spermatids and spermatocytes can usually be differentiated from leukocytes in a semen smear stained by the Papanicolaou procedure.[63] Identification can be based on staining coloration, nuclear size and shape (see Plates 6, 10, 11, 12, 13 and 14), absence of intracellular peroxidase, and lack of leukocyte-specific antigens. Multinucleated spermatids can easily be confused morphologically with polymorphonuclear leukocytes but stain a pinkish color, in contrast to the more bluish PMN leukocytes.[63] Round spermatids may be identified with stains specific for the developing acrosome,[70] lectins, or specific antibodies[65,71] (Figs. 19.14 and 19.15).

Nuclear size may also help in identification. Spermatogonia (very rarely seen in semen) have a nucleus of approximately 8µm, spermatocytes have a nucleus of approximately 10 µm, and spermatids have a nucleus of approximately 5 µm. These sizes are only guidelines, since degeneration and division affect the size of the nucleus (Fig 19.14).

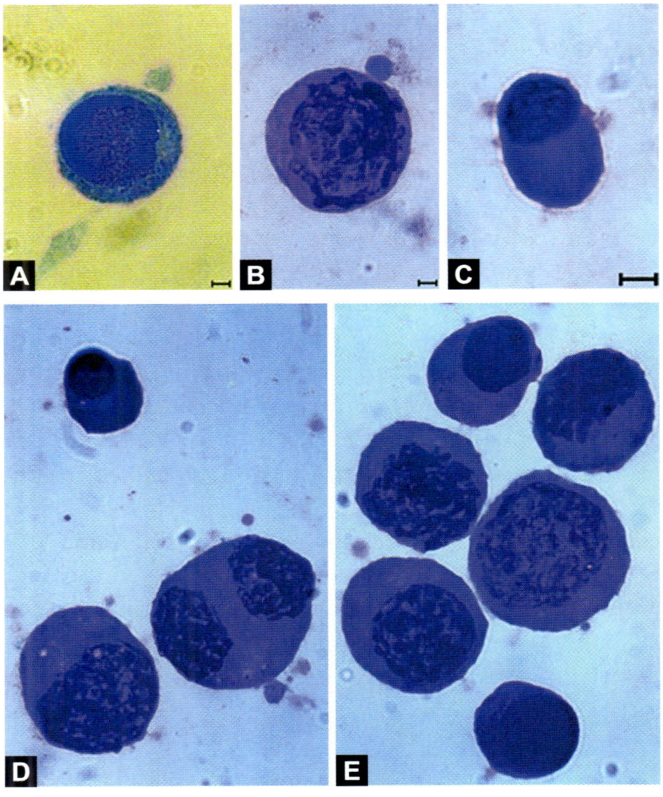

Figs. 19.14A to E: Immature germ cells isolated by semen using Percoll gradient, May–Grünwald–Giemsa staining: (A) spermatogonia; (B) primary spermatocyte; (C) spermatid; (D) primary spermatocyte, primary spermatocyte in meiotic division, spermatid; (E) group of spermatocytes and spermatids. Scale bars = 1 µm. https //www.researchgate.net/figure/30939046_Figure-1-Immature-germ-cells-isolated-by-semen-using-Percoll-gradient-May-Gruenwald-Giemsa-stain.

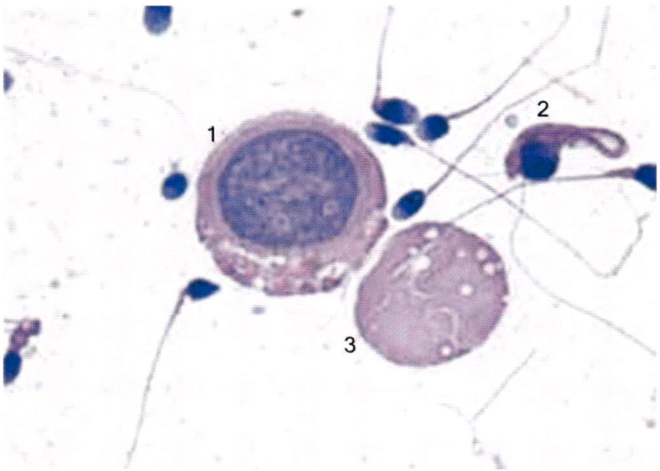

Fig. 19.15: (1) Macrophage; (2) Abnormal spermatozoon; (3) Cytoplasm.
Microphotograph by C Brazil: WHO Manual for Laboratory examination & procedures of Semen Analysis Ed. V; 2010: page 96.

Antisperm Antibody

If spermatozoa demonstrate agglutination (i.e., motile spermatozoa stick to each other head-to-head, tail-to-tail or in a mixed way), the presence of sperm antibodies may be the cause. Sperm antibodies can be present without sperm agglutination; equally, agglutination can be caused by factors others than sperm antibodies. The mere presence of sperm antibodies is insufficient for a diagnosis of sperm autoimmunity. It is necessary to demonstrate that the antibodies interfere severely with sperm function; this is usually done by a sperm–mucus penetration test. Antibodies can also interfere with zona binding and the acrosome reaction.

Anti-sperm antibodies (ASAs) in semen belong almost exclusively to two immunoglobulin classes: IgA and IgG. IgM antibodies, because of their larger size, are rarely found in semen. IgA antibodies may have greater clinical importance than IgG antibodies.[72] Both classes can be detected on sperm cells or in biological fluids in related screening tests.

Mixed Antiglobulin Reaction Test

The mixed antiglobulin reaction (MAR) test is an inexpensive, quick and sensitive screening test,[73] but it provides less information than the direct immunobead test.

In the MAR test, a "bridging" antibody (anti-IgG or anti-IgA) is used to bring the antibody-coated beads into contact with unwashed spermatozoa in semen bearing surface IgG or IgA. The direct IgG and IgA MAR tests are performed by mixing fresh, untreated semen separately with latex particles (beads) or treated red blood cells coated with human IgG or IgA. To the suspensions is added a monospecific antihuman-IgG or antihuman-IgA. The formation of mixed agglutinates between particles and motile spermatozoa indicates the presence of IgG or IgA antibodies on the spermatozoa. (Agglutination between beads serves as a positive control for antibody–antigen recognition.)

If spermatozoa have antibodies on their surface, the latex beads will adhere to them. The motile spermatozoa will initially be seen moving around with a few or even a group of particles attached. Eventually the agglutinates become so massive that the movement of the spermatozoa is severely restricted. Sperm that do not have coating antibodies will be seen swimming freely between the particles.

The goal of the assay is to determine the percentage of motile spermatozoa that have beads attached to them. A common problem occurs with NP spermatozoa that are close to beads, but are not attached. Whether the beads are bound can often be verified by lightly tapping the coverslip with a small pipette tip: the movement of beads in concert with active spermatozoa is indicative of positive binding.

There are currently no reference values for antibody-bound spermatozoa in the MAR test of semen from fertile men. Pending additional evidence, the WHO (2010) manual retains the consensus value of 50% motile spermatozoa with adherent particles as a threshold value.

Sperm penetration into the cervical mucus and *in vivo* fertilization tend to be significantly impaired when 50% or more of the motile spermatozoa have antibody bound to them.[74] Particle binding restricted to the tail tip is not associated with impaired fertility and can be present in fertile men.[75]

Direct Immunobead Test

This assay is more time-consuming than the MAR test but provides information about antibodies on spermatozoa that have been removed from possible masking components in seminal plasma.

In the direct immunobead (IB) test, beads coated with covalently bound rabbit anti-human immunoglobulins against IgG or IgA are mixed directly with washed spermatozoa. The binding of beads with anti-human IgG or IgA to motile spermatozoa indicates the presence of IgG or IgA antibodies on the surface of the spermatozoa.

There are currently no reference values for antibody-bound spermatozoa in the IB test of semen from fertile men. Therefore, like for MAR test, the consensus value of 50% motile spermatozoa with adherent particles is considered as a threshold value.

The diagnosis of immunological infertility is made when 50% or more of the motile spermatozoa (progressive and nonprogressive) have adherent particles.[76] Particle binding restricted to the tail tip is not associated with impaired fertility and can be present in fertile men.[75]

Limitations

Results are based on the analysis of motile sperm. Samples made using sperm with poor motility may give false-negative results. A positive finding of more than 50% of motile sperm with attached beads is considered to be clinically significant.

Semen Microbiology and Virology

Infection of the male reproductive tract can directly or indirectly cause infertility.[77] Inflammation caused by infection or various disorders can affect the secretary function of both the prostate and seminal vesicles. Asymptomatic infections of the prostate can cause partial or complete obstruction of the ejaculatory duct resulting in oligozoospermia or even azoospermia. Infection of the seminal vesicle often cause substantial reduction in ejaculate volume and a low seminal fructose concentration. Microbiological examination of the semen is required to differentiate a specific microbiological-induced pyospermia form other abnormalities that cause an increase in leukocytes.

Pyospermia

It's a laboratory finding categorized as abnormal presence of leukocytes in human semen ejaculate. When seminal concentration of WBCs is in the range between 5×10^5 / mL and 5×10^6 seminal fluid. Numerous studies have demonstrated that leukocytes in ejaculate have a physiological effect on sperm function, which may further impact male infertility.

The differential diagnosis of symptomatic pyospermia includes infection, autoimmune disease, and inflammation of the accessory sex glands and the lower male urogenital tract. Urogenital infections include acute and chronic prostatis, seminal vesicultis, epidydimo-orchitis, cystistis, urethritis, urethral stricture, stone disease, foreign bodies, upper urinary tract infections, retrograde ejaculation, and localized sepsis of the adjacent lower gastrointestinal tract and asymptomatic bacteriurea. Chronic infections that may result in pyospermia include fungal, mycobacterial, and congenital lesions that cause urogenital tract infection.

Organisms Found in Semen

Many organisms found in semen are actually contaminants from the patient's skin or from the air at the time of collection. Not all are associated with pyospermia. Hence, caution must be taken to interpret the positive cultures.

Ureaplasma and Mycoplasma

These species are common commensal inhabitants of the lower genitourinary tract in adolescents and adult men and women who are sexually active. The organisms can be transmitted venereal and vertically from mother to offspring. *Ureaplasma urealyticum* and to a lesser extent *Mycoplasma hominis* are therefore often found in semen of infertile patients. *Ureaplasma urealyticum* is part of the normal genital flora of both men and women and is found in about 70% of sexually active humans. Their presence is abnormal, and most authorities agree that the infection must be treated with antibiotics.

Chlamydia trachomatis

Chlamydia trachomatis is occasionally present in human semen. It is the cause of the most prevalent sexually transmitted bacterial disease worldwide and is responsible for an estimated 90 million infections. Considering the high prevalence *C. trachomatis* infection, artificial insemination using donor sperm is a potential route for the spread of *C. trachomatis* and has been reported as such. It cannot be cultured, since seminal plasma factor is toxic to the cell lines used for the culture. Treatment must extend to both the partners.

Neisseria gonorrhoeae

This organism causes severe symptoms in men. It can be identified in semen as gram-negative intracellular diplococci. Transmission is through sexual intercourse as well.

Trachomonas vaginalis and Escherichia coli

In men with urinary tract infections, *E. coli* can colonize the prostate and cause production of IgA leading to sperm agglutination. Other organism that form the normal flora of the reproductive tract may commonly be present, these include enterococci such as *Streptococcus faecalis* and staphylococci such as *Staphylococcus epidermidis*. Mycobacterium tuberculosis may be present in the absence of pyospermia.

Viruses

Many viruses can be isolated from semen, but the most important is human immunodeficiency virus (HIV). Its presence can be detected by either culture or polymerase chain reaction. Other viruses that could be present in semen are human T-cell lymphotrophic virus type I (HTLV-I), hepatitis B, hepatitis C, cytomegalovirus (CMV) and human papilloma virus (HPV). Gental herpes virus often is isolated from semen in infected patients.

Biochemical Assessment of Seminal Plasma, Prostate, Epididymis and Seminal Vesicles

The prostate, seminal vesicles, and epididymis produce components such as zinc, citric acid and α-glucosidase that are uniquely specific to each accessory gland.

Measurement of Zinc

A kit for measurement of serum zinc by spectrophotometric assay is commercially available and can be adapted for semen. The method described[78] below is modified for the use of a 96-well plate reader with sensitivity 4 µmol/L. The volumes of semen and reagents can be proportionally adjusted for spectrophotometers using 3- or 1-mL cuvettes. The appropriate corrections must be made in calculating the results.

Reagents:

1. Zinc kit: Chromogen solution is prepared by mixing color reagents A and B in 4:1 proportion. It is stable for 1 week at 4°C.
2. Zinc standard: 0.1 mM

Specimens:

1. Centrifuge semen at 1,000 g for 15 minutes. A 100 µL of semen is centrifuged to obtain 10 µL of neat seminal plasma.
2. A 10 µL aliquot of cell-free seminal plasma is diluted with 600 µL of water.

Procedure:

1. Set absorbance readings on the spectrophotometer to 560 nm, and allow adequate time for stabilization.
2. Prepare a standard curve in duplicate (100 µM diluted to give 80, 60, 40, 20, and 10 µM).
3. Set the spectrophotometer to zero with a cuvette containing reagent water.
4. Add 2.5 mL working chromogen solution (mix four parts of color reagent A with one part of color reagent B). Add 20 µL of color reagent to 40 µL of diluted semen samples, standard, and blank.
5. Leave at room temperature for 5 minutes.
6. Measure absorbance at 560 nm and calculate results.
7. Calculation: Multiply by dilution factor to obtain the concentration of zinc (mM) in undiluted seminal plasma. Multiply by ejaculate volume to obtain µmol/ejaculate.

Results: Zinc is a specific marker of prostate function. Normal range of seminal zinc is 1.2–3.8 mmol/L or more than 2.4 µmol per ejaculate.

Measurement of Citric Acid in Seminal Plasma

Citric acid is an indicator of prostatic gland function. Decreased citric acid levels may indicate either prostate dysfunction or prostatic duct obstruction. It can be measured using Boehringer Enzymatic, NADH-linked kit.

Reagents

1. *Boehringer Lit no. 130976:* Contains solution 1.3 × bottle 1 (mainly NADH), which is reconstituted by adding 12 mL reagent water and shaking well. 3 × bottle 2 (citrate-lyase), reconstituted by adding 0.3 mL reagent water and shaking well.
2. *Triethanolamine buffer (pH 7.7)*: Prepared by dissolving 14.9 g triethanolamine in 750 mL reagent water and adjusting the pH to 7.6 by adding 1N HCl. Dissolve 0.027 g $ZnCl_2$ in 250 mL reagent water and add it to the triethanolamine solution. Add 0.5 g of sodium azide and mix thoroughly.
3. *Trichloroacetic acid (TCA, 15%):* Dissolve 15 g of trichloroacetic acid in 100 mL reagent water.
4. *NaOH (6 N):* Dissolve 24 g NaOH pellets dissolved in 100 mL reagent water.
5. *Citric acid standard:* 0.174 g citric acid in 10 mL reagent water. Make a 1 + 57 dilution.

Specimens

1. Centrifuge 250 µL liquefied semen (cell and protein free) in an Eppendorf tube at 1,000 g for 15 minutes.
2. Add 100 µL of supernatant to 4.95 mL of 15% TCA in a small, capped vial and shake well.

3. Add 0.75 mL NaOH (6 N) and adjust the pH to 7.0.
4. Freeze three 0.5 mL aliquots of the extract in Eppendorf tubes at −20°C

Procedure

1. Set the spectrophotometer to 340 nm and allow adequate time for stabilization.
2. Mix 0.5 mL of solution 1, 2.3 mL TRA buffer and 0.2 mL sample, standard, or blank in a disposable cuvette. Prepare each set in duplicate.
3. Adjust the spectrophotometer reading to zero with a cuvette containing reagent water.
4. Measure initial absorbance (A1).
5. Add 20 μL of solution 2. Shake it well, wait exactly 5 minutes, and measure the absorbance again (A2).
6. Calculate and analyze the results according to the formula: $\Delta A \times (V \div V) \times DF \times MW \div E \div D + 100 = g/L$, where DF is the specimen dilution factor, V is the final volume (3.02 mL), MW is the molecular weight of the substance analyzed (192.1), E is the absorption coefficient of NADH at 340 nm (6.3 $cm^3/\mu mol$), V is the sample volume (0.2 mL) and $\Delta A \times 139.0$ is mmol citric acid/L

Results

The normal range of seminal plasma citric acid concentration is 9.4–43.4 mmol/L or 52 μmol per ejaculate. Decreased levels of citric acid may indicate either prostatic dysfunction or duct obstruction. Further evaluation must be done by a clinician.

Measurement of Neutral α-Glucosidase in Seminal Plasma

Seminal plasma contains both a neutral α-glucosidase isoenzyme, which originates in the epididymis, and an acid isoenzyme contributed by the prostate. The latter can be selectively inhibited by sodium dodecyl sulfate (SDS) to permit measurement of the neutral glucosidase, which reflects epididymal function. Accounting for nonglucosidase-related substrate breakdown, by using the inhibitor castanospermine, makes the assay more sensitive. The method described below is for use with a 96-well plate reader with sensitivity 1.9 mU/mL. The volumes of semen and reagents can be proportionally adjusted for spectrophotometers with 3- or 1-mL cuvettes. The appropriate corrections must be made in calculating the results.

Reagents

A kit for the estimation of epididymal neutral α-glucosidase in semen is commercially available. Only kits including SDS and castanospermine are recommended for measurement of this enzyme in semen. Alternatively, prepare the following reagents:

1. Buffer 1 (0.2 mol/L phosphate, pH 6.8): dissolve 4.56 g $K_2HPO_4.3H_2O$ in 100 mL of purified water. Dissolve 2.72 g of KH_2PO_4 in a separate 100 mL aliquot of purified water. Mix approximately equal volumes of each until the pH is 6.8.
2. Buffer 2: dissolve 1 g of SDS in 100 mL of buffer 1. SDS will precipitate on storage at 4°C, but redissolves on gentle warming.
3. Color reagent 1 (for stopping the reaction, 0.1 mol/L sodium carbonate): dissolve 6.20 g of $Na_2CO_3.H_2O$ in 500 mL of water.
4. Color reagent 2: dissolve 0.1 g of SDS in 100 mL of color reagent 1.
5. Substrate *p*-nitrophenol glucopyranoside (PNPG) (5 mg/mL): dissolve 0.1 g of PNPG in 20 mL of buffer 2 and warm the solution on a hotplate at about 50°C with stirring for about 10 minutes. A few crystals may remain undissolved. The solution should be kept at 37°C during use. Make a fresh solution for each assay.
6. Glucosidase inhibitor for semen blanks (castanospermine, 10 mmol/L): dissolve 18.9 mg of castanospermine in 10 mL of purified water. Dilute this 10-fold in purified water to give a 1 mmol/L working solution. Freeze approximately 1-mL aliquots at −20°C.
7. Standard curve of product *p*-nitrophenol (PNP) (5 mmol/L): dissolve 69.5 mg of PNP in 100 mL of purified water, warming the solution if necessary. Store at 4°C in the dark in an aluminum foil-covered or brown glass bottle. Make up a fresh standard solution every 3 months.
8. Prepare a standard curve (within the last hour of incubation): place 400 μL of 5 mmol/L stock PNP in a 10-mL volumetric fl ask and make up to 10 mL with color reagent 2 (200 μmol/L). Dilute the 200 μmol/L standard with color reagent 2 to yield four additional standards of 160, 120, 80 and 40 μmol/L PNP.
9. Frozen internal quality control pools of seminal plasma (step 1).

Procedure I

1. Buffer 1 (0.2 mol/L phosphate, pH 6.8): Dissolve 4.56 g $K_2HPO_4{\cdot}3H_2O$ in 100 mL of purified water.

Dissolve 2.72 g of KH_2PO_4 in a separate 100 mL aliquot of purified water. Mix approximately equal volumes of each until the pH is 6.8.

2. Buffer 2: dissolve 1 g of SDS in 100 mL of buffer 1. SDS will precipitate on storage at 4°C, but redissolves on gentle warming.
3. Color reagent 1 (for stopping the reaction, 0.1 mol/L sodium carbonate): dissolve 6.20 g of $Na_2CO_3{\cdot}H_2O$ in 500 mL of water.
4. Color reagent 2: dissolve 0.1 g of SDS in 100 mL of color reagent 1.
5. Substrate *p*-nitrophenol glucopyranoside (PNPG) (5 mg/mL): dissolve 0.1 g of PNPG in 20 mL of buffer 2 and warm the solution on a hotplate at about 50°C with stirring for about 10 minutes. A few crystals may remain undissolved. The solution should be kept at 37°C during use. Make a fresh solution for each assay.
6. Glucosidase inhibitor for semen blanks (castanospermine, 10 mmol/L): dissolve 18.9 mg of castanospermine in 10 mL of purified water. Dilute this 10-fold in purified water to give a 1 mmol/L working solution. Freeze approximately 1-mL aliquots at –20°C.
7. Standard curve of product p-nitrophenol (PNP) (5 mmol/L): dissolve 69.5 mg of PNP in 100 mL of purified water, warming the solution if necessary. Store at 4°C in the dark in an aluminum foil-covered or brown glass bottle. Make up a fresh standard solution every 3 months.
8. Prepare a standard curve (within the last hour of incubation): place 400 μL of 5 mmol/L stock PNP in a 10-mL volumetric flask and make up to 10 mL with color reagent 2 (200 μmol/L). Dilute the 200 μmol/L standard with color reagent 2 to yield four additional standards of 160, 120, 80, and 40 μmol/L PNP.
9. Frozen internal quality control pools of seminal plasma.

Procedure II

1. Centrifuge the semen sample remaining after analysis for 10 minutes at 1,000 g. Decant and store the sperm-free seminal plasma at –20°C until analysis. Sperm-free seminal plasma can be pooled with other samples to provide a quality control pool as an internal standard for future assays.
2. Thaw the sperm-free seminal plasma and mix well on a vortex mixer. Also thaw and mix an aliquot of pooled seminal plasma for internal quality control.
3. Place replicate samples of 15 μL of seminal plasma in each of two 1.5-mL tubes using a positive displacement pipette. Include replicate blanks (15 μL of water) and quadruplicate 15-μL internal quality control samples from semen pools.
4. To two of the internal quality control samples add 8 μL of 1 mmol/L castanospermine to provide the seminal plasma blank value.
5. Add 100 μL of PNPG substrate solution, at about 37°C, to each tube.
6. Vortex each tube and incubate at 37°C for 2 hours (exact temperature and time control are crucial).
7. Stop incubation after 2 hours by adding 1 mL of color reagent 1 and mix.
8. Transfer 250 μL of samples and standards to the 96-well plate.
9. Read the plate in a 96-well plate reader at 405 nm wavelength within 60 minutes, using the water blank to set the zero.

Calculation

1. Read the concentration of PNP produced by the sample from the standard curve (μmol/L) by comparing absorbance values.
2. Reject samples that lie above the top standard and reassay these samples after dilution (use buffer 1 to dilute).
3. Multiply by the correction factor (0.6194; see note) to obtain the activity of neutral glucosidase in undiluted seminal plasma (IU/L).
4. Subtract the activity (IU/L) of the castanospermine seminal plasma blank from each sample to obtain the corrected (glucosidase-related) activity.
5. Replicates should agree within 10%, i.e. difference between estimates/mean of estimates, 100 ≤10%. If they do not, repeat the assay on two new aliquots of seminal plasma.
6. Multiply the corrected glucosidase activity by the whole volume of semen (mL) to obtain the glucosidase activity (mU) of the ejaculate.

One international unit (IU) of glucosidase activity is defined as the production of 1 μmol of product (PNP) per minute at 37°C. In this assay the activity is derived from 15 μL of seminal plasma in a total volume of 1.115 μL over 120 minutes, so the correction factor is (1115/15)/120 = 0.6194.

Reference Limit

The lower reference limit for neutral α-glucosidase is 20 mU per ejaculate

Quantitative Seminal Fructose

Sperm in semen sample are lysed, and addition of resorcinol and subsequent heating at 70°C results in a salmon-pink color, which is read at 420 nm.

Reagents

1. Concentrated HCl;
2. Deionized water;
3. Fructose (0.32 mmol/L). Add 14.4 g of fructose to make 250 mL of deionized water (5.56 mg/dL);
4. Resorcinol 0.05%. Add 25 mg of resorcinol to 50 mL of ethanol (95%).

Freeze three aliquots (150 μL) in 1.5 mL Eppendorf tubes at –20°C.

Procedure

1. Turn on the 77°C water bath.
2. Set spectrophotometer absorbance at 420 nm.
3. Adjust the reading to zero with cuvette containing reagent water.
4. Label three beakers for patient, positive control (pooled seminal plasma from normal donors) and negative controls (no semen added).
5. Treat with acid: To a clean beaker add 7.5 mL of deionized water + 2.5 mL of HCl and 50 μL of semen or seminal plasma. Mix each patient and control sample carefully (200 times dilution).
6. Label beaker for each patient and control. Using a Whatman no. 1 filter paper, filter each patient and control mixture into appropriately labeled beaker.
7. Label in duplicate 13 × 100 mm glass tubes for each standard, control and patient sample. Add the following to appropriate tube.
8. Mix the tubes carefully and add 3.0 mL of conc. HCl to each tube under the fume hood. Mix carefully.
9. Add 1.9 mL of 0.05% resorcinol to each tube, cap and vortex carefully.
10. Place the tubes in the ice bath. Cool to room temperature. Transfer to disposable cuvettes and read the tubes at 420 nm.
11. Calculate the average OD from the standard. Multiply by dilution (200) to obtain the final results in mg/dL.

Reference Limit

Fructose is a marker for seminal vesicle function. Normal range for seminal fructose is more than 150 mg/dL.

Safety and Quality Control in the Andrology Laboratory

All general safety precautions related to electrical or chemical hazards, compressed gases, fire and physical injury must be observed in the laboratory. Safety precautions must be exercised when handling biological specimens in the laboratory. All semen samples must be treated as biological hazard, and extreme caution should be exercised. This includes use of protective clothing, eye protection, use of safety gloves, and any other protective measures necessary.

Strict quality control and appropriate training of technical staff performing semen analysis and other laboratory procedures are important. All andrology technicians must be periodically trained to ensure uniformity, accuracy and reproducibility, especially in sperm count, motility and sperm morphology. Internal quality controls, proficiency testing of slides for viability and morphology both by WHO and Kruger's strict criteria are available, and laboratories can enroll in a proficiency-testing program. Technicians score the slides in a blind fashion, and the results are mailed to the proficiency testing program. Adequate remedial measures should be in place to minimize inter- and intraobserver variations. In addition, strict quality control for monitoring all equipment in use is critical, and all solutions and reagents must be subjected to strict quality control measures to optimize performance and accuracy of results.

Semen Analysis: The Future

As can be gleaned from this discussion and the literature, some of the difficulty with ensuring that semen analysis reports are reliable and consist of meaningful data is adherence to standardized protocols for testing that aim to generate such data. An example was put forth earlier regarding automated analysis for hormone testing. Although there is still some variation, e.g., due to instrumentation, the points for variance are decreased by the removal of aspects of human intervention and observation. This is why, in some ways, the manually performed semen analysis is archaic. The level of scientific technology available today urges that the way in which the semen analysis is performed be modernized. A number of years ago computer-assisted sperm analyzers were introduced and there was a feeling of anticipation that these new instruments would advance the way in which semen analysis was performed. For numerous reasons this potential was only partially realized. Therefore, what current technologies are available that might offer not only the fidelity that automated analyzers afford but also the ability to integrate tests of sperm function into the same platform? Imagine a semen analysis either with the most up to date accessories or as a completely new model.

REFERENCES

1. World Health Organization. WHO Laboratory Manual for the Examination of Human Semen and Sperm-Cervical Mucus Interaction, 1st edition. Singapore: Press Concern; 1980.
2. World Health Organization. WHO Laboratory Manual for the Examination of Human Semen and Sperm-Cervical Mucus Interaction, 2nd edition. Cambridge: Cambridge University Press; 1987.
3. World Health Organization. WHO Laboratory Manual for the Examination of Human Semen and Sperm-Cervical Mucus Interaction, 3rd edition. Cambridge: Cambridge University Press; 1992.
4. World Health Organization. WHO Laboratory Manual for the Examination of Human Semen and Sperm-Cervical Mucus Interaction, 4th edition. Cambridge: Cambridge University Press; 1999.
5. World Health Organization. WHO Laboratory Manual for the Examination and Processing of Human Semen, 5th edition. Geneva: World Health Organization; 2010.
6. Björndahl L, Kvist U. Sequence of ejaculation affects the spermatozoon as a carrier and its message. Reprod Biomed Online. 2003;7:440-8.
7. Cooper TG. Cytoplasmic droplets: the good, the bad or just confusing? Hum Reprod. 2005;20:9-11.
8. Ng KK, Donat R, Chan L, Lalak L, Di Pierro I, Handelsman D.J. Sperm output of older men. Hum Reprod. 2004;19:1811-5.
9. De Jonge C, LaFromboise M, Bosmans E, Ombelet W, Cox A, Nijs M. Influence of the abstinence period on human sperm quality. Fertil Steril. 2004;82:57-65.
10. Tyler JP, Crockett NG, Driscoll GL. Studies of human seminal parameters with frequent ejaculation II. Spermatozoal vitality and storage. Clin Reprod Fertil. 1982;1:287-93.
11. Correa-Perez JR, Fernández-Pelegrina R, Aslanis P, Zavos PM. Clinical management of men producing ejaculates characterized by high levels of dead sperm and altered seminal plasma factors consistent with epididymal necrospermia. Fertil Steril. 2004;81:1148-50.
12. Cooper TG, Keck C, Oberdieck U, Nieschlag E.. Effects of multiple ejaculations after extended periods of sexual abstinence on total, motile and normal sperm numbers, as well as accessory gland secretions, from healthy normal and oligozoospermic men. Hum Reprod. 1993;8:1251-8.
13. Tyler JP, Crockett NG, Driscoll GL. Studies of human seminal parameters with frequent ejaculation. I. Clinical characteristics. Clin Reprod Fertil. 1982;1:273-85.
14. Holstein AF, Schulze W, Davidoff M. Understanding spermatogenesis is a prerequisite for treatment. Reprod Biol Endocrinol. 2003;1:107.
15. Handelsman DJ, Conway AJ, Boylan LM, Turtle JR. Testicular function in potential sperm donors: normal ranges and the effects of smoking and varicocele. Int J Androl. 1984;7: 369-82.
16. Behre HM, Yeung CH, Holstein AF, Weinbauer GF, Gassner P, Nieschlag E. Diagnosis of male infertility and hypogonadism. In: Nieschlag E, Behre HM (Eds). Andrology, Male Reproductive Health and Dysfunction. Berlin: Springer; 2000. p. 92.
17. Andersen AG, Jensen TK, Carlsen E, Jørgensen N, Andersson AM, Krarup T, et al. High frequency of sub-optimal semen quality in an unselected population of young men. Hum Reprod. 2000;15:366-72.
18. Baker HW, Kovacs GT. Spontaneous improvement in semen quality: regression towards the mean. Int J Androl. 1985;8:421-6.
19. Alvarez C, Castilla JA, Martínez L, Ramírez JP, Vergara F, Gaforio JJ (). Biological variation of seminal parameters in healthy subjects. Hum Reprod. 2003;18:2082-8.
20. Zavos PM, Goodpasture JC. Clinical improvements of specific seminal deficiencies via intercourse with a seminal collection device versus masturbation. Fertil Steril. 1989;51:190-3.
21. de la Taille A, Rigot A, Mahe A, Gervais A, Dumur A, Lemaitre A, et al. Correlation of genitourinary abnormalities, spermiogram and CFTR genotype in patients with bilateral agenesis of the vas deferens. Progress Urol. 1998;8:370-6.
22. Daudin M, Bieth E, Bujan L, Massat G, Pontonnier F, Mieusset R. Congenital bilateral absence of the vas deferens: clinical characteristics, biological parameters, cystic fibrosis transmembrane conductance regulator gene mutations, and implications for genetic counseling. Fertil Steril. 2000;74:1164-74.
23. von Eckardstein S, Cooper TG, Rutscha K, Meschede D, Horst J, Nieschlag E. Seminal plasma characteristics as indicators of cystic fibrosis transmembrane conductance regulator (CFTR) gene mutations in men with obstructive azoospermia. Fertil Steril. 2000;73:1226-31.
24. Weiske WH, Sälzler N, Schroeder-Printzen I, Weidner W. Clinical findings in congenital absence of the vasa deferentia. Andrologia. 2000;32:13-8.
25. Le Lannou D, Griveau JF, Le Pichon JP, Quero JC. Effects of chamber depth on the motion pattern of human spermatozoa in semen or in capacitating medium. Hum Reprod. 1992;7:1417-21.
26. Kraemer M, Fillion C, Martin-Pont B, Auger J. Factors influencing human sperm kinematic measurements by the Celltrak computer-assisted sperm analysis system. Hum Reprod. 1998;13:611-9.
27. Rose NR, Hjort T, Rümke P, Harper MJK, Vyazov O. Techniques for detection of iso- and auto-antibodies to human spermatozoa. Clin Experiment Immunol. 1976;23:175-99.
28. Jouannet P, Ducot B, Feneux D, Spira A. Male factors and the likelihood of pregnancy in infertile couples. I. Study of sperm characteristics. Int J Androl. 1988;11:379-94.
29. Larsen L, Scheike T, Jensen TK, Bonde JP, Ernst E, Hjollund NH, et al. Computer-assisted semen analysis parameters

as predictors for fertility of men from the general population. The Danish First Pregnancy Planner Study team. Hum Reprod. 2000;15:1562-7.
30. Zinaman MJ, Brown CC, Selevan SG, Clegg ED. Semen quality and human fertility: a prospective study with healthy couples. J Androl. 2000;21:145-53.
31. Chemes HE, Rawe YV. Sperm pathology: a step beyond descriptive morphology. Origin, characterization and fertility potential of abnormal sperm phenotypes in infertile men. Hum Reprod Update. 2003;9:405-28.
32. Wilton LJ, Temple-Smith PD, Baker HW, de Kretser DM. Human male infertility caused by degeneration and death of sperms in the epididymis. Fertil Steril. 1988;49: 1051-8.
33. Jeyendran RS, Van der Ven HH, Perez-Pelaez M, Crabo BG, Zaneveld LJ. Development of an assay to assess the functional integrity of the human sperm membrane and its relationship to the other semen characteristics. J Reprod Fertil. 1984;70:219-28.
34. Hossain AM, Rizk B, Barik S, Huff C, Thorneycroft IH. Time course of hypo-osmotic swellings of human spermatozoa: evidence of ordered transition between swelling subtypes. Hum Reprod. 1998;13:1578-83.
35. Carreras A, Ramirez JP, Mendoza C. Sperm plasma membrane integrity measurement: a combined method. Andrologia. 1992;24:335-40.
36. Slama R, Eustache F, Ducot B, Jensen TK, Jørgensen N, Horte A, et al. Time to pregnancy and semen parameters: a cross-sectional study among fertile couples from four European cities. Hum Reprod. 2002;17:503-15.
37. Bonde JP, Ernst E, Jensen TK, Hjollund NH, Kolstad H, Henriksen TB, et al. Relation between semen quality and fertility: a population based study of 430 first-pregnancy planners. Lancet. 1998;352:1172-7.
38. MacLeod J, Wang Y. Male fertility potential in terms of semen quality: a review of the past, a study of the present. Fertil Steril. 1979;31:103-16.
39. Eliasson R. Analysis of semen. In: Behrman SJ, Kistner RW (Eds). Progress in Infertility, 2nd edition. New York: Little, Brown; 1975. pp. 691-713.
40. Seaman EK, Goluboff E, BarChama N, Fisch H. Accuracy of semen counting chambers as determined by the use of latex beads. Fertil Steril. 1996;66:662-5.
41. Mahmoud AM, Depoorter B, Piens N, Comhaire FH. The performance of 10 different methods for the estimation of sperm concentration. Fertil Steril. 1997;68:340-5.
42. Brazil C, Swan SH, Tollner CR, Treece C, Drobnis EZ, Wang C, et al. Quality control of laboratory methods for semen evaluation in a multicenter research study. J Androl. 2004;25:645-56.
43. Douglas-Hamilton DH, Smith NG, Kuster CE, Vermeiden JP, Althouse GC. Particle distribution in low-volume capillary-loaded chambers. J Androl. 2005;26:107-14.
44. Douglas-Hamilton DH, Smith NG, Kuster CE, Vermeiden JP, Althouse GC. Capillary-loaded particle fluid dynamics: effect on estimation of sperm concentration. J Androl. 2005;26:115-22.
45. Björndahl L, Barratt CL. Semen analysis: setting standards for the measurement of sperm numbers. J Androl. 2005;26:11.
46. Sharif K. Re classification of azoospermia: the time has come? Hum Reprod. 2000;15:237-8.
47. Ezeh UI, Moore HM. Redefining azoospermia and its implications. Fertil Steril. 2001;75:213-4.
48. Eliasson R. Analysis of semen. In: Burger H, de Kretser D (Eds). The Testis. New York: Raven Press; 1981. pp. 381-99.
49. Lindsay KS, Floyd I, Swan R. Classification of a zoospermic samples. Lancet. 1995;345:1642.
50. Jaffe TM, Kim ED, Hoekstra TH, Lipshultz LI. Sperm pellet analysis: a technique to detect the presence of sperm in men considered to have a zoospermia by routine semen analysis. J Urol. 1998;159:1548-50.
51. Corea M, Campagnone J, Sigman M. The diagnosis of azoospermia depends on the force of centrifugation. Fertil Steril. 2005;83:920-2.
52. Mortimer D. Practical Laboratory Andrology. Oxford: Oxford University Press; 1994.
53. Cooper TG, Yeung CH. Computer-aided evaluation of assessment of "grade a" spermatozoa by experienced technicians. Fertil Steril. 2006;85:220-4.
54. Menkveld R, Wong WY, Lombard CJ, Wetzels AM, Thomas CM, Merkus HM, et al. Semen parameters, including WHO and strict criteria morphology, in a fertile and subfertile population: an effort towards standardization of in-vivo thresholds. Hum Reprod. 2001;16:1165-71.
55. Mortimer D, Menkveld R. Sperm morphology assessment—historical perspectives and current opinions. J Androl. 2001;22:192-205.
56. Gandini L, Lombardo F, Paoli D, Caponecchia L, Familiari G, Verlengia C, et al. Study of apoptotic DNA fragmentation in human spermatozoa. Hum Reprod. 2000;15:830-9.
57. Lee JD, Kamiguchi Y, Yanagimachi R. Analysis of chromosome constitution of human spermatozoa with normal and aberrant head morphologies after injection into mouse oocytes. Hum Reprod. 1996;11:1942-6.
58. Dadoune JP, Mayaux MJ, Guihard-Moscato ML. Correlation between defects in chromatin condensation of human spermatozoa stained by aniline blue and semen characteristics. Andrologia. 1988;20:211-7.
59. Devillard F, Metzler-Guillemain C, Pelletier R, DeRobertis C, Bergues U, Hennebicq S. Polyploidy in large-headed sperm: FISH study of three cases. Hum Reprod. 2002;17: 1292-8.
60. Martin RH, Rademaker AW, Greene C, Ko E, Hoang T, Barclay L, et al. A comparison of the frequency of sperm chromosome abnormalities in men with mild, moderate, and severe oligozoospermia. Biol Reprod. 2003;69:535-9.
61. Cooper TG, Barfield JP, Yeung CH. Changes in osmolality during liquefaction of human semen. Int J Androl. 2005;28: 58-60.
62. Tomlinson MJ, Barratt CL, Cooke ID. Prospective study of leukocytes and leukocyte subpopulations in semen suggests they are not a cause of male infertility. Fertil Steril. 1993;60:1069-75.

63. Johanisson E, et al. Evaluation of "round cells" in semen analysis: a comparative study. Hum Reprod Update. 2000;6:404-12.
64. Wolf DP. Semen cryopreservation. In: Keye WR et al. (Eds). Infertility Evaluation and Treatment. Philadelphia: WB Saunders; 1995. pp. 686-95.
65. Homyk M, Anderson DJ, Wolff H, Herr JC. Differential diagnosis of immature germ cells in semen utilizing monoclonal antibody MHS-10 to the intra-acrosomal antigen SP-10. Fertil Steril. 1990;53:323-30.
66. Eggert-Kruse W, Bellmann A, Rohr G, Tilgen W, Runnebaum B. Differentiation of round cells in semen by means ofmonoclonal antibodies and relationship with male fertility. Fertil Steril. 1992;58:1046-55.
67. Aitken RJ, Baker HW. Seminal leukocytes: passengers, terrorists or good Samaritans? Hum Reprod. 1995;10:1736-9.
68. Rossi AG, Aitken RJ. Interactions between leukocytes and the male reproductive system. The unanswered questions. Adv Experiment Med Biol. 1997;424:245-52.
69. Wolff H. The biologic significance of white blood cells in semen. Fertil Steril. 1995;63:1143-57.
70. Couture M, Ulstein M, Leonard J, Paulsen CA. Improved staining method for differentiating immature germ cells from white blood cells in human seminal fluid. Andrologia. 1976;8:61-6.
71. Ezeh UI, Martin M, Cooke ID, Moore HD. Correlation of testicular pathology and sperm extraction in azoospermic men with ejaculated spermatids detected by immunofluorescent localization. Hum Reprod. 1998;13:3061-5.
72. Kremer J, Jager S. Characteristics of anti-spermatozoal antibodies responsible for the shaking phenomenon, with special regard to immunoglobulin class and antigen reactive sites. Int J Androl. 1980;3:143-52.
73. Rajah SV, Parslow JM, Howell RJ, Hendry WF. Comparison of mixed antiglobulin reaction and direct immunobead test for detection of sperm-bound antibodies in subfertile males. Fertil Steril. 1992;57:1300-3.
74. Abshagen K, Behre HM, Cooper TG, Nieschlag E. Influence of sperm surface antibodies on spontaneous pregnancy rates. Fertil Steril. 1998;70:355-6.
75. Chiu WW, Chamley LW. Clinical associations and mechanisms of action of antisperm antibodies. Fertil Steril. 2004;82:529-35.
76. Barratt CLR, Dunphy BC, McLeod I, Cooke ID. The poor prognostic value of low to moderate levels of sperm surface-bound antibodies. Hum Reprod. 1992;7:95-8.
77. Mortimer D. Biochemistry of spermatozoa and seminal plasma. In: Practical Laboratory Andrology. Oxford: Oxford University Press; 1994. pp. 127-33.
78. Johnsen O, Eliasson R. Evaluation of a commercially available kit for the colorimetric determination of zinc in human seminal plasma. Int J Androl. 1987;10:435-40.

CHAPTER

Medical Management of Male Infertility

20

Chaitanya Nagori

INTRODUCTION

About 40–50% of infertility is partially or completely due to male factor. Though in today's era of *in vitro* fertilization (IVF) and intracytoplasmic sperm injection (ICSI), very little importance is given to its medical management. In India, majority of our patients cannot afford multiple attempts of IVF. They may with all difficulties manage one cycle, the success rate of which is barely 25–35%. If the amount that costs for one IVF/ICSI cycle is instead used for medical management of oligozoospermia, it will improve the sperm count permanently. This can give better pregnancy rates than a single IVF/ICSI cycle; moreover, can also give spontaneous pregnancies in future also. This is the reason why we insist on medical management of male subfertility as an important treatment option for couples with male factor infertility.

CRITERIA FOR MEDICAL MANAGEMENT IN MALE INFERTILITY

Semen analysis is still the gold standard for evaluation and management decision of infertile male. The normal semen parameters have been defined by world health organization (WHO) and are being revised from time to time.

These tables below present the normal semen parameters as defined by WHO in 1999 (Table 20.1) and in 2010 (Table 20.2). These tables clearly show that the parameters for normal semen analysis have changed over the years and according to 2010 WHO parameters it is claimed that with only 15 million/mL count, 30% motility and more than 4% normal sperms, spontaneous conceptions can occur. Sperm count, motility and normal sperm morphology, lower than these values mentioned above are considered abnormal. Low count is named as oligozoospermia and abnormal morphology named as asthenozoospermia. Depending on the severity of oligozoospermia, the treatment options for these subfertile males may vary. Mild oligozoospermia patients can be treated with IUI, moderate oligozoospermias with IVF and severe oligozoospermia patients may be treated with ICSI. (Table 20.3). The whole moto of medical management of a subfertile male is not to increase the sperm count 5–10 times or to achieve excellent semen parameters. The moto is to increase the count by a few million so that ICSI can be converted to IVF, IVF to intrauterine insemination (IUI) and perhaps IUI into natural conception.

Let us look into this case study which is an eye opener. It shows the importance and success of medical treatment of an infertile male and must be thought of before using high

Table 20.1: Normal reference values (WHO, 1999).

Volume	1.5–5 mL
pH	>7.2
Viscosity	<3 (scale 0–4)
Sperm concentration	>20 million/mL
Total sperm number	>40 million/ejaculate
Percent motility	>50%
Forward progression	>2 (scale 0–4)
Normal morphology	>14% normal
Round cells	<5 million/mL
Sperm agglutination	<2 (scale (0–3)

Table 20.2: Normal reference values (WHO, 2010).

Volume	1.5 mL
pH	7.2
Viscosity	<3 (scale 0–4)
Sperm concentration	15 million/mL
Total sperm number	39 million/ejaculate
Percent motility	40% total, 32% progressive
Forward progression	>2 (scale 0–4)
Vitality	58% sperms live/ejaculate
Normal morphology	>4% normal
Round cells	<5 million/mL
Sperm agglutination	<2 (scale 0–3)

Table 20.3: Mild, moderate, and severe oligozoospermia.

Normal count: >15 million/mL or 30 million/ejaculate
Mild oligospermia: 10–15 million/mL
Moderate oliogospermia: 5–10 million/mL
Severe oligospermia: <5 million/mL

end techniques for conception or after having failures with high end assisted reproductive technology (ART)—IVF-ICSI.

This was a case with 9 years of infertility that had undergone seven IVF/ICSI cycles and still had no success. The male was 32 years old and the female is 29 years old. Female factor was assessed and was normal. Husband's semen count was only 3 million/mL. He was evaluated for the hormones and varicocele and was all within limits. Instead of repeating another ICSI cycle, we considered treating the male medically considering this as a qualitative hormonal failure. The semen analysis was repeated at 3 and 6 months. At the sixth month, the sperm count reached 22 million/mL. And the couple conceived with timed intercourse. They had a second natural conception after 2 years.

MEDICAL TREATMENT OPTIONS FOR MALE INFERTILITY

1. Specific therapy
2. Empiric therapy

Specific Therapy

There is a definite cause of infertility and specific therapy should be given, which will be highly effective. This means the treatment is based on the cause of infertility.

Hypogonadotropic Hypogonadism

Estrogen is low because of low follicle stimulating hormone (FSH) and luteinizing hormone (LH). This is common in congenital Kallmann syndrome associated with anosmia, deafness, renal abnormalities and cleft palate. It may also be associated with trauma, tumor, panhypopituitarism, isolated gonadotropin deficiency, etc.

This can be treated by:

1. Clomiphene citrate
2. Gonadotropins

Clomiphene citrate (CC): It was a customary teaching that CC does not work in hypogonadotropic hypogonadism. But here are several recent papers that suggest that CC is very useful for spermatogenesis[1] in nonobstructive azoospermia and hypogonadotropic hypogonadism.[2] CC is an analog of nonsteroidal estrogen chlorotrianisene (TACE) and increases the serum gonadotropin levels. It became popular as a drug for subfertile males in 1977.[3]

The recommended dose is 25–75 mg on alternate days. The dose titration is done by morning serum testosterone estimation which should be between 600 and 800 ng/dL. This treatment is given for 3–9 months. In the same study, 64.3% patients showed sperms in ejaculate with mean density of 3.8 million/mL. In rest of the patients, sperms could be retrieved from testis.[1]

Gonadotropins: In patients with hypogonadotropic hypogonadism, follicle-stimulating hormone (FSH) and luteinizing hormone (LH) are very low and have to be supplied from outside. For initiation of spermatogenesis, testosterone is very useful. Therefore, human chorionic gonadotropin (hCG) in a dose of 2,000–3,000 iu twice a week or 5,000 iu every fifth day is given for 6–8 weeks till testosterone level comes to normal. Then, HMG/uFSH/rFSH 75 iu is added thrice a week. hCG is continued once a week but the dose may be adjusted if gynecomastia occurs.[4] We have found excellent results with this regime like other studies.[5]

Gonadotropin releasing hormone (GnRH) is a good alternative to hCG-HMG/FSH regime in hypogonadotropic hypogonadism, but its availability is still restricted. It is of no use in patients with disturbed spermatogenesis and high FSH.

Kallmann syndrome is also a type of hypogonadotropic hypogonadism, typically characterized by anosmia. It is commonly an X linked disease and is transmitted as autosomal dominant or recessive pattern. The therapy suggested in these cases is 2,000 iu of hCG sc thrice a week and if sperms are not present till 6 months of treatment, FSH therapy is started in the form of HMG 75 iu sc thrice weekly.[4] This therapy also is effective in only a small subgroup of patients with Kallmann syndrome as these patients have absent endogenous pulsatile gonadotropin release. GnRH infusion pumps may benefit these patients when GnRH is secreted in doses of 50 μg every 2 hours.

Hyperprolactinemia

Hyperprolactinemia (HPRL) leads to hypogonadism. In male, the commonest cause of increased prolactin is macroadenoma and it is to be surgically removed. Diagnosis is suspected with the history of loss of libido and pressure effects on optic chiasma and is confirmed by MRI.[6]

Macroadenomas (larger than 1 cm in diameter) show serum prolactin levels of more than 200 ng/mL.

But surgery should not be done for microadenoma. HPRL is between 100 and 200 μg/mL in these cases dopaminergic agonists such as bromocriptine or cabergoline is the treatment. Cabergoline is given 0.5—2 mg, in doses divided twice a week to maintain prolactin levels between 10 and 15 μg/mL. Cabergoline is found superior to bromocryptine.[6] Serum prolactin and testosterone levels are monitored every 6 months. Recently, this therapy is also tried in patients with macroadenomas.[7]

Genital Tract Infections

Chlamydia is most common and should be treated with doxycycline for 14 days. *Chlamydia* infections are often not diagnosed and therefore these patients may be thought of having unexplained infertility. *Chlamydia* leads to asthenospermia, by damaging the nuclear machinery of the sperms. In view of this, the evidence suggests that men with pyospermia, active urethral symptoms, or unexplained asthenospermia should be evaluated and if necessary treated for *Chlamydia*. In resistant cases, semen culture is done and treated accordingly. In patients with HIV wishing to become a father of a child, IUI is the treatment of choice. This has been discussed in Chapter 12 of this book.

Disorders of Ejaculation

Disorders of ejaculation has been discussed in detail in Chapter 24 of this book.

Immunological Causes

Nowadays, immunological cause in abnormal semen parameters is treated only with IUI. No steroids are given.[8]

Isolated Testosterone Deficiency

It is treated with hCG 2,000 iu, twice a week.

Congenital Adrenal Hyperplasia

This is treated with glucocorticoids-dexamethasone 0.5 mg at bedtime.

Empiric Therapy

Introduction

Empiric therapy is the treatment prior to final diagnosis, based on clinical concepts or theories without proven efficacy. About 25% of cases of male infertility are having idiopathic infertility. Empiric therapy is the only available form of treatment for them.[9,10] All proven drugs used now have been tried earlier as empiric drugs because when a new drug is tried there is no evidence base. Clinical trials are ahead of all evidence based medicine and this explains the place of empiric therapy in male infertility (Table 20.4).

Clomiphene Citrate

This is the cheapest available drug. It has been mentioned in the text book on infertility written by Insler, it has been mentioned that only a subgroup of patients is improved by CC therapy. But we do not know who all are in this subgroup and therefore this cheap, fairly safe drug can be tried in patients. It is given 12.5–25 mg for 25 days for 3–6 months.[3] He gave 40% pregnancy rate in a group of 32 subfertile men. The men with partial androgen resistance and mild hypogonadotropic hypogonadism are the best candidates to respond to this therapy.[11] Follow-up is done every month. This is especially required because an occasional patient may show worsening of the sperm count. Apart from semen analysis, FSH and testosterone are also monitored every month. The dose setting should be such that it should increase FSH and testosterone should be normal with drug. A study by Hussien et al. suggested considering a course of CC prior to sperm retrieval in patients with nonobstructive azoospermia.[1]

Men with either partial androgen sensitivity or mild hypogonadotropic hypogonadism may be the best candidates for this treatment.[11]

Table 20.4: List of drugs empirically used for male subfertility with the doses.

Drug	Dose
Clomiphene citrate	12.5–25 mg/day
hCG	2,000–5,000 iu twice a week
FSH	75 iu thrice a week + hCG 5,000 iu twice a week
Tamoxifen	40 mg + testosterone undeconate 120 mg daily
Zinc	100–200 mg bd
Ketotifen	1 mg bd
Cyproheptadine HCl	4 mg tds
Captopril	50 mg daily
Kallikrein	600 mg daily
Indomethacin	25 mg tds
Anastrazole	1 mg daily

Tamoxifen Citrate

First positive report after the use of tamoxifen in infertile male came in 1976.[12] This report showed 20% pregnancy rate in men with idiopathic oligospermia in the dose of 20 mg/day for 6–11 months. But no controlled studies reported a similar effect. A subgroup of patients in whom after tamoxifen therapy, there was no rise in FSH actually should improve sperm count.[13] Although a combination of tamoxifen citrate and testosterone undeconate has shown to have a significant improvement in the semen quality.[14] WHO recommends treatment with antiestrogens–tamoxifen for idiopathic oligozoospermia when motility and morphology are not significantly affected.[15] *If S. FSH is not elevated, tamoxifen is given 20 mg per day.*

Significant improvement in semen quality and increase in pregnancy rates (33.9% vs 10.3%) were found with use of 20 mg tamoxifen with testosterone undecanoate 120 mg for 6 months.[14] This regime has been mentioned later in this chapter.

Human Chorionic Gonadotropin

Human chorionic gonadotropin in a dose of 2,500–5,000 iu twice a week is a very useful regime in a patient of idiopathic oligozoospermia. This indicates the testosterone level. Intratesticular testosterone is 100 times higher than serum level. Therefore, exogenous hCG should be given rather than testosterone. The Leydig cells of the testis can respond positively to exogenous hCG and produces more amount of testosterone even under hypogonadotropic conditions. This suppresses endogenous gonadotropin level by negative feedback. The hCG-based hormonal therapy prior to a second micro-TESE attempt is effective in men with hypospermatogenesis.[16] Before the era of ICSI, we have very often used this drug with excellent results. We still use this drug for mild to moderate oligozoospermia.

This drug is very useful after varicocele ligation. The first reported studies showed 60% improvement in semen parameters.[17,18] Patients with relative androgen deficiency are more.[19]

FSH + hCG

This is a useful combination for idiopathic normogonadotropic oligozoospermia.[20] The argument in favor of this therapy by Prof. Ishidori (Sweden) is that these are the patients who have inadequate gonadotropin activity. Here RIA results are normal but the bioactivity is low. This bioactivity can be assessed by monoclonal antibody testing, but is not available in our country. To compensate for this deficient bioactivity, exogenous FSH and hCG are given for 3–6 months.[20] I have found this regime very useful for idiopathic, oligozoospermia. The case report described earlier in this chapter indicates efficacy of this regime.

Treatment protocol is:

- HMG/ rFSH 75–150 iu thrice a week
- hCG 5,000 iu once a week.

For maturation arrest at spermatid level, only FSH can be given for completion of spermatogenesis.[21]

A significant reduction in sperm aneuploidy levels has been detected after varicocele repair[22] and in men treated with rFSH.[23]

Androgen

Androgen level in testis is approximately 50-fold higher than that in the blood.[24] Testosterone has no role in improving spermatogenesis. On the contrary, exogenous testosterone therapy can produce azoospermia through inhibition of gonadotropin secretion. Stopping testosterone will resume spermatogenesis is a therapy called testosterone rebound therapy. Formerly, rebound therapy was given which is discarded because it causes permanent azoospermia in some patients. Testosterone is not a useful drug.[25,26]

Tamoxifen + Testosterone Undeconate

WHO recommends treatment with antiestrogens–tamoxifen for idiopathic oligozoospermia when motility and morphology are not significantly affected.[15] When S. FSH is not elevated, tamoxifen is given 20 mg/day.

When testosterone undeconate 120 mg is combined with 20 mg tamoxifen, there is significant improvement in semen quality and increase in pregnancy rate. Pregnancy rates increased from 10.3 to 33% as described in a study.[14]

Zinc

Zinc is very useful in low testosterone levels with zinc deficiency. Recommended dose is 120–220 mg twice a day for 3 months. It improves accessory glands function. It helps in exploration of immature cells. It helps in improving oligozoospermia as well as motility and maturation of spermatozoa.[27,28] But overdose may have a detrimental effect on sperm function.

Ketotifen

It inhibits histamine release from mast cells. It helps in blood testis barrier dysfunction. The dose is 1 mg bd for 3–6 months.[29] It has incompatibility with alchohol.[30]

Antiserotonin Agents

Cyproheptadine HCl (hydrochloride) 4 mg thrice a day for 90 days can be given in two courses. It improves count and motility in 33–50% of cases. Mechanism of action is that it reduces uptake of serotonin which reduces testicular damage.[31]

Captopril

It is ACE (Angiotensin converting enzyme) inhibitor. It inhibits kininase II and prevents degradation of kininogens to kinins. It is given in a dose of 50 mg per day for 3 months. It is contraindicated in presence of inflammation.[32]

Tissue Hormones

Pancreatic kallikrein converts kininogens to kinins which helps in cell proliferation. It has shown to play a role in regulation and stimulation of sperm motility.[32,33] It helps in oligo-astheno-teratozoospermia. It is given in a dose of 600 mg/day for 3–12 months.[34] But cumulative results are not promising.[35]

Anti-inflammatory Drugs

Chlamydia infection is very common in patients having male factor as a cause of infertility. It is extremely difficult to diagnose infection in genital tract and is very expensive also. Instead one course of doxycycline 100 mg bd for 14 days is cost effective as the incidence of infection has been quoted between 28 and 91%. It prevents occlusion of passage and local immunity is improved. Tetracycline and metronidazole are very effective. But antibiotic therapy does not necessarily improve conception rates.[36]

Indomethacin

Prostaglandins have inhibitory effect on testicular steroidogenesis and spermatogenesis.[37] Indomethacin and ketoprofen act as antiprostaglandins and raise FSH, LH and testosterone. Indomethacin 25 mg tds increases sperm count and motility.[38] It is inexpensive and non toxic and should be tried.

Aromatase Inhibitors

Teslac (testolactone) is tried for improving count and motility. It is well tolerated and improves testicular function. It prevents aromatization to estrogen. Therefore, patients having low T/E2 are potential candidates to improve with this drug. It should be considered for obese patients and those with elevated E2 levels. Anastrazole is a very potent drug and is used in a dose of 1 mg/day.[39] This is especially useful in patients with low testosterone levels. By preventing aromatization, it increases the testosterone and sperm production.[40]

Autocrine-Paracrine Mechanism

IgF1, IgF2, EGF and TGF are potent stimulants for spermatogenesis. Therefore, FSH + growth factors can improve spermatogenesis. CRF-β endorphins are inhibitors of spermatogenesis. Naltrexone is the drug which prevents CRF-β endorphin system. Therefore, FSH + Naltrexone can improve spermatogenesis.

ROLE OF ANTIOXIDANTS

Introduction

The definitive role of ROS testing in the diagnostic situation remains to be established, although detrimental effects of ROS on male reproductive potential is now well established.[41,42]

Therefore, systematic treatment of men with antioxidants has received great interest in recent years and it seems to have some clinical benefit, though the story remains somewhat confused[43] (Table 20.5).

8-Hydroxy-2'-deoxyguanosine, a biomarker of oxidative DNA damage highly correlated with sperm DNA fragmentation, in human sperm DNA has significant value in predicting the chance of a clinical pregnancy after IUI but not ICSI in ART.[44] Supplementing antioxidants (vitamin C, E and folate) and micronutrients (zinc) can also be helpful in producing sperms with less DNA damage in older man as well.[45]

Antioxidants are more useful as follow-up or complementary treatment to conventional treatment of varicocele, antibiotic treatment for infection or antiestrogenic treatment for idiopathic oligozoospermia. It has also been suggested that patients with asthenozoospermia should be advised to adhere to a diet rich in fruits, vegetables, poultry, skim milk and sea foods and low in processed meat and sweets.[46]

Table 20.5: List of antioxidants that can be used to treat male subfertility.

Tocopherol (vit E)	Glutathione
Ascorbic acid (vitamin C)	Arginine
Vitamin B_{12}	Carnitine
Folic acid	Coenzyme Q
Pentoxiflline	Vitamin D
Selenium	

According to Lipschutz, high doses of antioxidants have theoretical adverse effects and should be used in low or moderate doses (Table 20.6). With exception of patients with specific vitamin deficiency, efficacy of any vitamin therapy in normal men is questionable.

Vitamin E

Vitamin E improves motility of spermatozoa. The recommended dose is 300–600 mg daily for 6–12 weeks. Vitamin E improves sperm-oocyte fusion. Therefore, it is included in certain media preparations. Addition of vitamin E in media reduces the damaging effect of configuration during sperm preparation.[47] Astaxanthin is a carotenoid extracted from the algae *Haematococcus pluvialis*. The potency of this antioxidant is much higher as a singlet molecular oxygen quencher compared with vitamin E.[48] A positive effect of Astaxanthin on sperm parameters and fertility is seen in a study by Comhaire et al.[49]

Vitamin C

Low levels of vitamin C leads to infertility due to disturbed sperm functions. Vitamin C improves sperm quality. The dose is 1,000 mg daily.

Vitamin B_{12}

This is very useful for synthesis of DNA and RNA. It is useful for oligospermia and asthenospermia. Recommended dose is 1,000–1,500 μg/day for 6 months.[50]

Folic Acid

This is an additive drug and along with other drugs it helps to improve sperm functions. The dose required is 5 mg/day.[51]

Pentoxifylline

It improves microcirculation. The dose required is 1.2 mg/day for 3–6 months. It improves count and motility.[52] However, there are various reports that indicate that pentoxiflline, sildenafil and other methylxanthines when administered systematically give no response.[53]

Table 20.6: List of antioxidants used in male subfertility and their daily doses.

Vitamin E	300–600 mg/day
Vitamin C	1,000 mg/day
Vitamin B_{12}	1,000–15,000 μg daily
Folic acid	5 mg daily
Pentoxiflline	1–2 mg daily
Selenium	225 μg daily
Glutathione	6,000 mg IM daily
Arginine	4 g daily
L-Carnitine + LAC	3 g daily
Co-Q	100 mg bd

Selenium

It is an antioxidant as well as an anti-inflammatory agent. It is concentrated in male reproductive tract. Its highest concentration is in prostate and improves motility. The dose required is 225 μg/day. It is found that only 50% of patients improve as far as motility is concerned.[54]

Glutathione

It is a simple naturally occurring three aminoacid compound, acts as antioxidant and prevents lipid peroxidation. It has positive effect on sperm motility and is given in a dose of 600 mg IM daily. Daily injections are cumbersome and therefore this treatment has not gained popularity.[55]

Arginine

Improves sperm motility and recommended dose is 4 g/day.

L-Carnitine and L-Acetyl/Carnitine

L-Carnitine brings acetyl co-A into mitochondria. Therefore, its role is important in sperm cell metabolism. Concentration of L-carnitine is highest in epididymal fluid which is available to sperm cells. Combination of L-carnitine and L-acetylcarnitine are more effective in improving sperm motility than individual one in patients with lower baseline levels.[56] LC and LAC are useful in idiopathic OAT and low grade varicoceles. It is also useful in patients with prostate-vesiculo-epididymitis after treatment with NSAID.[57,58]

L-Carnitine 1 g bd + acetyl L-carnitine 500 mg bd + cinnoxicam 30 mg every four days showed significant reduction in aneuploid sperms and improved ICSI pregnancies a live births in severe OAT patients.[59] The fact is carnitine is not essential as it is synthesized in body. The exogenous source is nonvegetarian food. Deficiency occurs in patients with hemodialysis. However, there are several papers giving controversial opinion regarding its role as antioxidant. It has selective role in oligoasthenozoospermia.[60]

We must remember that positive effect of the drug does not last for a long time after therapy. Therefore, during the treatment for fertility, the drug is to be continued. We cannot prescribe the drug and wait for the results. Simultaneous superovulation with IUI or ART is a must.

Total oxyradical scavenging capacity (TOSC) assays differentiate different forms of ROS and its role for specific antioxidants. Therefore, in future, we will be able to decide which antioxidant is required for a particular patient.

Coenzyme Q 10

It is the component of mitochondrial respiratory chain. It has very important role in energy metabolism. It is biosynthesized in testis and has protective role as antioxidant for cell membranes and lipoprotein. The natural source of Co-Q 10 is broccoli, spinach, soyabean oil, palm oil, vitamins, minerals act as cofactors for producing Co-Q-10.

It is available as 50–100 mg soft gel capsules that has almost 100% absorption. Therapeutic application of Co-Q10 for 6 months increases its reduced form ubiquinol which improves kinetic property of sperm cells.[61]

Reduced Co-Q level is found in seminal plasma and sperm cells in infertile man with idiopathic oligospermia and varicocele associated with oligo-asthenospermia.

There is strong support as antioxidant by indirect medium. But there is no conclusion for improved pregnancy rates by this therapy. Like L-carnitine, its beneficial effect also does not last long.

Note: We must remember that we should prescribe the drug only in full therapeutic dose; otherwise it will not be useful. The combinations of drugs available in market should be fully studied well and should be prescribed to appropriate patients. Haphazard prescriptions simply add cost to the patients.

Vitamin D

Lately, vitamin D receptors are found in testis with vitamin D metabolizing enzymes. These enzymes are also found in epididymis and mature sperms.[62] Vitamin D can also be positively associated with testosterone and free androgen index and negatively with SHBG.[63] Still, another study has shown that 1,25$(OH)_2$ D_3 increases intracellular calcium concentration, sperm motility and induced the acrosome reaction in mature spermatozoa and vitamin D levels in serum were positively associated with sperm motility.[64] Combined treatment with taurine, cystiene and glutathione statistically significantly ameliorated the reduction in sperm motility during *in vitro* manipulation of human sperm.[65] However, other studies do not show that low vitamin D is a risk factor for poor semen quality in a population of young healthy men.[66]

Varicocele correction is to be offered to patients with palpable lesion with one or more abnormal semen parameters.[67] Though some workers have tried a documented improvement in males with oligozoospermia and azoospermia with acupuncture therapy, large and reliable studies are yet to be documented.

REFERENCES

1. Hussein A, Ozgok Y, Ross L, Niederberger C. Clomiphene administration for cases of nonobstructive azoospermia: a multicentre study. J Androl. 2005;26:787-91.
2. Whitten SJ, Nangia AK, Kolettis PN. Select patients with hypogonadotrophic hypogonadism may respond to treatment with clomiphene citrate. Fertil Steril. 2006;86: 1664-8.
3. Paulson DF, Hammond CB, de Vere White R, Wiebe RH. Clomiphene citrate: pharmacologic treatment of hypofertile male. Urology. 1977;9:419-21.
4. Sigman M, Jarow JP. Male infertility. In: Walsh PC, Retik AB, Vaughan ED, Wein AJ (Eds). Campbell's Urology, Vol. 2, 8th edition. St. Luois, MO: Saunders; 2002. pp. 1475-531.
5. Whitcomb RV Crowley WF Jr. Male hypogonadotrophic hypogonadism. Endocrinol metab Clin North Am. 1993;22:125-43.
6. Gillam MP, Molitch ME, Lombardi G, Colao A. Advances in treatment of prolactinomas. Endocr Rev. 2006;27: 485-534.
7. Shimon I, Benbassat C, Hadani M. Effectiveness of long-term cabergoline treatment for giant prolactinoma: study of 12 men. Eur J Endocrinol. 2007;156:225-31.
8. Lahteenmaki A, Rasanen M, Hovatta O. Low dose prednisolone does not improve the outcome of *in vitro* fertilization in male immunological infertility. Hum Reprod. 1995;10(12):3124-9.
9. Dubin L, Amelar RD. Etiologic factors in 1294 consecutive cases of male infertility. Fertil Steril. 1971;22:469-74.
10. Greenberg SH, Lipshultz LI, Wein AJ. Experience with 425 subfertile male patients. J Urol. 1978;119:507-10.
11. Akin JW. The use of clomiphene citrate in the treatment of azoospermia secondary to incomplete androgen resistance. Fertil Steril. 1993;59:223-4.

12. Comhaire F. Treatment of oligospermia with tamoxifen. Int J Fertil. 1976;21:232-8.
13. Schill WB, Schiilinger R. Selection of oligospermic men for tamoxifen treatment by an antioestrogen test. Andrologia. 1987;19:266-72.
14. Adamopoulos DA, Pappa A, Billa E, Nicopoulou S, Koukkou E. Michopoulos J. Effectiveness of combined tamoxifen citrate and testosterone undeconate treatment in men with idiopathic oligozoospermia. Fertil Steril. 2003;80:914-20.
15. Rowe PJ, Comhaire FH, Hargreave TB, Mahmoud AMA. WHO manual for the standardized investigation, diagnosis and management of the infertile male. Cambridge University Press; 2000. p. 91.
16. Shiraishi K, Ohmi C, Shimabukuro T, Matsuyama H. Human chorionic gonotrophin treatment prior to micro-dissection testicular sperm extraction in non-obstructive azoospermia. Hum Reprod. 2012;27:331-9.
17. Glass SJ, Holland HM. Treatment of oligospermia with large doses of human chorionic gonadotrophin. Fertil Steril. 1963;14:500-6.
18. Mehan DJ, Chehval MJ. Human chorionic gonadotrophin in the treatment of the infertile man. J Urol. 1982;128:60-3.
19. Lunenfield B, Mor A, Mani M. Treatment of male infertility. I. Human gonadotropins. Fertil Steril. 1967;18:581-92
20. Acosta AA, Khalifa E, Oehninfer S. Pure human follicle stimulating hormone has a role in the treatment of severe male infertility by assisted reproduction: Norfolk's total experience. Hum Reprod. 1992;7:1067-72.
21. Schwarzstein L, Aparicio NJ, Schally AV. D-tryptophan-6-leutinizing hormone-releasing hormone in the treatment of normogonadotrophic oligoasthenozoospermia. Int J Androl. 1982;5:172-8.
22. Bacetti BM, Bruni E, Capitani S, Collodel G, Mancini S, Piomboni P, et al. Studies on varicocoele III: ultrastructural sperm evaluation and 18, X and Y aneuploidies. J Androl. 2006;27:94-101.
23. Piomboni P, Serafini F, Gambera L, Musacchio C, Collodel G, Morgante G, et al. Sperm aneuploidies after human recombinant follicle stimulating hormone therapy in infertile males. Reprod Biomed Online. 2009;18:622-9.
24. Turner TT, Jones CE, Howards SS, Ewing LL, Zegeye B, Gunsalus GL. On the androgen microenvironment of maturing spermatozoa. Endocrinology. 1984;115:1925-32.
25. Charny CW. The use of androgens for human spermatogenesis. Fertil Steril. 1959;10:557-70.
26. Charny CW, Gordon JA. A testosterone rebound therapy: a neglected modality. Fertil Steril. 1978;29:64-8.
27. Ebish IM, Pierik FH, De Jong FH, Thomas CMG, Steegers-Theunissen RPM. Does folic acidand zinc sulphate intervention affect endocrine parameters and sperm characteristics in men? Int J Androl. 2006;29:339-45.
28. Wong WY, Merkus HM, Thomas CM, Menkveld R, Zielhuis GA, Steegers-Theunissen RP. Effects of folic acid and zinc sulphate on male factor subfertility: a double blind, randomized placebo-controlled trial. Fertil Steril. 2002;77(3):491-8.
29. Matsuki S, Sasagawa I, Suzuki Y, Yazawa H, Tateno T, Hashimoto T, et al. The use of ebastine, a mast cell blocker, for treatment of oligozoospermia. Arch Androl. 2000;44:129.
30. Schill WB, Michalopoulos M. Treatment of male fertility disturbances current concepts. Drugs. 1984;28(3):263-80.
31. Schill WB, Parsch EM, Miska W. Inhibition of angiotensin-converting enzyme: a new concept of medical treatment of male infertility? Fertil Steril. 1994;61(6):1123-8.
32. Schill WB. Improvement of sperm motility in patients with asthenozoospermia by kallikrein treatment. Andrologia. 1975;20:61-3.
33. Schill WB, Braun-Falco O, Haberland GL. The possible role of kinins in sperm motility. Int J Fertil. 1974;19:163-7.
34. Kamidono S, Hazama M, Matsumoto O, Takasa KI, Tomioka O, Ishigami J. Kallikrein and male subfertility: usefulness of high-unit kallikrein tablet. Andrologia. 1981;13(2): 108-20.
35. Keck C, Behre HM, Jockenhovel F, Nieschlag E. Ineffectiveness of kallikrein in treatment of idiopathic male infertility: a double-blind, randomized, placebo-controlled trial. Hum Reprod. 1994;9(2):325-9.
36. Haidl G. Management strategies for male actor infertility. Drugs. 2002;62:1741.
37. Bartke A, Kupfer D, Dalteiro S. Prostaglandins inhibit testosterone secretion by mouse testis *in vitro*. Steroids. 1976;28:81-8.
38. Barkay J, Harpaz-Kerpel S, Ben-Erza S, Gordon S, Zuckerman H. The prostaglandin inhibitor effect of anti-inflammatory drugs in therapy of male infertility. Fertil Steril. 1984;42(3):406-11.
39. Schlegel PN, Raman JD. Aromatase inhibitors for male infertility. J Urol. 2002;167:624-9.
40. Schlegel PN. Aromatase inhibitors for male infertility. Fertil Steril. 2012;98(6):1359-62.
41. Saleh RA, Agrawal A. Oxidative stress and male infertility: from research bench to clinical practice. J. Androl. 2002;23:737-52.
42. Agrawal A, Saleh RA, Bedaiwy MA. Role of reactive oxygen spices in the pathophysiology of human reproduction. Fertil Steril. 2003;79:829-43.
43. Agrawal A. Role of antioxidants in treatment of male infertility: an overview of the literature. Reprod Biomed Online. 2004;8:616-27.
44. Thomson LK, Zieschang JA, Clark AM. Oxidative DNA damage in sperm has a negative impact on clinical pregnancy rate in intrauterine insemination but not in intracytoplasmic sperm injection cycles. Fertil Steril. 2011;96:843-7.
45. Schmid TE, Eskenazi B, Marchetti F, Young S, Weldon RH, Baumgartner A, et al. Micronutrients intake is associated with iproved sperm DNA quality in older men. Fertil Steril. 2012;98(5):1130-7.
46. Elsamian G, Amirjannati N, Rashidkhani B, Sadeghi MR, Hekmatdoost A. Intake of food groups and idiopathic asthenozoospermia: a case control study. Hum Reprod. 2012;27(11):3328-36.

47. Keskes-Ammar L, Feki-Chakroun N, Rebai T, Sahnoun Z, Ghozzi H, Hammami S. Sperm oxidative stress and the effect of an oral vitamin E and selenium supplement on semen quality in infertile male. Arch Androl. 2003;49(2):83-94.
48. Di Mascio P, Devasagayam TP, Kaiser S, Sies H. Carotenoids, tocopherols and thiols as biological singlet molecular oxygen quenchers. Biochem Soc Trans. 1990;18:1054-6.
49. Comhaire FH, Garem YE, Mahmoud A, Eertmans F, Schoonjans F. Combined conventional/antioxidant "Astaxanthin" treatment for male infertility: a double blind randomised trial. Asian J Androl. 2005;7:257-62.
50. Sandler B, Faragher N. Treatment of oligozoospermia with vitamin B12. Infertility. 1984;7:133.
51. Ebisch IM, van Heerde WL, Thomas CM, van der Put N, Wong WY, Steegers-Theunissen RP. C677T methylenetetrahydrofolate reductase polymorphism interferes with the effect of folic acid and zinc sulphate on sperm concentration. Fertil Steril. 2003;80(5):1190-4.
52. Schill WB. Therapy of idiopathic astheno- and oligozoospermia with pentoxifylline. Fortschr Med. 1982;100:696 (German).
53. Burger M, Sikka SC, Bivalacqua TJ, Lamb DJ, Hellstrom WJ. The effect of sildenafil on human sperm motion and function from normal and infertile men. Int J Impot Res. 2000;12(4):229-34.
54. Scott R, MacPherson A, Yates RW, Hussain B, Dixon J. The effect of oral selenium supplementation on human sperm motility. Br. J Urol. 1998;82(1):76-80.
55. Lenzi A, Culasso F, Gandini L, Lombardo F, Dondero F. Placebo controlled double-blind, cross-over trial of glutathione therapy in male infertility. Hum Reprod. 1993;8:1657-62.
56. Lenzi A, Sgrò P, Salacone P, Paoli D, Gilio B, Lombardo F, et al. A placebo-controlled double-blind randomized trial of the use of combined-carnitine and L-acetyl carnitine treatment in men with asthenozoosprmia. Fertil Steril. 2004;81(6):1578-84.
57. Cavallini G, Ferraretti AP, Gianaroli L, Biagiotti G, Vitali G. Cinnoxicam and L-cartinine/acetyl-L-carnitine treatment for idiopathic and varicocoele associated oligoasthenospermia. J Androl. 2004;25:761-70.
58. Vicari E, La Vignera S, Calogero AE. Antioxidant treatment with carnitines is effective in infertile patients with prostatovesiculaoepididymitis and elevated seminal leukocyte concentrations after treatment with non-steroidal anti-inflammatory compounds. Fertil Steril. 2002;78:1203-8.
59. Cavallini G, Magli MC, Crippa A, Ferraretti AP, Gianaroli L. Reduction in sperm aneuploidy levels in severe oligoasthenoteratospermic patients after medical therapy: a preliminary report. Asian J Androl. 2012;14:591-8.
60. Lenzi A, Lombardo F, Sgro P, Salacone P, Caponecchia L, Dondero F, et al. Use of carnitine therapy in selected cases of male factor infertility: a double-blind cross-over trial. Fertil Steril. 2003;79:292-300.
61. Balercia G, Buldreghini E, Vignini A, Tiano L, Paggi F, Amoroso S, et al. Coenzyme Q10 treatment in infertile men with idiopathic asthenozoospermia: a placebo-controlled, double-blind randomized trial. Fertil Steril. 2009;91(5): 1785-92.
62. Bloomberg JM, Nielson JE, Jorgenson A, Rajpert De ME, Kristensen DM, Jorgenson N, et al. Vitamin D receptors and vitamin D metabolizing enzymes are expressed in the human male reproductive tract. Hum Reprod. 2010;25:1303-11.
63. Wehr E, Pilz S, Boehm BO, Marz W, Obermayer-Pietsch B. Association of vitamin D status with serum androgen levels in men. Clin Endocrinol (Oxf). 2010;73:243-8.
64. Bloomberg JM, Bjerrum PJ, Jessen TE, Nielson JE, Joenson UN, Oleson IA, et al. Vitamin D is positively associated with sperm motility and increases intracellular calcium in human spermatozoa. Hum Reprod. 2011;26(6):1307-17.
65. Yun JI, Gong SP, Song YH, Lee ST. Effects of combined antioxidant supplementation on human sperm motility and morphology during sperm manipulation *in vitro*. Fertil Steril. 2013;100:373-8.
66. Ramlau-Hansen CH, Moeller UK, Bonde JP, Oslen J, Thulstrup AM. Are serum levels of vitamin D associated with semen quality? Results from a cross-sectional study in young healthy men. Fertil Steril. 2011;95(3):1000-4.
67. Sharlip ID, Jarow JP, Belkar AM, Lipshultz LI, Sigman M, Thomas AJ, et al. Best practice policies for male infertility. Fertil Steril. 2002;77:873-82.

CHAPTER

Surgical Management of Male Infertility

21

Sunil K Jindal

INTRODUCTION

Over the past couple of years, the indications for and techniques of surgery for male infertility have been significantly refined, resulting in substantially increased success in the management of male-factor infertility. These advances include (1) refined microsurgical techniques for sperm retrieval combined with *in vitro* fertilization (IVF) with intracytoplasmic sperm injection (ICSI) for men with nonobstructive azoospermia; (2) improved techniques for microsurgical reconstruction for obstruction; (3) the use of varicocelectomy for enhancement of spermatogenesis in azoospermic or severely oligospermic men, for prevention of future infertility and androgen deficiency in young men, and for treatment of androgen deficiency in men of all ages;[1] and (4) increasing use of genetic and molecular biologic markers to better select patients for surgical treatment. Even men with nonobstructive azoospermia caused by Klinefelter syndrome, once regarded as hopeless cases, can now father biologic offspring with assisted reproductive techniques.

Infertility is a common complaint at urologists' offices and affects approximately 8% of reproductive-age men. Among them, 1–10% present with conditions that affect their reproductive potential. The conditions which can be corrected with surgical procedures were identified in approximately one third of the male partners.[2] Azoospermic males who were not candidates for surgery or who remained azoospermic after surgical reconstruction could benefit from sperm retrieval techniques and assisted conception. Thus, surgical management may be offered to more than 50% of the infertile male patient population.

IVF with ICSI has expanded our ability to treat even the most severe forms of male-factor infertility such as unreconstructable reproductive tract obstruction and nonobstructive azoospermia.

On the other hand, recent analyses clearly indicate that specific treatments for male-factor infertility, such as microsurgical reconstruction for obstructive azoospermia and varicocelectomy for impaired testis function, in properly selected patients remain the safest and most cost-effective ways of managing infertile men and also can be complimentary. Specific treatment aimed at correcting or enhancing male infertility can upgrade a couple from intensive levels of assisted reproduction to simpler methods such as intrauterine insemination (IUI) or even to naturally conceived pregnancies.

When surgery for male infertility is undertaken, only rarely is the life (or death) of the patient at stake. What is at stake when the surgery described in this chapter is undertaken is new life, with the potential for altering not only the quality of a couple's life but the future of our species. The responsibilities assumed by the surgeon in these circumstances demand the utmost in judgment and skill.

AVAILABLE SURGICAL TREATMENT

Varicocele Repair

Varicocele can be diagnosed in up to 35% of infertile men. It is currently recommended that treatment should be offered to couples with documented infertility whose male partner has a clinically palpable varicocele associated with an abnormal semen analysis.[3]

Repair of varicocele will halt any further damage to testicular function[4] and in a large percentage of men will result in improved spermatogenesis[5] as well as enhanced Leydig cell function. The potentially important role of urologists in preventing future infertility and/or androgen deficiency underscores the importance of using a varicocelectomy technique that minimizes the risk of complications and recurrence. Table 21.1 summarizes the pros and cons of various methods of varicocele repair.

Preoperative Evaluation

A preoperative hormone profile that includes an analysis of follicle-stimulating hormone (FSH) and testosterone, a testicular volume assessment using a measurement

Table 21.1: Technique of varicocelectomy.[6]

Technique	*Artery preserved*	*Hydrocele (%)*	*Failure (%)*	*Potential for serious morbidity*
Retroperitoneal	No	7	15–25	No
Conventional inguinal	No	3–30	5–15	No
Laparoscopic	Yes	12	3–15	Yes
Radiographic	Yes	0	15–25	Yes
Microscopic inguinal or subinguinal	Yes	0	0.5–1.0	No

instrument such as the Prader orchidometer or a pachymeter, and the results of at least two semen analyses should be obtained.[7] Men with clinical varicoceles presenting with azoospermia may be candidates for surgical repair, but genetic evaluation including Giemsa karyotyping and polymerase chain reaction screening for Yq microdeletion of the AZFa, AZFb, and AZFc regions is recommended. A testis biopsy (open or percutaneous) provides testicular histology, which has been shown to be the only significant prognostic factor for the restoration of spermatogenesis in azoospermic individuals with varicocele.[8] The benefit of varicocelectomy in azoospermic men with genetic abnormalities is doubtful and the procedure should be carefully considered. The same caution must be used for patients with atrophic testes and/or a history of cryptorchidism, testicular trauma, orchitis, or systemic or hormonal dysfunction; varicocele may be coincidental in these cases rather than the cause of infertility.

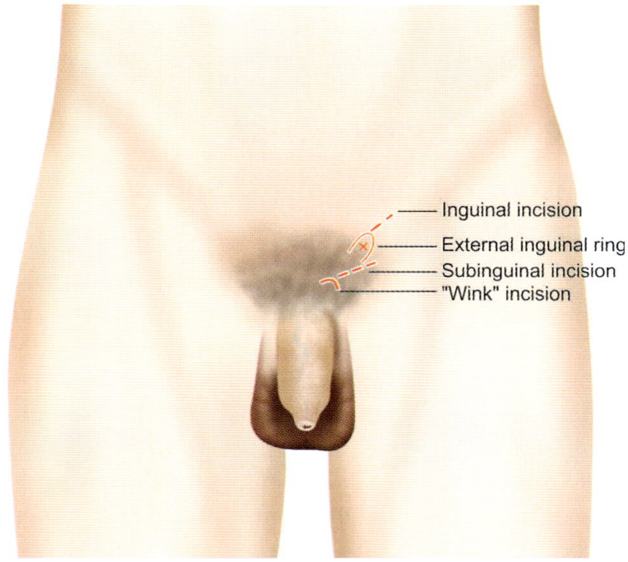

Fig. 21.1: Different incisions for inguinal or subinguinal approach of varicocele repair.

Scrotal Approach

A variety of surgical approaches have been advocated for varicocelectomy.

The earliest recorded attempts at repair of varicocele date to antiquity and involved external clamping of the scrotal skin, including the enlarged veins. In the early 1900s an open scrotal approach was used, involving the mass ligation and excision of the varicosed plexus of veins. At the level of the scrotum, however, the pampiniform plexus of veins are intimately entwined with the coiled testicular artery. Therefore, scrotal operations are to be avoided because damage to the arterial supply of the testis frequently results in testicular atrophy and further impairment of spermatogenesis and fertility.

Retroperitoneal Approach

Retroperitoneal repair of varicocele involves incision at the level of the internal inguinal ring. At this level, only one or two large veins are present, and in addition, the testicular artery has not yet branched and is often distinctly separate from the internal spermatic veins. Retroperitoneal approaches involve ligation of the fewest number of veins. A disadvantage of a retroperitoneal approach is the high incidence of varicocele recurrence, especially in children and adolescents, when the testicular artery is intentionally preserved. Recurrence rates after retroperitoneal varicocelectomy are in the range of 15%[9] (Fig. 21.1).

Laparoscopic Approach

Laparoscopic repair is in essence a retroperitoneal approach, and many of the advantages and disadvantages are similar to those of the open retroperitoneal approach.[10] The magnification provided by the laparoscope allows visualization of the testicular artery. With experience, the lymphatics may be visualized and preserved as well. With laparoscopic varicocelectomy the internal spermatic veins are ligated at the same level as with the retroperitoneal approach.

The potential complications of laparoscopic varicocelectomy (injury to bowel, vessels, or viscera; air embolism; peritonitis) are significantly more serious than those associated with the open techniques. Furthermore, laparoscopic varicocelectomy requires a general anesthetic. The microsurgical techniques described next can be performed with local or regional anesthesia and use an incision of 2–3 cm for unilateral repair.

This is often no greater than the sum of incisions used for a laparoscopic approach. Postoperative pain and recovery from the laparoscopic technique are the same as those associated with subinguinal varicocelectomy.

PREFERRED APPROACHES

Microsurgical Inguinal and Subinguinal Approaches

Subinguinal varicocelectomy is currently the most popular approach. It has the advantage of allowing the spermatic cord structures to be pulled up and out of the wound so that the testicular artery, lymphatics, and small periarterial veins may be more easily identified. An inguinal or subinguinal approach allows access to the testis for biopsy or examination of the epididymis for obstruction or repair of hydrocele. Traditional approaches to inguinal varicocelectomy involve a 5-cm incision made over the inguinal canal, opening of the external oblique aponeurosis, and encirclement and delivery of the spermatic cord. An attempt is made to identify and preserve the testicular artery and, if possible, the lymphatics. In addition, the cord is elevated, and any external spermatic veins that are running parallel to the spermatic cord or perforating the floor of the inguinal canal are identified and ligated. Conventional inguinal operations are associated with an incidence of postoperative hydrocele formation varying from 3% to 15% with an average incidence of 7%. The introduction of microsurgical technique to varicocelectomy has resulted in a substantial reduction in the incidence of hydrocele formation. This is because the lymphatics can be more easily identified and preserved. Furthermore, the use of magnification enhances the ability to identify and preserve the 0.5- to 1.5-mm testicular artery, thus avoiding the complications of atrophy or azoospermia.

Anesthesia

If the testis is delivered as described later, regional or light general anesthesia is preferred. If only the cord is delivered, local anesthesia with a 50–50% combination of 0.25% bupivacaine and 1% lidocaine is satisfactory with adjunctive intravenous heavy sedation. After infiltration of the skin and subcutaneous tissues the cord is infiltrated before delivery. Blind cord block carries with it a small risk of inadvertent testicular artery injury. A 26-gauge needle should therefore be used for cord block to minimize the risk of injury and hematoma.

Inguinal and Subinguinal Approaches

In the subinguinal approach, just below the external inguinal ring, we do not open any fascial layer and is associated with less pain and a rapid recovery comparable to laparoscopic procedures. At the subinguinal level, however, significantly more veins are encountered, the artery is more often surrounded by a network of tiny veins that must be ligated, and the testicular artery has often divided into two or three branches, making arterial identification and preservation more difficult.

In general, it is best to use a subinguinal approach in men with a history of any prior inguinal surgery. Under these circumstances the cord is usually stuck to the undersurface of the external oblique, and opening the fascia risks injury to the cord. A subinguinal approach is easier in obese men in whom opening and closing the fascia is difficult through a small incision. A subinguinal approach is easier in men with high, lax, capacious external rings and in men with long cords and low-lying testes. In these men, the level of the external ring is fairly proximal to the testis, and opening the fascia will not result in a significant diminution in the number of veins to be ligated or in the branching of the testicular artery.

Consider opening the fascia in men with prior failed subinguinal varicocelectomy to dissect proximal to the prior scarred ligation area. The microdissection will be quicker and easier. A subinguinal operation is significantly more difficult than a high inguinal operation and should be used only by surgeons who perform the operation frequently.

If the decision is made to perform an inguinal operation and thus to open the fascia, the incision is begun at the external ring and extended laterally 2–3.5 cm along the Langer lines.

Dissection of the Cord

The operating microscope is then brought into the field. Under 6× to 10× magnification, the external spermatic fascia is opened with an electrocautery instrument in the direction of the cremasteric fibers to avoid injury to the cremasteric arteries. A Vicryl suture is placed at the apex of the opening to facilitate later closure. The relatively avascular internal spermatic fascia is opened with scissors as high as possible and held open with the straight mosquito forceps. The magnification is increased to 10× to 25× and, after irrigation with 1% papaverine solution; the cord is inspected for the presence of pulsations revealing the location of the testicular artery. Micro-Doppler is extremely useful in identifying arteries. Once the testicular artery has been identified, it is dissected free of all surrounding tissue, tiny veins, and lymphatics, using a fine-tipped nonlocking micro needle holder and microforceps. The artery is encircled with a vessel loop for positive identification and gentle retraction. The suspected artery is tested by elevating the artery with the tips of the micro needle holder until it is completely occluded and then slowly lowering it until a pulsating blush of blood appears just over the needle holder. If the artery is not immediately identified, the cord is carefully dissected beginning with the largest veins. The veins are stripped clean of adherent lymphatics and the undersides of the largest veins inspected for an adherent artery. In approximately 50% of patients, the testicular artery is adherent to the undersurface of a large vein.[11] All veins within the cord, with the exception of the vasal veins, are doubly ligated. The vasal veins are preserved, providing venous return. If the vas deferens is accompanied by dilated veins greater than 2.5 mm in diameter, they are dissected free of the vassal artery and ligated. The vas deferens is always accompanied by two sets of vessels. As long as at least one set of deferential veins remains intact, venous return will be adequate. At the completion of the dissection, the cord is run over the index finger and inspected to verify that all veins have been identified and ligated.

The external oblique aponeurosis, if opened, is reapproximated with continuous suturing using the previously placed 3-0 suture. The Scarpa and Camper fasciae are reapproximated with a single or continuous 3-0 plain catgut suture, and the skin is approximated with a 3-0 to 5-0 monofilament absorbable subcuticular suture.

Postoperative Care

Local dressing and scrotal support are maintained for 48–72 hours and 1 week, respectively. Patients are counseled to refrain from physical activity and sexual intercourse for 2–3 weeks. Oral analgesics usually suffice to control postoperative pain. Follow-up aims to evaluate improvement in semen parameters, complications and spontaneous or assisted conception. Semen analysis should be performed every 3 months until the semen parameters stabilize or pregnancy occurs.

TREATMENT

Several treatments are available for varicocele. The type of intervention chosen depends mainly on the experience of the therapist. Although laparoscopic varicocelectomy is feasible, it must be justified in terms of cost-effectiveness. Current evidence indicates that microsurgical varicocelectomy is the most effective and least morbid method among the varicocelectomy techniques.

Conclusions and recommendations for varicocele as per EAU guidelines (2016).

Conclusions	*LE*
Current information supports the hypothesis that the presence of varicocele in some men is associated with progressive testicular damage from adolescence onwards and a consequent reduction in fertility	2a
Although the treatment of varicocele in adolescents may be effective, there is a significant risk of overtreatment	3
Varicocele repair may be effective in men with subnormal semen analysis, a clinical varicocele and otherwise unexplained infertility	1a
Recommendations	*GR*
Varicocele treatment is recommended for adolescents with progressive failure of testicular development documented by serial clinical examination	B
No evidence indicates benefit from varicocele treatment in infertile men who have normal semen analysis or in men with subclinical varicocele. In this situation, varicocele treatment cannot be recommended	A
Varicocele repair should be considered in case of a clinical varicocele, oligospermia, infertility duration of ≥2 years and otherwise unexplained infertility in the couple	A

Insight into the Surgical Treatment of Varicocele

In a recent systematic review comparing surgical modalities used to treat varicocele, open microsurgical inguinal or subinguinal varicocelectomy techniques resulted in higher spontaneous pregnancy rates and fewer recurrences and postoperative complications than laparoscopic, radiologic embolization, and macroscopic inguinal or retroperitoneal techniques. A study by Cayan showed that hydrocele formation was the most common complication of varicocelectomy, and the incidence ranged from 0 to 10%. Recurrences were reported in the range of 0–35%. Overall recurrence rates were lower for microsurgical varicocelectomy and higher for retroperitoneal and macrosurgical inguinal approaches. The rate of accidental testicular artery ligation during microsurgical varicocelectomy has been reported to be about 1%, and this may cause testicular atrophy. Recently, a study demonstrated that the concomitant use of intraoperative vascular Doppler monitoring during microsurgical varicocelectomy allows for more arterial branches to be preserved, and more internal spermatic veins are likely to be ligated.

Varicocelectomy studies have reported significant improvements in one or more semen parameters in approximately 65% of men. Higher preoperative semen parameters or varicocele repair for large varicoceles are more likely to show postoperative improvements in semen parameters. The mean time for semen improvement and spontaneous pregnancy after surgery is approximately 5 and 7 months, respectively. Studies have also reported that the surgical treatment of clinical varicoceles is highly effective in decreasing seminal oxidative stress and increasing seminal concentrations of antioxidants. Conversely, reduced preoperative testicular volume, elevated serum FSH levels, diminished testosterone concentrations, subclinical varicocele and the presence of Y chromosome microdeletions seem to be negative predictors for fertility improvement after surgery. The management of infertility in men with a unilateral clinical varicocele and a subclinical varicocele on the contralateral side is a matter of debate. For example, Zheng et al. found that bilateral varicocelectomy had no benefit over left clinical varicocelectomy. Elbendary et al., however, observed that the magnitude of change in sperm count and motility and the spontaneous pregnancy rates were significantly higher in the group of men who had bilateral varicocele repair. Several guidelines propose that varicoceles should be treated if palpable and if abnormal semen analyses are observed. A recent meta-analysis of varicocelectomy conducted by Marmar et al. (2007) demonstrated the benefit of the surgical treatment of clinical varicoceles in infertile men with abnormal semen analyses.[7] The authors showed that the chances of spontaneous conception were 2.8-times higher in the varicocelectomy group compared with the group of patients who either did not receive treatment or received medication.

Interestingly, the reference values for semen parameters normalcy are lower in the newly released edition of the World Health Organization (WHO) manual for examination of human sperm than in previous editions. According to these new reference values, several patients with clinical varicoceles who had been previously categorized as having abnormal semen parameters would be reclassified as having normal semen and would not be eligible for treatment under the current guidelines for varicocele treatment. The question is not simply whether a man should undergo repair of clinical varicoceles if he has normal semen variables. Indeed, what we are really interested in determining is what the semen parameters of the same individual would have been if varicocele had been treated. It would be very informative to reanalyze the meta-analysis studies of varicocelectomy to determine the magnitude of sperm quality improvement in the subgroup of patients that is now classified as having "normal" semen. This information will certainly come, but emerging evidence seems to indicate the benefits of treatment for men with clinical varicocele and so-called "normal" semen parameters according to the new WHO reference values.

Surgical correction of the varicocele would only be offered when adolescents have already crossed into the infertile range, even though initial evaluation had already shown that their seminal profiles were significantly lower than their counterparts without varicocele. Due to the progressive nature of varicocele, it is to be expected that treatment of varicocele halts deterioration of sperm quality and prevents individuals with "normal" semen analysis from crossing into the infertile range. Moreover, improvements in sperm quality after varicocele repair may also increase the male reproductive potential even if pre- and post-treatment values are within the newly proposed reference values. Adolescents and adults with palpable varicoceles may present with a normal semen analysis, but elevated DNA fragmentation rates and oxidative stress levels show they already have altered sperm function. Studies have shown that men who achieved a postoperative total motile sperm count greater than 20 million and sperm DNA fragmentation decrease after varicocelectomy were more likely to initiate a pregnancy either spontaneously or via assisted reproductive technology (ART).

It is still unclear why fertility potential does not always improve after surgery (Table 21.2).

A recent meta-analysis reported the appearance of sperm in the ejaculates of 39% of azoospermic individuals whose varicoceles had been treated. In addition, testicular

Table 21.2: Recurrence and complication rates associated with treatments for varicocele as per European Association of Urology (EAU) guidelines (2016).

Treatment	*Recurrence/persistence (%)*	*Complication rates*
Antegrade sclerotherapy[12]	9	Complication rate 0.3–2.2%: testicular atrophy, scrotal hematoma, epididymitis, left-flank erythema
Retrograde sclerotherapy[13]	9.8	Adverse reaction to contrast medium, flank pain, persistent thrombophlebitis, vascular perforation
Retrograde embolization[14,15]	3.8–10	Pain due to thrombophlebitis, bleeding hematoma, infection, venous perforation, hydrocele, radiological complication (e.g. reaction to contrast media), misplacement or migration of coils, retroperitoneal hemorrhage, fibrosis, ureteric obstruction
Open operation		
Scrotal operation	–	Testicular atrophy, arterial damage with risk of devascularization and testicular gangrene, scrotal hematoma, postoperative hydrocele
Inguinal approach[16]	13.3	Possibility of missing out a branch of testicular vein
High ligation[17]	29	5–10% incidence of hydrocele (<1%)
Microsurgical inguinal or subinguinal[18,19]	0.8–4	Postoperative hydrocele arterial injury, scrotal hematoma
Laparoscopy[20]	3–7	Injury to testicular artery and lymph vessels; intestinal, vascular and nerve damage; pulmonary embolism; peritonitis; bleeding; postoperative pain in right shoulder (due to diaphragmatic stretching during pneumoperitoneum); pneumoscrotum: wound infection

histopathology results were predictive of success. Moreover, the postoperative appearance of sperm in the ejaculates increased 9.4-fold in patients with biopsy-proven HS or MA compared with SCO syndrome. Although the use of motile ejaculated sperm is preferred for ICSI, persistent azoospermia after varicocele repair is still a potential problem, and sperm extraction before ICSI will be inevitable for many individuals. In the case of persistent azoospermia after varicocelectomy, successful sperm retrieval rates of 60% have been reported using micro-TESE sperm extraction. Interestingly, one study suggested that varicocele repair may maximize the chances of retrieving sperm for ICSI in azoospermic men with clinical varicoceles.

Transurethral Resection of the Ejaculatory Duct (TURED)

Ejaculatory duct obstruction (EDO) is a cause of male infertility that can potentially be corrected by surgery. Congenital obstructions are caused by atresia or stenosis of the ejaculatory ducts as well as utricular, Müllerian, and wolffian duct cysts. Acquired obstructions may be secondary to trauma or infection/inflammation. Traumatic damage to the ejaculatory ducts may occur after the removal of seminal vesicle cysts, pull-through operations for an imperforate anus or even prolonged urethral catheterization or instrumentation. Genital or urinary infection and prostatic abscess may cause stenosis or complete obstruction of the ducts.[21]

Diagnosis

Ejaculatory duct obstruction is suspected in azoospermic or severely oligospermic and/or asthenospermic men with at least one palpable vas deferens, a low semen volume, acidic semen pH, and negative, equivocal or low semen fructose levels. If these men have normal serum levels of FSH and testis biopsy reveals normal spermatogenesis, the diagnosis of ejaculatory duct obstruction is entertained.

Transrectal sonography is a key to the diagnosis and treatment of ejaculatory duct obstruction. A midline cystic lesion or dilated ejaculatory ducts and seminal vesicles can be visualized sonographically.

Transrectal ultrasound-guided aspiration of the cystic or dilated ejaculatory ducts or seminal vesicles is performed. The aspirate is examined microscopically; if motile sperm are found, they are cryopreserved and 2–3 mL of indigo carmine diluted with water-soluble radiographic contrast is instilled. If a radiograph confirms a potentially resectable lesion, TURED is performed without the need for prior vasography because the presence of sperm in the seminal vesicles indicates that at least one epididymis is patent and that the cyst or dilated ejaculatory duct communicates with a nonobstructed vas. The instillation of indigo carmine assists in localizing the opening of the ejaculatory duct and confirms when resection has successfully opened the obstructed system. Transrectal sonography with aspiration should be performed immediately before anticipated surgery and uses the same bowel preparation and antibiotic prophylaxis as for transrectal prostate biopsy.

If no sperm are found in either vas when the vasotomy is made and vasography reveals ejaculatory duct obstruction, it is best to abandon attempts at reconstruction and simply perform microsurgical epididymal sperm aspiration and cryopreservation for future IVF and ICSI.

Technique

Cold knife incision alone almost always leads to reobstruction. The resectoscope, with the 24-Fr cutting loop, is engaged with a finger placed in the rectum providing anterior displacement of the posterior lobe of the prostate. The ejaculatory ducts course between the bladder neck and the verumontanum and exit at the level of and along the lateral aspect of the verumontanum. Resection of the verumontanum will often reveal the dilated ejaculatory duct orifice or cyst cavity. Resection should be carried out in this region with great care to preserve the bladder neck proximally, the striated sphincter distally, and the rectal mucosa posteriorly. Efflux of indigo carmine from dilated orifices confirms adequate resection. Avoid excessive coagulation. If formal vasography was performed, the hemivasotomies are carefully closed using microsurgical technique. A Foley catheter is left overnight and the patient receives an additional 7 days of oral antibiotics.

Results

TURED results in increased semen volume about two-thirds of the time and appearance of sperm in the ejaculate in about 50% of previously azoospermic men. Pregnancy rates are based on case reports and small series.[22] If viable sperm appear in the ejaculate but the quality is poor, IVF with ICSI is recommended and currently yields delivery rates of up to 38.5% per attempt. Because of the potential for serious complications, TUR should be performed only in azoospermic men or in severely oligoasthenospermic men and only after the male and female partners have stated they are unwilling to undergo IVF and have been fully apprised of the risks of TUR.

Reconstructive Surgery of the Vas Deferens and Epididymis

Vasovasostomy (VV) and vasoepididymostomy (VE) are designed to bypass an obstruction in the male genital tract.

Preoperative Planning

A detailed medical history must be taken, and prognostic factors should be identified. Obstruction intervals after vasectomy play a major role in determining surgical outcomes. Vasoepididymostomy is more likely to be required after long-interval obstructions because they are associated with a higher incidence of epididymal obstruction. Small and soft testes may indicate impaired spermatogenesis. Indurate, irregular epididymides, and the presence of hydrocele are often associated with epididymal obstruction and may indicate the need for VE.[23] The presence of a granuloma in the vas deferens should be interpreted as a favorable prognostic sign because this means that sperm have leaked from the vasectomy site. Serum FSH is only recommended as a marker of testicular reserve if testicular damage is suspected on physical examination.

A longitudinal scrotal incision is made in the anterior aspect of the scrotum on each side. The incision is made onto the palpable granuloma or onto the identified vasal gap, and only the vas ends are delivered through the skin incision. In cases where the vasectomy was performed high in the scrotum or a large segment was removed or repeat reconstructions were performed with difficult vasal mobilization, the incision may be extended to the inguinal region. Microsurgical dissection is carried out in the region of the prior vasectomy site to free the vas and its vascular pedicle from the surrounding scar tissue. Hemostasis is obtained with great care using either bipolar or hand-held thermal cautery units. After the vas has been mobilized and its scarred ends excised, patency of the abdominal vas end is confirmed with the introduction of a 24-gauge blunt tipped angiocatheter into the lumen and the injection of sterile saline. Fluid from the testicular vas end is examined for the presence of sperm. Copious, clear, watery or cloudy fluid and motile sperm has been shown to be associated with an excellent patency rate of 94%, which is compared with 60% when no sperm is found in the vasal fluid.[19] Thick, toothpaste-like vasal fluid is suggestive of epididymal obstruction. The most important factors in determining the type of reconstructive technique are the quality of sperm found in the intravasal fluid and the surgeon's microsurgical skills. Indeed, attention to surgical details directly affects the success of reconstructive microsurgeries. Important surgical details include the accurate mucosa-to-mucosa approximation, a water-tight tension-free anastomosis, preservation of the vasal blood supply and healthy tissue (mucosa and muscularis), and an adequate microscopic atraumatic technique. Several techniques have been described for VV: (1) the modified one-layer technique, which has been described by Sharlip, (2) the two-layer technique, which has been described by Belker, and (3) the multilayer microdot technique, which was originally described by Goldstein.[1] Recent reports have shown that it is possible to perform classical techniques using robotic assistance. Robots can offer the benefits of enhanced imaging (up to 100× magnification) and control of tremor. Vasoepididymostomy is a challenging surgical procedure that should only be attempted by experienced microsurgeons. Meticulous microsurgical technique and high magnification are required for a precise anastomosis of the vas (luminal diameter of 300–400 mm) to the epididymal tubule (150–250 mm). Intraoperative sperm harvesting and cryopreservation can be offered during VE. The VE procedure starts with the placement of a longitudinal incision in the upper scrotum. The testis is delivered, and the testis and epididymis are thoroughly inspected. The site of obstruction can often be grossly visible as an area where the epididymis transitions from a firm, wide caliber to a smaller, softer structure. The distal end of the vas deferens is mobilized in a similar fashion to the VV procedure, but a longer length is generally required to perform an epididymal anastomosis. Anastomosis is performed under an operating microscope. Currently, three variations of the technique have been used for precise approximation of the vas deferens lumen to a single epididymal tubule: end-to-end, end-to-side, and end-to-side intussusception techniques. Prior to the anastomosis, a dilated epididymal tubule must be identified immediately above the level of obstruction. The tubule must be opened, and the fluid should be inspected for the presence of motile sperm. If no sperm are identified, a more proximal site of the epididymis will be required for the anastomosis. Microsurgical techniques are clearly superior than macrosurgical or loupe-assisted anastomoses. The likelihood of sperm appearance in the semen and of pregnancy after microsurgical vasectomy reversal are inversely related to the duration of time since the vasectomy. Other factors that are related to success rates include the gross appearance of vas fluid at the time of surgery, the presence or absence of sperm in the vas fluid (and sperm quality), the length of the remaining segment adjacent to the epididymis, the age of the female partner, and the experience of the microsurgeon.

Postoperative follow-up should evaluate improvement in semen parameters, complications and spontaneous or assisted conception. Semen analysis should be performed every 2 months after surgery until the semen parameters stabilize or pregnancy occurs.

Summary of evidence and recommendations for vasectomy reversal as per EAU guidelines (2016). Summary of evidence and recommendations for male contraception

Summary of evidence	*LE*
Vasectomy meets best the criteria for the male contribution to contraception, with regard to efficacy, safety and side effects	1a
All available data indicate that vasectomy is not associated with any serious, long-term side-effects	1b
Microsurgical vasectomy reversal is a low-risk and (cost-) effective method of restoring fertility	1a
Methods of male contraception other than vasectomy are associated with high failure rates or are still experimental (e.g., hormonal approach)	3
Recommendations	*GR*
Vasectomy is the gold standard for the male contribution to permanent contraception	B
Cauterization and fascial interposition are the most effective techniques for the prevention of early recanalization	A
Inform patients seeking vasectomy about the surgical method, risk of failure, potential irreversibility, the need for post-procedure contraception until clearance, and the risk of complications	A*
To achieve pregnancy, MESA/PESA/TESE – together with ICSI is a second-line option for men who decline a vasectomy reversal and those with failed vasectomy reversal surgery	B

*Upgraded following panel consensus.
MESA, microsurgical epididymal sperm aspiration; PESA, percutaneous epididymal sperm aspiration; TESE, testicular sperm extraction; ICSI, intracytoplasmic sperm injection.

SPERM RETRIEVAL TECHNIQUES

Azoospermia, which is defined as the absence of spermatozoa in the ejaculate after centrifugation, is found in 1–3% of the male population and approximately 10% of infertile males. In obstructive azoospermia (OA), spermatogenesis is normal, but a mechanical blockage in the genital tract, somewhere between the epididymis and the ejaculatory duct, or the absence of the epididymis and vas deferens prevents spermatozoa from being expelled in semen. Acquired

OA may be secondary to vasectomy or result from a failed vasectomy reversal, postinfectious diseases, surgical procedures in the scrotal, inguinal, pelvic or abdominal regions, or trauma. Congenital causes of OA include cystic fibrosis, congenital absence of the vas deferens (CAVD), ejaculatory duct or prostatic cysts, and Young's syndrome.[24] Nonobstructive azoospermia (NOA) comprises a spectrum of testicular histopathology resulting from various causes, such as environmental toxins, medications, cryptorchidism, genetic and congenital abnormalities, varicocele, trauma, viral orchitis, endocrine disorders, or idiopathic causes. In both OA and NOA, pregnancy may be achieved through *in vitro* fertilization (IVF) associated with ICSI. Several surgical methods have been developed to retrieve epididymal and testicular sperm from azoospermic men. Either percutaneous epididymal sperm aspiration (PESA) or microsurgical epididymal sperm aspiration (MESA) can be successfully used to retrieve sperm from the epididymides in men with obstructive azoospermia. In addition, testicular sperm aspiration (TESA) can be used to retrieve sperm from the testes in men with OA who fail PESA and in men with NOA. Moreover, testicular sperm extraction (TESE) using single or multiple open biopsies and, more recently, microsurgery (micro-TESE) are indicated for men with NOA. The goals of surgical sperm retrieval are (1) to retrieve an adequate number of sperm for both immediate use and for cryopreservation, (2) to obtain the best quality sperm possible and (3) to minimize damage to the reproductive tract to avoid jeopardizing future sperm retrieval attempts or testicular function. Sperm can be easily obtained from infertile men with OA, whereas individuals exhibiting NOA have historically been the most difficult to treat.

Summary of evidence and recommendations for nonobstructive azoospermia as per EAU guidelines (2016).

Summary of evidence	*LE*
The WHO laboratory manual proposes reference values based on fertility hence, these reference values do not allow classifying a man as being infertile	2a
Impaired spermatogenesis is often associated with elevated FSH concentration	3
For patients with NOA who have spermatozoa in their testicular biopsy, ICSI with fresh or cryopreserved spermatozoa is the only therapeutic option. Spermatozoa are found by a TESE procedure in about 50% of patients with NOA	2a
Pregnancies and live births are eventually obtained in 30–50% of couples with NOA, when spermatozoa have been found in the testicular biopsy	3
Recommendations	*GR*
For men who are candidates for sperm retrieval, give appropriate genetic counseling – also when testing for genetic abnormalities was negative	A
In men with NOA, perform simultaneous testicular biopsy with multiple TESE (or micro TESE) to define spermatogenesis and diagnose ITGCNU	A

ICSI, intracytoplasmic sperm injection; ITGCNU, intratubular germ cell neoplasma of unclassified type; TESE, testicular sperm extraction; NOA, nonobstructive azoospermia.

Summary of evidence and recommendations for obstructive azoospermia as per EAU guidelines (2016)

Summary of evidence	*LE*
Obstructive lesions of the seminal tract are frequent in azoospermic or severely oligozoospermic patients with normal-sized testes and normal reproductive hormones	3
Recommendations	*GR*
For azoospermia caused by vasal or epididymal obstruction, perform microsurgical vasovasostomy or tubulovasostomy	B
Use sperm retrieval techniques, such as MESA, TESE, and PESA only when cryostorage of the material obtained is available	B

The pregnancy rates of ICSI using testicular sperm extracted by TESA or micro-TESE in NOA are significantly lower than those obtained with either ejaculated or epididymal/testicular sperm from men with OA.[25] Testicular spermatozoa of men with severely impaired spermatogenesis have decreased fertility potential and may have a higher tendency to carry deficiencies (e.g., related to the centrioles and genetic material), which ultimately affect the capability of the male gamete to activate the egg and trigger the formation and development of a normal zygote and a viable embryo. Although there is limited available data, studies have suggested that the sperm retrieval technique itself has no impact on ICSI success rates. Nonetheless, frozen-thawed surgically retrieved sperm from NOA men have significantly impaired reproductive potential compared with fresh sperm. Meta-analysis results have shown that fertilization rates by ICSI remain similar, but implantation was significantly higher (by 73%) with the use of fresh compared with frozen thawed testicular sperm. The question of whether ICSI using sperm retrieved from men with either OA or NOA might be associated with an increased risk of birth defects is still unresolved. In general, IVF techniques are associated with multiple gestations and an increased risk of congenital abnormalities (including hypospadias). ICSI in particular carries an increased

Table 21.3: Surgical techniques for sperm retrieval.[26] (Figs. 21.2 and 21.3)

	Advantages	*Disadvantages*
Microsurgical epididymal sperm aspiration (MESA)	Microsurgical procedure allows lower complication rate. Epididymal sperm has better motility than testicular sperm. Large number of sperm can be harvested for cryopreservation of multiple vials in a single procedure.	Requires anesthesia and microsurgical skills. Not indicated for nonobstructive azoospermia.
Percutaneous epididymal sperm aspiration (PESA)	No microsurgical skill required. Local anesthesia. Epididymal sperm has better motility than testicular sperm.	Complications include hematoma, pain, and vascular injury to testes and obstruction of the epididymis. Variable success in obtaining sperm. Smaller quantity of sperm obtained than with MESA. Not indicated for nonobstructive azoospermia.
Testicular sperm aspiration (TESA)	No microsurgical skill required. Local anesthesia. Can be used for obstructive azoospermia.	Immature or immotile testicular sperm. Small quantity of sperm obtained. Poor results in nonobstructive azoospermia. Complications include hematoma, pain, and vascular injury to testes and epididymis.
Testicular sperm extraction (TESE)	Low complication rate if performed microsurgically. Preferred technique for nonobstructive azoospermia.	Requires anesthesia and microsurgical skills.

risk of endocrine abnormalities and epigenetic imprinting effects. Although the absolute risk of any of these conditions remains low, current data is limited, and study populations are heterogenic. Therefore, well-defined groups of ICSI with ejaculated sperm, ICSI with epididymal sperm, ICSI with testicular sperm, and a control group of naturally conceived children should be closely monitored.

Percutaneous Sperm Retrieval Techniques

PESA is carried out under local anesthesia only or in association with intravenous sedation. In both cases, a 10 mL solution of 2% lidocaine is injected around the spermatic cord near the external inguinal ring (Table 21.3).

PESA Indications

PESA is indicated in obstructive azoospermia cases only.

Technique

After anesthetic blockade of the spermatic cord, epididymis is stabilized between the index finger, thumb and forefinger while the testis is held with the palm of the hand. Normally in the left hand if you are a right hander. A 26-gauge needle attached to a 1 mL tuberculin syringe is inserted into the epididymis through the scrotal skin. Alternatively you can use a 26–28 gauge butterfly with a 5 mL syringe. The hub of the syringe or about 500–600 μL of sperm medium is taken in the tubing of the butterfly.

Negative pressure is created and the tip of the needle is gently moved in and out within the epididymis until fluid enters the syringe. The amount of epididymal fluid obtained during aspiration is often minimal (~0.1 mL), except in cases of CAVD, in which 0.3–1.0 mL may be aspirated. The needle is withdrawn from the epididymis and the aspirate is flushed with the fluid which is in the hub or the tubing into a petri dish at 37°C. The dish containing the epididymal aspirate is transferred to the laboratory for

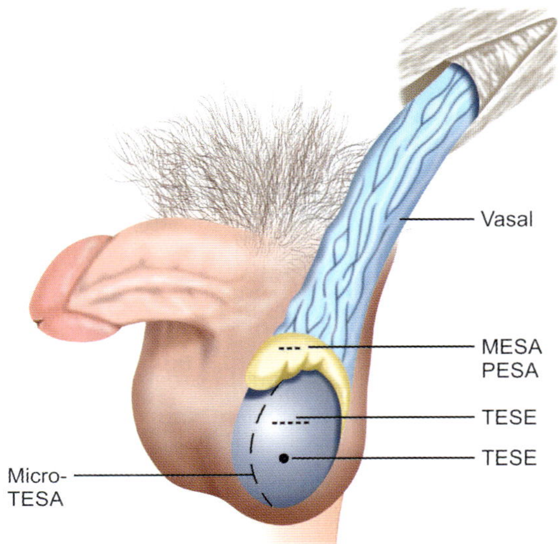

Fig. 21.2: Diagram demonstrating different sites for sperm retrieval

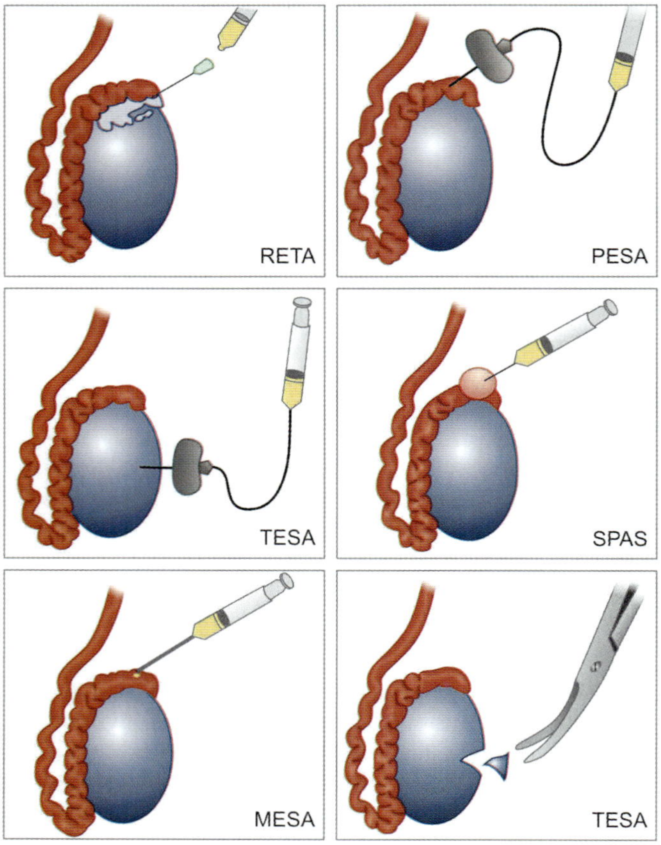

Fig. 21.3: Diagrammatic demonstration of various techniques of surgical sperm retrieval.

microscopic examination. PESA is repeated at a different site of the same epididymis (from cauda to caput) and/or at the contralateral one until adequate number of motile sperm is retrieved. If PESA fails to retrieve motile sperm for ICSI, TESA is performed at the same sitting.

Testicular Sperm Aspiration (TESA)

Indications

TESA may be performed in either OA or NOA cases. In OA, TESA is carried out after a failed PESA, but may be also used as a primary retrieval procedure in cases of absent epididymis or intense epididymal fibrosis. In NOA, TESA may be used as a diagnostic tool to obtain testicular parenchyma for histology analysis and sperm search previous to the ICSI cycle. In addition, it is indicated for sperm retrieval in cases of favorable prognosis, such as the ones with a previously successful TESA attempt or those with testicular biopsy result showing hypospermatogenesis.

Technique

After anesthetic blockade of the spermatic cord, epididymis is stabilized between the index finger, thumb, and forefinger while the anterior scrotal skin is stretched.

A 18–21 gauge needle attached to a 20 mL syringe is connected to a syringe holder and is inserted through the stretched scrotal skin into the anteromedial or anterolateral portion of the superior testicular pole, in an oblique angle toward the medium and lower poles. Alternatively, a 18–21 gauge butterfly is used with suction being developed by a 20 mL attached syringe. About 0.5–1.0 mL of sperm medium is taking into the syringe or the butterfly.

Negative pressure is created by pulling the syringe holder while the tip of the needle is moved in and out within the testis in an oblique plane to disrupt the seminiferous tubules and sample different areas. When a small piece of testicular tissue is aspirated, the needle is gently withdrawn from the testis while the negative pressure is maintained.

A pair of microsurgery forceps is used to grab the seminiferous tubules that exteriorize from the scrotal skin, thus aiding in the removal of the specimen. The specimen is flushed into a tube containing 0.5–1.0 mL warm sperm medium, and is transferred to the laboratory for microscopic examination. TESA or TESE may be performed at the contralateral testis if insufficient or no sperm are obtained.

Microsurgical Sperm Retrieval Techniques

Microsurgical sperm retrieval may be performed under either local anesthesia in association with intravenous sedation or epidural anesthesia.

MESA Indications

MESA is indicated in obstructive azoospermia cases only.

Technique

Atransverse 2 cm incision is made through the layers, and the testis is exteriorized. The epididymis is examined and its tunica is incised. An enlarged tubule is dissected and opened with sharp microsurgical scissors.

Fluid exuding from the tubule is aspirated with a silicone tube or blunted needle attached to a 1-mL tuberculin syringe. The aspirate is flushed into a 0.5–1.0 mL 37°C sperm medium.

The tube containing the epididymal aspirate is transferred to the laboratory for microscopic examination.

MESA is repeated at a different site of the same epididymis (from cauda to caput) and/or at the contralateral one until adequate number of motile sperm is retrieved. If MESA fails to retrieve motile sperm, TESA or TESE may be performed at the same operative time.

Microsurgical Testicular Sperm Extraction (Micro-TESE)

Indications

Micro-TESE is indicated in NOA cases only.

Technique

After anesthetic blockade of spermatic cord, the anterior scrotal skin is stretched and the skin and tunica vaginalis are infiltrated with 2 mL of 2% lidocaine. A transverse 2 cm incision is made through the anesthetized layers, and the testis is exteriorized.

A single, large, midportion incision is made in an avascular area of the tunica albuginea under 6–8× magnification, and the testicular parenchyma is widely exposed.

Dissection of the testicular parenchyma is carried out at 16–25× magnification searching for enlarged seminiferous tubules (more likely to contain germ cells and eventually normal sperm production). The superficial and deep testicular regions may be examined, if necessary, and microsurgical-guided testicular biopsies are performed by removing enlarged tubules. If enlarged tubules are not seen, then any tubule different than the remaining ones in size is excised. If all tubules are identical in appearance, random microbiopsies (at least three at each testicular pole) are performed.

Each excised testicular tissue specimen is placed at the outer-well dish containing sperm media. Specimens are washed grossly to remove blood clots and are sent to the laboratory for processing and search for sperm.

Albuginea and scrotal layers are closed using nonabsorbable and absorbable sutures, respectively.

Conventional Testicular Sperm Extraction (Conventional TESE)

Indications

Single or multiple open testicular biopsies may be taken to obtain sperm in both OA and NOA, but TESE is used mainly in cases of NOA. In OA, TESE may be used after failed PESA or TESA. In NOA, TESE may also be used as a diagnostic tool to obtain testicular parenchyma for histology analysis and search of sperm previous to the ICSI cycle. TESE may be performed under either local anesthesia with or without intravenous sedation or regional anesthesia.

Technique

After anesthetic blockade of spermatic cord, the anterior scrotal skin is stretched and the skin and tunica vaginalis are infiltrated with 2 mL of 2% lidocaine. A transverse 2 cm incision is made through the anesthetized skin, cremaster, and parietal tunica vaginalis. Conventional TESE is carried out without magnification.

A small self-retaining eyelid retractor is placed to improve exposure of the tunica albuginea, since the testis is not exteriorized.

The tunica albuginea is incised for approximately 1 cm. Gentle pressure is made on the testis to extrude testicular parenchyma.

A fragment of approximately 5 × 5 × 5 mm is excised with sharp scissors and placed promptly in sperm culture medium. Specimen is sent to the laboratory for processing and microscopic examination.

Albuginea is closed using nonabsorbable sutures. Procedure may be repeated if multiple biopsies are selected for preference.

Sperm Retrieval Rates

PESA and TESA were highly effective methods for retrieving sperm in the group of men with OA. Successful sperm retrieval (SRR) was achieved in over 85% of the cases using PESA, but more than one aspiration was required in several cases. In cases of failed PESA, TESA was adequate to obtain sperm in practically all cases. Motile spermatozoa was obtained in approximately 73% of the cases after the first or second PESA aspirations, and TESA was carried out as a rescue procedure after failed PESA in about 14% of the individuals. Successful sperm retrieval using percutaneous techniques appears to be independent of the cause of obstruction, since SRR rates did not differ among groups. In the group of men with NOA, SRR rates were in the range of 50–70% in most etiology-specific causes of NOA. Testicular histopathology results were predictive of sperm collection using both TESA and micro-TESE. According to our data involving 176 individuals, overall SRR rates by TESA were 64.4%, but only 20.7% and 33.3% in cases of Sertoli cell only and maturation arrest, respectively. On the other hand, SRR by TESA was 100% and 82.3% in NOA men presenting with either hypospermatogenesis on testicular histology or a history of a previous successful TESA attempt. Using micro-TESE, overall SRR rates were 52.3%, but higher than TESA in cases of maturation arrest and Sertoli cell-only.

CONCLUSION

Varicocele treatment based on the presence of clinically palpable varicocele and abnormal semen parameters should be reconsidered in light of the newly proposed WHO reference values for laboratory semen analysis. Open microsurgical inguinal or subinguinal techniques are currently the best treatment modalities because they result in higher spontaneous pregnancy rates and fewer recurrences and postoperative complications. Surgical repair of varicocele improves semen parameters and functional markers of oxidative stress and DNA integrity. Testicular histopathology is predictive of success, and men with MA and HS are more likely to ejaculate motile spermatozoa after surgery.

Men with OA may father children either by surgical correction of the obstruction, which may allow the couple to conceive naturally. The return of sperm to ejaculate after microsurgical reconstructions is achieved in 70–95% of cases, and 30–75% of couples achieve unassisted pregnancy.

TURED is the treatment of choice for EDO. After TURED, sperm return to the ejaculate in approximately 50–75% of men, and approximately 20% of couples achieve pregnancy. In OA, sperm production is normal and gametes can be easily retrieved from the epididymides or testicles in approximately 100% of cases, irrespective of the technique.

In NOA, successful sperm retrieval is approximately 50%. The use of microsurgery during TESE may improve the efficacy of sperm extraction with significantly less tissue removed, which ultimately facilitates sperm processing. Children conceived using sperm retrieved from men with OA or NOA should be monitored because it is still unclear if there is an increased risk of birth defects when ICSI is carried out with nonejaculated sperm.[27]

REFERENCES

1. Goldstein M. Surgical Management of Male Infertility. Campbell-Walsh Urology, 11th edition. Philadelphia: Elsevier; p. 580:12.
2. Vital and Health Statistics, Series 23, No. 26, CDC. http://www.cdc.gov.
3. Esteves S. Infertilidade masculina. In: Rhoden EL (Ed). Urologia no consultó rio, 1a. ed. Porto Alegre, RS: Artmed Editora; 2009: pp. 470-500.
4. Kass EJ, Belman AB. Reversal of testicular growth failure by varicocele ligation. J Urol. 1987;137(3):475-6.
5. Marmar JL, Agarwal A, Prabakaran S, Agarwal R, Short RA, Benoff S. Reassessing the value of varicocelectomy as a treatment for male subfertility with a new meta-analysis. Fertil Steril. 2007;88(3):639-48.
6. Goldstein M. Surgical management of male infertility. Campbell-Walsh Urology, 11th edition. Philadelphia: Elsevier; p. 604:25.5.
7. Esteves SC, Glina S. Recovery of spermatogenesis after microsurgical subinguinal varicocele repair in azoospermic men based on testicular histology. Int Braz J Urol. 2005;31: 541-8.
8. Weedin JW, Khera M, Lipshultz LI. Varicocele repair in patients with nonobstructive azoospermia—a meta-analysis. J Urol. 2010;183:2309-15.
9. Watanabe M, Nagai A, Kusumi N, Tsuboi H, Nasu Y, Kumon H. Minimal invasiveness and effectivity of subinguinal microscopic varicocelectomy: a comparative study with retroperitoneal high and laparoscopic approaches. Int J Urol. 2005;12(10):892-8.
10. Riccabona M, Oswald J, Koen M, Lusuardi L, Radmayr C, Bartsch G. Optimizing the operative treatment of boys with varicocele: sequential comparison of 4 techniques. J Urol. 2003;169(2):666-8.
11. Beck EM, Schlegel PN, Goldstein M. Intraoperative varicocele anatomy: a macroscopic and microscopic study. J Urol. 1992;148(4):1190-4.
12. Tauber R, Johnsen N. Antegrade scrotal sclerotherapy for the treatment of varicocele: technique and late results. J Urol. 1994;151:386-90.
13. Sigmund G, Bähren W, Gall H, Lenz M, Thon W. Idiopathic varicoceles: feasibility of percutaneous sclerotherapy. Radiology. 1987;164:161-8.
14. Lenk S, Fahlenkamp D, Gliech V, Lindeke A. Comparison of different methods of treating varicocele. J Androl. 1994;15(suppl):34S-7S.
15. Seyferth W, Jecht E, Zeitler E. Percutaneous sclerotherapy of varicocele. Radiology. 1981;139:335-40.
16. Ivanissevich O. Left varicocele due to reflux; experience with 4,470 operative cases in forty-two years. J Int Coll Surg. 1960;34:742-55.
17. Palomo A. Radical cure of varicocele by a new technique; preliminary report. J Urol. 1949;61:604-7.
18. Goldstein M, Gilbert BR, Dicker AP, Dwosh J, Gnecco C. Microsurgical inguinal varicocelectomy with delivery of the testis: an artery and lymphatic sparing technique. J Urol. 1992;148:1808-11.
19. Jungwirth A, Gögüs C, Hauser G, Gomahr A, Schmeller N, Aulitzky W, et al. Clinical outcome of microsurgical subinguinal varicocelectomy in infertile men. Andrologia. 2001;33:71-4.
20. Miersch WD, Schoeneich G, Winter P, Buszello H. Laparoscopic varicocelectomy: indication, technique and surgical results. Br J Urol. 1995;76:636-8.

21. Netto NR Jr, Esteves SC, Neves PA. Transurethral resection of partially obstructed ejaculatory ducts: seminal parameters and pregnancy outcomes according to the etiology of obstruction. J Urol. 1998;159:2048-53.
22. Yurdakul T, Gokce G, Kilic O, et al. Transurethral resection of ejaculatory ducts in the treatment of complete ejaculatory duct obstruction. Int Urol Nephrol. 2008;40(2): 369-72.
23. Parekattil SJ, Kuang W, Agarwal A, Thomas AJ. Model to predict if a vasoepididymostomy will be required for vasectomy reversal. J Urol. 2005;173:1681-4.
24. Jarow JP, Espeland MA, Lipshultz LI. Evaluation of the azoospermic patient. J Urol. 1989;142:62-5.
25. Goldstein M. Surgical management of male infertility. Campbell-Walsh Urology, 11th edition; Philadelphia: Elsevier; p. 601:25.3.
26. Nicopoullos JD, Gilling-Smith C, Almeida PA, Norman-Taylor J, Grace I, Ramsay JW. Use of surgical sperm retrieval in azoospermic men: a meta-analysis. Fertil Steril. 2004;82: 691-701.
27. Woldringh GH, Besselink DE, Tillema AH, Hendriks JC, Kremer JA. Karyotyping, congenital anomalies and follow-up of children after intracytoplasmic sperm injection with non-ejaculated sperm: a systematic review. Hum Reprod Update. 2010;16:12-9.

CHAPTER 22

Effect of Environment and Infections on Semen Quality

Natachandra Chimote

INTRODUCTION

Male reproductive function in the general population has drawn increasing attention due to reports indicating increased occurrence of testicular cancer, cryptorchidism and hypospadias across some time periods in some populations in the past 50 years.[1,2] Reports indicating declining sperm counts in some regions[3,4] have also greatly stimulated hypotheses that environmental pollutants may impair male fertility.[5]

The decline in semen quality in men of reproductive age is a controversial issue. The debate began when a review highlighted a decrease in sperm counts of up to 50% during the period 1940–1990[4] and continued with several meta-analyses reporting a decline in semen quality[6,7] around the world. Some recent studies have corroborated this decline in semen quality,[8-10] whereas others have found no such changes.[11-13] Among the hypotheses proposed to explain this phenomenon is that of exposure to endocrine-disrupting environmental pollutants, such as certain persistent organic pollutants (POPs).[14] Environmental contaminants, such as POPs are man-made bioaccumulative and lipophilic compounds, with long half-lives, that are found throughout the world as a result of widespread use in a variety of consumer products during the last century. As a consequence, all populations worldwide bear a body burden of POPs, with large interindividual and interpopulation differences.[15]

The discovery in 1977 of the severe spermatotoxic effect of the nematocide dibromochloropropane (DBCP) among workers at a chemical plant[16] initiated several studies of occupational and environmental risks to male reproductive function. Although for several decades, semen quality has been used as a marker of male reproductive function in case of environmental exposure, the data are still limited.[17,18]

An obvious consequence of exposure to reproductive toxicants is infertility. Infertility is defined as inability to conceive after a year of sexual intercourse without the use of contraceptives. A male contributory factor is involved in approximately half of these cases,[19] but most of the causes of reduced semen quality and other disturbances of male reproductive function are unknown.[20]

Studies in the immediate past, as reviewed by Sheiner et al. (2003)[21] and Jensen et al. (2006)[22] show that variety of environmental and occupational exposures may impair male fertility. These exposures and conditions include air pollution and drinking water pollutants, biopersistent organochlorines, trihalomethanes, phthalates and high frequency electromagnetic radiation related to use of mobile phones.

Endocrine Disruptor Compounds (EDCs), such as some polychlorinated biphenyls (PCBs), organochlorine compounds (pesticides) or phthalate esters (PEs), several heavy metals and polycyclic aromatic hydrocarbons (PAHs) may compromise semen quality.

Chemicals could adversely affect male reproductive system by, either disrupting the gonadal endocrine axis,[14,23] or the spermatogenesis process. Any of those mechanisms would result in poor semen quality.[24-26] Recent studies suggest that sperm DNA integrity may be altered by environmental exposure to some toxic chemicals.[27,28] DNA fragmentation may be an excellent marker for exposure to potential reproductive toxicants and a diagnostic tool for male infertility.[29-31]

In this chapter, we review the current evidence of on the association between the main occupational and lifestyles exposures and male infertility.

ENDOCRINE DISRUPTOR COMPOUNDS (EDCs)

EDCs not only might cause the "testicular dysgenesis syndrome" (TDS) but also disturb meiosis in developmental germinal cells.[5,14] It was suggested that the male reproductive system is most vulnerable to estrogenic agents during the critical period of cell differentiation and organ development in fetal and neonatal life.[14] In this period, the testes are structurally organized, establishing Sertoli cell and spermatogonia numbers to support spermatogenesis that will be initiated at puberty. The maintenance of tightly regulated estrogen levels is essential for its completion.

It has also been described that these compounds cross a blood–tissue barrier similar to that of the testis, suggesting that intratubular germ cells might be exposed.[32,33] Genistein, the principle soy isoflavone, has estrogen activity and is widely consumed. Doerge et al.[32] measured placental transfer of genistein in rats as possible route of developmental exposure. Pregnant Sprague–Dawley rats were administered genistein orally. Concentration of genistein aglycone and conjugates were measured in maternal and offspring serum and brain. Although fetal or neonatal serum concentrations of total genistein were approximately 20-fold lower than maternal serum concentrations, the biologically active genistein aglycone concentration was only fivefold lower, and the fetal brains contained predominantly genistein aglycone at levels similar to the maternal brain. These studies show that genistein aglycone crosses the rat placenta and can reach significant levels in fetal brains.

It was investigated that the hypothesis that farmers that have a high intake of organically grown commodities would have a high semen quality due to their expected lower levels of dietary pesticides intake.[34] In their conclusions, authors reported that estimated dietary intake of 40 groups of pesticides did not seem to entail a risk of impaired semen quality, but as they recommended, caution should be taken in trying to generalize these negative results to populations with higher dietary exposure levels or intakes of different groups of pesticides.

Endogenous hormones have a vital role in fetal life and ensure future fertility. Exposure to wrong hormones (male fetus exposed to female hormones) or inadequate amounts of these, could affect the reproductive system and genitalia may not develop properly resulting in fertility problems in adulthood.[35,36]

In the recent past, a review published[37] about a sensitivity of the child to sex steroids and the possible impact of exogenous estrogens. Some of the conclusions were that children are extremely sensitive to estradiol and may respond with increased growth and breast development even at serum levels below the current detection limits, and that those changes in hormone levels during fetal and prepubertal development may have several effects on adult life. The authors concluded that a cautionary approach should be taken to avoid unnecessary exposure of fetuses and children to exogenous sex steroids and endocrine disruptors, even at very low levels. The caution includes food intake, as possible adverse effects on human health may be expected by consumption of meat from hormone treated animals.

One more study[38] in the recent past carried out by Swan et al. suggests that the maternal beef consumption and possibly xenobiotics (anabolic steroids) in beef may alter testicular development in uterus and adversely affect reproductive capacity. Sperm concentration was adversely related to mother's weekly beef intake. In sons of "high consumers" (>7 beef meals/week), sperm concentration was 24.3% lower than that of men whose mother ate less beef.[37]

General population is exposed to many potential endocrine disruptors concurrently. Studies, both *in vitro* and *in vivo*, have shown that the action of estrogenic compounds is additive[39,40] but little is known about the possible synergistic or addictive effects of these compounds in human beings.

A recent work published by the Nordic Cryptorchidism Study Group studied the association between maternal exposure to 27 groups of pesticides and cryptorchidism among male children. In a nested case control study within a prospective birth cohort, researchers compared 62 milk samples from mothers of cryptorchid boys and 68 from mothers of healthy ones and significant differences were found for any individual chemical. However, combined statistical analysis of the eight most abundant and persistent pesticides showed that pesticide levels higher in boys with cryptorchidism.[41]

Consequently, it is being speculated that male reproductive anomalies (hypospadias, cryptorchidism) and global fall in sperm counts have both a causal link in the marked increase of phytoestrogens in our diet brought about by the western adoption of a fast food culture.[42]

HEAVY METALS

Exposure to metals (mainly lead and cadmium) has been long associated with low sperm motility and density, increased morphological anomalies and male infertility.[43,44] Males working in metal industry had a decreased fertility when compared to other workers as shown by delayed pregnancy and reduced semen quality.[45-51] It was observed that while comparing seminal plasma concentrations of cadmium in 60 infertile males with 40 normozoospermic males, seminal plasma levels of Cd were significantly higher than serum levels in all subjects ($p < 0.001$). A statistically significant inverse correlation was observed between serum Cd levels and all biophysical semen parameters except sperm volume. The result of that study[50] support previous findings concerning cadmium toxicity and male infertility.

Naha et al.[51] studied the blood and semen lead level concentration among battery and paint industry workers. Their results included oligozoospermia, concomitant lowering of sperm protein and nucleic acid content and increased percentage of sperm DNA haploids ($p < 0.001$), suggesting a diminution of sperm cell production after occupational lead exposure. Additionally, there was a decreased sperm velocity, reduced gross and forward progressive motility with high stationary motile spermatozoa ($p < 0.001$) suggesting retarded sperm activity among exposed workers. Finally, they also found increased incidence of teratozoospermia associated with high blood and seminal fluid lead levels ($p < 0.001$). Other reports also have shown a significantly negative correlation between blood lead concentration and semen quality.[52,53]

In the recent past, Telisman et al.[53] reported reproductive toxicity of low-level lead exposure in men with no occupational exposure to metals. In this study, semen quality, seminal plasma indicators of secretory function of the prostate and seminal vesicles, sex hormones in serum, and biomarkers of lead, cadmium, copper, zinc, and selenium body burden were measured in 240 Croatian men of age group 19–52 years. After adjustment in multiple regressions, a significant associations were found between blood lead and reproductive parameters, such as immature sperm concentration, percentage of pathologic sperm, wide sperm, round and short sperm, serum levels of testosterone and estradiol and a decrease in seminal plasma zinc and in serum prolactin ($p < 0.05$). These reproductive effects were observed at low-level lead exposures (median BPb 49 μg/L, range 11–149 μg/L in 240 objects) that are similar to those of the general population worldwide.

AIR POLLUTION

The major air pollutants in the whole world are sulfur dioxide (SO_2), nitrogen oxides (NO_x), particulate matter (PM) and ozone (O_3). Air pollutants can be in the form of solid particles, liquid droplets or gases. In addition, they may be natural or man-made. Sources of air pollution refer to the various locations, activities or factors, which are responsible for the releasing of pollutants into the atmosphere.

Several studies addressing links between ambient air pollution and semen quality have been published past few years.[54-57] The authors observed a reduced percentage of sperm with normal morphology and proportionately more sperm with abnormal chromatin in men. Significantly, increased frequency of sperm with abnormal morphology and reduced motility was observed in men with medium and high exposure to air pollution. More intensively exposed males also had significantly higher frequency of disomy in chromosomes X, XY and Y.[55]

A significant association was found between exposure to periods of high air pollution and the percentage of sperm with DNA fragmentation according to sperm chromatin structure assay (SCSA). Other semen measures were not associated with air pollution.[56]

The relationship between air pollutant levels and semen quality was also evaluated over 2-year period by analyzing repeated semen samples collected by sperm donors. Semen analysis data derived from 48 semen samples provided by sperm donors were correlated with air pollution level (ozone, nitrogen dioxide, carbon monoxide, particulate matter). There was a significant negative correlation between ozone levels at 0–9, 10–14 and 70–90 days before donation and average sperm concentration, which was adjusted for donor's birth date, age at donation, temperature and seasonality.[57]

Summing up, although some studies suggest a link between ambient air pollutants and various semen characteristics like reduced percentage of sperm with normal morphology and proportionately more sperm with abnormal chromatin and reduction of motility, additional research is needed to corroborate this association and to establish the causal agents.

ORGANOCHLORINE CONTAMINANTS, DIOXINS AND POLYCHLORINATED BIPHENYLS

Organochlorines were widely used worldwide from 1940 through 1970s, but most have been eliminated or restricted in use after recognition of their persistence in the environment, bioaccumulation in animals and humans and toxicity in laboratory animals and wildlife.

Exposure mainly occurs through ingestion of contaminated food, but can also occur through dermal contact and inhalation. A time-related deterioration in male reproductive function caused by exposure to persistent organochlorines (POCs) has been hypothesized. In animal studies, POCs were found to have adverse effects on male reproductive function. The studies on exposure to organochlorine compounds and semen quality suggested association between polychlorinated biphenyls (PCBs) exposure and poor sperm quality.

The total motile sperm counts were inversely proportional to the PCB concentrations and were significantly lower among infertile male than those of the controls.[58]

A strong and monotonically increasing DNA fragmentation index with increasing serum levels of 2,2′,4,4′,5,5′-hexachlorobiphenyl (CB-153) was found in a study performed by Spanò et al.[59] Sperm motility was also inversely related to the lipid adjusted serum concentration of CB-153 among men in each of four regions (Greenland, Sweden, Warsaw and Ukrania), which is consistent with several earlier findings and results of animal studies.[60] Thus, there is fairly strong evidence to suggest that persistent organic pollutants interfere with sperm motility, although the causal agent cannot be identified because of a strong correlation in serum concentration of a wide number of biopersistent pollutants.[61]

The results of the presented studies suggest that there is an association between exposure and poor sperm quality, especially an inverse relationship was found between sperm motility and the concentration of PCBs, whereas other effects (sperm count and morphology) are rather uncertain. Increasing DNA fragmentation index with increasing serum levels of CB-153 was also found. On the other hand, no effects of concentration of CB-153 and *p,p′*-DDE on sperm concentration and prostate-specific antigen (PSA) were observed.

TRIHALOMETHANES IN TAP WATER

Trihalomethanes (THMs) are a by-product of the water treatment process. They are formed when natural organic material reacts with chlorine used to treat the water. This reaction produces "disinfection by-products" (DBPs), the most common of which are trihalomethanes (THMs). THMs, such as chloroform, bromoform, chlorodibromomethane and bromodichloromethane, are the most prevalent and routinely measured class of DBPs found in the water.[62] Routes of exposure to THMs include dermal absorption during hand washing and bathing, inhalation during showering and ingestion of drinking water.[63]

Animal studies have consistently demonstrated an association between oral exposure to DBPs including haloacetic acids (HAAs) and trihalomethanes and adverse effects in male reproductive system: acute spermatoxicity, impaired reproductive competence, sperm quality,[64] delayed spermiation and distorted sperm motility and morphology,[65] histopathologic changes in testis and epididymis,[66] transient subfertility,[67] altered sperm production and epididymal tubule changes.[68] Contrary to large amount of evidences on the detrimental effects of DBPs on male reproductive function in animals, two so far completed human studies have not supported these findings.[69,70] Based on the presented results, there seems to be no association between exposure to THMs and poor semen quality (sperm concentration and sperm count). As the number of studies is limited, further studies of the effect of THMs on semen quality are needed.

PESTICIDES

Pesticides form a large group of heterogeneous chemicals, which are used to kill insects, weed, fungi and rodents. On the one hand, these substances bring a significant public health benefit by increasing productivity in the food industry and decreasing the incidence of diseases.

Pesticides in general may directly damage spermatozoa, alter Steroli cell or Laydig cell function, or disrupt the endocrine function in any stage of hormone regulation (hormone synthesis, release, storage, transport and clearance, receptor recognition and binding).[71] Clear effects on male fertility have been demonstrated for some pesticides, such as dibromochloropropane,[4] ethylene dibromide,[72] organophosphorus,[73,74] alochlor, metochlor, 2,4-D, atrazine,[75] fenvalerate,[76] carbaryl and chlorpyrifos.[77]

Among Danish greenhouse workers exposed to pesticides, the median values of sperm concentration and proportion of normal spermatozoa were lower by 60% and 14%, respectively, in the high- and low-level exposure groups. The median sperm concentration was lower by 40% for men with over 10 years work experience in a greenhouse than for those with experience below 5 years.[78] Also, significantly lower sperm count was found in pesticide plant workers exposed to fenvalerate compared with nonexposed controls in the study performed in China.[76]

Some studies assessed the levels of reproductive hormones. Farmers exposed to pesticides in Argentina had higher serum oestradiol concentrations and lower luteinizing hormone (LH) concentrations than nonexposed men.[79] In Japan, pesticide sprayers had the serum testosterone concentration in winter higher than the controls ($p < 0.05$), though luteinizing hormone and follicle-stimulating hormone concentrations were not significantly different. The sperm counts and vitality were comparable between the groups, but detailed sperm motility analysis in summer revealed that the percentages of slow progressive and non-progressive motile sperm were twice as high in the sprayers ($p < 0.05$), and that of rapid progressive sperm tended to be lower ($p = 0.06$). Such differences were not observed in winter.[80] Semen quality and reproductive hormones across a spraying season were examined among Danish farmers (using and not using pesticides) and controls (non farmers) that were asked to give two semen samples.[81] The median sperm concentration declined significantly from the first to the second sample in both groups, but there was no statistical difference in the decline between the two groups. It was concluded that semen quality did not change across a spraying season as a result of pesticide exposure. Sprayers and nonsprayers had an equal decline in sperm concentration from the first to the second semen sample.[81]

In China and Mexico, studies of the prevalence of sperm aneuploidy[73,74] in agricultural workers exposed to organophosphorous pesticides, such as ethyl parathion, methamidophos or endosulfan were conducted. In China, male workers at a large pesticide-manufacturing plant had an excess risk of aneuploidy and the risk of specific chromosome abnormalities: disomy for chromosome 18 and the three different types of sex chromosome disomy (XX, XY, YY).[74] In the Mexico study, aneuploidies were found in 0.67% of total sperm nuclei. The authors concluded that exposure to organophosphates could interfere with sperm chromosome segregation and increase the risk of Turner's syndrome.[73] The next study performed in Mexico showed the poorest semen quality among the subjects with the highest OP exposure and the highest urinary OP levels. Seasonal variations in sperm concentration and sperm count were registered. The results showed a significant decrease in total sperm count among subjects with the highest exposure to OP.[82]

Men with high exposure level of alachlor (>0.15 μg/g creatinine) had poorer semen parameters (concentration, percentage sperm with normal morphology, percentage motile sperm) than those less exposed. In addition, The exposure to herbicide 2,4-D, metolachlor and atrazine was associated with poorer sperm quality.[75] The next study where the exposure to carbaryl and chlorpyrifos was analyzed by detecting the urinary metabolites showed an associated between exposure and lower sperm concentration and motility among men attending an infertility clinic.[77]

Yucra et al.[83] reported a significant reduction of semen volume and an increase in semen pH in men with organophosphate metabolites in urine in the study performed in Peru.[83] The poorest semen quality was found among farmers with the highest OP exposure and the highest urinary OP levels. The results showed a significant decrease in total sperm count among subjects with the highest exposure to OP.[83]

In summary, there are several indications that some pesticides may impair semen quality in humans, but weak exposure assessment in most studies precludes proper identification of responsible agents and evaluation of exposure–response relations.

PHTHALATES

Phthalates are among the most widely used man-made chemicals released to the environment over the last several decades.[84] Phthalates are used as plasticizers to increase the flexibility of PCV products, such as toys, vinyl flooring and electricity cables or medical devices. The main plasticizer used in PVC based medical devices is di(2-ethylhexyl) phthalate (DEHP). Phthalates are also used as solvents or fixing agents in perfumes, body lotions and other cosmetics. Humans are mainly exposed to these compounds through the diet, medical devices and consumer products. In spite of short half times in the organism, the compounds or their metabolites have been detected in urine in more than 95% of men and women that have been investigated.[85]

Several recent epidemiological studies have addressed the male reproductive toxicity of phthalates.[86-92] They observed an inverse dose–response relationship between 2 phthalate metabolites [monobutyl- and monobenzyl phthalate (MBP, MbzP)] on the one side and sperm concentration and motility on the other. Also in a study performed in India, a negative correlation between semen phthalate level (DEHP) and sperm concentration, motility, percentage of abnormal sperm was found in a population of men that visited an infertility clinic.[91]

Duty et al.[86] to explore the association between environmental levels of phthalates and altered reproductive hormone levels in adult men showed that an interquartile range (IQR) change in monobenzyl phthalate (MBzP) exposure was significantly associated with a 10% decrease in follicle-stimulating hormone (FSH) concentration. Additionally, an IQR change in monobutyl phthalate (MBP) exposure was associated with a 4.8% increase in inhibin B, but this was of borderline significance.[86]

On other hand, in a Swedish study, Jonsson et al.[88] reported that only subjects within the highest quartile for monoethyl phthalate (MEP) had fewer motile sperms, more immotile sperms and lower luteinizing hormone values, but there was no suggestion of harmful effects for most other endpoints. In the study in China, there was no significant difference between phthalate concentrations of semen and sperm density and liveability, while there was a significant positive association between liquefied time of semen and phthalate concentrations of semen.[92]

Summing up, results of few studies of subfertile men demonstrate associations between phthalate levels commonly experienced by the public and impaired sperm quality (impact on sperm concentration, morphology, motility), but findings have not been corroborated in studies of men from the general population.

MOBILE PHONES

There has been a tremendous increase in the use of mobile phones in the past decade and concerns are growing about the possible detrimental effects of high-frequency electromagnetic fields (EMF) emitted by these devices on human health.

In a small prospective study involving 13 men with normal sperm, GSM phone usage in 5 days for 6 hours per day decreased the rapid progressive motility of sperm.[93] Interesting results were obtained in a pilot study performed in Australia; men who carried their mobile phone in their hip pocket or on their belt had lower sperm motility than men who did not carry a mobile phone or who carried their mobile phone elsewhere on the body.[94]

Electromagnetic radiation (EMR) exposure caused a subtle decrease in the rapid progressive and slow progressive sperm movement. It also caused an increase in the no-motility category of sperm movement. There was no statistically significant difference in the sperm concentration between two groups.[95] Samples exposed to radiofrequency electromagnetic waves (RF-EMW) showed a significant decrease in sperm motility and viability, increase in reactive oxygen species (ROS) level, and decrease in ROS-total antioxidant capacity (TAC) score. Levels of TAC and DNA damage showed no significant differences from the non-exposed group.[96]

The results of the presented studies provide limited support to the hypothesis that use of mobile phones may adversely affect semen quality, but most of the presented studies are small,[93-96] only three[97-99] were conducted on the sample of about 300 men. Therefore, future studies are needed in this area.

SUMMARY

Exposure to environmental factors (air pollution, pesticides, phthalates, PCB and the use of mobile phones) may affect semen quality. However, when reviewing the epidemiological studies on the influence of environmental hazards on semen quality, it is important to take into account the current limitations of these studies resulting from inadequacies in semen analysis, exposure evaluation and design of studies. The studies conducted in the general population are very rare mainly because of the difficulties in collecting the semen samples. The fact that most of the studies are drawn from infertility clinics may introduce a selection bias.

The results from the presented studies suggest that there are strong and rather consistent indications that some pesticides beside DBCP (as DDT/DDE, ethylenedibromide, organophosphates) affect sperm count. PCBs are detrimental to sperm motility; those findings are derived from small pilot studies, but are confirmed also by bigger studies. In case of air pollution, studies suggest a link between ambient air pollutants and various semen characteristics. Additional research is needed to corroborate this association and to establish the causal agents. Results of few studies of subfertile men demonstrate associations between phthalate levels commonly experienced by the public and impaired sperm quality (impact on sperm concentration, morphology, motility), but findings have not been corroborated in studies of men from the general population. Mobile phones might adversely affect the quality of semen by decreasing mostly motility but also the sperm counts, viability and morphology. In spite of their consistent results, most of the studies are rather small; only two big studies were performed in this area.

No association between exposure to THMs and poor semen quality was observed.

Presented studies usually used classical human semen parameters (concentration, motility and morphology). The assessment of exposure was performed in most of the studies (PCBs, THMs, air pollution), and only in a few of the pesticide and phthalate exposure studies. The studies conducted in the general population are very rare, mainly because of the difficulties in collecting the semen samples. This has caused also that some works are small pilot studies. The fact that most of the subjects are drawn from infertility clinics may introduce a selection bias. In addition, the most commonly used study design is cross sectional, which does not allow to make inferences on cause-effect mechanisms. Also, chronic exposures to reproductive toxins are not well documented and mechanisms of toxicity are either poorly understood or unknown. Therefore, it is necessary to conduct longitudinal studies with exposure assessment that should focus more on the explanation of the biological mechanisms.

In spite of their limitations, epidemiological studies suggest awareness of environmental factors which may affect semen quality, and both in case of well proven and disputable hazards, it is necessary to reduce the exposure of parents (including future ones) to those factors.

REFERENCES

1. Huyghe E, Matsuda T, Thonneau P. Increasing incidence of testicular cancer worldwide: a review. J Urol. 2003;170:5-11.
2. Paulozzi LJ, Erickson JD, Jackson RJ. Hypospadias trends in two US surveillance systems. Pediatrics. 1997;100(5):831-4.
3. Auger J, Kunstmann JM, Czyglik F, Jouannet P. Decline in semen quality among fertile men in paris during the past 20 years. New Eng J. 1995;332:281-5.
4. Carlsen E, Giwercman A, Keiding N, Skakkebaek NE. Evidence for decreasing quality of semen during past 50 years. BMJ. 1992;305:609-13.
5. Sharpe RM, Skakkebaek NE. Are oestrogens involved in falling sperm counts and disorders of male reproductive tract? Lancet. 1993;341:1392-5.
6. Swan SH, Elkin EP, Fenster L. Have sperm densities declined? A reanalysis of global trend data. Environ Health Perspect. 1997;105:1228-32.
7. Swan SH, Elkin EP, Fenster L. The question of declining sperm density revisited: an analysis of 101 studies published 1934–1996. Environ Health Perspect. 2000;108:961-6.
8. Jørgensen N, Vierula M, Jacobsen R, Pukkala E, Perheentupa A, Virtanen HE, et al. Recent adverse trends in semen quality and testis cancer incidence among Finnish men. Int J Androl. 2011;34:37-48.
9. Mendiola J, Jørgensen N, Mínguez-Alarcón L, Sarabia-Cos L, López-Espín JJ, Vivero-Salmerón G, et al. Sperm counts may have declined in young university students in Southern Spain. Andrology. 2013;1:408-13.
10. Rolland M, Le Moal J, Wagner V, Royère D, De Mouzon J. Decline in semen concentration and morphology in a sample of 26,609 men close to general population between 1989 and 2005 in France. Hum Reprod. 2013;28:462-70.
11. Fisch H, Goluboff ET, Olson JH, Feldshuh J, Broder SJ, Barad DH. Semen analyses in 1,283 men from the United States over a 25-year period: no decline in quality. Fertil Steril. 1996;65:1009-14.
12. Thorup J, McLachlan R, Cortes D, Nation TR, Balic A, Southwell BR, et al. What is new in cryptorchidism and hypospadias—a critical review on the testicular dysgenesis hypothesis. J Pediatr Surg. 2010;45:2074-86.
13. Fisch H, Braun SR. Trends in global semen parameter values. Asian J Androl. 2013;15:169-73.
14. Skakkebaek NE, Rajpert-De ME, Main KM. Testicular dysgenesis syndrome: an increasingly common developmental disorder with environmental aspects. Hum Reprod. 2001;5:972-8.
15. Porta M, Puigdomènech E, Ballester F, Selva J, Ribas-Fitó N, Llop S, et al. Monitoring concentrations of persistent organic pollutants in the generalpopulation: the international experience. Environ Int. 2008;34:546-1.
16. Whorton D, Krauss RM, Marshall S, Milby TH. Infertility in male pesticide workers. Lancet. 1977;2(8051):1259-61.
17. Bonde JP, Giwercman A. Occupational hazards to male fecundity. Reprod Med Rev. 1995;4:59-73.
18. Bonde JP, Giwercman A, Ernst E. Identifying environmental risk to male reproductive function by occupational sperm studies: logistics and design options. Occup Environ Med. 1996;53:511-9.
19. Irvine D. Epidemiology and aetiology of male infertility. Hum Reprod. 1998;13(Suppl 1):33-44.
20. Skakkebaek NE, Giwercman A, de Kretser D. Pathogenesis and management of male infertility. Lancet. 1994;343: 147-9.
21. Sheiner EK, Sheiner E, Hammel RD, Potashnik G, Carel R. Effects of occupational exposures on male fertility: literature review. Ind Med. 2003;41:55-62.
22. Jensen TK, Bonde JP, Joffe M. The influence of occupational exposure on male reproductive function. Occup Med. 2006;56:544-53.
23. Sharpe RM, Irvine DS. How strong is the evidence of a link between environmental chemicals and adverse effects on human reproductive health? BMJ. 2004;328:447-51.
24. Robins TG, Bornman MS, Ehrlich RI, Cantrell AC, Pienaar E, Vallabh J, et al. Semen quality and fertility of men employed in South Africa lead acid battery plant. Am J Ind Med. 1997;32:369-76.
25. AssennatoG, Paci C, Baser ME, Molinini R, Candela RG, Altamura BM, et al. Sperm count suppression without endocrine dysfunction in lead exposed men. Arch Environ Health. 1987;42:124-7.
26. Wyrobek AJ, Schrader SM, Perreault SD, Fenster L, Huszar G, Katz DF, et al. Assessment of reproductive disorders and birth defects in communities near hazardous chemical sites. III. Guidelines for field studies of male reproductive disorders. Reprod Toxicol. 1997;11:243-59.
27. Stronati A, Manicardi GC, Cecati M, Bordicchia M, Ferrante L, Spanò M, et al. Relationship between sperm DNA fragmentation, sperm apoptotic markers and serum levels of CB-153, and p,p′-DDE in European and Inuit populations. Reproduction. 2006;132:949-58.
28. Aitken RJ, De Luiis GN. Origin and consequences of DNA damage in male germ cells. Reprod Biomed Online. 2007;14:727-33.
29. Evenson DP, Wixon R. Environmental toxicants cause sperm DNA fragmentation as detected by the sperm

Chromatin structure Assay (SCSA). Toxicol Appl Pharmacol. 2005;207(Suppl 2):532-7.

30. Ozmen B, Caglar GS, Koster F, Schopper B, Diedrich K, Al-Hasani S. Relationship between sperm DNA damage, induced acrosome reaction and viability in ICSI patients. Reprod Biomed Online. 2007;15:208-14.
31. Mortensen JT. Risk for reduced sperm quality among metal workers, with special reference to welders. Scand J Work Environ Health. 1988;14:27-30.
32. Doerge DR, Churchwell MI, Chang HC, Newbold RR, Delclos KB. Placental transfer of the soy isoflavone genistein flowing dietary and gavage administration to Sprague Dawley rats. Reprod Toxicol. 2001;15:105-10.
33. West MC, Anderson L, McClure N, Lewis SEM. Dietary estrogens and male fertility potential. Hum Fertil. 2005;8:197-207.
34. Juhler RK, Laren SB, Meyer O, Jensen ND, Spanò M, Giwercman A, et al. Human semen quality in relation to dietary pesticide exposure and organic diet. Arch Environ Contam Toxicol. 1999;37:415-23.
35. Sharpe RM. Pathways of endocrine disruption during male sexual differentiation and masculinization. Best Pract Res Clin Endocrinol Metab. 2006;20:91-110.
36. Sharpe RM, Franks S. Environment, lifestyle and infertility—an intergenerational issue. Nat Cell Biol. 2002;4(Suppl):s33-40.
37. Aksglaede L, Juul A, Leffers H, Skakkebaek NE, Andersson AM. The sensitivity of the child to sex steroids: possible impact of exogenous estrogens. Hum Reprod Update. 2006;12:341-9.
38. Swan SH, Liu F, Overstreet JW, Brazil C, Skakkebaek NE. Semen quality of fertile US males in relation to their mother's beef consumption during pregnancy. Hum Reprod. 2007;22:1497-502.
39. Rajapakse N, Silva E, Kortenkamp A. Combining xenoestrogens at levels below individual no-observed-effects concentrations dramatically enhances steroid hormone action. Environ Health Perspect. 2002;110:917-21.
40. Tinwell H, Ashby J. Sensitivity of the immature rat uterotrophic assay to mixtures of estrogens. Environ Health Perspect. 2004;112:575-82.
41. Toppari J, Skakkebaek NE. Sexual differentiation and environmental endocrine disrupters. Baillieres Clin Endocrinol Metab. 1998;12:143-56.
42. O'Donnell L, Robertson KM, Jones ME, Simpson ER. Estrogens and spermatogenesis. Endocr Rev. 2001;22:289-318.
43. Wagner U, Schlebusch H, Van der Ven H, van der Ven K, Diedrich K, Krebs D. Accumulation of pollutants in the genital tract of sterility patients. J Clin Chem Clin Biochem. 1990;28:683-8.
44. Umeyama T, Ishikawa H, Takeshima H, Yoshii S, Koiso K. A comparative study of seminal plasma trace elements in fertile and infertile men. Fertil Steril. 1986;46:494-9.
45. Xuezhi J, Youxin L, Yilan W. Studies of lead exposure on reproductive system: a review of work in China. Biomed Environ Sci. 1992;5:266-75.
46. Gennart JP, Buchet JP, Roels H, Ghyselen P, Ceulemans E, Lauwerys R. Fertility of male workers exposed to cadmium, lead or manganese. Am J Epidemol. 1992;135:1208-19.
47. Chia SE, Chan OY, Sam CT, Heng BH. Blood cadmium levels in non-occupationally exposed adult subjects in Singapore. Sci Total Environ. 1994;145:119-23.
48. Spinelli A, Figa-Talamanca, Osborn J. Time to pregnancy and occupation in a group of Italian women. Int J Epidemiol. 1997;26:601-9.
49. Danadevi K, Rozati R, Reddy PP, Grover P. Semen quality of Indian welders occupationally exposed to nickel and chromium. Reprod Toxicol. 2003;17:451-6.
50. Akinloye O, Arowojolu AO, Shittu OB, Anetor JI. Cadmium toxicity: a possible cause of male infertility in Nigeria. Reprod Biol. 2006;6:17-30.
51. Naha N, Chowdhuri AR. Inorganic lead exposure in battery and paint factory: effect on human sperm structure and functional activity. J UOEH. 2006;28:157-71.
52. Benoff S, Hurley IR, Millan C, Napolitano B, Centola GM. Seminal lead concentrations negatively affect outcomes of artificial insemination. Fertil Steril. 2003;80:517-25.
53. Telisman S, Cvitkovic P, Jurasovic J, Pizent A, Gavella M, Rocić B. Semen quality and endocrine function in relation to biomarkers of lead, cadmium, zinc and copper in men. Environ Health Perspect. 2000;108;45-53.
54. Selevan SG, Borkovec L, Slott VL, Zudova Z, Rubes J, Everson DP, et al. Semen quality and reproductive health of young Czech men exposed to seasonal air pollution. Environ Health Perspect. 2000;108:887-94.
55. Rubes J, Zudova Z, Vozdova M, Hajnova R, Urbanova J, Borkovec L, et al. Air pollution and sperm quality. Cas Lek Cesk. 2000;139(6):174-6.
56. Rubes J, Selevan SG, Evenson DP, Zudova D, Vozdova M, Zudova Z, et al. Episodic air pollution is associated with increased DNA fragmentation in human sperm without other changes in semen quality. Hum Reprod. 2005:20(10): 2776-83.
57. Sokol R, Kraft P, Fowler IM, Mamet R, Kim E, Berhane KT. Exposure to environmental ozone alters semen quality. Environ Health Perspect. 2006;114(3):360-5.
58. Rozati R, Reddy PP, Reddanna P, Mujtaba R. Xenoestrogens and male fertility: myth or reality? Asian J Androl. 2000;2(4):263-9.
59. Spanò M, Toft G, Hagmar L, Eleuteri P, Rescia M, Rignell-Hydbom A, et al. Exposure to PCB and p,p'-DDE in European and Inuit populations: impact on human sperm chromatin integrity. Hum Reprod. 2005;20(12):3488-99.
60. Toft G, Rignell-Hydbom A, Tyrkiel E, Shvets M, Giwercman A, Lindh CH, et al. Semen quality and exposure to persistent organochlorine pollutants. Epidemiology. 2006;17(4):450-8.
61. Bonde JP, Toft G, Rylander L, Rignell-Hydbom A, Giwercman A, Spano M, et al. Fertility and markers of male reproductive function in Inuit and European populations spanning large contrasts in blood levels of persistent organochlorines. Environ Health Perspect. 2008;116(3):269-77.
62. Richthoff J, Rylander L, Jönsson BAG, Akesson H, Hagmar L, Nilsson-Ehle P, et al. Serum levels of 2,2',4,4',5,5'-hexachlorobiphenyl (CB-153) in relation to markers of reproductive function in young males from the general Swedish population. Environ Health Perspect. 2003;111(4):409-13.

63. Graves CG, Matanoski GM, Tardiff RG. Weight of evidence for an association between adverse reproductive and developmental effects and exposure to disinfection by-products: a critical review. Regul Toxicol Pharmacol. 2001;34:103-24.
64. Linder RE, Klinefelter GR, Strader LF, Narotsky MG, Suarez JD, Roberts NL, et al. Dibromoacetic acid affects reproductive competence and sperm quality in male-rat. Fundam Appl Toxicol. 1995;28(1):9-17.
65. Linder RE, Klinefelter GR, Strader LF, Suarez JD, Roberts NL. Spermatotoxicity of dichloroacetic acid. Reprod Toxicol. 1997;11(5):681-8.
66. Linder RE, Klinefelter GR, Strader LF, Veeramachaneni DNR, Roberts NL, Suarez JD. Histopathologic changes in the testes of rats exposed to dibromoacetic acid. Reprod Toxicol. 1997;11(1):47-56.
67. Luft JC, Garges JB, Rockett JR, Dix DJ. Male reproductive toxicity of bromochloroacetic acid in mice. Biol Reprod. 2000;62(1):246-7.
68. Christian MS, York RG, Hoberman AM, Frazee J, Fisher LC, Brown WR, et al. Oral (drinking water) two-generation reproductive toxicity study of dibromoacetic acid (DBA) in rats. Int J Toxicol. 2002;21(4):237-76.
69. Luben T, Olshan AF, Herring AH, Jeffay S, Strader L, Buus RM, et al. The healthy men study: an evaluation of exposure to disinfection by-products in tap water and sperm quality. Environ Health Perspect. 2007;115(8):1169-76.
70. Fenster L, Waller K, Windham G, Henneman T, Anderson M, Mendola P, et al. Trihalomethane levels in home tap water and semen quality. Epidemiology. 2003;14(6):650-8.
71. Bretveld R, Brouwers M, Ebisch I, Roeleveld N. Influence of pesticides on male fertility. Scand J Work Environ Health. 2007;33(1):13-28.
72. Ratcliffe JM, Schrader SM, Steenland K, Clapp DE, Turner T, Hornung RW. Semen quality in papaya workers with long term exposure to ethylene dibromide. Br J Ind Med. 1987;44:317-26.
73. Recio R, Robbins WA, Ocampo-Gómez G, Borja-Aburto V, Morán-Martinez J, Froines JR, et al. Organophosphorous pesticide exposure increases the frequency of sperm sex null aneuploidy. Environ Health Perspect. 2001;109(12):1237-40.
74. Padungtod C, Hassold TJ, Millie E, Ryan LM, Savitz DA, Christiani DC, et al. Sperm aneuploidy among Chinese pesticide workers: scoring by the FISH method. An abstract. Am J Ind Med. 1999;36(2):230-8.
75. Swan S, Kruse R, Liu F, Barr DB, Drobnis E, Redmon J, et al. Semen quality in relation to biomarkers of pesticide exposure. Environ Health Perspect. 2003;111(12):1478-84.
76. Lifeng T, Wang S, Ji J, Sun X, Li Y, Wang Q, et al. Effects of fenvalerate exposure on semen quality among occupational workers. Contraception. 2006;73:92-6.
77. Meeker JD, Ryan L, Barr DB, Herrick RF, Bennett DH, Bravo R, et al. The relationship of urinary metabolites of carbaryl/naphthalene and chlorpyrifos with human semen quality. Environ Health Perspect. 2004;112(14):1665-70.
78. Abell A, Ernst E, Bonde JPE. Semen quality and sexual hormones in greenhouse workers. Scand J Work Environ Health. 2000;26(6):492-500.
79. Oliva A, Spira A, Multigner L. Contribution of environmental factors to risk of male infertility. Hum Reprod. 2001;16(8):1768-76.
80. Kamijima M, Hibi H, Gotoh M, Taki K, Saito I, Wang H, et al. A survey of semen indices in insecticide sprayers. J Occup Health. 2004;46(2):109-18.
81. Larsen SB, Giwercman A, Span M, Bonde JPE. Seminal characteristics following exposure to pesticides among agricultural workers. Scand J Work Environ Health. 1999;25(Suppl 1):74-5.
82. Recio-Vega R, Ocampo-Gómez G, Borja-Aburto VH, Moran-Martínez J, Cebrian-Garcia ME. Organophosphorus pesticide exposure decreases sperm quality: association between sperm parameters and urinary pesticide levels. J Appl Toxicol. 2008;28(5):674-80.
83. Yucra S, Gasco M, Rubio J, Gonzales GF. Semen quality in Peruvian pesticide applicators: association between urinary organophosphate metabolites and semen parameters. Environ Health. 2008;7(59):1-10.
84. Rastogi SK, Kesavachandran C, Mahdi F, Pandey A. Phthalate exposure and health outcomes. Indian J Occup Environ Med. 2006;10:111-5.
85. Wittassek M, Wiesmüller GA, Koch HM, Eckard R, Dobler L, Müller J, et al. Internal phthalate exposure over the last two decades—a retrospective human biomonitoring study. Int J Hyg Environ Health. 2007;210(3-4):319-33.
86. Duty SM, Silva MJ, Barr DB, Brock JW, Ryan L, Chen Z, et al. Phthalate exposure and human semen parameters. Epidemiology. 2003;14:269-77.
87. Duty SM, Calafat AM, Silva MJ, Ryan L, Hauser R. Phthalate exposure and reproductive hormones in adult men. Hum Reprod. 2005;20(3):604-10.
88. Hauser R, Meeker JD, Duty S, Silva MJ, Calafat AM. Altered semen quality in relation to urinary concentrations of phthalate monoester and oxidative metabolites. Epidemiology. 2006;17:682-91.
89. Jönsson BAG, Richthoff J, Rylander L, Giwercman A, Lars H. Urinary phthalate metabolites and biomarkers of reproductive function in young men. Epidemiology. 2005;6(4):487-93.
90. Wirth JJ, Rossano MG, Potter R, Puscheck E, Daly DC, Paneth N, et al. A pilot study associating urinary concentrations of phthalate metabolites and semen quality. Syst Biol Reprod Med. 2008;54(3):143-54.
91. Pant N, Shukla M, Patel KD, Shukla Y, Mathur N, Gupta YK, et al. Correlation of phthalate exposures with semen quality. Toxicol Appl Pharmacol. 2008;231:112-6.
92. Zhang Y, Zheng L, Chen B. Phthalate exposure and human semen quality in Changhai: a cross-sectional study. Biomed Environ Sci. 2006;19(3):205-9.
93. Davoudi M, Brossner C, Kuber W. The influence of electromagnetic waves on sperm motility. Urol Urogynaecol. 2002;19:18-22.
94. Kilgallon JS, Simmons LW. Image content influences men's semen quality. Biol Lett. 2005;1(3):253-5.
95. Erogul O, Oztas E, Yildirim I, Kir T, Aydur E, Komesli G, et al. Effects of electromagnetic radiation from a cellular phone

on human sperm motility: an *in vitro* study. Arch Med Res. 2006;37(7):840-3.

96. Agarwal A, Desai NR, Makker K, Varghese A, Mouradi R, Sabanegh E, et al. Effects of radiofrequency electromagnetic waves (RF-EMW) from cellular phones on human ejaculated semen: an *in vitro* pilot study. Fertil Steril. 2009;92(4):1318-25.
97. Agarwal A, Deepinder F, Sharma RK, Ranga G, Li J. Effect of cell phone usage on semen analysis in men attending infertility clinics: an observational study. Fertil Steril. 2008;89(1):124-8.
98. Fejes I, Závaczki Z, Szöllosi JS, Daru J, Kovács L, Pál A. Is there a relationship between cell phone use and semen quality? Arch Androl. 2005;51(5):385-93.
99. Wdowiak A, Wdowiak L, Wiktor H. Evaluation of the effect of using mobile phones on male fertility. Ann Agric Environ Med. 2007;14:169-72.

CHAPTER

Genetic and Chromosomal Anomalies in Male Infertility

23

Parth S Shah, Sandip C Shah, Mandava V Rao

INTRODUCTION

Male infertility is one of the common problems of health. Despite prevalence and significance of the health problem, resources and focus have not been sufficiently paid on this issue. About 15% of couples of reproductive age are affected by it and in some 50% the male is a main contributor. It is likely that majority of these patients have genetic abnormalities that are the cause of their infertility. During past 20–25 years, significant improvements in technology have made to identify and treat it. After completion of Human Genome Project (HGP), a new era of unprecedented momentum and ability to tackle the complex issue in the genetics of male infertility. New tools include *in vitro* methodologies, in silico technologies and new model organisms.[1] Few technologies to mention are karyotyping fluorescence in-situ hybridization (FISH), PCR types, gene sequencers, microarray, and next generation sequencer (NGS) of various types. Digital PCR is for correct identification of genetic abnormalities from chromosome to gene level. The etiology, treatment, classification and management are well understood to assist a patient; however, 50% of cases still remain unclassified.

There are different types to classify the genetic basis of male infertility.[2,3] In some text books, various forms are divided into pre-testicular, testicular and post-testicular forms.[4,5] Genetic and chromosomal disorder that impair hormonogenesis or stimulate spermatogenesis (pre-testicular event) or can affect spermatogenesis (testicular event). Others that affect sperm transport (post-testicular event). However, we classify the following scheme of genetic basis of infertility in the male: (1) male infertility with a gene defect and (2) infertility with chromosomal aberrations numerically and structurally.[6,7]

MALE INFERTILITY WITH GENE DEFECTS

These disorders are due to a mutation at a gene level and can occur de novo or are inherited as autosomal (dominant or recessive) or X-linked. It is known that about 10,000 human diseases are monogenic. The global prevalence of single gene diseases is approximately 10/1,000 at birth. A list is provided, which is incomplete, but includes the genetic conditions potential for clinical challenges[8] with slight modifications (Table 23.1).

Kallman's Syndrome (KS)

Kallman's syndrome (KS) possesses hypogonadism with small testes, anosmia and delayed puberty. The gene responsible for it is X-linked form of KS, KAL-1 encodes a protein, anosmia-1, playing a key role in the migration of GnRH neurons and olfactory nerves to the hypothalamus. As a consequence of failed neuronal migration, the hypothalamus and pituitary failed to stimulate the testes leading to subfertility. In addition to X-linked autosomal dominant and recessive types of KS have also been reported.[9] Autosomal dominant KAL-2 in 8P12 (FGFR-1 fibroblast growth factor receptor-1) and autosomal recessive KAL-3 are associated with nonreproductive failure including cleft palate, mirror movements and dental agenesis. Recent studies revealed that mutations in KAL-1 gene occur in minority of KS cases. Majority of these are familial/sporadic caused by other autosomal genes.[10]

Congenital Adrenal Hyperplasia (CAH)

CAH results from inherited defects in one of the five enzymatic steps necessary for synthesis of cortisol from the precursor, cholesterol. The most common form of CAH (95%) is due to a deficiency of 21 hydroxylase located on 6P21.3.[11,12]

Mutation in cytochrome p450 21-hydroxylase gene (CPY21) tend to be transmitted in an autosomal recessive pattern. Deficiency of these enzymes occurs in three forms: (1) simple virilizing, (2) salt wasting and (3) nonclassical. The simple virilizing and salt wasting forms of 21-hydroxylase deficiencies are characterized by excess adrenal androgen biosynthesis in utero. This disorder in males is not recognized at birth. It is diagnosed later. Cortisol and aldesterone production is low, but testosterone

Table 23.1: Genetic defects and male infertility modified from Patrizio et al. (2008).

Condition	*Gene involved(mapping)*	*Incidence*	*Phenotype*	*Inherited*	*Diagnosis*
Androgen insensitivity syndrome	AR (Xq11-q12)	1:60,000	Partial/ complete testicular feminization	X–linked recessive	Clinical, hormonal & DNA analysis
5α-Reductase deficiency	SRD5A1(5p15) SRD5A2(2p23)	Unknown	Male pseudoherma-phroditism, severe hypospadias	Autosomal recessive	Enzyme assay & DNA analysis
Autosomal dominant polycystic kidney disease	PKD1 (16p21.3) PKD2 (4q.2.1.23) PKD3 (11q12.3)	1:1,000	Multiple cysts (kidney, liver, spleen, pancreas, testis,epididymis, seminal vesicle)	Autosomal dominant	DNA analysis
Bartet-Biedl syndrome	BBS(11q13, 16q21, 3p12-q13, 15q22.3, 2q31, 20p12, 4q27, 14q32.11)	1:160,000	Retinal degeneration, obesity, cognitive impairment, GU malformations, polydactyly, hypogonadism	Autosomal recessive	Clinical & DNA analysis
Cerebellar ataxia	CLA1 (9q34-9) CLA3 (20q11-q13)	1:50,000	Eunuchoid phenotype, cerebellar impairment, atrophic testes	Autosomal recessive	Clinical & DNA analysis
Congenital adrenal hyperplasia	P450C21(6p21.3) 21-hydroxylase deficiency(most common)	1:5,000	Variable, elevated ACTH, inhibited FSH/LH Secretion, azoospermia	Autosomal recessive	Endocrine & DNA analysis
Cystic fibrosis	CFTR (7q31.2)	1:2,500	Respiratory infections,Wolffian duct anomaly, pancreatic insufficiency	Autosomal recessive	DNA analysis
Hemochromatosis	HFE (6p21.3) HFE (1q21-juvenile)	1:500	Organ failure (liver and testes) by iron overload	Autosomal recessive	DNA analysis
Immotile cilia syndrome	DNAI1(9p21-p13) DNAH5(5p) 19q13.2,16p2,15q13	1:35,000	Sinusitis,bronchiectasis, immotile sperm	Autosomal recessive	Clinical, sperm study by EM and DNA analysis
Kallaman's syndrome	KLA1 (Xp22.3)[1] KLA2 (8p12)[2] KLA3 (20p13)[3]	1:30,000	Hypogonadotropic hypogonadism, anosmia	[1]X-linked recessive [2]Autosomal dominant [3]Autosomal recessive	Clinical and DNA analysis
LH/FSH hormone and receptor mutations	LHβ (19q13.32) FSHβ(11p13)	Few male cases reported	Delayed puberty, arrested spermatogenesis	Autosomal recessive	Endocrine & DNA analysis
Mixed gonadal dysgenesis	WT1 (11p13) DAX1 (Xp21.3) Testatin(20p11.2)	Rare	Unilateral testis (most common with SCO) and contralateral streak gonad, ambiguous external genitalia	Autosomal dominant X-linked recessive cytogenetic	DNA analysis
Mytonic dystrophy	DMPK(19q.13.23)	1:8,000	Muscle wasting, cataracts, atrophic testes	Autosomal dominant	Clinical & DNA analysis
Persistent Müllerian duct syndrome	AMH (19P13.3-P13.2) AMHR(12q13)	<200 cases reported	Incomplete involution of Müllerian structures	Autosomal X-linked	Clinical & DNA analysis
Prader–Willi syndrome	SNRPN(15q11q13)	1:20,000	Obesity, muscular hypotonia, mental retardation, hypogonadotropic hypogonadism	Autosomal dominant	Clinical & DNA analysis
Sickle cell anemia	HBB(11p15.5) (mutation)	1:58,000	RBC sickle shape, testicular microinfractions	Autosomal recessive	Hb and DNA analyses

(contd…)

Table 23.1: Genetic defects and male infertility modified from Patrizio et al. (2008). (*contd...*)

Condition	*Gene involved(mapping)*	*Incidence*	*Phenotype*	*Inherited*	*Diagnosis*
Sex reversal syndrome	SRY(Yp11.3)	1:25,000	46, XX SRY (+) 46, XY SRY (–)	Y-linked	DNA analysis
Usher's syndrome	USH1 (14q32) USH2 (1q41) USH3 (3q21-q25)	1:17,000	Low sperm motility, hearing loss, retinitis pigmentosa	Autosomal recessive	Sperm & DNA analyses
β-Thalassemia	HBB(11p15) (deletion/mutation)	1:1140,000	Anemia; iron overload (pituitary and testis)	Autosomal recessive	Hb & DNA analyses

ACTH, adrenocorticotrophic hormone; FSH, follicle-stimulating hormone; GU, genitourinary; Hb, hemoglobin; LH, luteinizing hormone; RBC, red blood cell; SCO, sertoli cell-only syndrome.

production is normal. Gradually elevated ACTH causes augmented adrenal androgen secretion in male CAH patients may suppress FSH and LH production with resultant small testes, decreased spermatogenesis and testicular androgen production.[12,13]

Prader–Willi Syndrome (PWS)

It was the first human disorder attributed to genome imprinting where the genes are expressed differentially based on parent of origin. PWS results from the loss of gene SNRPN on the parental 15q11.2-13 locus with autosomal dominant pattern. The loss of maternal genomic material of same locus results in another imprinted disorder (Angelman's syndrome). Characteristics include neonatal hypotonia, childhood-onset hyperphagia obesity, mental retardation and short stature. A deficiency of GnRH is postulated cause for the hypogonadism.[14]

Bardet–Biedl Syndrome (BBS)

It is a genetically heterogeneous genetic disorder with linkage to eight loci, i.e. BBS1–BBS8.[15] It is a recessive defect, but controversy exists about the presence of a recessive pattern with variable penetrance. Their mapping is 11q13, 16q21, 3p12-q13, 15q22.3, 2q31, 20p12, 4q27 and 14q32.11, respectively.[16] Cardinal features are obesity, retinitis pigmentosa polydactyly, hypogonadotropic hypogonadism, renal cystic dysplasia and developmental delay. Others in BBS patients are diabetes, hypertension and congenital heart defects. At least, four of these clinical symptoms are necessary for its disease. Some BBS genes are also involved in the function of cilia and flagella formation, which can impair sperm motility to cause sterility.[17,18]

Hereditary Hemochromatosis (HH)

It is an autosomal disorder, which is characterized by excessive absorption of dietary iron, which may result parenchymal iron overload and then leads to tissue damage. Hypogonadotropic hypogonadism is associated with HH, secondary to iron deposition in pituitary gonadotrophs leading to loss of libido, impotence and body hair loss.[19] These are four types of HH (HH1, HH2, HH3, and HH4). HH1 is common, their loci are 6p21, 1q21, 7q22, and 2q32. The other types are rare and have been identified in small member of families.[20]

Cerebellar Ataxia and Hypogonadism

It is a rare autosomal recessive type most commonly observed in consanguineous marriages with onset at 20 years old. Features include cerebellar impairment (speech and gait abnormalities and eunuchoid phenotype with atrophic testis and low libido. Infertility is secondary to hypothalamic–pituitary dysfunction, possibly because of brain atrophy or hypoplasia. The genes are CLA1 (9q34-9) for adult onset and CLA3 (20q11-q13) for infant onset.[21,22]

Other Idiopathic Hypogonadotropic Hypogonadism (IHH)

Other forms of HH are idiopathic hypogonadotropic hypogonadism (IHH) have recently been linked with genetic mutations. One such type is DAX1 gene, which encodes a nuclear transcription factor leading to X-linked IHH joined with CAN. Another mutation in the prohormone convertase 1 gene (PC1) has been linked to HH and deficient conversion of proinsulin to insulin.[23] Homozygous mutations in a gene encoding G-protein coupled receptor-54 (GPR54) is reported as another cause of HH.[24]

Immotile Cilia Syndrome (ICS)

It is a group of heterogeneous diseases with impaired or absent ciliary motility and most common is Kartagener's syndrome. Anomalies in motor apparatus or axoneme, due to either loss or short dynein arms cause a deficiency in sperm motility. Clinical manifestations are chronic cough, sinus, infection and infertility with asthenozoospermia. It is autosomal recessive and is caused by mutations in genes encoding dynein axoneme chain (DNA1).[25]

Autosomal Dominant Polycystic Kidney Disease

Numerous large cysts of the kidneys, liver, pancreas and spleen including brain mark this disorder. It is asymptomatic till adulthood, affected men may initially present with infertility. Cysts in epididymis, seminal vesicles or ejaculatory ducts can obstruct the ductal system and cause infertility. Three separate genes have been associated with autosomal dominant polycystic kidney disease (ADPKD). PKD1 accounts 85% of the disease and is mapped onto chromosome 16p15.3. It encodes a receptor like integral membrane protein involved in cell-cell and cell-matrix interaction. The PKD2, a mild form is mapped to chromosome 4q21-23 and encodes a nonspecific Ca^{2+} permeable channel. The another one, PKD3 is unmapped. An association with ICS and ADPKD diseases is noticed.[26]

Cystic Fibrosis Transmembrane Regulatory Mutations (CFTR Mutations)

CF is the most common fatal autosomal recessive disease in Caucasians with an incidence of 1:2,500 births and a carrier frequency of 1:25. Clinical features include chronic pulmonary obstruction and infection, exocrine pancreatic insufficiency and male infertility. The CF gene cystic fibrosis transmembrane regulator (CFTR; 7q31.2), encodes a protein that regulates the CAMP chloride channel that controls the transport of electrolytes in many secretory epithelia. More than 1,000 mutations have been identified in the CFTR gene, encompassing about 90% cases of CF.[27] This gene also influences the SV, vas deferens and epididymis.[28]

Congenital Bilateral Absence of the Vas Deferens (CBAVD)

This condition occurs in 1–2% of infertility men. These patients exhibit a spectrum of Wolffian duct defects as found in those with cystic fibrosis. It lacks pulmonary, pancreatic and intestinal problems. Spermatogenesis is normal in 90% of men with CBAVD. The corpus and caput epididymis and seminal vesicles (SV) may be present.[29,30] It is that CBAVD is based on allele patterns similar to CF, but with less severe mutations.[31] It is better to include the 5T (thymidines) variants (intron 8) in the genetic screening for CF in patients and their patterns before using assisted reproductive technologies (ARTs).

Congenital Unilateral Absence of the Vas Deferens (CUAVD)

Another male infertility phenotype probably linked with CFTR mutations. It affects 0.5% of general population and only rarely presents with infertility.[32] Almost 40% of patients with CUAVD have been reported to have at least one mutation in CFTR. CUAVD is more frequent in left side (70%).

Androgen Receptor Gene Mutation

The androgen receptor (AR) is a large steroid receptor whose gene is located on X-chromosome (Xq11-q12) and is essential for masculinization and virilization in the foetus. AR mutations result in absent or structurally altered causing complete or partial resistance to androgen.[33] The phenotype is variable, ranging from complete insensitivity (female phenotype) to normally virilized, but infertile males. Clinical features include ambiguous genitalia, testicular atrophy, micropenis and hypospadias.[33,34] About 300 distinct mutations have been identified in AR. Complete androgen insensitivity syndrome (CAIS) is also called testicular feminization syndrome (TFS) or mom's syndrome. Similarly partial androgen insensitivity syndrome (PAIS) is also known as male pseudohermaphroditism/Lub's syndrome, Refenstein's syndrome/Gilbert-Dreyfus syndrome.

Myotomic Dystrophy (MD)

It is the most common cause of adult onset muscular dystrophy and usually presents with cataracts, muscle weakness and wasting hypogonadism, ECG changes, diabetes and cholelithiasis. The gene is located in the long arm of chromosome 19q13.2-3 (D M PK gene) that encodes serine/threonine/protein kinase family (myotonin-1). In MD, there is an expansion of CTG repeats. In normal cases the repeats of CTG ranges from 5 to 35 copies, mildly affected persons have between 50 and 80 copies and severely affected have 2,000 or more copies. About 30% of subjects have infertility. A recent report claimed an association between MD and defective sperm capacitation and the acrosome reaction.[35]

Usher's Syndrome

This is the most common cause of deafness and blindness in men. This autosomal recessive defect maps on three chromosomes and results three different phenotypes [US_1(14q32), US_2(1q41) and US_3(3q21-q25)]. Recently, an association between US and infertility has been documented.[36]

β-Thalassemia and Sickle-cell Anemia

β-Thalassemia is caused by mutations in HBB gene mapped on chromosome 11p15.4. Depending upon types of β-thalassemia (minor, intermedia, major types), clinical features differ in intermedia and major conditions, blood transfusion is required.[37,38] Infertility results from deposition of iron load in pituitary, hypothalamus and testes. At molecular level, iron over-load may induce ROS, sperm DNA oxidation and altered sperm membranes.[39]

Sickle cell anemia is an autosomal recessive genetic disease occurring due to gene/point mutation, where substitution of valine for glutamic acid joined at 11p15.5 of the HBB responsible for defective form of HbS. Pituitary and testes microinfarcts from this disease account for secondary hypogonadism and infertility.[40]

SRY Gene Defects

Sex determining region on Y chromosome (SRY) is located on short arm of the "Y" chromosome (Yp11.3) and plays a pivotal role in male sex determination. It encodes SRY protein that binds to a membrane of the HMG-box family for testis formation in the fetus. Mutation in this gene gives rise to XY females (Xp22.11-p12.2) with gonadal dysgenesis, i.e. Swyer's syndrome. Translocation of SRY to the X chromosome causes the XX male phenotype, who are (46, XX) sterile due to absence of long arm of "Y" chromosome containing AZF region necessary for normal spermatogenesis. These conditions are called sex reversals.[41]

5-Alpha Reductase Deficiency

A deficiency in the 5-alpha reductase type-2 isozyme produces a form of male pseudohermaphroditism (autosomal recessive) due to lack of conversion of testosterone to dihydrotestosterone (DHT). Two genes are involved to encode 5α reductase, i.e., type-1 is mapped on chromosome 5, whereas type-2 on chromosome 2p23. Infertility results from structural abnormalities of the external genitalia. Although spermatogenesis has been noted in descended testes, natural fertility has not been resulted.[42,43]

Mixed Gonadal Dysgenesis

In male and females, it is a heterogeneous state characterized by a unilateral testis on one side and a streak gonad on the opposite side. The phenotype ranges from normal males to patients with ambiguous external genitalia or females, depending upon the amount of testosterone secreted by the testis. Genotypically, these cases are usually 46,XY or 45,X/46,XY mosaicism. The patients are associated with impaired gonadal development.[44]

Polymorphisms

The analysis of polymorphisms in genes involved in spermatogenesis represents in most exciting area of research in this issue of male infertility. The pathogenesis of testicular failure remains undefined and is referred as 'idiopathic infertility'. Idiopathic testicular failure is likely to be genetic origin because the number of gene involved in human spermatogenesis is possibly thousand or more. Few are identified and screened in infertile men,[45] which require further elucidation.

CHROMOSOMAL ABERRATIONS AND MALE INFERTILITY

Chromosomal disorders are defined as the loss, gain or abnormal arrangement of genetic material at the chromosome level. These can be of numerical and structural chromosomal anomalies. Structural chromosomal disorders occur in single (deletions, duplications and inversions) or multiple (translocations) chromosomes. These usually result as a consequence of breakage that occurs during meiosis leading to male infertility. Translocations are more frequent contributing factor ranging to 15% of azoospermic and 5% of oligospermic men.[46]

Numerical Aberrations

Klinefelter's syndrome (1:1,000) is the most common genetic reason in 14% of cases with azoospermia. Clinical features include small, firm testes, with germ cells azoospermia and gynecomastia. The phenotype can vary from a normal/virilized man with androgen deficiency. Testicular histology shows hyalinized seminiferous tubules and Leydig cell hyperplasia.[43] It may also be associated tall stature, low IQ, female hair distribution, diabetes, leukemia and extragonadal germ-cell tumors.[47] About 90% cases have classic 47,XXY genotype and remaining 10% have mosaicism with a combination of XXY/XY chromosomes.

XXY Syndrome

The XXY Syndrome has an incidence of 1:1,000 live births. About 2% of men with the 47,XXY karyotype may be infertile. The extra Y originates through chromosomal nondisjunction (86%). The remain cases are due to postzygotic events.[48] The phenotypic character includes tall stature, aggressive and antisocial behavior/criminals. They have a high risk of leukemia.[49]

Noonan's Syndrome (NS)

This syndrome has an incidence of 1:1,000–2,500 live births. Noonan's syndrome patients are phenotypically equivalent to those of Turner's syndrome (XO). These patients have webbed neck, short stature, cardiovascular disorder, and pulmonary stenosis. This syndrome is autosomal dominant pattern with karyotype 46, XY/XO mosaicism. A gene notified at 12q24.2–q24.31 (PTPN/candidate gene) which is involved to encode a protein-tyrosine phosphatase that plays a role in cellular response to extracellular signaling.[50] A second type of NS (type 2) appears to be transmitted in autosomal recessive patterns. These have hypertrophic obstructive cardiomyopathy.[51] The fertility impairment is related to abnormal spermatogenesis with cryptorchidism (77%) at birth and elevated FSH.[52]

Translocations

Translocations are classified as Robertsonian (incidence 1:900) or reciprocal (incidence 1:625). The former type involves chromosome 13, 14, 15, 21 and 22 and the other one involves in any chromosome. If there is no loss or no gain the translocation is called balanced (unaffected phenotype) but the reproductive risk with a balanced translocation is that the sperm may carry an unbalanced chromosome leading pregnancy loss. Reciprocal translocation can lead to reduced fertility, spontaneous abortions, or birth defects depending on the chromosomes involved and nature of translocations.[52] Many other translocations have been associated with male infertility. The most called Robertsonian translocation observed in infertile males is t (13q:14q), where autosomal rearrangement in meiosis causes spermatogenesis impairment. Carrier of other Robertsonian translocation between 14 and 21 are at risk for pregnancy loss and offspring with Down's syndrome and birth defects.[53]

Inversions

An inversion occurs when a chromosome breaks in two places and the material between break points rotates 180°, hence reversing the order chromatin material (genes). The incidence is 1:1,000. Such rearrangements may either interrupt important genes at the break point or interfere with normal chromosome pairing during meiosis, because of imbalance in chromosome mass. Autosomal inversion of chromosome 9, in particular, occurs in more in infertile than in normal fertile men. This type of chromosomal rearrangements tends to be balanced and result in phenotypically normal males, but with severe azoospermia or oligoasthenozoospermia.[54,55]

Chromosome Microdeletions

Structural changes (microdeletions) of the short or long arm of the "Y" chromosome could result in impairment of normal spermatogenesis. The microdeletion is one of the second most frequent genetic causes of infertility.[56]

The Yq11 region of long arm of "Y" chromosome is associated with spermatogenesis. It is called azoospermia region (AZF), divided into AZFa, AZFb and AZFc. Loss of any part of these regions can result in a variety of spermatogenic phenotypes causing infertility. AZFd is a part of AZFb+c regions. These regions contain candidate genes to regulate spermatogenesis. The AZFa region has USPAY,DBY, UTY, TB4Y; the AZFb regions has RBMY, SMCY, HSF4, CD4 and the AZFc contains PRY,DA2, TTY_2, BPYZ candidate genes. AZFa contributes to deletion frequency of 2–5% and is associated with Sertoli cell only syndrome (SCOS). AZFb region has the deletion frequency of

Table 23.2: Characteristics of AZF candidate genes.[57]

AZF Region	*Length (Mb)*	*Candidate genes*	*Deletion frequency (%)*	*The most common STSs*	*Phenotype*
AZFa	1–3	USP9Y, DBY, UTY, TB4Y	4.9	sY84: 324 bp	SCO syndrome
				sY86: 326 bp	Partial spermatogenic arrest
AZFb	6–7.7	HSFY, eIF-1Y, CDY, SMCY, BPY2, DAZ, RBMY, PRY	16.00	sY127: 274 bp	Maturation arrest of germ cells and Azoospermia
				sY134: 301 bp	
AZFc	3.5	DAZ, CDY1, BPY2, PRY, TTY2	60	sY254: 400 bp sY255: 126 bp	Mild or severe oligozoospermia, Azoospermia
AZFb+c	7.0–7.7		14		SCOs to meiotic arrest

STS, sequence tagged site.

16% leading to maturation arrest of germ cells. Azoospermia and AZFc region contribute to 50–60% deletion frequency associating with mild or severe oligospermia and AZFd (b+c) region has deletion frequency of 14% associated with SCOS and meiotic arrest as listed in Table 23.2.[57] Thus, infertile men with nonobstructive azoospermia (NOA) and those with sperm concentration <5–10 × 10^6/mL can be offered testing for micro deletion of "Y" chromosome.[1,58]

CONCLUSION

The cause of male infertility is associated with various factors. Genetic factors are one of them. To evaluate these genetic defects several techniques are underway including karyotyping, genetic analysis using gene sequencing, NGS, PCR, Fluorescence in situ hybridization (FISH), in silico techniques after completion of human genome project (HGP). Based on genetic evaluation of patients within impaired fertility in the male using latest scientific technologies till now, men with NOA with severe oligozoospermia could be tested for microdeletions. Patients with obstructive azoospermia (OA) owing to congenital anomalies of vas deferens epididymis, idiopathic infertility, microsurgery and others are tested for genetic and chromosomal defects after female partners are screened. Such cases are further subjected to genetic counseling before adopting testicular sperm-extraction (TESE), intracytoplasmic sperm injection (ICSI) and preimplantation genetic diagnosis (PGD) methodologies.

ACKNOWLEDGMENTS

Assistance rendered from Ms Mudra H Kansara and Mrs Aparna Satapathy, Department of Zoology, Biomedical Technology and Human Genetics, School of Sciences, Gujarat University, Ahmedabed, is well appreciated. The authors are also grateful to Dr Ketan K Vaghasia and Mr Hari S Ray of Supratech-Genopath Laboratory and Research Institute, Ahmedabad, for their support in the manuscript preparation.

REFERENCES

1. Carrell, DT. The Genetics of Male Infertility. New Jersey: Humana Press; 2007.
2. Oehninger SC, Kruger TF. Male Infertility: Diagnosis and Treatment. London: Informa (Healthcare); 2007.
3. Mak V, Jarvi KA. The genetics of male infertility. J Urol. 1996;156(4):1245-57.
4. Hargreave TB. Genetics and male infertility. Curr Opin Obstetric Gynecol. 2000;12:207.
5. Nudell DM, Turek PJ. Genetic causes of male infertility: current concepts. Curr Urol Rep. 2000;1:273.
6. WHO. The World Health Report: Changing History. Geneva, Switzerland: WHO; 2004.
7. Patrizio P, Broomfield D. The genetic basis of male infertility. In: Glover TD, Barrat LR (Eds). Male Fertility and Infertility. Cambridge: Cambridge University Press; 1999. p. 162.
8. Patrizio P, Sepulveda J, Mehri S. Chromosomal and genetic abnormalities in male infertility. In: Oehninger SC, Kruger TF (Eds). Male Infertility: Diagnosis and Treatment. London: Informa (Healthcare); 2007. pp. 239-54.
9. Pitteloud N, Acierno Jr JS, Meysing AU, Dwyer AA, Hayes FJ, Crowley Jr WF. Reversible Kallmann syndrome, delayed puberty, and isolated anosmia occurring in a single family with a mutation in the fibroblast growth factor receptor 1 gene. J Clin Endocrinol Metab. 2005;90(3):1317-22.
10. Oliveira LM, Seminara SB, Beranova M, Hayes FJ, Valkenburgh SB, Schipani E, et al. The importance of autosomal genes in Kallmann syndrome: genotype-phenotype correlations and neuroendocrine characteristics. J Clin Endocrinol Metab. 2001;86(4):1532-8.

11. Forest MG. Recent advances in the diagnosis and management of congenital adrenal hyperplasia due to 21-hydroxylase deficiency. Hum Reprod Update. 2004;10:469.
12. Burtis CA, Bruns DE. Tietz Fundamentals of Clinical Chemistry and Molecular Diagnostics. London: Elsevier Health Sciences; 2014.
13. Yang RM, Fefferman RA, Shapiro CE. Reversible infertility in man with 21-hydroxylase deficiency congenital adrenal hyperplasia. Fertil Steril. 2005;83:223.
14. Kim JC, Ou YY, Badano JL, Esmail MA, Leitch CC, Fiedrich E, et al. MKKS/BBS6, a divergent chaperonin-like protein linked to the obesity disorder Bardet–Biedl syndrome, is a novel centrosomal component required for cytokinesis. J Cell Sci. 2005;118(5):1007-20.
15. Mykytyn K, Mullins RF, Andrews M, Chiang AP, Swiderski RE, Yang B, et al. Bardet–Biedl syndrome type 4 (BBS4)-null mice implicate BBS4 in flagella formation but not global cilia assembly. Proc Natl Acad Sci U S A. 2004;101(23):8664-9.
16. Burghes A, Vaessin H, Chapellea A. The land between mendelian and multifractional inheritance. Science. 2001;293:2213.
17. Katsanis N. The oligogenic properties of Bardet–Biedl syndrome. Hum Mol Genet. 2004;13:65.
18. Beales P. Lifting the lid on Pandoras box: the Bardet–Biedl syndrome. Curr Opin Genet Develop. 2005;15:315.
19. Walsh CH. Non-diabetic endocrinopathy in hemochromatosis. In: Barton JC, Edward CQ (Eds). Hemochromatosis: Genetics, Pathophysiology, Diagnosis and Treatment. Cambridge: Cambridge University Press; 2000. p. 278.
20. Worwood M. Iron regulatory protein 1 and 2 in human monocytes, macrophages and duodenum: expression and regulation in hereditary hemochromatosis and iron deficiency. Haematologica. 2006;91(3):289B.
21. Delague V, Bareil C, Bouvagnet P, Salem N, Chouery E, Loiselet J, et al. Nonprogressive autosomal recessive ataxia maps to chromosome 9q34-9qter in a large consanguineous Lebanese family. Ann Neurol. 2001;50(2):250-3.
22. Tranebjaerg L, Teslovich TM, Jones M, Barmada MM, Fagerheim T, Dahl A, et al. Genome-wide homozygosity mapping localizes a gene for autosomal recessive non-progressive infantile ataxia to 20q11-q13. Hum Genet. 2003;113(3):293-5.
23. Silveira LF, MacColl GS, Bouloux PM. Hypogonadotropic hypogonadism. Semin Reprod Med. 2002;20(4):327-38.
24. Semple RK, Achermann JC, Ellery J, Farooqi IS, Karet FE, Stanhope RG, et al. Two novel missense mutations in g protein-coupled receptor 54 in a patient with hypogonadotropic hypogonadism. J Clin Endocrinol Metab. 2005;90(3): 1849-55.
25. Chemes HE. Phenotypes of sperm pathology: genetic and acquired forms in infertile men. J Androl. 2000;21(6):799-808.
26. Al-Bhalal L, Akhtar M. Molecular basis of autosomal dominant polycystic kidney disease. Adv Anat Pathol. 2005;12(3):126-33.
27. Quinzii C, Castellani C. The cystic fibrosis transmembrane regulator gene and male infertility. J Endocrinol Invest. 2000;23(10):684-9.
28. Patrizio P, Salameh WA. Expression of the cystic fibrosis transmembrane conductance regulator (CFTR) mRNA in normal and pathological adult human epididymis. J Reprod Fertil Suppl. 1988;53:261.
29. Silber SJ, Patrizio P, Asch RH. Quantitative evaluation of spermatogenesis by testicular histology in men with congenital absence of the vas deferens undergoing epididymal sperm aspiration. Hum Reprod. 1990;5:89.
30. Patrizio P, Ord T, Silber SJ, Asch RH. Correlation between epididymal length and fertilization rate in men with congenital absence of the vas deferens. Fertil Steril. 1994;61(2):265-8.
31. Phillipson GTM, Petrucco OM, Matthews CD. Congenital bilateral absence of the vas deferens, cystic fibrosis mutation analysis and intracytoplasmic sperm injection. Hum Reprod. 2000;15(2):431-5.
32. Casals T, Bassas L, Egozcue S, Ramos MD, Giménez J, Segura A, et al. Heterogeneity for mutations in the CFTR gene and clinical correlations in patients with congenital absence of the vas deferens. Hum Reprod. 2000;15(7):1476-83.
33. Rao MV, Hydrabadi VR, Chandel D. Complete androgen insensitivity in three generations of a family. Int J Hum Genet. 2008;8(4):361-3.
34. Gottlieb B, Beitel LK, Wu JH, Trifiro M. The androgen receptor gene mutations database (ARDB): 2004 update. Hum Mutat. 2004;23(6):527-33.
35. Hiort O, Holterhus PM, Horter T, Schulze W, Kremke B, Bals-Pratsch M, et al. Significance of mutations in the androgen receptor gene in males with idiopathic infertility. J Clin Endocrinol Metab. 2000;85(8):2810-5.
36. Hortas ML, Castilla JA, Gil MT, Molina J, Garrido ML, Morell M, et al. Decreased sperm function of patients with myotonic muscular dystrophy. Hum Reprod. 2000;15(2):445-8.
37. Shah PS, Shah ND, Ray HP, Khatri NB, Vaghasia KK, Shah SC, et al. Mutational analysis of East-Western population of India: a recent report. Appl Clin Genet. May 2017;10:27-35.
38. Rao MV, Shah SR, Patel AR. β-Thalassemia. In: Gupta PD, Srivastav LM (Eds). Essentials of Inborn Metabolic and Genetic Disorders. Chennai: PUG Publication Pvt. Ltd.; 2015. pp. 169-79.
39. Perera D, Pizzey A, Campbell A, Katz M, Porter J, Petrou M, et al. Sperm DNA damage in potentially fertile homozygous β-thalassaemia patients with iron overload. Hum Reprod. 2002;17(7):1820-5.
40. Barden EM, Kawchak DA, Ohene-Frempong K, Stallings VA, Zemel BS. Body composition in children with sickle cell disease. Am J Clin Nutrit. 2002;76(1):218-25.
41. Shah VC, Smart V. The human Y chromosome and SRY. Cell Biol Int. 1988;20:3-8.
42. Hédia S, Mohamed S, Insaf HA, Houda G, Yamina F, Myrvat K, et al. Male pseudo-hermaphroditism due to partial 5 alpha-reductase deficiency, a case report. La Tunisie Medicale. 2001;79(4):261-5.
43. Turek PJ, Pera RAR. Current and future genetic screening for male infertility. Urol Clin North Am. 2002;29(4):767-92.

44. Álvarez-Nava F, Soto M, Borjas L, Ortiz R, Rojas A, Martínez S, et al. Molecular analysis of SRY gene in patients with mixed gonadal dysgenesis. Annales De Génétique. 2001;44(3): 155-9.
45. Krausz C, Forti G, McElreavey K. The Y chromosome and male fertility and infertility. Int J Androl. 2003;26(2): 70-5.
46. Nudell DM, Pagani R, Lipshultz LI. Indications for genetic evaluation of men in a reproductive medicine program. J Braz Soc Urol. 2001;27(2):105-19.
47. Brugh VM, Maduro MR, Lamb DJ. Genetic disorders and infertility. Urol Clin North Am. 2003;30(1):143-52.
48. Rives N, Joly G, Machy A, Simeon N, Leclerc P, Mace B. Assessment of sex chromosome aneuploidy in sperm nuclei from 47, XXY and 46, XY/47, XXY males: comparison with fertile and infertile males with normal karyotype. Mol Hum Reprod. 2000;6(2):107-12.
49. Maduro MR, Lamb DJ. Understanding new genetics of male infertility. J Urol. 2002;168(5):2197-205.
50. Tartaglia M, Mehler EL, Goldberg R, Zampino G, Brunner HG, Kremer H, et al. Mutations in PTPN11, encoding the protein tyrosine phosphatase SHP-2, cause Noonan syndrome. Nat Genet. 2001;29(4):465.
51. Van der Burgt I, Brunner H. Genetic heterogeneity in Noonan syndrome: evidence for an autosomal recessive form. Am J Med Genet. 2000;94(1):46-51.
52. Griffin DK, Finch KA. The genetic and cytogenetic basis of male infertility. Hum Fertil. 2005;8(1):19-26.
53. Antonelli A, Gandini L, Petrinelli P, Marcucci L, Elli R, Lombardo F, et al. Chromosomal alterations and male infertility. J Endocrinol Investig. 2000;23(10):677-83.
54. Shah K, Sivapalan G, Gibbons N, Tempest H, Griffin DK. The genetic basis of infertility. Reproduction. 2003;126(1):13-25.
55. Vaghasia KK, Shah ND, Bhatt VM, Shah PS, Shah SC, Rao MV. Karyotypic analysis of chromosomal polymorphism in relation to reproductive failure. Int J Pharm Pharmaceut Sci. 2017;9(4):140-143.
56. Rao MV, Patel TA, Pandya H, Bavishi H. Prevalence of "Y" chromosome microdeletions in infertile males in Gujarati Population India. Unpublished data. 2017.
57. Ghorbian S. Routine diagnostic testing of Y chromosome deletions in male infertile and subfertile cases. Gene. 2012;503(1):160-4.
58. Thangaraj K, Gupta NJ, Pavani K, Reddy AG, Subramainan S, Rani DS, et al. Y chromosome deletions in azoospermic men in India. J Androl. 2003;24(4):588-97.

CHAPTER

Ejaculatory Dysfunctions: Diagnosis and Management

24

Tejanshu P Shah, Mihir Shah

INTRODUCTION

Ejaculation is a complex biphasic process involving the coordination of an intricate sequence of neurophysiological events and the contraction of numerous muscle groups eventuating in the expulsion of seminal fluid bolus through the urethra in the antegrade direction.[1] Process of ejaculation is associated with two important aspects namely sexual satisfaction and fertility potential of man. Though biological paternity can be achieved in men suffering from ejaculatory dysfunction with variety of treatment modalities, whenever possible restoration of ejaculatory function should be aimed, as it bring back normalcy to married life. This requires thorough knowledge of anatomy and neurophysiology of ejaculatory apparatus, understanding of diseases and iatrogenic factors that disrupt this function and the best modality of treatment in a given situation.

ANATOMY

Beside the structures derived from paired mesonephric ducts, namely epididymis, vasa, seminal vesicles and ejaculatory ducts, the other midline constituents of ejaculatory apparatus includes prostate, bladder neck, external urethral sphincter, Cowper's and litter's glands, urethra and periurethral musculature.

Testicular sperms coming out from efferent ductules enters epididymis which is 3–4 cm long and begin as caput(head) later to form body and tail, finally to transit into vas deference. It measures 30–40 cm in length and join with seminal vesicle to form ejaculatory duct. Last 5 cm of vas which is slightly dilated called ampulla and stores most of sperms. Seminal vesicles are lobulated structures situated lateral to ampullary portion of vas deference and about 1.5 cm × 4 cm and it contributes 70% of ejaculate, whereas 20% come from prostate and 10% from vasa. Ejaculatory duct passes through prostatic parenchyma to open in the prostatic urethra on the verumontanum. During ejaculation, components of seminal fluid are deposited in the prostatic urethra. The bladder neck serves as a physiologic sphincter during emission and ejaculation. Contraction of the bladder neck, especially during emission is under sympathetic neural control (alpha1 adrenergic).[2] Closure of bladder neck prevents semen from flowing back into bladder (retrograde ejaculation). External urethral sphincter which belongs to deep transverse perineal muscle and bulbocavernosus which surrounds corpus spongiosum and urethra has somatic innervations from perineal nerve (via the pudendal nerve, S 2–4).

PHYSIOLOGY OF EJACULATION

Ejaculation reflex leads to two sequential events: emission and ejaculation proper. This highly integrated and coordinated reflex arc has its control center located in lower thoracic and upper lumber spinal cord (T12-L1) in anterolateral gray column which is sympathetic outflow. It is known as spinal ejaculation generator (SEG). It acts as coordinator center to integrate afferent inputs from various sources like genital sensory from penile stimulation and cerebral cortical inputs. Cortical input to SEG may be both excitatory and inhibitory but the exact location of cortical foci is poorly understood. Genital sensory input passes via pudendal nerve to S2-4 spinal cord region, then ascend to SEG. On threshold excitation of SEG, sympathetic discharge starts to bladder neck, vasal ampulla, seminal vesicles and prostate. Secretions of vasal ampulla, seminal vesicle and prostate are deposited in posterior urethra with closure of bladder neck. SEG simultaneously prompts closure of external urethral sphincter via efferent somatic outflow through motor fibers of pudendal nerve. This leads to high intraprostatic urethral pressure causing ejaculatory inevitability. SEG causes activation of Onuf's nucleus in the ventral horn of S2-4 leading to somatic outflow generated simultaneously with sympathetic discharge leading to rhythmic contraction of bulbospongiosus synchronized with intermittent opening of external urethral sphincter coupled with closure of bladder neck

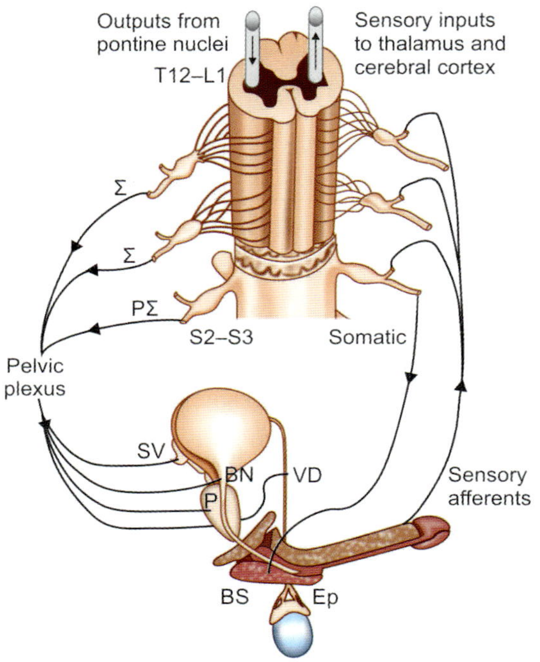

Fig. 24.1: Neurophysiology of ejaculation.

allow antegrade and rhythmic expulsion of seminal fluid.[3] Thus, ejaculation is an intricate neurophysiological event with contraction of numerous muscle groups both striated and smooth (Fig. 24.1).

Interruption of afferent input from penis increases latency of ejaculation but will not result in total loss of ejaculation response as long as cortical afferents and sympathetic efferents are not affected.[4]

DISORDERS OF EJACULATION

1. Premature ejaculation (too fast or rapid)
2. Anejaculation (absent, dry sex, ejaculatory failure)
   - Primary or absent orgasm
   - Secondary or absent emission
3. Retrograde ejaculation (backward)

Both anejaculation and retrograde ejaculation are associated with absence of semen during intercourse, also known as aspermia.

PREMATURE EJACULATION (PE)

- Most common ejaculatory problems involve 30% of adult men.
- Definition is unclear; however, man is considered suffering from PE when he is unable to control ejaculation long enough to satisfy his partner in at least 50% of his coital opportunity. In normal situation, average time from vaginal penetration to ejaculation is 5–10 minutes. Hence, practically, PE exists if this time is less than 1 minute or ejaculation occurs prior to 10 pelvic thrusts. The most severe form ejaculation occurs before interomission and is responsible for infertility.

CAUSES

- Psychogenic: excessive sensitivity or anxiety or stress
- Prolonged abstinence
- Associated with ED or fear of losing erection
- Prostatitis or seminal vesicular pathology, rarely.

TREATMENT

Goal is to increase control over ejaculation process by reducing genital sensitivity, adjusting behavioral response leading to better cortical control of ejaculatory center.

1. Behavioral therapy
   - Start-stop technique: Approach climax but stop before ejaculatory inevitability to reduce stimulation.
   - Squeeze-pullout: before ejaculatory inevitability withdraw penis from vagina and squeeze glans penis.
   - Mind distraction.
2. Local therapy: Local anesthetic prilocaine and lidocaine 2.5% to reduce sensitivity of penis.
3. Oral medications: Dapoxetine or paroxetine, short acting SSRI are not good enough for depression but useful in PE Sildenafil or tadalafil are used if underlying erectile dysfunction is present.

ANEJACULATION (EJACULATORY FAILURE)

Commonest cause of aspermia or dry sex, it may be primary or secondary.

Primary Ejaculatory Failure (PEF)

Here anejaculation is due to failure to reach climax or orgasm. Such anorgasmic anejaculation is mostly psychological. It is commonly associated with significant parental suppression or conservative thinking about sex. These patients had never masturbated nor had ejaculation during sex; however, nocturnal ejaculation is present which rules out other pathology. Careful history determines that intercourse last for 5–30 minutes or even longer, at the end patient gets tired or looses erection without orgasm or ejaculation.

It is important to take careful history to avoid unrequired investigations, wrong diagnosis, treatment or surgery.

Treatment is directed toward measures to enable the patient to reach climax which he has never experienced so far. Painstaking efforts should be made. Psychosexual therapy, reassurance, visual sexual stimulation including teaching to masturbate and ejaculate are vital for obtaining success. Correct use of penile vibratory stimulation (PVS) at frenulum of erect penis to provide strong and prolonged penile stimulation gives success in over 75% cases. Use of yohimbin 10–20 mg and tadalafil 10 mg if associated mild ED, given 3 hours prior will aid to success.

Secondary Ejaculatory Failure (SEF)

Patient had normal ejaculation in past. SEF occurs due to failure of sympathetic innervation due to RPLND for testicular cancer, aortoiliac reconstruction, colorectal excision, anterior approach lumbar spine surgery, neurological diseases such as MS, transverse myelitis, neural tube defects, autonomic neuropathy due to diabetes mellitus, traumatic spinal cord injury (SCI). Patient does reach orgasm but unable to deposit spermatic fluid into urethra due to failure of sympathetic innervation for emission. Many medications having sympatholytic property may cause similar problem.

Treatment Strategy

By understanding which neurological arm or what anatomic structure of ejaculatory apparatus is involved, suitable treatment options needs to be found.

Therapeutic options are

1. Oral sympathomimetic drugs
2. Penile vibratory stimulation (PVS)
3. Rectal probe electroejaculation (RPE)
4. Sperm retrieval technique for ICSI

Oral Sympathomimetic Drugs

Oral sympathomimetic drugs (Alpha agonist compounds) act by augmenting sympathetic tone to vas, seminal vesicles and bladder neck. This is especially true when there is partial surgical disruption of sympathetic plexus or functional disturbance in diabetic autonomic neuropathy. Pseudoephedrine 60 mg given 1 hour before intercourse helps restore antegrade ejaculation. In patients with this type of history, alpha agonist therapy is always tried initially.[5,6]

Penile Vibratory Stimulation (PVS)

In normal man, ejaculation reflex is triggered by two factors: (1) afferent sensory inflow from genital stimulation and (2) cortical augmentory influence; a learned condition reflex. In SCI patients, connection with higher center is absent, whereas in PEF cortical augmentory influence is not properly learned.

By providing overwhelming supraphysiological sensory stimulation to the spinal ejaculation generator through application of a vibrator to the penile frenulum, activation of the ejaculatory reflex can be initiated in the absence of cortical augmentory influence.[7]

PVS can also be successfully applied to SCI male where injury to cord is above sympathetic outflow (above T12-L1) and cord structures below lesion are viable, demonstrated by intact bulbocavernosus reflex (BCR) and hip flexor reflex (HR). In appropriate case of SCI, above T10 chances of success will be approximately 80% and hence is the first-line treatment and not surgical sperm retrieval.

PVS involves the use of a vibrator or vibrator having multiple stimulation points, which is created specifically for this purpose. Device is placed on frenum or glans. Stimulation is done for 2 minutes, if ejaculation is not elicited another attempt can be made for 3 minutes after period of rest and gradually increasing period up to 30 minutes. Once ejaculation occurs, specimen is collected in wide mouthed jar. Great caution should be exercised in patient with SCI above T6 while undergoing PVS as enhanced sympathetic tone from T6 segment can cause constriction of blood vessels leading to hypertension due to autonomic dysreflexia. Under such circumstances procedure should be terminated immediately. Repeat PVS session is kept after couple of days and 5–10 mg sublingual nifedipine is given before beginning treatment (Fig. 24.2).

PVS is not applicable to those men who are having SCI below L1 or with disruption of peripheral sympathetic outflow as in RPLND or pelvic surgery.

Rectal Probe Electroejaculation (RPE)

First line therapy for men with lower spinal cord (lumber) lesions with flaccid lower extremities and absent bulbocavernosus and hip flexor reflexes. As these patients are

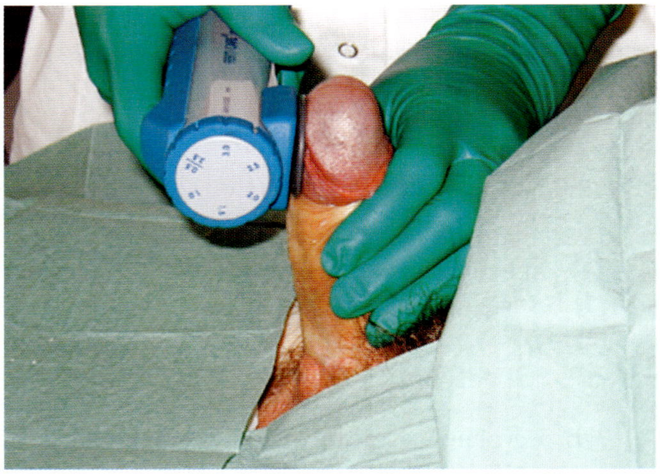

Fig. 24.2: Use of penile vibrator for erection

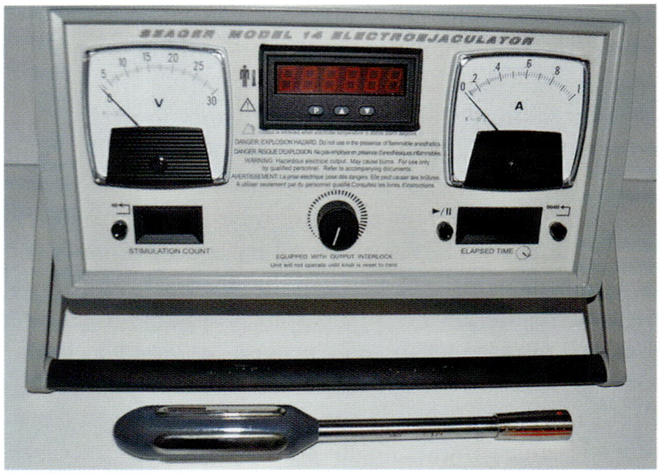

Fig. 24.3: Rectal probe electroejaculation in SCI patient.

associated with loss of sensations, RPE can be performed without anesthesia (Fig. 24.3).

Patient with thoracic SCI in whom PVS has failed are considered for RPE. Requirement of anesthesia depends upon presence or absence of sensation and autonomic dysreflexia. Patient with cervical SCI usually have significant AD, hence general anesthesia is the safest option. RPE may be ineffective if terminal vas has become aperistaltic as in long-standing diabetes.

Presently, Seager electroejaculator (Model 14) is the only FDA USA approved device.

Procedure

General anesthesia is given to all patients having rectal sensation (e.g., post-RPLND) or likely to have significant AD (e.g., SCI cervical level quadriplegic). Bladder is emptied using 14F catheter and 10 mL of buffer is instilled to optimize retrieval of sperm going in retrograde direction. Left lateral position is given and rectal probe is inserted with stimulating electrode facing anteriorly to prostate and seminal vesical. Electrical current is started at 3–5 V for 5 seconds and stopped for 20 seconds and increased in 1–5 V increments till ejaculation occurs or maximum 20–30 V reached.[8] Current is terminated abruptly after each wave. Stimulation is continued till seminal fluid is seen dribbling from meatus. Bladder is catheterized to obtain retrograde specimen. When specimen is obtained without anesthesia in office setup and is of good quality, it may be used for IUI. Whereas patients in whom specimen can be obtained only under GA with relatively few motile sperm, cryopreservation with ICSI is a better option. Success rates in different patient population by RPE is 75–90%

Surgical Sperm Retrieval

When PVS and RPE have failed, sperms are retrieved by TESA, PESA or micro surgical sperm harvesting is done but it should not routinely be the first choice.

RETROGRADE EJACULATION (RE)

In RE, there is emission of seminal fluid into the posterior urethra but it flow back into bladder due to failure of bladder neck closure. Causes of RE are congenital wide bladder neck, bladder neck surgery including TURP which do not respond to medical treatment. In contrast, other causes like neurological condition such as diabetes mellitus, multiple sclerosis and retroperitoneal surgery. Affecting sympathetic plexus may respond to medical therapies. The third group of patients are those receiving sympatholytic or adrenergic blocking drugs most common are tamsulosin, alfuzosin used to treat BPH. This group responds well to withdrawal of offending drug, if it is feasible for the period of 8–12 weeks and ejaculation usually resume back.

Pharmacotherapy for retrograde ejaculation is likely to be effective in patients who do not have surgical changes of bladder neck. Pseudoephedrine 60 mg qid and imipramine 25 mg bid is given for at least 7 days before planned ejaculation timed to wife's ovulatory cycle and continued for maximum 2 weeks. Continuous administration is not recommended as tolerance may develop.

Recovery of sperm from bladder urine is done in patients who are unresponsive to medical therapy or who have undergone surgical ablation of bladder neck. Deposition of pH adjusted media in the bladder or alkalinization of urine by profuse water intake with sodium bicarbonate 650 mg qid or acetazolamide 250 mg qid are mandatory. Sperms are recovered by gentle centrifugation and then washed in appropriate insemination media.

Surgical reconstruction of bladder neck was used in past but operation is major and not always successful. With advancement in semen processing technique, this surgery is hardly ever advised today.

In future, stem cell therapeutics in SCI and purine agonist may be useful in patients of ejaculatory failure.

REFERENCES

1. Muller A, Mulhall JP. The epididymis and accessory sex organs erection, emission and ejaculation: mechanisms of control. In: Lipshultz LI, Nagler HS, Niederberger CS (Eds). Infertility in the Male, 4th edition. Cambridge (United Kingdom): Cambridge University Press; 2009. pp. 132-52.
2. Michel MC, Barendrecht MM. Physiological and pathological regulation of the autonomic control of urinary bladder contractility. Pharmacol Ther. 2008;117(3):297-312.
3. Shafik A. Response of the urethral and intracorporeal pressures to cavernosus muscle stimulation: role of the muscles in erection and ejaculation. Urology. 1995;46(1)85-8.
4. Comarr AE. Sexual concepts in traumatic cord and cauda equine lesions. J Urol. 1971;106(3):375-8.
5. Gilja I, Parazajder J, Radej M, Cvitković P, Kovacić M. Retrograde ejaculation and loss of emission: possibilities of conservative treatment. Eur Urol. 1994;25(3):226-8.
6. Kamischke A, Nieschlag E. Update on medical treatment of ejaculatory disorders. Int J Androl. 2002;25(6):333-44.
7. Oates RD, Kasabian N. The use of vibratory stimulation for ejaculatory abnormalities. In: Nagker HM, Whitehead ED (Eds). Management of impotence and infertility. Philadelphia: JB Lippincott Co; 1994. pp. 314-20.
8. Ohl DA, Wolf LJ, Menge AC, Christman GM, Hurd WW, Ansbacher R, et al. Electroejaculation and assisted reproductive technologies in the treatment of anejaculatory infertility. Fertil Steril. 2001;76(6):1249-55.

CHAPTER

25

Recurrent Miscarriage

Mala Arora, Surekha Tayade

INTRODUCTION

Recurrent miscarriage (RM) is a profound personal tragedy experienced by couples seeking parenthood and is an equally challenging task for the attending physician. Miscarriage is defined as the spontaneous loss of pregnancy before the fetus reaches viability and therefore, includes all pregnancy losses from the time of conception until 20 weeks of gestation.[1] Recurrent miscarriage may also be referred as recurrent pregnancy loss (RPL) and recurrent spontaneous miscarriage (RSM).

DEFINITION

Recurrent miscarriage is classically defined as three or more consecutive pregnancy losses at 20 weeks or less or with fetal weight of less than 500 g.[2] Recently, ACOG defined it as two or more spontaneous miscarriages for clinical purposes.[3] American Society of Reproductive Medicine (ASRM) defines recurrent pregnancy loss as two or more failed clinical pregnancies, which should be documented by either ultrasound or histopathological examination. None of the definitions include biochemical pregnancies, ectopic pregnancies or pregnancy of uncertain location.[4]

Sporadic miscarriages occur in 25% of pregnancies. A woman may have three sporadic miscarriages during her obstetric career, but if these are interspersed with viable births they are not classified as recurrent miscarriages.

Primary aborters are women who have no previous pregnancy that progressed to viability and *secondary aborters* are women who have one or more pregnancies that have proceeded beyond 20 weeks of gestation.

For research purposes, the definition of RM is three or more consecutive losses and Royal College of Obstetricians and Gynecologists (RCOG) recommends investigations after three consecutive losses. However, ASRM practice guidelines state that, in the clinical scenario, evaluation should be considered following two consecutive miscarriages, especially with advanced maternal age.[5] One sporadic miscarriage does not warrant detailed investigations as the chances of a subsequent normal birth are high.

INCIDENCE

Although spontaneous abortion occurs in around 15–25%[6] of pregnancies, recurrent miscarriages (as per the classic definition of three or more consecutive pregnancy losses) affects 0.4–1% of couples.[7]

RECURRENT RISK

The risk of recurrence is influenced by various factors, which includes maternal age, parental and fetal karyotypes, gestation age of previous loss and various laboratory parameters. The risk of miscarriage is higher (25–57%) in less than 6 weeks of gestation and reduces to 2–3% in gestation above 10 weeks.[8] Chromosomal analysis offers an explanation in 50% of cases.[9] Table 25.1 shows the risk of miscarriage with number of prior miscarriages.

ETIOLOGY

The causes of recurrent miscarriage are listed in Table 25.2.[10] The list is exhaustive and investigations are expensive. More than one factor may operate in successive

Table 25.1: Risk of miscarriage with number of prior miscarriages.[10]

	No. of prior miscarriages	*% risk of recurrence in next pregnancy*
Women with one live born infant	0	12
	1	24
	2	26
	3	32
	4 or more	40–50
Women with no live infant	2 or more	40–45

Table 25.2: Causes of recurrent miscarriage.

Lifestyle factors	Uterine synechiae and polyps
Maternal age >35 years	T-shaped uterus
Maternal obesity, BMI >30	Cervical incompetence
Paternal age	Inherited thrombophilia
Immunological-autoimmune	Antithrombin III deficiency
Primary antiphospholipid syndrome	Deficiency of protein C and protein S
Secondary antiphospholipid syndrome – SLE, autoimmune thyroiditis	Activated protein C resistance
Immunological-alloimmune (classified as unexplained)	Factor V Leiden mutation
Abnormalities of cytokine production-lack of shift of Th1 to Th 2 response	Methyl tetrahydrofolate gene homozygosity and Hyperhomocysteinemia
Lack of alpha V beta 3 integrin	Prothrombin gene mutation
Increased levels of tumor necrosis factor alpha (TNF) in the endometrium	Plaminogen activator inhibitor
Increased uterine natural killer cells	Semen factors
Abnormal timing and duration of implantation window	High sperm DNA fragmentation index
Genetic	Male urogenital infections
Fetal trisomy, polyploidy, monosomy	Infections
Parental balanced translocations, inversions, deletions, duplications	Genital bacterial vaginosis, tuberculosis
Skewed inactivation of X chromosome	Systemic syphilis, Lyme's disease, toxoplasmosis, brucellosis
Single gene defects, e.g. alpha thalassemia major, Retts syndrome, etc.	Systemic conditions
Hormonal	Hypertension
Polycystic ovarian syndrome	Chronic renal disease
Luteal phase defects	Chronic pulmonary disease
Hyperandrogenism	Heart disease
Hypothyroidism/hyperthyroidism	Severe rhesus sensitization
Hyperprolactinemia	Miscellaneous
Low AMH/poor ovarian reserve	Endocrine disrupters
Adrenal hyperplasia/Addison's disease	Smoking, alcohol, drugs
Deficiency of vitamin D	Exposure to irradiation
Uncontrolled diabetes mellitus	Exposure to environmental toxins, pesticides, DDT, dry cleaning chemicals
Anatomical	Exposure to anesthetic gases
Müllerian abnormalities, septate uterus	Idiopathic
Fibroids – submucous, intramural	Cytokine abnormalities
	Increased uterine natural killer cells
	Lack of pinopode formation

pregnancies, e.g., early miscarriages due to any cause may be coupled with a late miscarriage due to cervical incompetence. On the other hand, early miscarriages may be coupled with a late fetal demise in patients with either congenital or acquired thrombophilia.

The mechanism of pregnancy loss in various conditions is discussed below:

Genetic Causes

Genetic Abnormalities in Karyotypically Normal Parents

Various studies demonstrate that at least 50% of clinically recognized pregnancy loss results from a cytogenetic

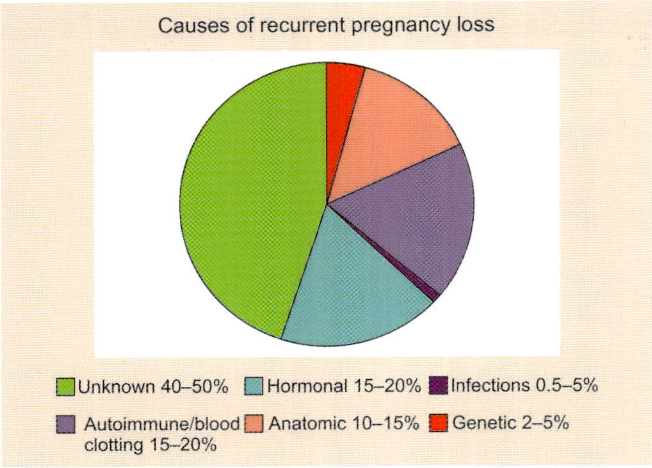

Fig. 25.1: Percent distribution of etiology of recurrent miscarriages.

abnormality,[11] of which 51% show autosomal trisomies, 22% show polyploidy, 19% show monosomy, 4% show translocations, and the rest are unclassified genetic defects. The autosomal trisomies commonly encountered are those of chromosomes 3, 4, 9, 13–16, 19, 21 and 22.[12] (Fig. 25.1).

Genetic Abnormalities in Karyotypically Abnormal Parents

Women may have structural chromosomal abnormality in the following forms.

- Deletions and duplications produce large chromosomal defects, which may cause severe phenotypic anomalies, thus individuals with these anomalies rarely reproduce.
- Dicentric and ring chromosomes are mitotically unstable, therefore the chances of offspring acquiring these anomalies are very small.
- In balanced translocations in men, the reproductive fitness is only slightly diminished.[13] In spite of their good reproductive performance, these individuals show a significant decrease in live births, and a significant increase in both fetal death and interval infertility; hence they will present with recurrent miscarriage.
- In unbalanced translocations in men, not only is there productive fitness greatly decreased but the risk of abnormal offspring is also increased.[13]
- In single gene defects, diagnosis can only be made by a detailed family history coupled with fluorescent PCR testing.

Hormonal Disorders

A multitude of endocrinal disorders can cause recurrent miscarriage.

Polycystic ovarian syndrome is one of the most common endocrinal abnormalities affecting female reproductive performance. Besides infertility, it presents higher risks of first- and second-trimester miscarriages.[14]

Factors associated with a high-miscarriage rate are *hyperandrogenism, hyperinsulinemia* and/or *ovulatory dysfunction* that accompany high levels of luteinizing hormone and low levels of progesterone.

Women with poorly controlled *type 1 (insulin-dependent) diabetes mellitus* with glycosylated (HbA1C) hemoglobin levels greater than four standard deviations above the mean had a higher pregnancy loss rate. Well-controlled diabetes had pregnancy loss rates similar to those of nondiabetics. Apart from frank diabetes, syndrome X,[15] which comprises impaired glucose tolerance test (GTT), hypertension, hypertriglyceridemia and a procoagulant state with increased coronary heart disease, could also potentially cause recurrent pregnancy loss.

Abnormal maternal thyroid functions have been implicated as a cause of recurrent miscarriage.[16] However, mild or subclinical thyroid dysfunction is not associated with recurrent miscarriage, as it more often leads to infertility, but increased levels of thyroid peroxidase and/or microsomal antibodies have been associated with recurrent miscarriage.[17] In autoimmune thyroid disease (AITD), the risk of miscarriage was the same whether the status was hypothyroid or euthyroid, indicating that AITD negatively affects fetal implantation. Hence all women with positive thyroid antibodies should be treated with a low dose of thyroxine replacement to suppress thyroid autoimmunity and achieve a favorable maternal and perinatal outcome.[18]

Hyperprolactinemia usually causes infertility due to luteolysis; however, in partially treated cases, the picture may change to early pregnancy loss due to corpus luteum deficiency.

Although rare, the patient with an untreated late onset *congenital adrenal hyperplasia* may have an increased chance of recurrent miscarriage owing to hyperandrogenism. On the other hand, incipient *Addison's disease* will also cause recurrent miscarriages; the patient often has low blood pressure and hyperpigmentation.

Poor ovarian reserve, diagnosed by low levels of anti-Müllerian hormone (AMH) and a poor antral follicle count, remains an important factor responsible for

Table 25.3: Frequency of various anatomical abnormalities.[21]

	Comparison of uterine anomalies		
	Primary RM compared with secondary RM		
	Primary RM (*n* = 479)	**Secondary RM (*n* = 425)**	***p***
All uterine anomalies	22.8 (109)	15.8 (67)	0.009
Congenital anomalies	8.8 (42)	4.5 (19)	0.011
Bicornuate uterus	1.0 (5)	0.5 (2)	ns
Didelphic uterus	0.2 (1)	0.2 (1)	ns
Septate uterus	6.3 (30)	3.1 (13)	0.028
T-shaped uterus	0.4 (2)	0.2 (1)	ns
Unicornuate uterus	0.8 (4)	0.5 (2)	ns
Acquired anomalies	14.6 (70)	11.8 (50)	ns
Adhesions	4.0 (19)	4.2 (18)	ns
Fibroid(s)	7.3 (35)	5.4 (23)	ns
Polyp (s)	4.0 (19)	2.4 (10)	ns
Values are % occurrence (*n*)	Jaslow and Kutteh, 2013:99;1916-22		

recurrent miscarriage, owing to increased rate of aneuploidy in oocytes. Women with AMH levels below 1 ng/mL not only experience difficulty in conceiving but also have a higher rate of pregnancy loss due to a higher rate of aneuploidy in the embryo.

Anatomic Abnormalities

Anatomic abnormalities of the uterus and cervix are amenable to surgery. An estimated 15% of couples (one in six) with recurrent miscarriage have an anatomic abnormality of the uterus as the primary cause. These abnormalities include the following:

- Defects of Müllerian fusion, which include septate uterus, unicornuate uterus and bicornuate uterus with unequal uterine horns.
- Acquired anatomical defects, such as submucous or intramural myomas, endometrial polyps and uterine synechiae.
- Small tubular uterine cavity: this may be congenital, secondary to diethylstilboestrol exposure in utero or genital tuberculosis.
- Cervical incompetence, which is diagnosed by visualizing the cervix with an empty bladder on transvaginal ultrasound scan and assessing the width at the internal os as well as the cervical length from internal to external os.[19,20] It may be a congenital weakness or secondary to repeated cervical dilatation. It is also associated with unicornuate or bicornuate uteri.

Although women with primary recurrent miscarriages are more likely to have anatomical abnormalities, recent study indicates that the uterus needs evaluation even in cases of secondary recurrent miscarriages (Table 25.3).[21]

Immunological Causes

Antiphospholipid antibody syndrome (APS) is the most common immunological cause of recurrent miscarriage. Antibodies are directed against negatively charged phospholipids, which are the major constituents of trophoblast. These antibodies can cause placental thrombosis, infarction, impaired trophoblastic function and abnormal placentation, and thus may lead to pregnancy-induced hypertension, intrauterine growth retardation (IUGR), intrauterine fetal death and recurrent miscarriage. Pregnancy loss usually occurs in the midtrimester between 14 and 18 weeks; however, both early first-trimester losses and late third-trimester losses can occur. There is usually an ultrasound confirmation of a viable pregnancy prior to the pregnancy loss in most first trimester losses.

The diagnosis of APS is made by the presence of *one clinical criterion and one-laboratory criterion, which must be positive on two occasions 3 months apart.*

Clinical criteria include the following:[22,23]

- one or more unexplained deaths of a morphologically normal fetus of more than 10 weeks of gestation documented by ultrasonography or direct examination;

- one or more preterm births at or before 34 weeks of gestation due to severe preeclampsia or placental insufficiency with evidence of IUGR;
- three or more consecutive abortions before 10 weeks of gestation with no maternal hormonal, anatomic abnormalities, normal maternal and paternal chromosomes and other causes of recurrent losses being ruled out.

Laboratory criteria include detection of any of the following:

1. Lupus anticoagulant by DRVVT, APTT or PTT
2. Anticardiolipin antibodies
3. Antiphospholipid antibodies
4. Antibeta 2 glycoprotein antibodies

Autoimmune disorders, such as systemic lupus erythematosus, systemic sclerosis, and autoimmune thrombocytopenia are associated with recurrent miscarriage, and are often classified as secondary antiphospholipid syndrome (or SAPS). The mechanism of loss and the treatment are the same as those for primary APS.

Treatment with steroids is not recommended based on current evidence. A combination of low dose aspirin and unfractionated/low molecular weight heparin currently gives the best pregnancy outcome. Heparin is not only an anticoagulant; it has a potent complement inhibitory action which is beneficial in preventing complement mediated damage in APS syndrome. Aspirin should be started preconceptually and heparin after a positive pregnancy test and continued until the time of delivery. Postpartum thromboprophylaxis is recommended for 2 weeks to prevent deep vein thrombosis.

Thrombophilias

These are rare inherited disorders that predispose an individual to venous and arterial thrombosis. They cause inadequate placental circulation owing to thrombosis in the placental vasculature, and lead to adverse pregnancy outcomes like IUGR, intrauterine fetal death and placental abruption. They are not commonly associated with recurrent early miscarriages. However Congenital thrombophilias include the followings:

- Activated protein C resistance (APCR)[1] due to Factor V Leiden mutation: A single missense mutation of the factor V gene can cause 90% cases of APCR and is present in 5% of the UK population.
- Deficiency of antithrombin III: This occurs in 32–51% patients with thrombophilia.[24]
- Deficiency of protein C and protein S: In patients with thrombophilia, 22–26% have protein C deficiency, while 12–17% have protein S deficiency.[25]
- Prothrombin gene mutation G 20210A leads to elevated levels of prothrombin and is present in 2% of the UK population.[24]
- Homozygosity for the thermolabile mutation of methylene tetrahydrofolate reductase (MTHFR) causing hyperhomocysteinemia.

Homozygous genotype for plasminogen activator-1 is also associated with recurrent miscarriages.

Hyperhomocysteinemia

Homocysteine is an amino acid that is synthesized in the body from methionine. Its normal levels are 4–15 μmol/L. High homocysteine levels result from genetic mutations that cause enzyme deficiency, or dietary deficiency of vitamin B6, B12 and folic acid that are cofactors essential for the functioning of the enzyme that metabolizes it to cysteine. Homocysteine levels normally decrease during pregnancy, but high levels are associated with placental vascular thrombosis and placental abruption.[26]

Homocysteine levels may be lowered by administration of vitamin B6, B12 and folic acid. Its association with recurrent miscarriages is not proved but when levels are more than 30 μmol/L it may cause a thrombogenic state and result in recurrent miscarriages.

The risk of adverse pregnancy outcomes in thrombogenic states is depicted in Table 25.4.

Systemic Conditions

Severe maternal illness, such as essential hypertension, cardiac disease, chronic pulmonary disease and chronic nephritis are important causes of recurrent miscarriages. Pregnancy in a rhesus-sensitized woman with a high titer of anti-D antibodies will also result in RPL.

Systemic infections like syphilis were an important cause of recurrent miscarriages in the past and are re-emerging in the HIV positive population. Currently, Lyme's disease and toxoplasmosis can result in repetitive losses. Bacterial infections acquired from dairy products, like *Brucella abortus*, also causes recurrent miscarriage.

Genital Infections

Genitourinary tuberculosis is classically associated with infertility, but in its latent form, can also cause recurrent

Table 25.4: Thrombophilias

High risk	*Medium risk*	*Low risk*
Antiphospholipid syndrome	Protein C deficiency	Heterozygosity for Factor V Leiden mutation
	Protein S deficiency	Heterozygosity for prothrombin gene mutation
Antithrombin deficiency	Homozygosity for Factor V Leiden mutation	Hyperhomocysteinemia 13–30 µmol/L
Hyperhomocysteinemia >30 µmol/L	Homozygosity of Prothrombin gene mutation	
	Combined heterozygosity for Factor V Leiden and prothrombin gene mutation	

ectopic pregnancy biochemical pregnancies as well as miscarriages. Bacterial vaginosis is now implicated in recurrent miscarriages, recurrent preterm labor and preterm premature rupture of membranes.

Miscellaneous Causes

Excessive smoking, alcohol intake and the use of recreational drugs will cause recurrent miscarriage. Other factors include prolonged exposure to irradiation and anesthetic gases, pesticides and other environmental toxins. Of increasing importance is the presence of endocrine disrupters that are emanated by plastic devices in our environment.

Idiopathic Causes

In 50% of cases, the cause of recurrent miscarriages is not clearly elucidated at present. Implantation is a complex process that involves synchronization of endometrial maturity with fertilization. Successful implantation involves expression of *HOX A 10* genes in the endometrium, formation of pinopodes, as well as the presence of cytokines of the anti-inflammatory kind, such as interleukins 4, 6 and 10, leukemia inhibiting factor (LIF) and transforming growth factor beta (TGF-β). A disturbance in any of the above processes will lead to early pregnancy losses. Absence of the cytokine LIF in the endometrium is associated with recurrent miscarriages in the knockout mouse model but its exact role in humans is yet to be elucidated. Other cytokine abnormalities, such as increased levels of inflammatory cytokines, i.e., TNF alpha in the endometrium are the subject of current research in recurrent miscarriages. Measurement of levels of TNF alpha in the peripheral blood, during the luteal phase of the cycle or during early pregnancy, has been recommended by some. These are classically raised in graft rejection and may be marginally raised in fetal rejection. However, the test is not standardized for clinical use during pregnancy yet.

An increased number of natural killer cells in the endometrium will lead to embryolysis. Increased numbers of natural killer cells result from an abnormal maternal immune response to the foreign antigenic makeup of the embryo and are hence termed *alloimmune* cause of RM. Measurement of natural killer cell subsets in peripheral blood has also been recommended by some. However, its correlation to the uterine natural killer cell population is still not established. Immune potentiation may help a small subset of these patients with alloimmune causes or immune rejection of the fetal allograft.

Autoimmunity is also known to affect embryogenesis by altering the endometrial environment. In a recent study, 515 patients with idiopathic recurrent miscarriages and no overt autoimmune disease, and a control group, were screened for autoantibodies. The results were as follows: antithyroglobulin antibody was positive in 21.2% in RM group vs. 7.8% in the control group. Antimitochondrial antibody was positive in 4.8% in RM group vs. 0.5% in control group. In short, any one antibody was positive in 28.3% in RM group vs. 14.5% in the control group. Similarly, another study reported deficiency of IgG subclass in women with RM compared with controls,[27] while yet another study reported micro-RNA mutations diagnosed by PCR amplification in the idiopathic RM group ($n = 200$) vs. fertile controls ($n = 300$) with an odds ratio of 2.98 and CI of 1.40–2.81 and a p value of 0.0001.[28]

These studies point out that a variety of unrelated pathologies may be responsible for idiopathic RM and investigating this group fully may not be clinically feasible at present but will be possible in the near future.

Hence recurrent miscarriages may occur due to a variety of causes, some well understood and others less so.[1] Some are treatable, such as immunological, hormonal, anatomical causes as well as thrombophilias. An abnormal cytokine environment may be responsible for some of the hitherto unexplained recurrent miscarriages and enhancing maternal immune modulation may be beneficial.

EVALUATION AND WORKUP

Ideally, the couple should be seen together at a dedicated recurrent miscarriage clinic and given accurate information to facilitate decision-making about future pregnancies. Clearly written patient leaflets are recommended to provide written information that the couple can take home. Various guidelines have been proposed for the evaluation of recurrent miscarriages by various academic societies. However, it is important to understand that it might be difficult to categorize a particular case of RPL into one homogenous condition; hence individualization should be done when managing such a condition.

History

A careful history should include details of the previous losses (pattern, trimester, characteristics), preceding infertility and its management, past history suggestive of acute or chronic infections, endocrinological disorder (thyroid dysfunction, hyperprolactinemia, diabetes mellitus, thrombosis) APLAS and other autoimmune disorders should be noted. Prior medication history, consumption of recreational drugs, caffeine, alcohol, cigarette smoking should be noted. Prior gynecological surgery is relevant.

Physical Examination

Obesity, hirsutism, acanthosis, thyroid enlargement and galactorrhea are obvious indicators of the cause. A pelvic examination should be carried out to exclude infection and to look for possible anatomic abnormalities.

Transvaginal Ultrasound Scan

Uterine evaluation is required in all patients with recurrent miscarriages. This will diagnose Müllerian abnormalities, submucous myomas, adenomyosis and endometrial hyperplasia. If indicated, further evaluation is performed with the help of transvaginal 3D and 4D scan which diagnoses all uterine abnormalities comfortably. It is noninvasive and has a high sensitivity and specificity in experienced hands. Sonohysteroscopy is the procedure of scanning after saline infusion of the uterine cavity. This will help diagnose intra cavity lesions like polyps and adhesions. Hysterosalpingography involves exposure of the ovaries to radiation but provides a visual record of the uterine cavity and tubal patency. It is valuable in confirming Müllerian anomalies like unicornuate uterus. Hystero/laparoscopy is not only the gold standard for diagnosis but also allows remedial action at the same time like excision of polyp, adhesions, submucous myomas and uterine septum. Difficult cases may be performed under laparoscopic vision to avoid perforations.

Algorithm for Workup

Checking for hormonal abnormalities, screening for antiphospholipid syndrome and evaluation of the uterine cavity is recommended after two consecutive miscarriages. Fetal karyotype evaluation is recommended after the second or third consecutive miscarriage. Products of conception obtained from early nonviable pregnancies via a dilatation and evacuation may not be suitable for karyotyping but can be analyzed by fluorescent in situ hybridization (FISH) analysis. This analyzes five chromosomes, i.e., 13,18,21,X and Y. Flowchart 25.1 shows the algorithm for genetic workup in RM.

For a full workup all the possible causes have to be looked into (Flowchart 25.2).

TREATMENT

Anatomical Causes

The treatment often involves corrective hysteroscopic surgery. Resection of the septum may be done with the use of cautery or rarely with hysteroscopic scissors. Excision of submucous myoma is performed with the resectoscope. Adhesion bands and polyps are excised with the help of hysteroscopic scissors rarely correction of bicornuate uterus requires a Strassman operation. Repeated implantation in the smaller horn of a bicornuate uterus may require excision of the rudimentary horn by laparoscopy/laparotomy. Disabling implantation in a rudimentary horn by placing an IUCD in it may also be a viable noninvasive treatment option to prevent miscarriages.[30]

Cervical Insufficiency

Prenatal diagnosis can be done with a hysterosalpingogram. Serial cervical sonographic surveillance should be

Flowchart 25.1: Initial evaluation of recurrent miscarriage.[29]

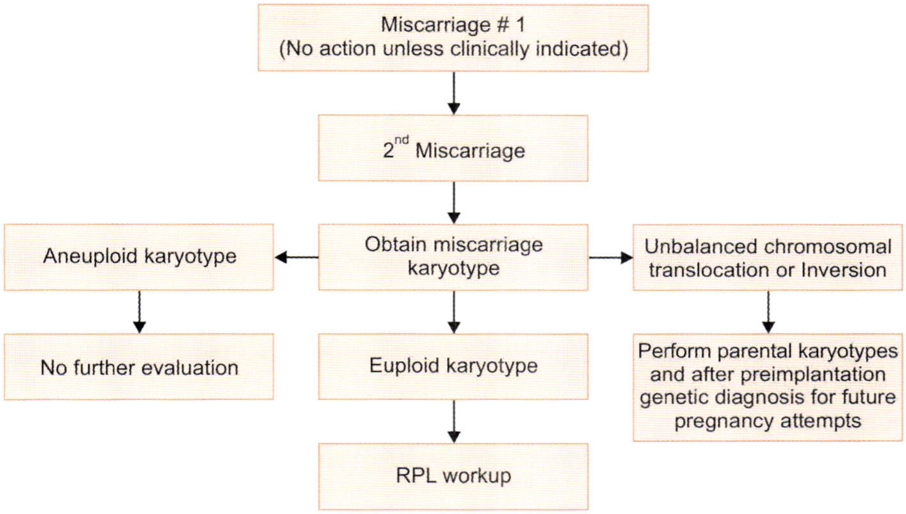

Flowchart 25.2: Full RPL workup.[29]

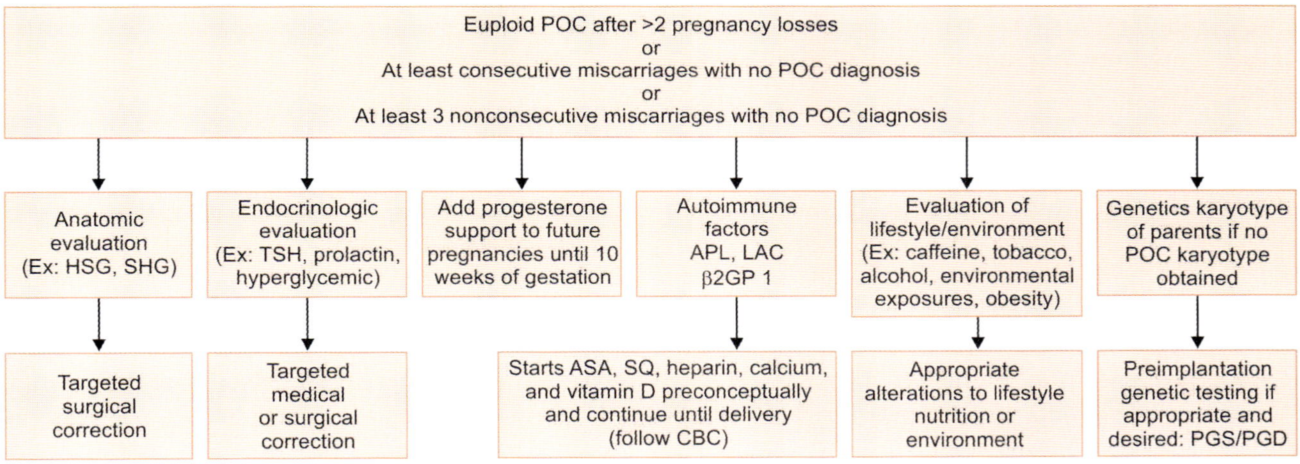

offered in the pregnant women with history of second trimester pregnancy loss and a cervical length of less than 25 mm is considered significant. Progesterone therapy (vaginal or parenteral) is recommended and cervical cerclage may be offered if cervical length is less than 1.5 cm.[20] However, there is no conclusive evidence that prophylactic cerclage reduces the risk of pregnancy loss and preterm delivery in women at risk of preterm birth or midtrimester loss due to infective causes or multiple gestations. Most often cervical dilatation may be the result of a sterile inflammatory response (SIRS) at the decidual membrane interface that causes release of prostaglandins. Cervical dilatation may be prevented by diagnosing and treating subclinical endocervical infection and bacterial vaginosis. Probiotics may be more effective than antibiotics in many instances as there is an overgrowth of vaginal commensals that do not grow on routine cultures.

HORMONAL CAUSES

Luteal Phase Deficiency

There is controversy whether this entity actually exists. Absence of corpus luteum formation at the 6 weeks scan is sometimes documented. Earlier the diagnosis

Table 25.5: Frequency of abnormal tests in 1,020 women with RPL.[21]

Control	*Of prior losses*	*2* *n = 447*	*3* *n = 343*	*≥4* *n = 230*	*p value* *2, 3, or 4*
0.4%	Parental genetics	2.8%	5.4%	5.2%	NS
7.5%	Anatomy	18.7 %	18.2%	16.7%	NS
0.5%	Lupus anticoagulant	5.0%	2.9%	1.9%	NS
6.7%	Anticardiolipin	15.6%	13.1%	17.1%	NS
3.9%	TSH	8.1%	6.5%	6.2%	NS
6.9%	HgbA1c	14.1%	16.3%	17.4%	NS

is based on result of a phased endometrial biopsy; however, this is not recommended as a diagnostic modality any more. Poor echogenic change in the endometrium, low levels of serum progesterone in the mid luteal phase (<10 ng/mL) is considered diagnostic. A recent Cochrane review evaluating 15 trials concluded that routine administration of progesterone to all women with RPL had considerable benefit.[31] However, recently concluded randomized multicentric PROMISE study concluded that pregnancy outcome was not affected by progesterone administration.[32]

Thyroid Dysfunction

The American Thyroid Association recommends serum thyroid stimulating hormone (TSH) measurement for targeted screening and includes history of preterm delivery or miscarriage as one of the indication. TSH values more than 2.5 IU/L are considered abnormal during pregnancy. The Endocrine society recommends that patients with RPL be treated to maintain TSH levels between 1.0 and 2.5 mIU/mL in first trimester and up to 3 and 3.3 mIU/mL in second and third trimester, respectively. For TSH levels between 2.5 and 10 mIU, levothyroxine is recommended in the starting dose of 50 ug/day.[33] The mechanism of pregnancy loss may be autoimmune rather than a hormonal deficiency.

Abnormal Glucose Metabolism

Screening with HbA1c levels is recommended for all women with recurrent miscarriages. This has replaced the oral GTT in the first trimester. Weight reduction, diet alteration and lifestyle modification are first steps in the management. Oral hypoglycemic agents like metformin are safe to prescribe during pregnancy in borderline cases. However, strict glycemic control is required in the first trimester to prevent congenital anomalies and insulin is often required. Patient education and counseling and initiation of self blood glucose monitoring (SBGM) along with self-injections of insulin improves pregnancy outcome. Maintaining a diary of weekly blood sugar series fasting and post prandial with insulin dosage administered helps the clinician fine tune the glycemic control.

Strict glycemic control is desirable prior to pregnancy with HbA1c levels less than 7 in patients with overt diabetes (Table 25.5).

Infections

The role of infection in RPL is unclear. Toxoplasmosis, rubella, cytomegalovirus, herpes and listeria infections are not implicated in RPL and hence routine TORCH test is not recommended. Most patients with RPL are not benefitted by extensive workup for detecting infective etiology. Bacterial vaginosis is a risk factor for preterm delivery and a strong risk factor for late miscarriages. In symptomatic women testing and treatment of bacterial vaginosis is indicated by checking the vaginal pH, which will be greater than 6 and looking for clue cells in vaginal secretions. The results of screening and treatment trials in asymptomatic women however are inconsistent.

Genetic Causes

Most early miscarriages show genetic abnormalities in the implanting embryo. Although this may be a sporadic event in embryogenesis and is not often repeated, patients with advanced maternal age and poor ovarian reserve will benefit by fast tracking to IVF with the possibility of trophectoderm biopsy of the blastocyst which will confirm the genetic makeup of the embryo. Chromosomal analysis may be performed with FISH for five chromosomes (13,18,21,X&Y), Complete genomic hybridization (CGH) for all 23 chromosomes or next generation sequencing (NGS) for quicker results.

In cases where there are no normal embryos formed, the option of donor oocytes or embryos should be explored. In cases of balanced translocations in the parents, substitution with donor gametes may be required, although many cases of spontaneous normal embryogenesis and pregnancy are reported after multiple miscarriages.

Unexplained Recurrent Miscarriage

A significant proportion of cases of recurrent miscarriage remain unexplained despite detailed workup. Supportive care without pharmacological intervention in a dedicated RPL care offers an excellent prognosis for future pregnancy outcome in women with unexplained recurrent miscarriage. These women can be reassured that the prognosis for a successful future pregnancy with supportive care alone is in the region of 75%. The value of psychological support in improving pregnancy outcome cannot be overemphasized.[10]

Immune potentiation may be achieved by the following methods:

- Lymphocyte immune therapy (LIT): This involves injection of husbands/third party leucocytes subcutaneously in the mother. This therapy does not have the approval of US FDA, and its benefits are to date unproven. Besides it carries the potential hazard of transmitting communicable diseases as well as a small risk of graft versus host reaction. Hence LIT therapy is not recommended.
- Correction of low vitamin D levels: Vitamin D deficiency is endemic in India. Besides contributing positively to bone health, vitamin D is a potent immunopotentiator, hence its deficiency should be corrected in all individuals.[34]
- Intravenous immunoglobulins (IVIG): In women with isolated IgG subclass 1–4 deficiency, these were measured in 160 patients of RM and 160 controls. In the RM group, 16 patients showed a deficiency of IgG which when corrected with IgG administration 200 mg/kg/month throughout pregnancy. This resulted in a successful pregnancy outcome in more than 90% of cases.[35] Use of IvIG in other autoimmune/alloimmune conditions is largely empirical.
- Intralipid: An extract of soy lecithin that was developed in Sweden for total parenteral nutrition. It demonstrated effective immune modulation in mice and has been used in a small number of humans with recurrent implantation failure and idiopathic RM with promising results.[36] However, there are no randomized controlled trials as yet to prove its superiority over placebo.
  A Cochrane review of immunotherapy for RM by Porter, which was conducted in 2006, and included 28 trials of high quality that used paternal cell immunization, third party donor leucocytes, trophoblast membrane and IVIGs, concluded that various forms of immunotherapy did not show significant benefit over placebo.[37] There has been no review on vitamin D and intralipid use.
- Granulocyte colony stimulating factor (GCSF): In a randomized controlled trial subcutaneous administration of GCSF in a dose of 1 μg/kg body weight/day administered from sixth postovulatory day and repeated every alternate day has shown to improve clinical pregnancy rates in unexplained recurrent miscarriages.[38]
- TNF alpha blockers: Although the diagnostic test for high TNF alpha levels as the cause of miscarriage is not robust, some people have tried using TNF alpha blockers with a variable response in patients with RM associated with high TNF alpha levels in the peripheral blood. These are expensive molecules with no data on fetal safety as yet and need to be used with extreme caution. However, in patients with rheumatoid arthritis with high TNF alpha levels, these drugs have been used successfully. Ratio of interferon (IFN) beta to IFN alpha, if high will predict a poor response to TNF alpha inhibitors.[39] These are classified as category B drugs in pregnancy. The molecules that have been used during pregnancy are
  1. Infliximab
  2. Etanercept
  3. Adalimumab
  4. Cetrolizumab

However, its use in pregnancy is limited to a few patients suffering from severe inflammatory bowel disease. Certolizumab is used and its use is stopped in the second trimester as it crosses the placenta and will cause IUGR.[40]

In a review of use of anti TNF alpha blockers during pregnancy of rheumatology patients, 58 case reports/case series were analyzed and the review concluded that the use of TNF alpha blockers does not increase the rate of congenital malformations nor does it increase the chances of any other adverse pregnancy outcomes.[41]

Prognostic Factors in Early Pregnancy Transvaginal Scan

Abnormalities of the gestational sac between 4 and 6 weeks of pregnancy will be predictive of pregnancy outcome. Some abnormal features that may be encountered are:[42]

- No gestational sac visible with a serum beta hCG level of 1,500 IU/L or more signifies pregnancy of uncertain location.
- No visible yolk sac with a mean sac diameter (MSD) of 8 mm or more signifies a pseudosac which is seen in ectopic pregnancy.
- No visible fetal pole with a MSD of 16 mm or more signifies anembryonic pregnancy.
- Irregular shape of gestational sac is associated with missed miscarriage.
- Thin choriodecidual reaction less than 3 mm signifies poor implantation.
- Large yolk sac more than 10 mm or calcification in the yolk sac is associated with fetal demise.
- Sac position too low in the cavity may be seen in scar ectopic/cervical ectopic pregnancy.
- Oligo amniotic sac MSD - CRL = <5 mm signifies poor trophoblastic invasion.
- Early growth retardation MSD - CRL = <4 mm
- Slow increase in sac diameter less than 0.7 mm/day. Normal increase is 1.2 mm/day.
- Absent fetal cardiac activity with a fetus of CRL 6 mm or more.
- Fetal bradycardia of less than 85 beats per minute at 6 weeks or more.
- Subchorionic hemorrhage of more than 40% of the sac volume.

Corrective action can be taken if above abnormalities are diagnosed in early pregnancy. This includes progesterone support and other treatment modalities indicated.

Prognosis

With appropriate medical therapy and continued psychological support, the prognosis for women with recurrent miscarriage is good. Lund,[43] in his study on 987 women with RPL, found that the chances of achieving a live birth within 5 years of initial evaluation was 80% in women less than 30 years of age and around 60–70% for women aged 31–40 years (Fig. 25.2).

- 20–40 years of age at first consultation
- 25–29 years of age at first consultation
- 30–34 years of age at first consultation
- 35–39 years of age at first consultation
- 40 years of age or older at first consultation.

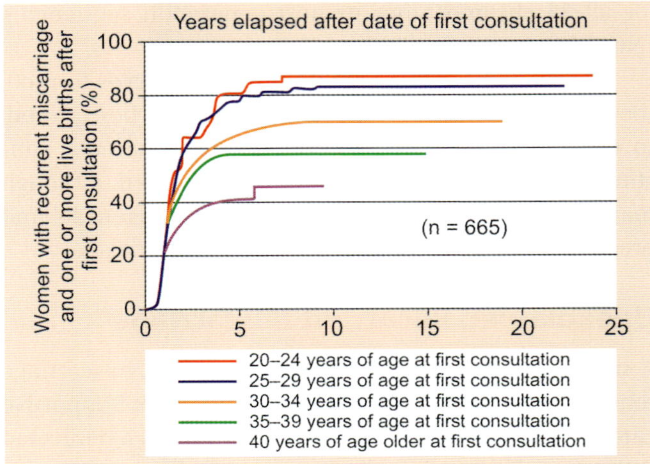

Fig. 25.2: Prognosis of RPL based on maternal age and current diagnostic and treatment strategies.[43]

SUMMARY

Majority of miscarriages are sporadic and thought to result from genetic abnormalities of the embryo, which are influenced by maternal age. Dilemmas exist in defining RPL; however, most researchers are of the opinion that for epidemiological purposes it should be defined as three consecutive losses. In the clinical setting though, a thorough physical examination and testing is recommended after two consecutive miscarriages. In almost 50% cases of RPL, the cause remains unexplained and pharmacological intervention is not recommended. Immunotherapy needs to be evaluated by multicentric randomized controlled trials. Tender loving care, reassurance and stress relieving therapies like acupressure, acupuncture, yoga and meditation are supportive therapies that go a long way in reducing stress and should be the mainstay for all patients with RPL.

REFERENCES

1. Royal College of Obstetricians and Gynecologists. The investigation and treatment of couples with recurrent first-trimester and second-trimester miscarriage. Green-top Guideline No. 17; April 2011. www.rcog.org.uk.
2. Bhattacharya S. Recurrent miscarriage: should the definition be revised? In: Arora M (Ed). World Clinics Obstetrics & Gynecology. New Delhi: Jaypee; 2011.

3. ACOG 2013 FAQ100. www.acog.org.
4. Practice Committee of the American Society for Reproductive Medicine. Definitions of infertility and recurrent pregnancy loss. Fertil Steril. 2008;89:1603.
5. Practice Committee of the American Society for Reproductive Medicine. Aging and infertility in women. Fertil Steril. 2006;86(5 Suppl):S248-52.
6. Stirrat GM, Recurrent miscarriage. Lancet. 1990;336: 673-5.
7. Salat-Baroux J. Recurrent spontaneous abortions. Reprod Nutr Dev. 1988;28:1555-68.
8. Wilcox AJ, Weinberg CR, O'Connor JF, Baird DD, Schlatterer JP, Canfield RE, et al. Incidence of early loss of pregnancy. N Engl J Med. 1988;319(4):189-94.
9. Lathi RB, Gray Hazard FK, Heerema-McKenney A, Taylor J, Chueh JT. First trimester miscarriage evaluation. Semin Reprod Med. 2011;29:463-9.
10. Arora M, Konje J (Eds). Recurrent Pregnancy Loss. New Delhi: Jaypee; 2007.
11. Boui J, Boui A, Lazar P. Retrospective and prospective epidemiological studies of 1500 karyotyped spontaneous human abortions. Teratology. 1975;12:11.
12. Papa Dopoulos G, Templeton AA, Fisk N, Randall J. The frequency of chromosomal anomalies in human preimplantation embryos after *in vitro* fertilization. Hum Reprod. 1987;4:91.
13. Jacobs PA. Structural rearrangements of chromosomes in men. In: Hook EB, Porter IM, (Eds). Population Cytogenetics. New York: Academic Press; 1977. pp. 81-97.
14. Regan L, Owen EJ, Jacobs HS. Hypersecretion of luteinizing hormone, infertility and miscarriage. Lancet. 1990;336: 1141-4.
15. Zaveroni I, Bonini L, Fantuzzi M, Dall'Aglio E, Passeri M, Reaven GM. Hyperinsulinemia, obesity and AQ Syndrome X. J Intern Med. 1994;235:51-6.
16. Gilnoer D, Soto MF, Bourdoux P, Lejeune B, Delange F, Lemone M, et al. Pregnancy in patients with mild thyroid abnormalities: maternal and neonatal repercussion. J Clin Endocrinol Metab. 1991;73:421-7.
17. Bussen S, Steck T. Thyroid antibodies in euthyroid non pregnant women with recurrent spontaneous abortions. Hum Reprod. 1995;10:2938-40.
18. Lata K, Dutta P, Sridhar S, Rohilla M, Srinivasan A, Prashad GR, et al. Thyroid autoimmunity and obstetric outcomes in women with recurrent miscarriage: a case control study. Endocr Connect. 2013;2(2):118-24.
19. Gomez R. Ultrasonographic examination of uterine cervix is better than cervical digital examination as a predictor of the likelihood of premature delivery in patients with preterm labor and intact membranes. Am J Obstet Gynecol. 1994;171:956-64.
20. O'Brien J. Cervical causes of preterm labor. In: Arora M (Ed). World Clinics Obstetrics & Gynecology, Vol. 2. New Delhi: Jaypee; 2012.
21. Jaslow CR, Kutteh WH. Effect of prior birth and miscarriage frequency on the prevelance of acquired and congenital uterine anomalies in women with recurrent miscarriages: a cross sectional study. Fertil Steril. 2013;99(7):1916-22.
22. Rai RS. Antiphospholipid syndrome and recurrent miscarriages. J Postgrad Med. 2002;48:3-4.
23. Ernest JM, Marshburn PB, Kutteh WH. Obsteric antiphospholipid antibody syndrome: an update on pathophysiology and management. Semin Reprod Med. 2011;29:522-39.
24. Robertson L, Wu O, Langhorne P, Twaddle S, Clark P, Lowe GD, et al. Thrombophilia in pregnancy: a systematic review. Br J Haematol. 2006;132:171-96.
25. Nelson Piercy C. Thromboembolic disease. In: Obstetric Medicine, Vol. 1. London: Martin Dunitz; 2002. pp. 42-4.
26. Arora M (Ed). Hyperhomocysteinemia in pregnancy. Elsevier, ECAB; 2012.
27. Mumusoglu S, Beksac MS, Ekiz A, Ozdemir P, Hascelik G. Does presence of antibodies without autoimmune disease have an effect on RPL? J Matern Fetal Neonatal Med. 2016;29(14):2352-7.
28. Praveen F, Agrawal S. Recurrent miscarriage and micro RNA among North Indian women. Reprod Sci. 2015;22(4):410-5.
29. Brezina PR, Ke RW, Kutteh WH. Preimplantation genetic screening: a practical guide. Clin Med Insights Reprod Health. 2013;7:37-42.
30. Arora M, Basu HK. Non-surgical management of uterus didelphus. Saudi Med J. 1989:10(1):141-2.
31. Haas DM, Ramsy PS. Progestogen for preventing miscarriage. Cochrane Database Syst Rev. 2013;(10):CD003511.
32. Coomarasamy A, Williams H, Truchanowicz E, Seed PT, Small R, Quenby S, et al. PROMISE trial: A randomized trial of progesterone in women with recurrent miscarriages. N Eng J Med. 2015;373:2141-8.
33. De Groot L, Abalovich M, Alexander EK, Amino N, Barbour L, Cobin RH, et al. Management of thyroid dysfunction during pregnancy and postpartum: an endocrine society clinical practice guideline. J Clin Endocrinol Metab. 2012;97:2543-65.
34. Ota K, Dambaeva S, Han AR, Beaman K, Gilman-Sachs A, Kwak-Kim J. Vitamin D deficiency may be a risk factor for recurrent pregnancy losses by increasing cellular immunity and autoimmunity. Hum Reprod. 2014;29(2):208-19.
35. Manfredi G, Dell'Aera L, Ligouri R. Overcoming RSM in women suffering from IgG subclass deficiency: high efficiency of low dose IvIg treatment. Eur Ann Allergy Clin Immunol. 2015;47(3):91-4.
36. Clark DA. Intralipid as treatment for recurrent unexplained abortion? Am J Reprod Immunol. 1994;32(4):290-3.
37. Porter TF, La Coursiere Y, Scott JR. Immunotherapy for recurrent miscarriage. Cochrane Database Syst Rev. 2006;(2):CD000112.
38. Scarpellini F, Sbracia M. Use of granulocyte colony stimulating factor for the treatment of unexplained recurrent miscarriage: a randomized controlled trial. Hum Reprod. 2009;24(11):2703-8.

39. Harrison P. Blood test predicts TNF inhibitor response in RA patients. American College of Rheumatology (ACR) 2014 annual meeting.
40. Gispert JP Chaparro M. Safety of anti TNF agents during pregnancy and breast feeding in women with inflammatory bowel disease. Am J Gastroenterol. 2013;108(9): 1426-38.
41. Nielson OH, Loftus EV Jr, Jess T. Safety of TNF alpha inhibitors during IBD pregnancy: a systematic review. BMC Med. 2013;11:174.
42. Valia A. Practical tips for ultrasound. In: Arora M, Sharma A (Eds). A Practical Guide to First Trimester of Pregnancy. New Delhi: Jaypee; 2014.
43. Lund M, Kamper-Jorgensen M, Nielsen HS, Lidegaard Ø, Andersen AM, Christiansen OB. Prognosis for live birth in women with recurrent miscarriage: what is the best measure of success. Obstet Gynecol. 2012;119:37-43.

CHAPTER

26

Gamete Banking

Keshav Malhotra, Narendra Malhotra, Jaideep Malhotra, Neharika Malhotra

INTRODUCTION

The availability of viable functionally normal gametes is an essential prerequisite to successful fertilization both *in vivo* and *in vitro* and is therefore critical to the implementation of a broad range of reproductive technologies, such as artificial insemination, *in vitro* fertilization, embryo transfer and genetic engineering. By eliminating the constraints of time and location on the availability of gametes and embryos, cryopreservation of these specialized and otherwise short lived cells has become an essential complimentary procedure in the application of most technology requiring their use.

The types of gamete banking are:

1. Semen banking
2. Oocyte banking

SEMEN BANKING

With the discovery of cryopreservation for gametes and embryos reproductive medicine has reached unimaginable heights. Cryopreservation is now one of the most crucial aspects of any ART laboratory. Cryopreservation means storing cells at sub-zero temperatures to stop all biological activity and preserve them for future use. Initial trials were ineffective as the cells suffered from concentration changes, ice crystal formation, and dehydration. Thus, it was clear that some form of protection was required. The concept of cryopreservation is quite old; some studies suggest that it date back to 200 years ago. Recording and publishing evidence though for cryopreservation only started in the early 19th century, when B. J. Luyet brought forward new concepts for cryopreservation in the 1930s, in the 1940s more research on cryoprotectants led to the discovery of glycerol as a penetrating cryoprotectant. Subsequently, more cryoprotectants were discovered and by late 1970s we had protocols for freezing gametes and embryos. In the same era, programmable slow cooling devices were also enveloped and these advances led to the birth from the first cryopreserved semen sample in 1953, from the first cryopreserved embryo in 1984 and from the first cryopreserved oocyte in 1986.[1]

Cryopreservation of semen does cause quite a significant decrease in most semen parameters ranging from vitality of the sample to motility rates and recent literature shows that even the DNA and mitochondria of the sperm is affected. The cause of this effect is still largely unknown and is being studied by various researchers and we still do not have the ability to predict how the quality of the sample would be post thawing. Thus, cryopreservation of semen samples is basically suitable to be used only for a selected pool of patients.[1]

Human semen cryobanking can be divided into two broad categories: autologous banking for personal fertility preservation and donor sperm banking. Semen banking is useful in many situations and can be considered a safeguard against unforeseen future circumstances. These may include prior to chemotherapy or radiation therapy; prevasectomy; before certain types of pelvic or testicular surgery; in cases of degenerative illnesses such as diabetes or multiple sclerosis, spinal cord disease or injury; high risk occupations or sports; and preparation for future fertility treatment.[2] Usually several steps are required prior to initiation of semen storage. Most sperm banks only accept patients referred by their physician; however, sometimes self-referral is possible. Patients have to be screened by the collection of blood, urine and semen samples to ensure that their samples are contaminated with other infectious diseases when placed into the storage. Consent for freezing and storage of semen has to be signed and witnessed. It is important that patients should have a clear understanding of the process of banking and that they provide clear instructions on who is responsible for the disposition of the specimens in the event of their demise.[2-4] Similarly, costs associated with banking and long-term storage need to be clearly defined and assigned in case the patient becomes incapacitated. When samples are either used for procreation, transported to another facility or storage is to be discontinued, the patient or designate must complete specific consent forms allowing the bank to comply with their wishes. In most countries, it is assumed or stated by law that the semen belongs to the individual who produced the sample, and he is the individual who must sign all consents, unless the sample was designated for donation (e.g., in the case of anonymous sperm donation). If possible, multiple donations are usually recommended to ensure an adequate sperm reserve for future procreation, depending on the quality of the sample, individual circumstances and reason for sperm banking.[2-4]

SEMEN FREEZING: TECHNIQUES AND PROTOCOLS

Cryoprotectants

Most cells would not survive cryopreservation without cryoprotective agents (CPAs), which can minimize cryoinjury of cells. CPAs are low-weight chemicals that serve to shield spermatozoa from solidifying harm or ice crystallization by diminishing the point of solidification of materials.[5] There are two classifications of CPAs and they vary in their capacity to enter the plasma layer. First, penetrating CPAs, for example, dimethyl acetaldehyde, dimethyl sulfoxide (DMSO), glycerol, glycol, ethylene and methanol, settle cell plasma layer proteins and decrease groupings of electrolytes.[8] Second, nonpermeating CPAs, for example, albumins, dextrans, egg yolk citrate, hydroxyethyl, polyethylene glycols, polyvinylpyrrolidone and sucrose, minimize intracellular crystallization by expanding consistency of the specimen.[5,6] CPAs themselves can be hazardous if utilized at high focuses and spermatozoa are defenseless against osmotic changes instigated by these.[9] In spite of the utilization of CPAs, plasma layers can in any case be harmed or can burst because of the underlying broad lack of hydration took after by cell swelling and osmotic stress.[6] Continuous acquaintance of CPAs with the cell suspension or stepwise increment in their fixation, with a restricted holding period preceding solidifying, is used to minimize the potential negative impacts of these operators.[10]

There are two customary freezing strategies utilized as a part of sperm cryopreservation: slow freezing and rapid freezing.

Slow Freezing

This method proposed by Behrman and Sawada comprises dynamic sperm cooling over a time of 2–4 hours in a few stages, either physically or naturally utilizing a semi-programmable cooler.

The manual strategy is performed by decreasing the temperature of the semen while adding a cryoprotectant in a stepwise way and subsequently plunging the specimens into liquid nitrogen. It has been demonstrated that the ideal beginning cooling rate of the example from room temperature to 6°C is 0.5–1°C/minute. The specimen is then frozen at a temperature of 6°C to –80°C at a rate of 1–10°C/minute. The sample is then submerged into nitrogen at –196°C.[11]

Regardless of reports demonstrating fruitful sperm freezing with manual systems, the reproducibility of this strategy could represent a few issues. Thus, programmable coolers have been researched.[12] These coolers utilize a plate to hold the straws, which in turn are cooled by liquid nitrogen held in a capacity tank under the plate. Liquid nitrogen is filled in the tank, and the machine, which is preprogrammed, the software data logging helps to obtain cooling from 20°C to –80°C at rate of 1.5°C/minute and then at 6°C/minute; at completion of the freezing, the straws are removed and stored into liquid nitrogen at –196°C. This takes around 40 minutes.[12] Programs are simple to use and allow for a cooling combination which does not require continuous operator intervention and have been used to increase the reproducibility of the freezing operations.[12]

A few researchers contend that ordinary slow freezing, either manual or automated, causes broad physical harm to the sperm most likely in light of ice crystallization.[13]

Rapid Freezing

Rapid freezing was initially proposed by Sherman.[5] This system requires direct contact between the straws and the nitrogen vapors for 8–10 minutes and then submersion in liquid nitrogen at –196°C. The sample is first mixed with equivalent volume of cryoprotectant in dropwise manner; the blend is then stacked into the straws and kept at 4°C for 10 minutes. The straws are then set at a separation of 15–20 cm over the level of liquid nitrogen (–80°C) for 15 minutes; after this stage, the straws are submerged in liquid nitrogen. This system has a few downsides such as low reproducibility,[17] to be sure, the temperature drop bend cannot be controlled, and the solidifying temperatures may change from –70°C, –80°C and –99°C.[7]

Thawing

The thawing strategy is an equally essential step. The cell must be permitted to recoup its natural activity while attempting to avoid any unexpected thermal stress. As a rule, the cryopreservation protocols utilize a thawing temperature of 37°C. Even though higher thawing temperatures allow for more rapid heating, they are not used because of the risks associated to cell damage.

At the present time, a few thawing protocols are utilized, such as

- thawing at room temperature for 10 minutes and at 37°C for another 10 minutes,
- thawing at 37°C for 10 minutes in a water bath, and
- thawing at room temperature for 15 minutes.

Once the semen is thawed, it is isolated from the cryopreservation medium by washing in a preferred culture medium and centrifuging.[7]

Adverse Effects of Cryopreservation on Sperm Integrity

Compared to other cell sorts, spermatozoa appear to be less sensitive to cryopreservation harm as a result of the high fluidity of the membrane and the low water content (around half). In spite of this, cryopreservation may prompt injurious changes of sperm structure and capacity.[5] It was, to a great extent, reported that few harming procedures could happen amid freezing and thawing of human spermatozoa, for example, heat shock with arrangement of intracellular and extracellular ice crystals within the spermatozoa, cell dehydration and osmotic shock.[15]

The essential driver of cell injury amid cryopreservation is the development of intracellular or extracellular ice crystals. Amid the freezing procedure, the cooling rate assumes an imperative part in deciding the degree of cryoinjury to the spermatozoa.[16]

A quick cooling rate causes serious intracellular ice crystallization, because the efflux of water over the layer is disrupted. Ice crystals rupture the layers and disrupt the organelle capacity. This condition prompts hindered cell survival.

A slow cooling rate decides the efflux of water from the interior to the outside environment, increasing the concentration of solutes and the osmotic pressure. This condition prompts cell volume changes associated with the displacement of water, dehydration and toxic injury because of high solute fixation.[16] Cryoinjury is not constrained to the feeling procedure but rather may likewise happen amid the thawing procedure as the ice liquefies or rather recrystallizes.[9] The marvel of recrystallization of both intracellular and extracellular ice, in frozen samples, happens in the form of smaller ice crystals which have a rate of recrystallization that increases with temperature.[13]

It has to a great extent been accounted for that chilling injury can alter the structure and integrity of plasma layers[18] chiefly created by phospholipids and cholesterol.[18]

The plasma and mitochondrial layers have the same susceptibility to cryopreservation.[26] Mitochondria are set along the midpiece between the plasma layer and the nine fibrous segments, to form a covering that is vitality important for sperm motility.[19] The ATP produced by oxphos in the inward mitochondrial layer is exchanged to the microtubules, to drive motility.[19] Therefore, a weakness of mitochondrial function may be the reason behind the decrease in motility and vitality of thawed samples.[19] Moreover, cryopreservation appears to reduce the antioxidant action in spermatozoa making them more vulnerable to ROS harm. High concentration of ROS and fall of antioxidative agent lead to cell apoptosis.[20]

Although the impacts of cryopreservation on the fertilization potential, motility, morphology, and integrity of spermatozoa are very much recorded, the topic of the conceivable increase of sperm DNA fragmentation subsequent to freezing/thawing is still open. There is no agreement in the literature neither on whether cryopreservation induces DNA damage nor on the amount of damage. In a few studies, researchers have reported noteworthy changes of sperm DNA integrity after cryopreservation/warming,[6] whereas different studies have communicated an alternate sentiment.[21,22] This debate between one study and the other could as a matter of first importance be clarified by the way that the discoveries do not allude to an extensive number of tests and is likewise because of the utilization of (1) distinctive cryopreservation methodology, (2) unique tests to assess the DNA integrity, and (3) diverse semen preparation systems before cryopreservation (i.e., swimup or density centrifugation). For instance, Donnelly and associates[6] examined precryopreservation and postcryopreservation DNA integrity of both semen and prepared sperm samples in 50 men. They reported that freezing sperm in seminal plasma enhances post-thaw DNA integrity. Sperm-frozen unprepared in seminal fluid seems to be more resistant to freezing damage than frozen prepared sperm; further improvement can be achieved by preparing sperm and freezing after addition of seminal plasma. This may be due to the presence of abundant antioxidants in seminal plasma. Concerning the variability linked to different freezing procedures, Petyim et al.[23] evaluated cryodamage on sperm chromatin comparing two different procedures: liquid nitrogen vapor versus computerized program freezer. They analyzed 50 semen samples using acridine orange and concluded that DNA damage was significantly higher following freezing with liquid nitrogen. Even if the opinions on the issue of "cryopreservation and DNA damage" are still highly controversial, the evaluation of the impact of cryopreservation on sperm chromatin is of extreme importance. Likewise, sperm DNA integrity is an important factor for the success of ART.

Cryopreservation and Reproductive Outcomes

Cryopreservation is broadly known to hinder sperm motility and reduce fertilization rates through negative impacts on membranes, acrosomal structure, and acrosin activity and chromatin structure,[24] leading to a potential danger of decondensation of the sperm nucleus after entering into the oocyte, in this manner, diminishing fertilization rate.[25] Considering the decline in sperm fertilization potential affected by cryopreservation, it can be easily comprehended that intrauterine insemination and traditional *in vitro* preparation (IVF) with frozen samples result in lower pregnancy rates contrasted and insemination with fresh sperm.[14]

The contemplations are distinctive for intracytoplasmic sperm infusion (ICSI), on the grounds that this system requires just a little number of motile spermatozoa for effective treatment. Subsequently, the current question is whether utilizing fresh as opposed to cryopreserved sperm cells has the same impact on fertilization with ICSI. To date, just a couple of substantial scale studies talk on comparative result contrasting fresh and frozen samples and they have not been conclusive as of now.

OOCYTE BANKING

Cryopreservation means storing cells at subzero temperatures to halt all biological activity and preserve them for future use.[26] The practical use of cryopreservation started around the mid-20th century. Initial trials were ineffective, as cells could not survive the concentration changes, ice crystal formation and dehydration and it was clear that some form of protection was needed. It was not until the 1940s that the first penetrating cryoprotectant, glycerol, was discovered.[27] Penetrating cryoprotectants work by displacing water within the cell. It was found that glycerol could protect sperm throughout the process of cryopreservation.[27] Research in the early 1970s led to the discovery of various cryoprotectants such as ethylene glycol (EG), propanediol (PrOH) and DMSO, which protected the cells from damaging effects of cooling. Along with these, programmable slow cooling machines were developed so that cooling could occur at a slower pace and sufficient cell dehydration could occur leading to lesser ice crystal formation.[28] These major improvements led to the first birth from a cryopreserved embryo in 1984 and from a cryopreserved oocyte in 1986. In the effort to improve on the success rates seen with slow cooling, another form of cryopreservation was developed termed "vitrification" which is derived from the Latin word "vitreum" meaning "glass." The process of slow cooling as the name suggests required an initial slow but controlled rate of cooling, which was followed by rapid cooling as the sample is plunged into liquid nitrogen (LN_2) for storage,[29] vitrification on the other hand involves using ultra-fast rates of cooling much higher than 1,000°C/minute and sometimes even more than 10,000°C/minute.[28,29] It also utilizes higher concentrations of cryoprotectants; typically the vitrification protocol requires cryoprotectants in concentrations of 30–50% approximately compared with 5–10% for slow freezing.[29] The rapid rates of cooling along with higher concentrations of cryoprotectants lead to the cells being stored in a glass like state bypassing the damage due to ice crystal formation seen in slow freezing. Initially cryopreservation was limited to embryos and sperm.[30] The oocyte, being the largest cell in the human body, was relatively more difficult to cryopreserve than sperm due to larger internal volumes of water, but in the last decade or so a large number of studies have developed various techniques for oocyte cryopreservation.[31] A disproportionately large amount of data on freezing oocytes has emerged from Italy, due to their enforcement of strict laws on assisted reproductive technology and practice[32] (Tables 26.1 and 26.2) Oocyte cryopreservation has always been permitted under Italian law, however, cryopreservation of embryos has not, due to pressure from the Catholic Church regarding the status of the embryo and their interpretation of where life begins. Many of these laws have recently been amended, but the techniques developed for freezing oocytes have found other niches where their adoption can be beneficial. Oocyte cryopreservation brings forward an option in managing female fertility that avoids the requirement of first creating an embryo. This can be used if there is failure of the male partner to produce sperm, it can ensure safer oocyte donation strategies, and it can be used in the preservation of fertility as well.

Table 26.1: Total embryos per warmed oocyte (Levi Setti et al., 2014)

Year	*SF*	*%*	*VT*	*%*
2007	4,173/12,573	33.2	1,049/2,317	45.3
2008	4,536/13,592	33.4	1,155/2,949	39.2
2009	3,868/10,821	35.7	2,507/5,707	43.9
2010	2,393/6,068	39.4	2,951/6,906	42.7
2011	1,904/4,860	39.2	3,695/8,625	42.8
Overall	16,874/47,914	35.2	11,357/26,504	42.9

OOCYTE CRYOPRESERVATION OVERVIEW

The success of oocyte cryopreservation considering survival rate, fertilization rate and pregnancy rate was initially low.[30] The success of oocyte cryopreservation was limited by many factors such as maturity of the oocyte, size, water content and chromosomal arrangement. M-II stage oocyte is now the gold standard stage of freezing.[35] It is well documented that cryopreservation causes hardening of the zona, reducing the success of conventional *in vitro* fertilization and increasing the need to perform intracytoplasmic sperm injection (ICSI) instead.[33] Over the last few years, there have been many modifications in the cryopreservation techniques, such as a refinement in the composition of cryoprotectant in slow cooled protocols, and these seem to have improved the survival rate.[33] A change in the initial temperature of cryoprotectant and the seeding temperature, also seem to have a positive effect on oocyte survival rates. Various factors determine the efficacy of a cryopreservation protocol and these can be classified into "intrinsic" and "extrinsic." Intrinsic factors are the cryobiological properties of the cell whereas extrinsic factors relate to technical practice such as the type of device that is used during the procedure. To improve existing protocols, certain factors must be taken into consideration (Fig. 26.1). Though the successful thawing of oocytes has improved for both slow cooling and vitrification, most studies in recent times suggest that vitrification of oocytes give better survival rates and better pregnancy rate as compared to slow freezing.[30]

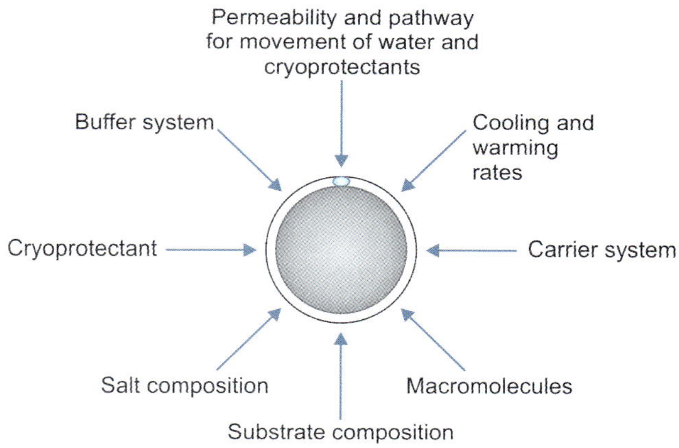

Fig. 26.1: Factors affecting oocyte cryopreservation.

OOCYTE CRYOBIOLOGY

Cryopreservation subjects a cell to significant thermal as well as biophysical changes. Successful cryopreservation requires a comprehensive understanding of the cryobiology of the cell to optimize the technique.[33] A large volume of the oocyte is made up of water, with estimates of about 80% being reported. This was one of the initial hurdles that many faced while performing oocyte cryopreservation. The difficulty that arises with larger water content is that the oocyte requires a higher concentration of cryoprotectant and/or a longer time submersed in the toxic compounds used.[34]

The large size of the oocyte and its water content makes it more susceptible to biophysical damage during the process, which can be caused by intracellular ice crystals, concentration of the solutions and possibly osmotic shock.[33] This could severely impair oocyte quality-survival, fertilization and developmental potential. It is also found that

Table 26.2: Pregnancy rates per cycle (Levi Setti et al., 2014)

Year	*SF*	*VT*	*(SF = 1) vs. VT*	*P value*
2007	10.5 (254/2,426)	12.9 (73/568)	1.26 (0.96–1.67)	.101
2008	11.9 (312/2,625)	13.7 (90/659)	1.17 (0.91–1.51)	.215
2009	12.4 (238/1,916)	16.5 (196/1,186)	1.40 (1.14–1.71)	.001
2010	13.8 (151/1,097)	13.7 (184/1,344)	0.99 (0.79–1.25)	.958
2011	13.8 (119/863)	14.2 (233/1,644)	1.03 (0.81–1.31)	.793
All	12.0 (1,074/8,927)	14.4 (776/5,401)	1.23 (1.11–1.35)	<.001

cryopreservation of oocytes leads to a rise in the intracellular calcium levels, which could be the cause of zona hardening usually seen with cryopreserved oocytes.[30,33] Furthermore, it was determined that different cryoprotectants had different effects on calcium oscillations in the oocyte.[33] The analysis of calcium oscillations in mouse oocytes showed that the least increase was seen with EG, whereas propanediol and DMSO had a more sustained effect. Furthermore, these were tested in calcium-free media and it was found that in both EG and propanediol protocols calcium oscillations were reduced while DMSO had the same effect.[33] This suggesting the fact that propanediol and EG caused an influx of extracellular calcium, but DMSO caused increase in the intracellular calcium stores possibly by affecting the endoplasmic reticulum.[33] This evidence does not support the use of DMSO as a good option for oocyte cryopreservation, and that calcium levels in cryopreservation media need further evaluation.[33] More recent studies have established that premature calcium oscillations do affect oocyte quality and improvements to the cryopreservation system may be required to prevent this; the use of calcium free media is a suggested solution.[33] The success of oocyte cryopreservation is not restricted to water content, zona pellucida hardening or cortical granules. With recent advances in imaging technology more information is being shown on what exactly is going on in the oocytes after freeze/thawing. In a mature oocyte, chromosomes are held together by microtubules forming what is known as the meiotic spindle.[36] The spindle is required to correctly segregate the chromosomes during the second polar body extrusion, as well as downregulating the M-phase promoting factor. In short, correct spindle formation is essential in completion of meiosis. Cryopreservation has been shown to disrupt the spindle by depolymerizing the microtubule structure.[30,33] Earlier studies that have investigated spindle formation and function have typically utilized different staining techniques, such as labeling with fluorescent conjugated antibodies and other fluorochromes.[37] Newer techniques allow visualization of the spindle without actually disrupting the viability of the oocytes. Most of the studies done in the early 2000s suggested that during the process of vitrification the spindle remained intact,[33] but more recent investigation has shown that the spindle was vulnerable even with vitrification are vulnerable to the vitrification process[33,38] (Fig. 26.2)

A more recent study suggests that vitrification does not affect the spindle structure.[39] However, the study used the fixatives deuterium oxide (D_2O) and taxol,[39] which are known to promote microtubule polymerization,[30] so the observations may not be particularly relevant. Four antibodies which were anti-β-tubulin, anti-γ-tubulin, anti-pericentrin and anti-NEDD1 were utilized in another study, and found that the spindle microtubules as well as its components did undergo a dynamic change during the process of vitrification. Most studies also report that spindle restores itself during incubation at 37°C post thaw, though the recovery time varied among studies.[30,38] The above-mentioned study also showed that the restoration of spindle was highly complex and dynamic, but it did restore itself after 2 hours post thaw. Modifications in media composition and protocols did improve the survival rates after thawing but the fertilization rate and cleavage rates did not improve by much, in the early 2000s ongoing pregnancy rates were still below the 35% success rate. Therefore, it was hypothesized by various research groups that mitochondrial potential of the oocyte might be involved in the predicting the developmental competence of the oocyte. Studies showed that cryopreservation did affect mitochondrial distribution by affecting the cytoplasmic microtubule structure and thus lead to abnormal ATP distribution which could hinder the development of the oocyte.[40] To study mitochondria, the common stains used are JC-1 and Mitotracker. JC-1 is a fluorescent probe mainly used to detect the function of mitochondria through its membrane potential. Under the influence of a number of factors, JC-1 forms a monomer or polymer and produces distinct wave-lengths of fluorescence. When the mitochondrial membrane potential is low, the efficiency of energy supply by oxidative phosphorylation will drop. Mitotracker on the other hand detects mitochondrial distribution, which can be useful to know in a range of other situations. Freezing protocols could decrease the mitochondrial membrane potential, though it may not be accompanied by early apoptotic changes. Vitrification on the other hand has been shown to affect mitochondrial distribution, but this may be due to poor vitrification practice, rather than the technique itself. Compared to control group where mitochondrial distribution was polar, thawing of vitrified oocytes yielded evenly distribution patterns of mitochondria in a more recent study.[41] (Fig. 26.3)

SLOW FREEZING

Since the use of the first slow cool protocol for oocyte cryopreservation, major changes have been trialed, with most being related to the amount of sucrose and other nonpenetrating cryoprotectants in the media. In the beginning,

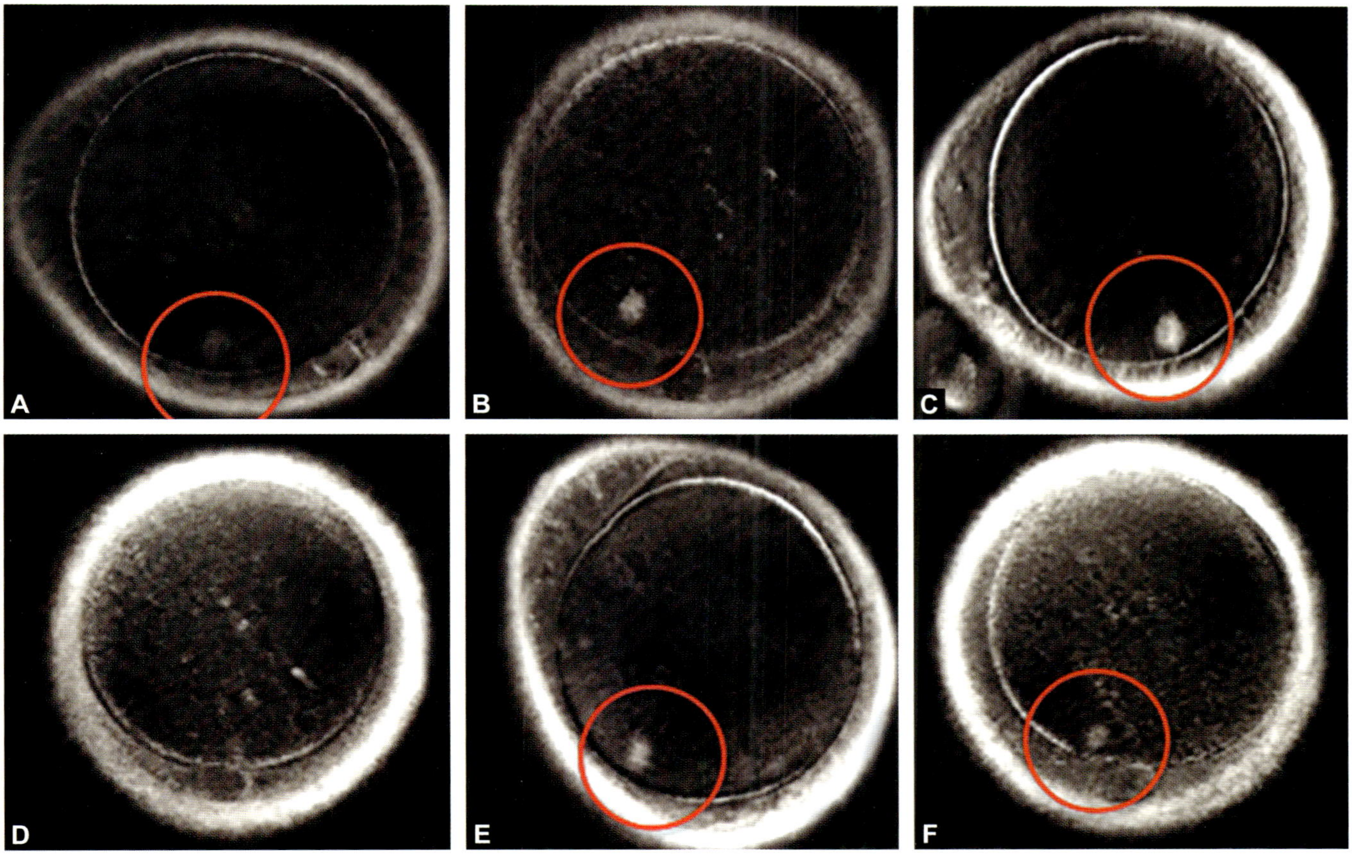

Figs. 26.2A to F: Effect of oocyte cryopreservation on meiotic spindle viewed under polarized light. (A and B) Noncryopreserved human oocytes. (C and D) Vitrified and slow cooled oocyte. (E and F) Vitrified and slow cooled oocyte after 2 hours.[33]

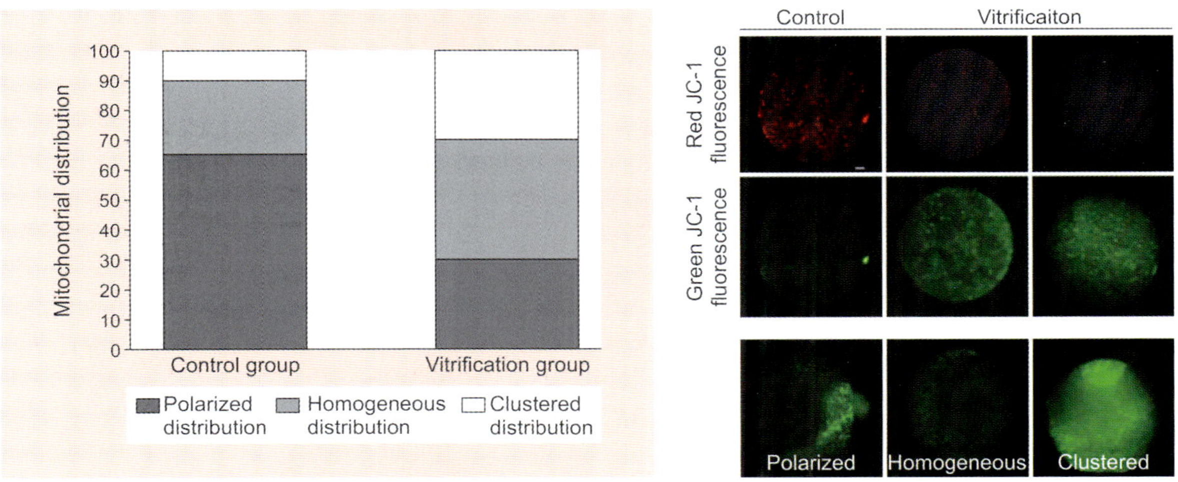

Fig. 26.3: Effect of vitrification on Mitochondrial potential evaluated by JC-1 (Lei et al., 2014).

Table 26.3: Comparative studies of various cooling systems.

	Cryoprotectants	Survival rate (%)	Cryopreservation IR (%) Cleavage stage ET	Blastocyst ET	Fresh IR (%)
Optimal slow cooling					
Gook and Edgar (2011)	1.5 M PROH, 0.2 M sucrose	75.8	30.0 (<38 years)		26.0 (<38 years)
Yang *et al.* (2002), donor	1.5 M PROH, 0.2 M sucrose	70.9	25.3		43.4
Bianchi *et al.* (2007)	1.5 M PROH, 0.2 M sucrose	75.1	16.7		17.3
Konc *et al.* (2008b)	1.5 M PROH, 0.3 M sucrose	76	15.4[a]		18
Ferraretti *et al.* (2010)	1.5 M PROH, 0.3 M sucrose	71.8	18.9 (≤34 years)		
Parmegiani *et al.* (2009)	1.5 M PROH, 0.3 M sucrose	71.6	15.1		
Optimal vitrification					
Antinori *et al.* (2007)	15% EG, 15% DMSO, 0.5 M sucrose	99.4	13.2		10.3
Rienzi *et al.* (2010)	15% EG, 15% DMSO, 0.5 M sucrose	96.7–89.7	27.3 (≤34 years)		30.0 (≤34 years)
Ubaldi *et al.* (2010) Almodin *et al.* (2010)	15% EG, 15% DMSO, 0.5 M sucrose	84.9	14.9		21.3
Cobo *et al.* (2010a), donor	15% EG, 15% DMSO, 0.5 M sucrose	92.5	39.9		40.9
Trokoudes *et al.* (2011), donor	15% EG, 15% DMSO, 0.5 M sucrose	91.4	24.7		25.6
Cobo *et al.* (2008a), donor	15% EG, 15% DMSO, 0.5 M sucrose	96.9		40.8	
Nagy *et al.* (2009), donor	15% EG, 15% DMSO, 0.5 M sucrose	89		55.3	47.4
Garcia *et al.* (2011), donor	15% EG, 15% DMSO, 0.5 M sucrose	89.4		43.9	42.9
Comparison of slow cooled and vitrified (vit)					
Smith *et al.* (2010), slow	1.5 M PROH, 0.3 M sucrose	65	13[a,b]		
Smith *et al.* (2010), vit	15% EG, 15% DMSO, 0.5 M sucrose	75	38[a,b]		
Noyes *et al.* (2010), slow	1.5 M PROH, 0.3 M sucrose	85	NR (mixed transfers)		
Noyes *et al.* (2010), vit	15% EG, 15% DMSO, 0.5 M sucrose	88	NR (mixed transfers)		
Fadini *et al.* (2009), slow	1.5 M PROH, 0.3 M sucrose	57.9	4.3		
Fadini *et al.* (2009), vit	EG, PROH, sucrose (Medicult)	78.9	9.3		

addition of sucrose was found to lead to better survival rates; however, few reported the additional, ultra structural changes caused by excessive dehydration[42] (Table 26.3). It was seen that oocyte survival increased[42] due to excessive shrinkage of the cell but viability was reduced.[43] More research on cell permeability led to a decrease in sucrose concentration in the freezing solutions and eventually produced better survival rates and pregnancy rates. Modified freezing solutions which now contained 0.2 M sucrose, and thawing solution 0.3 M, lead to greater survival rates, with 76% fertilization, and 93.7% cleavage of fertilized zygotes,[44] which was later confirmed using the same technique.[44] At the ALPHA consensus on cryopreservation it was stated that the modified slow-freeze protocol maintained survival of the oocyte, fertilization potential, embryo formation and embryo quality, as reported by previous protocols, as well as an improved implantation and pregnancy rate.[43] Therefore, slow freezing of oocyte with more recently developed protocols can return better outcomes than previously developed techniques, with more consistent outcomes.[45]

VITRIFICATION

Vitrification did suffer disappointing outcomes in the beginning but with recent advances in oocyte cryobiology the quality of oocytes produced with vitrification protocols has also produced good substantial results.[31] Although it is cheaper than the programmable freezing protocols, vitrification does require a higher skill level. A large number of studies have reported good results with vitrification.[36,46] A randomized prospective clinical trial compared the outcome of vitrified oocytes to fresh with 300 patients randomized per group.[31] The ongoing pregnancy rates achieved were 43.7% vs 41% vitrified and fresh, respectively. There was no significant difference to fresh embryos and the odds ratio of the ongoing pregnancy rate (0.921) slightly favored the vitrification group.[31] Studies like this open a whole new range of possibilities for ART, be it oocyte donation programs, cancer patients and fertility preservation.[47]

SLOW FREEZING VERSUS VITRIFICATION

The bulk of comparative data received from Italy during the period of 2004–2009, where there was a ban on embryo cryopreservation. This resulted in Italy producing large amounts of data in the field of oocyte cryopreservation.[32] Survival of the oocyte was definitely better in the vitrification group compared to slow freezing, but in the fertilization rate there was no significant difference due to a skill bias that existed during 2007–2009; however, comparing the survival and implantation rates during the period between 2010 and 2011, the results were statistically significant.

The data does to some extent suggest that vitrification is a better modality to cryopreserve oocytes. For comparing both techniques, ideal studies would be those utilizing both techniques using similar number and same standards for both, although attempts to control for all affecting factors have been conducted.[46]

SUMMARY

Oocyte cryopreservation is a beneficial tool for optimizing ART protocols and the scope for improvement of technology is immense. Currently, due to the high success rate, vitrification has become the standard procedure for oocyte cryopreservation but this does not mean that slow cooling is inferior, newer modified protocols have shown good results for slow cooling as well, and further studies are required to delineate between all of the factors involved.

Donor Selection and Screening

Selection and screening of semen donors involves two major activities. The initial screening is based on the donor's history, including family medical and genetic history, as well as sexual and social history. The purpose of interview screening is to eliminate donors who have a history of certain medical and genetic conditions, including but not limited to alcoholism, autoimmune diseases, significant heart disease, and certain neurological conditions. Furthermore, donors are eliminated if they report a sexual and social history that places them at risk for sexually transmitted infections, factors include drug use, multiple sexual partners, etc. The second screening step includes a physical examination, with specific examination of the urogenital tract. A physical examination could reveal conditions that may not have been reported in the history assessment, including sexually transmitted infections. Finally, specific blood tests and cultures using approved testing methodology by licensed clinical laboratories are performed prior to semen donation, cryopreservation, and quarantine. Blood tests and cultures are repeated after a 6-month quarantine period and before any specimens are released for use in artificial insemination or assisted reproductive technology programs.

ICMR GUIDELINES FOR SPERM DONATION

- The individual must be free of HIV and hepatitis B and C infections, hypertension, diabetes, sexually transmitted diseases, and identifiable and common genetic disorders such as thalassemia.
- The age of the donor must not be below 21 or above 45 years.
- An analysis must be carried out on the semen of the individual, preferably using a semen analyzer, and the semen must be found to be normal according to WHO method manual for semen analysis, if intended to be used for ART.
- The blood group and the Rh status of the individual must be determined and placed on record.
- Other relevant information in respect of the donor, such as height, weight, age, educational qualifications, profession, color of the skin and the eyes, record of major

Table 26.4: Screening tests for semen donors

	Initial	*Six-month Prerelease*
Physical examination	X	
Genetic testing	X*	
Gonorrhea	X	X
Syphilis serology (RPR)	X	X
Hepatitis B surface antigen	X	X
Hepatitis B core antibody	X	X
Hepatitis C virus	X	X
HIV 1 and HIV 2	X	X
HTLV 1	X	X
Chlamydia trachomatis	X	X
Cytomegalovirus (IgG, IgM)	X	X

*Karyotyping is not required by any accrediting or licensing organization. However, testing for certain genetic diseases, when available, such as cystic fibrosis, Tay-Sachs, beta thalassemia, and sickle cell (for certain ethnic groups) is strongly recommended, and in some cases, mandatory. HIV, human immunodeficiency virus; HTLV, human T-cell lymphoma/leukemia virus; Ig, immunoglobulin; RPR, rapid plasma reagin.

diseases including any psychiatric disorder, and the family background in respect of history of any familial disorder, must be recorded in an appropriate proforma[48] (Table 26.4)

ICMR GUIDELINES FOR OOCYTE DONATION

- The individual must be free of HIV and hepatitis B and C infections, hypertension, diabetes, sexually transmitted diseases, and identifiable and common genetic disorders such as thalassemia.
- The blood group and the Rh status of the individual must be determined and placed on record.
- Other relevant information in respect of the donor, such as height, weight, age, educational qualifications, profession, color of the skin and the eyes, and the family background in respect of history of any familial disorder, must be recorded in an appropriate proforma.
- The age of the donor must not be less than 21 or more than 35 years.[48]

Psychological Consultation

The clinician should strongly recommend psychological counseling by a qualified mental health professional to all donors, donor gamete recipients, and their partners.

Screening and Testing of Oocyte and Sperm Donors

1. Age:
   - Sperm donors between the ages of 18–40.
   - Oocyte donors between the ages of 21 and 34 years. If a prospective oocyte donor is over 34 years of age, the age of the donor should be revealed to the recipient as part of the informed consent discussion concerning cytogenetic risks and the effect of donor age on pregnancy rates.
2. Established fertility is desired, but not required.
3. Medical, social, and psychological evaluation is required.
4. Genetic evaluation:
   - Genetic screening for heritable diseases should be performed in potential donors.
   - Chromosomal analyses on all donors are not required.
5. Person who has received any transfusion of blood or blood components or human organ or tissue transplants or treatment with human extracts cannot act as donor.
6. Before acceptance, and every 6 months while remaining an active donor, donors should undergo a complete physical examination.
7. A complete personal and sexual history should be obtained to exclude as donors individuals who might be at high risk for HIV, STIs, or other infections.
8. Semen testing:
   - It is suggested that more than one sample be examined.
   - The minimum criteria for normal semen quality can be applied the minimum criteria for normal semen quality can be applied.

Choosing Donor Characteristics

Race and/or ethnic group, height, body build, complexion, eye color, and hair color and texture. Consideration should be given to blood type and Rh factor, particularly for Rh-negative recipients.

- The ASRM recommends that all directed donor semen specimens be frozen and quarantined for a minimum of 180 days, with the donor then retested.[49]
- All potential recipient couples should be offered the option of cryopreserving and quarantining embryos derived from donor oocytes for 180 days, with release of embryos only after the donor has been retested with confirmed negative results.

- No owner, operator, laboratory director or employee of a facility performing TDI may serve as a donor in that practice.
- Neither the patient's physician nor the individual performing the actual insemination can be the donor.

ICMR GUIDELINES FOR SEMEN BANKS

- Either an ART clinic or a law firm or any other suitable independent organization may set up a semen bank. If it is a set up by an ART clinic, it must operate as a separate identity.
- The bank will ensure that all criteria mentioned in the guidelines are met.
- Requirements for a sperm donor are met and a suitable record of all donors is kept for 10 years after which, or if the bank is wound up during this period, the records shall be transferred to an ICMR repository.
- A bank may advertize suitably for semen donors who may be appropriately compensated financially.
- On request for semen by an ART clinic, the bank will provide the clinic with a list of donors (without the name or the address but with a code number) giving all relevant details.
- The semen bank shall not supply semen of one donor for more than ten successful pregnancies.
- It will be the responsibility of the ART clinic or the patient, as appropriate, to inform the bank about a successful pregnancy.
- The bank shall keep a record of all semen received, stored and supplied, and details of the use of the semen of each donor. This record will be liable to be reviewed by the accreditation authority.
- The bank must be run professionally and must have facilities for cryopreservation of semen, following internationally accepted protocols. Each bank will prepare its own standard operating procedures (SOP) for cryopreservation.
- Semen samples must be cryopreserved for at least 6 months before first use, at which time the semen donor must be tested for HIV and hepatitis B and C.
- The bank must ensure confidentiality in regard to the identity of the semen donor.
- A semen bank may store a semen preparation for exclusive use on the donor's wife or on any other woman designated by the donor. An appropriate charge may be levied by the bank for the storage. In the case of nonpayment of the charges when the donor is alive, the bank would have the right to destroy the semen sample or give it to a bonafide organization to be used only for research purposes. In the case of the death of the donor, the semen would become the property of the legal heir or the nominee of the donor at the time the donor gives the sample for storage to the bank. All other conditions that apply to the donor would now apply to the legal heir, excepting that he cannot use it for having a woman of his choice inseminated by it. If after the death of the donor, there are no claimants, the bank would have the right to destroy the semen or give it to a bonafide research organization to be used only for research purposes.

REFERENCES

1. McLaughlin EA. Cryopreservation, screening and storage of sperm—the challenges for the twenty-first century. Hum Fertil. 2002;5(Suppl 1):S61-5.
2. Sanger WG, Olson JH, Sherman JK. Semen cryobanking for men with cancer—criteria change. Fertil Steril. 1992;58(5):1024-7.
3. Jensen JR, Morbeck DE, Coddington III CC. Fertility preservation. Mayo Clin Proc. 2011;86(1):45-9.
4. Anger JT, Gilbert BR, Goldstein M. Cryopreservation of sperm: indications, methods and results. J Urol. 2003;170 (4 Pt 1);1079-84.
5. Sherman J. Cryopreservation of human semen. In: Keel B, Webster BW (Eds). Handbook of the Laboratory Diagnosis and Treatment of Infertility, Boca Raton, FL: CRC Press; 1990.
6. Abdelhafez F, Bedaiwy M, El-Nashar SA, Sabanegh E, Desai N. Techniques for cryopreservation of individual or small numbers of human spermatozoa: a systematic review. Hum Reprod Update. 2009;15(2):153-64.
7. Royere D, Barthelemy C, Hamamah S, Lansac J. Cryopreservation of spermatozoa: a 1996 review. Hum Reprod Update. 1996;2(6):553-9.
8. Carpenter JF, Crowe JH, Arakawa T. Comparison of solute-induced protein stabilization in aqueous solution and in the frozen and dried states. J Dairy Sci. 1990;73(12):3627-36.
9. Gao DY, Ashworth E, Watson PF, Kleinhans FW, Mazur P, Critser JK. Hyperosmotic tolerance of human spermatozoa: separate effects of glycerol, sodium chloride, and sucrose on spermolysis. Biol Reprod. 1993;49(1):112-23.
10. McGann LE, Farrant J. Survival of tissue culture cells frozen by a two-step procedure to –196°C: I. Holding temperature and time. Cryobiology. 1976;13(3):261-8.
11. Thachil JV, Jewett MAS. Preservation techniques for human semen. Fertil Steril. 1981;35(5):546-8.
12. Holt WV. Basic aspects of frozen storage of semen. Anim Reprod Sci. 2000;62(1-3):3-22.
13. Mazur P, Rall WF, Rigopoulos N. Relative contributions of the fraction of unfrozen water and of salt concentration to the survival of slowly frozen human erythrocytes. Biophys J. 1981;36(3):653-75.
14. Watson PF. The causes of reduced fertility with cryopreserved semen. Anim Reprod Sci. 2000;60-61:481-92.

15. Stanic P, Tandara M, Sonicki Z, Simunic V, Radakovic B, Suchanek E. Comparison of protective media and freezing techniques for cryopreservation of human semen. Eur J Obstetric Gynecol Reprod Biol. 2000;91(1):65-70.
16. Said TM, Gaglani A, Agarwal A. Implication of apoptosis in sperm cryoinjury. Reprod Biomed Online. 2010;21(4):456-62.
17. Sherman JK. Synopsis of the use of frozen human semen since 1964: state of the art of human semen banking. Fertil Steril. 1973;24(5):397-412.
18. Giraud MN, Motta C, Boucher D, Grizard G. Membrane fluidity predicts the outcome of cryopreservation of human spermatozoa. Hum Reprod. 2000;15(10):2160-4.
19. O'Connell M, McClure N, Lewis SEM. The effects of cryopreservation on sperm morphology, motility and mitochondrial function. Hum Reprod. 2002;17(3):704-9.
20. Wang X, Sharma RK, Sikka SC, Thomas Jr AJ, Falcone T, Agarwal A. Oxidative stress is associated with increased apoptosis leading to spermatozoa DNA damage in patients with male factor infertility. Fertil Steril. 2003;80(3):531-5.
21. Duru NK, Morshedi MS, Schuffner A, Oehninger S. Cryopreservation-thawing of fractionated human spermatozoa is associated with membrane phosphatidylserine externalization and not DNA fragmentation. J Androl. 2001;22(4):646-51.
22. Isachenko E, Isachenko V, Katkov II, Rahimi G, Schöndorf T, Mallmann P, et al. DNA integrity and motility of human spermatozoa after standard slow freezing versus cryoprotectant-free vitrification. Hum Reprod. 2004;19(4):932-9.
23. Petyim S, Choavaratana R. Cryodamage on sperm chromatin according to different freezing methods, assessed by AO test. J Med Assoc Thailand. 2006;89(3):306-13.
24. Royere D, Hamamah S, Nicolle JC, Lansac J. Chromatin alterations induced by freeze-thawing influence the fertilizing ability of human sperm. Int J Androl. 1991;14(5):328-32.
25. Sakkas D, Urner F, Bianchi PG, Bizzaro D, Wagner I, Jaquenoud N, et al. Sperm chromatin anomalies can influence decondensation after intracytoplasmic sperm injection. Hum Reprod. 1996;11(4):837-43.
26. Oktay K, Cil AP, Bang H. Efficiency of oocyte cryopreservation: a meta-analysis. Fertil Steril. 2006;86(1):70-80.
27. Polge C, Smith AU, Parkes AS. Revival of spermatozoa after vitrification and dehydration at low temperatures. Nature. 1949;164(4172):666.
28. Leibo SP, Pool TB. The principal variables of cryopreservation: solutions, temperatures, and rate changes. Fertil Steril. 2011;96(2):269-76.
29. Liu J, Phy J, Yeomans E. Theoretic considerations regarding slow cooling and vitrification during cryopreservation. Theriogenology. 2012;78(8):1641-52.
30. Edgar DH, Gook DA. A critical appraisal of cryopreservation (slow cooling versus vitrification) of human oocytes and embryos. Hum Reprod Update. 2012;18(5):536-54.
31. Cobo A, Diaz C. Clinical application of oocyte vitrification: a systematic review and meta-analysis of randomized controlled trials. Fertil Steril. 2011;96(2):277-85.
32. Levi Setti PE, Porcu E, Patrizio P, Vigiliano V, de Luca R, d'Aloja P, et al. Human oocyte cryopreservation with slow freezing versus vitrification. Results from the National Italian Registry Data, 2007-2011. Fertil Steril. 2014;102(1):90-5.
33. Gardner DK, Sheehan CB, Rienzi L, Katz-Jaffe M, Larman MG. Analysis of oocyte physiology to improve cryopreservation procedures. Theriogenology. 2007;67(1):64-72.
34. Ruffing NA, Steponkus PL, Pitt RE, Parks JE. Osmometric behavior, hydraulic conductivity, and incidence of intracellular ice formation in bovine oocytes at different developmental stages. Cryobiology. 1993;30(6):562-80.
35. Clark NA, Swain JE. Oocyte cryopreservation: searching for novel improvement strategies. J Assist Reprod Genet. 2013;30(7):865-75.
36. Noyes N, Knopman J, Labella P, McCaffrey C, Clark-Williams M, Grifo J. Oocyte cryopreservation outcomes including pre-cryopreservation and post-thaw meiotic spindle evaluation following slow cooling and vitrification of human oocytes. Fertil Steril. 2010;94(6):2078-82.
37. Morato R, Izquierdo D, Albarracin JL, Anguita B, Palomo MJ, Jimenez-Macedo AR, et al. Effects of pre-treating *in vitro*-matured bovine oocytes with the cytoskeleton stabilizing agent taxol prior to vitrification. Mol Reprod Dev. 2008;75(1):191-201.
38. Koutlaki N, Schoepper B, Maroulis G, Diedrich K, Al-Hasani S. Human oocyte cryopreservation: past, present and future. Reprod Biomed Online. 2006;13(3):427-36.
39. Porcu E, Fabbri R, Damiano G, Giunchi S, Fratto R, Ciotti PM, et al. Clinical experience and applications of oocyte cryopreservation. Mol Cellular Endocrinol. 2000;169(1-2):33-7.
40. Hu W, Marchesi D, Qiao J, Feng HL. Effect of slow freeze versus vitrification on the oocyte: an animal model. Fertil Steril. 2012;98(3):752-60.e3.
41. Lei T, Guo N, Tan MH, Li YF. Effect of mouse oocyte vitrification on mitochondrial membrane potential and distribution. J Huazhong Univ Sci Technol Med Sci. 2014;34(1): 99-102.
42. Fabbri R, Porcu E, Marsella T, Rocchetta G, Venturoli S, Flamigni C. Human oocyte cryopreservation: new perspectives regarding oocyte survival. Hum Reprod. 2001;16(3): 411-6.
43. Borini A, Levi Setti PE, Anserini P, De Luca R, De Santis L, Porcu E, et al. Multicenter observational study on slow-cooling oocyte cryopreservation: clinical outcome. Fertil Steril. 2010;94(5):1662-8.
44. Bianchi V, Lappi M, Bonu MA, Borini A. Oocyte slow freezing using a 0.2–0.3 M sucrose concentration protocol: is it really the time to trash the cryopreservation machine? Fertil Steril. 2012;97(5):1101-7.
45. Alpha Scientists in Reproductive Medicine. The Alpha consensus meeting on cryopreservation key performance indicators and benchmarks: proceedings of an expert meeting. Reprod Biomed Online. 2012;25(2):146-67.
46. Kuwayama M. Highly efficient vitrification for cryopreservation of human oocytes and embryos: the Cryotop method. Theriogenology. 2007;67(1):73-80.
47. Domingo J, Guillen V, Ayllon Y, Martinez M, Munoz E, Pellicer A, et al. Ovarian response to controlled ovarian hyperstimulation in cancer patients is diminished even before oncological treatment. Fertil Steril. 2012;97(4):930-4.
48. icmr.nic.in/About_Us/Guidelines.html.
49. https://www.asrm.org/Guidelines/.

CHAPTER

Contraceptive Practice in Adolescent

27

Matan Elami-Suzin, Joseph G Schenker

INTRODUCTION

Choosing a contraceptive method in adolescents may not be an easy task. The features of an ideal contraceptive method would be that it is cheap, highly effective, have no side effects, independent of intercourse, does not require a regular action on the part of the user, is acceptable to all cultures and religions, and is easily distributed and administered by non-healthcare personnel.

There is no other method that fits all of these criteria and one must choose from a variety of available methods, each with its own advantages and disadvantages. Female teens perceive cost, lack of information and lack of access to confidential healthcare services, as significant barriers. Additional barriers include concerns regarding potential pelvic examination and fear from side effects.

ORAL CONTRACEPTIVES

Especially in the adolescent age group there are various adherence problems with oral contraceptives (OCs), such as:

1. Not refilling the prescription,
2. Forgetting to take the pill,
3. Starting next pack late,
4. Using pills inconsistently and sporadically,
5. Not using a back-up method when needed.

Therefore, the adolescent should be provided clear verbal and written instructions. The clinician should ascertain that she has sufficient reading skills to interpret labels and instructions.

To optimize the adolescent's adherence to OCs, we suggest giving her only the following instructions:

1. When to start the pill.
2. Take the pill every day at the same time, especially when doing something else regularly, like teeth brushing.
3. Call the clinic if there are any questions.

Oral contraceptives can be started at any time. In adolescents, they are typically started on the first day of the next menstrual period or the Sunday after the onset of the menstrual period ("Sunday start method"). The rationale for this delayed start date is to make sure that the adolescent is not pregnant. However, as many as 25% of adolescents who seek OCs from family planning clinics never take the first pill.[1,2]

It is also, in our opinion, important to give teenage girls the regiments with less hormone-free interval (i.e., 24/4 preparations instead of 21/7) because these preparations allows the adolescent to simply take a pill every day and to start the next pack immediately after finishing the previous one. This makes things easy on her and she will be less likely to forget.

EXTENDED-CYCLE OR CONTINUOUS PILL USE

The desire to avoid monthly periods may be related to participation in athletic events or summer camps, or to the general discomfort and "hassle" of monthly periods. A schedule that involves continuous pill use for 84 days followed by a week of pill-free days may help to increase adherence in adolescents who wish to avoid a monthly period. In addition, an OC that provides continuous, year-round contraception has been approved by the FDA. It contains levonorgestrel 90 μg and ethinyl estradiol 20 μg.

Until studies are conducted in adolescents, information on extended-cycle and continuous, year-round pills must be drawn from studies and clinical experience in adults. One-half to two-thirds of adult women report a decrease in breakthrough spotting or bleeding (BTB) in the second half compared with the first half of the extended or year-long regimen. To manage BTB, a 3-day, hormone-free interval was more beneficial than continuous pills.[3]

A systematic review of continuous use of OCs in adult women found that other menstrual symptoms including headaches, genital irritation, tiredness, bloating and dysmenorrhea also improved with extended-cycle pill use.[4]

Adolescents have specific fears and concerns regarding the use of contraception because of the following potential side effects:

- Weight gain: Many teenagers fear of gaining weight with the use of hormonal contraception. However, they should be reassured that available evidence does not support this regarding OCs. In the case of depot-medroxyprogesterone acetate (DMPA), weight gain might be a concomitant event, but no causal relationship has been established. Factors other than DMPA may contribute to weight gain.
- Bone density: Ultra-low dose estrogen (20 µg) OCs and DMPA might interfere with achieving peak bone mass in teenagers and young adults. Rare cases of osteoporosis, including fractures, have been reported in patients taking DMPA, and the prescribing information for DMPA includes a boxed warning that DMPA should be used as a long-term birth control method (e.g., longer than 2 years) only if other birth control methods are inadequate.[5]

  It is vital to share information with the adolescent regarding the potential effects of DMPA on bone density. There is a general agreement that DMPA should be avoided early puberty, but there is lack of evidence to limit its use in older adolescents. In fact, some experts argue that for adolescents in whom DMPA is the only acceptable contraceptive option, the benefit of pregnancy prevention outweighs the potential risk to bone health.

  The Society for Adolescent Health and Medicine has published a position paper regarding the boxed warning for DMPA.[6] This paper suggests that:
  - With adequate explanation of benefits and potential risks, *DMPA may continue to be prescribed to adolescent girls* who need contraception.
  - Decisions regarding bone density monitoring of adolescents using DMPA for contraception should be individualized; the decisions should be made by the clinician in concert with the adolescent, and potentially the adolescent's guardian.
  - *Duration of use of DMPA need not be restricted to 2 years.*
  - *Adolescents using DMPA should be encouraged to take 1,300 mg of elemental calcium and 400 international units vitamin D and to exercise each day.*
  - *Estrogen supplementation should be considered for girls who are doing well on DMPA and have osteopenia or are at risk for osteopenia and who have no contraindications to estrogen.*
- Thromboembolism: Probably one of the most feared negative consequence of combined estrogen–progestin hormonal contraception is venous thromboembolism (VTE). Use of combined OCs increases VTE risk by two- to fourfold compared to nonusers. *However, this should be put readily in perspective, because the absolute risk is still very low* (increases from 2 to 3:10,000 nonusers to 8–12:10,000 current users) *and much lower than the VTE risk during pregnancy and postpartum period* (60–80:10,000). It is, indeed, safer to prevent an unwanted pregnancy than terminating or continuing carrying it!

  Although reducing the estrogen dose had improved the safety and side effects profile of OCs, it did not eliminate completely the increased risk of VTE.[7-9] There are several factors which influence the risk:
  - Progestin type: Several studies and meta-analyses have reported a greater VTE risk with some of the third-generation OCs (desogestrel and gestodene, but not norgestimate) when compared with levonorgestrel, a second-generation progestin.
  - In addition, two antiandrogenic progestins (drospirenone and cyproterone acetate) have been associated with a similar increase in VTE risk. However, the absolute excess risk is small, and is considered medically acceptable given the many benefits of combined hormonal contraceptives.

    In 2011, the European Medicines Agency also concluded that drospirenone-containing birth control pills carry a higher risk of VTE, but noted the overall risk of blood clot from any birth control method remains small and stopped short of advising women to stop taking pills containing drospirenone.[10]

    Acquired resistance to activated protein C has been suggested as one mechanism by which the third-generation OCs could predispose to VTE.[11,12] In addition, third-generation and second-generation progestins have different effects on the anticoagulant pathway.[13,14] It has been suggested that second-generation progestins, such as levonorgestrel, are more effective than third-generation progestins, such as desogestrel, in counteracting the thrombotic effects of estrogen.[15]

- Obesity: Among OC users in two case-control studies, obese women had a 2-[16] to 24-fold[17] higher risk of VTE than nonobese women. In a third case-control study of 454 consecutive patients with a first episode of objectively diagnosed deep vein thrombosis (DVT), the risk of thrombosis among those with both obesity and OC use was increased 10-fold compared with women with neither risk factor; the increase in risk was lower (2.3- to 4.6-fold) with either risk factor alone.[18]
- Age: In a pooled analysis of two case-control studies, the risk of VTE rose sharply after age 39 years among women taking estrogen–progestin OCs. The estimated incidence in women over age 39 years, when compared with adolescents, was 100 versus 25 cases of VTE per 100,000 person per years, respectively.[19]
- *According to this analysis, the risk of VTE in adolescents who use OCs is actually the same as for nonusers.*

TRANSDERMAL CONTRACEPTIVE PATCH

Data are conflicting on whether the risk of VTE is higher in users of the transdermal contraceptive patch (Ortho Evra) than users of OCs.

Oral and Injectable Progestin

Oral and injectable progestin-only preparations for contraception do not appear to be associated with an increased risk of thromboembolism.

In order to prevent thromboembolism, it is important to take a comprehensive and thorough history from the adolescent regarding personal and family history of VTE, for risk-stratification purposes.

- Pelvic inflammatory disease (PID): The relationship between OCs and PID is complex. Whereas some studies indicate that the use of OCs increases the risk of PID, others suggest that OCs increase the risk for cervicitis and endometritis, but not salpingitis, thereby decreasing the severity of PID.[20-23] No association was found between DMPA and PID.[24]

INTRAUTERINE DEVICE

Usually, most physicians are reluctant to insert an IUD to an adolescent, and even to nulliparous adult patient. This practice stems from several reasons including[25] history of negative publicity, disinformation about the risk of ectopic pregnancy, infection and infertility, misconceptions about the mechanism of action of the IUD, lack of provider training, and fears of litigation.

In the 1970s, the IUD was used by 10% of women in the United States. When the Dalkon Shield (a common IUD used in that era) was linked to PID, utilization of all IUDs fell and litigation rose.

One probable explanation for the increases infectious morbidity in the 1970s is the construction of the IUD tail, which were multifilament and braided and acted like "ropes" that allowed bacteria to ascend upward from the lower genital tract. Coupled with the fact that no test had yet been developed to detect asymptomatic *Chlamydia* infection.

Current IUDs, which have monofilament tail strings, have not been associated with an elevated infection risk, beyond the first 2–3 weeks after insertion. In 2005, the US Food and Drug Administration (FDA) approved liberalized package labeling for the copper T380A (Paragard), removing any proscription against its use in nulliparous women or in those with more than one sexual partner. Initial studies with the newest levonorgestrel releasing IUD (LNg14 IUD; Jaydess*, Skyla*) include nulliparous women. Based on the results of these trials, the product label contains no recommendation against use in nulliparous women. Although the LNg20 IUD (Mirena*) package label contains a recommendation for its use in parous women, the LNg20 has been studied in nulliparous women and found to be safe. The American College of Obstetrics and Gynecologists (ACOG) states that IUDs are safe and appropriate for most women, including nulliparous women and adolescents, and that use of IUDs should be encouraged as a first-line approach to pregnancy prevention.[26,27] The IUD is an attractive option for adolescents and adolescent mothers who desire long-term, uninterrupted contraception. It lasts 3–10 years depending on the type of device. Parous adolescents may be better candidates for the IUD than nulliparous adolescents because higher expulsion rates have been reported in nulliparous adolescents. However, the 3- and 5-year devices have been successfully used in nulliparous adolescents. This has been shown in a large study based on medical records of 1,177 female teenagers aged 13–24 years old.[28] In this study, the first-attempt success rate was 95.8% for nulliparous women and 96.7% for parous women. The first-attempt success rate was 95.5% (n = 169) for women aged 13–17 years compared with 96.3% (n = 963) for women aged 18–24 years.

The World Health Organization (WHO) suggests:[29]

- The IUD is an unacceptable risk in a woman with PID or purulent cervicitis currently or in the past 3 months.
- The risks outweigh the advantages of inserting an IUD in a woman with multiple partners or a partner with multiple partners.
- There is no restriction on IUD placement when there is a past history of PID and no current sexually transmitted infection.

Mechanisms of Action

There are several possible mechanisms of action for IUD,[30-34] including changes in cervical mucus that inhibit sperm transport (e.g., increased copper concentration, thickening, glandular atrophy or decidualization); chronic inflammatory changes of the endometrium and fallopian tubes, which have spermicidal effects and inhibit fertilization and implantation; thinning and glandular atrophy of the endometrium, which inhibits implantation; and direct toxic effects on the oocyte. It is important to stress that *the IUD is not an abortifacient* (defined as interruption of an implanted pregnancy).[30]

Absolute and Relative Contraindications

- Absolute contraindications for any IUD placement include possible or confirmed pregnancy; severe distortion of the uterine cavity (such as by fibroids or anatomic anomalies) that precludes IUD insertion; acute, recent (within 3 months) or recurrent uterine infection (includes sexually transmitted, postpartum and postabortion infections); untreated cervicitis; Active genital actinomycoses.
- Absolute contraindications for copper IU include Wilson's disease and known copper allergy.
- Absolute contraindications for levonorgestrel IUD include known allergy to levnorgestrel, acute liver disease or liver tumor, and known or suspected carcinoma of the breast.
- Relative contraindications for any IUD placement include patients at high risk for STIs (sexually transmitted infections) (multiple sexual partners, past infections); previous IUD problem (perforation, significant cramps); unresolved abnormal uterine bleeding; known severe vasovagal reactions.
- Relative contraindications for copper IUD include current anemia or menorrhagia-associated anemia.
- Relative contraindications for levonorgestrel IUD include past intolerance to progestin and patient unwilling to accept a change in menstrual pattern (hypomenorrhea or amenorrhea).

Complications

Uterine Perforation

This occurs in about 1:1,000 interval IUD insertions. The risk factors include cervical stenosis, inexperienced provider, postpartum period, breastfeeding and fixed or retroverted uterus. If perforation by the sound or the IUD is suspected, the adolescent must be monitored for tachycardia, hypotension, syncope or an acute abdomen. Even though these rarely occur after perforation, they warrant a transfer to hospital for further management. If perforation is suspected in a stable patient (which usually is the case), IUD removal can be attempted by placing gentle traction on the string. If the string is not visible, the location of the IUD can usually be determined by ultrasound examination.

Depending on the location, the IUD can then be retrieved using a hysteroscope or laparoscope. Removing the IUD under direct vision helps prevent injury to pelvic organs that could be snagged by the device. Laparotomy is required if laparoscopic or hysteroscopic removal is difficult, if perforation of intraabdominal organs is suspected or with ongoing intraperitoneal hemorrhage. Immediate intervention is not essential if the patient is stable. A uterine perforation caused by a sound or an IUD is not a contraindication for future vaginal delivery.

Vasovagal Response

Sometimes, the IUD insertion causes transient syncope or presyncope, hypotension, bradycardia and/or nausea. These typically resolve by stopping the procedure, placing the adolescent in a recumbent position, and giving supportive care.

Postinsertion Patient Counseling

We teach the adolescent to feel the IUD strings and to verify periodically and especially after the menses that the IUD is retained. We guide her, that if she does not feel the strings, she should schedule an appointment and use a back-up contraceptive method until her healthcare provider confirms whether or not the IUD is in place. Even with absent problems we schedule a follow-up visit in

1–3 months, because it was shown to increase continuation of the method.

CONTRACEPTIVE PROGESTIN IMPLANT

These were also suggested (together with the IUD) as a first-line contraceptive method in adolescents.[26,31] The contraceptive implant is potentially an attractive option for adolescents and adolescent mothers who desire long-term contraception. It provides pregnancy protection within 24 hours of insertion, and fertility returns quickly after its removal. Unexpected and prolonged bleeding can be a problem and can trigger request for premature removal. One should reliably exclude pregnancy before implant insertion.

DEPO MEDROXY PROGESTERONE ACETATE (DMPA) INJECTIONS

Typically, the first injection is given during the menstrual period to ensure absence of pregnancy. If DMPA is initiated more than 7 days after the first day of the menstrual period and she has had unprotected intercourse during the cycle, clinicians and patients must recognize that there is a small chance of preimplantation or early pregnancy despite a negative pregnancy test prior to the injection. We suggest that in these cases to receive emergency contraception (EC) if intercourse occurred within the previous 120 hours, and we advise to use back-up contraception for 7 days after DMPA injection since ovulation may occur within 24 hours of the initial injection, and we counsel them to repeat the pregnancy test in 2–3 weeks.

Adolescents who are late for injection should not be turned away solely because of that. After a 150 mg injection, ovulation does not occur for at least 14 weeks. Therefore, a 2-week "grace period" (repeat injection without pregnancy testing) is appropriate for adolescent women receiving injections every 3 months (13 weeks). For adolescents more than 2 weeks late for their injection (>15 weeks from the last injection), we suggest a pregnancy test before administering DMPA and back-up contraception (or abstinence) for 7 days.

As a result of a study showing that contraceptive efficacy is maintained with a "grace period" as long as 4 weeks,[32] the WHO adopted a longer grace period in its updated guidelines. A limitation of these data is that more than one third of the women in the study were lactating, placing them at low baseline risk for conception.

Therefore, in high-resource countries, we continue to encourage women to return on time and allow a 2-week grace period, and require documentation of a negative pregnancy test in women who present more than 2 weeks (>15 weeks from their last injection).

PROS AND CONS OF DMPA INJECTIONS

- Advantages of DMPA injections include reversibility, privacy, lasts 12 weeks, effective in obese adolescents, reduces risk of ectopic pregnancy, menses decreases or ceases, reduces dysmenorrhea and other menstrual symptoms, few drug interactions, less seizures in epileptics, less pain crises in adolescents with sickle cell anemia, reduction in endometriosis related pelvic pain, reduction in abnormal uterine bleeding associated with leiomyomas, possible reduction in the incidence of PID.
- Disadvantages of DMPA injections include increase in unscheduled bleeding, possible increase in weight gain, possible induction of depression, a decrease in bone density that is *usually reversible*, small risk of severe allergic reaction, a delay in return to fertility, repeated injection is needed every 12 weeks.

VAGINAL CONTRACEPTIVE RING

For some adolescents, this is a very attractive option because it needs to be changed only every 3 weeks. However, some adolescents do not feel comfortable in insertion of things into their vaginas. Those who use tampons might be better candidates for this method.

If the ring remains in place more than 3-5 weeks, it is removed and a new one is inserted after a 1-week ring-free interval; if the ring is left in place for more than 5 weeks, back-up contraception is recommended until a new ring has been in place for 7 days. The ring remains effective when left in place for up to 5 weeks, as the ring contains sufficient steroids to maintain stable blood concentrations for this period of time.[33] Thus, inhibition of ovulation is sufficiently maintained if an adolescent forgets to remove the ring after the usual 3-week use period. Adolescents who desire fewer days of withdrawal bleeding and are willing to tolerate some spotting can safely use an extended ring regimen whereby the ring is changed every 3 weeks, omitting the hormone-free week for up to 1 year.[34-38] Extended use is effective and does not worsen bothersome side effects, except for unscheduled bleeding.

Unplanned removal or expulsion of the contraceptive ring can occur. The ring should not be removed during intercourse. If it accidentally falls out, it may be rinsed with cool or warm (not hot) water and reinserted into the vagina within 3 hours. From our own experience, many teenagers do not feel "clean" with the vaginal ring and have a need to wash it frequently. Frequent washing decreases effectiveness and may cause intermittent bleeding or spotting.

If the ring is out of the vagina for more than three consecutive hours, subsequent steps depend on the week of the cycle that the ring is out:

- During the first 2 weeks of the cycle, the ring is reinserted as soon as possible. Pregnancy may not be prevented if the ring is out for more than 3 hours during this time, so an additional form of contraception, such as condoms with spermicide, is used until the reinserted ring has been in place for seven continuous days. The ring should subsequently be removed according to the original schedule, after which the adolescent can expect to have her normal period.
- During week three of the cycle, the adolescent discards the ring. She then chooses one of two different restart options:
  - Option one: Insert a new ring and begin a new 3-week cycle. Back-up contraception or abstinence is recommended until the new ring has been used continuously for 7 days. The adolescent may not have a regular period until she reaches her next ring-free week, but she may have vaginal spotting or bleeding prior to that point.
  - Option two: Insert a new ring and begin a new 3-week cycle. Back-up contraception or abstinence is recommended until the new ring has been used continuously for 7 days. The adolescent may not have a regular period until she reaches her next ring-free week, but she may have vaginal spotting or bleeding prior to that point.

These steps are consistent with recommendations from the manufacturer.

TRANSDERMAL PATCH

The fact that the transdermal patch does not require daily attention makes it an attractive option for adolescents. However, the need for weekly change also may promote decreased adherence. The patch is applied to the buttock, abdomen, upper arm, or upper torso (but not the breast, as it might cause breast tenderness due to high local estrogen concentration). A different site is used each time a new patch is applied. The patch is changed once a week for 3 weeks (21 total days), followed by 1 week that is patch-free. It should always be changed/applied on the same day of the week.

Reminder systems are useful to ensure appropriate weekly changes. The consequences of failing to change the transdermal contraceptive patch at the appropriate time should be addressed with the adolescent.

- *Delay in beginning the first patch in a cycle:* When a new patch cycle is delayed beyond the scheduled start day, users are instructed to apply a patch as soon as they remember and use back-up contraception (or avoid sex) for at least 1 week. The day they apply the new patch becomes the new patch change day.
- *Delay in beginning the second or third patch in a cycle:* There is a 2-day (48 hours) period of continued release of adequate contraceptive steroid levels when the patch is left on for two extra days. If users change the patch within this window, the patch change day remains the same and there is no need for back-up contraception. After this 2-day (48 hours) time period, failure to replace the second or third patch in a cycle increases the risk for contraceptive failure. Therefore, users will need to use back-up contraception (or avoid sex) for 7 days and, in some instances, use EC, if this occurs. The day the patient remembers to apply the patch becomes the new change day.
- *Delay in removing the third patch in a cycle:* Forgetting to remove the third patch on time carries less risk than forgetting to remove the first or second patch. The user is instructed to remove the patch when she remembers; the patch change day is not altered.

Strategies to promote weekly changes should be reviewed with adolescents using the transdermal patch. These include using a wall, computer, or cell phone calendar; a cell phone weekly alarm; or a sticker designating the change day on the bathroom mirror.

If a patch becomes partially or completely detached for less than 24 hours, it should be reapplied at the same location (if it has not lost its stickiness: ancillary adhesives or tape should not be used), or replaced with a new patch immediately. If detachment lasts longer than 24 hours, a new patch should be applied, and this day of the week becomes the new patch change day. An additional method of contraception (e.g., condoms, spermicides) should be used for the first 7 days of this cycle or the patient should avoid sex.

In various trials, 1.8% of transdermal patches required replacement for complete detachment and 2.9% became partially detached.[39] Living in a warm, humid climate did not increase the risk of detachment. The quality of adherence was illustrated in a study in which 30 women were subjected to various conditions over several 7-day time periods during transdermal patch use.[39] The conditions included normal activity, use of a sauna, immersion in a whirlpool bath, use of a treadmill followed by showering, cool water immersion, and a combination of these activities. Only one patch became detached during the 87 cycles that were evaluated, suggesting that skin adherence is not adversely affected by a vigorous, athletic lifestyle.

CONDOMS

We always stress the benefit of dual-protection against both pregnancy and STI. Girls planning to use condoms should receive them before leaving the office or clinic, if possible, to ensure availability and promote adherence.

EMERGENCY CONTRACEPTION

Emergency contraception (also known as postcoital contraception and the morning-after pill) refers to the use of drugs or a device as an emergency measure to prevent pregnancy. As adolescents are particularly prone to have unprotected intercourse, they are potential candidates for EC. It is intended for occasional or back-up use, not as a primary contraceptive method for routine use.

In most of the developed countries, some form of orally given EC is available as over-the-counter drug. Both oral and intrauterine EC are *only effective before implantation.*

Orally available EC are:

- Levonorgestrel: 0.75 mg given twice daily, 12 hours apart up to 72 hours, efficiency 60–94%.
- Mifepristone: single dose 600 mg, up to 5 days, efficiency 99–100%.
- Ulipristal: single oral dose of 30 mg, up to 72 hours, efficiency 99–100%.

It is recommend that ulipristal acetate be avoided in women using enzyme-inducing drugs or who have taken them within the last 28 days. Patients should also be advised to avoid ulipristal if they are currently taking drugs that increase gastric pH (e.g., antacids, histamine H2 antagonists and proton pump inhibitors).

Although the Centers for Disease Control and Prevention (CDC) and the WHO Medical Eligibility Criteria for Contraceptive Use applies contraindications to daily use of hormonal contraceptives in some women based on their medical history, these contraindications do not apply to adolescents and women seeking EC. In particular, cardiovascular disease, thrombophilic disorders, migraine, liver disease and breastfeeding are considered conditions where the advantages of using the method generally outweigh the theoretical or proven risks.

Some data suggest levonorgestrel and ulipristal EC may be less effective in overweight or obese women. A 2015 study reported that levonorgestrel EC was less effective at preventing pregnancy as weight and body mass index increased.[40] The women in the 80 kg group had a pregnancy risk of 6%, which was similar to the pregnancy risk as if no contraceptive had been used. At least one pharmaceutical package insert for levonorgestrel EC warns of reduced contraceptive efficacy in women weighing more than or equal to 75 kg. However, the European Medicines Association concluded that the available data were too limited and not robust enough to be certain the contraceptive efficacy of levonorgestrel or ulipristal EC is reduced with increased body weight and that the benefits of taking these medications outweigh any risks.[41]

Copper intrauterine device, inserted up to 5 days, efficiency at least 99%.

Contraindications to copper IUD use include severe uterine distortion, active pelvic infection, copper allergy and suspected pregnancy.

RESUMING OR INITIATING HORMONAL CONTRACEPTION

The duration of effectiveness of EC has not been determined. Thus, it is not clear when regular contraception should be resumed or initiated within the menstrual cycle of emergency contraceptive use.[42] The safest approach is to advise adolescents using EC pills that a risk of pregnancy still exists if they have unprotected sexual intercourse after the emergency contraceptive pills have been taken; therefore, they should immediately initiate an effective contraceptive method.

For those taking levonorgestrel or combined estrogen-progestin EC, any regular contraceptive method can be started immediately after the use of the emergency contraceptive.[43] Backup methods of contraception (e.g., condom or diaphragm) or abstinence are required during the first 7 days of use. Although efficacy is not compromised by immediate initiation, it is prudent to avoid starting longer-acting hormonal methods (e.g., DMPA, etonogestrel implant, Levonorgestrel-releasing intrauterine devices) until it is certain that pregnancy has not occurred. However, this concern should be balanced against risk of unintended pregnancy if initiation of one of these methods is delayed.

For those taking ulipristal for EC, there is theoretical concern that starting a hormonal method after taking ulipristal could make either the ulipristal or the hormonal method less effective by competitive binding to the progestin receptors. In 2015, the US Food and Drug Administration amended the package insert and stated that progesterone-containing contraceptives should not be used with ulipristal or for 5 days following ulipristal use.[44] The ulipristal package insert recommends using a barrier method for the remainder of the cycle to avoid any potential drug interactions with a hormonal contraceptive. Some experts advise waiting 7 days after ulipristal to start a hormonal method. A guideline from the United Kingdom recommends that additional precautions be taken for 14 days after taking ulipristal (9 days if using or starting the progestogen-only pill, 16 days, for estradiol valerate/dienogest pill).[45]

REPEATED EMERGENCY CONTRACEPTION

There is no contraindication to giving a second dose of hormonal EC if a second episode of unprotected intercourse occurs any time after the first dose was administered. In contrast, there is no support for use of ulipristal more than once per cycle or if there has been another episode of unprotected sexual intercourse outside the treatment window (>120 hours).[43]

CONCLUSION

Adolescents are a vulnerable population in terms of unintended pregnancies and sexually transmitted infections. In this review, we have specifically regarded issues relevant to correct and successful use of different contraceptive methods in adolescents. The important "take-home" messages are:

1. We should provide counseling and ensure access for a range of contraceptive methods. We should allow sufficient time during the medical encounter to dispel myths and provide reassurance about the general safety of various contraceptive methods.
2. Age per se is not a contraindication to any type of contraceptive and neither nulliparity.
3. The LARC methods should be considered first-line choice for adolescents.
4. There is no need for a pelvic exam before prescribing hormonal contraception in asymptomatic healthy adolescents.
5. Always encourage "dual-protection" with condom use in every sexual intercourse.
6. We should remember and stress the noncontraceptive benefits of hormonal contraception.
7. Adolescents with disabilities and chronic illnesses have sexual health and contraception need that are similar to their healthy peers.

REFERENCES

1. Polaneczky M, Slap G, Forke C, Rappaport A, Sondheimer S. The use of levonorgestrel implants (Norplant) for contraception in adolescent mothers. N Engl J Med. 1994;331(18):1201-6.
2. Lara-Torre E. "Quick Start", an innovative approach to the combination oral contraceptive pill in adolescents. Is it time to make the switch? J Pediatr Adolesc Gynecol. 2004;17(1):65-7.
3. Coffee AL, Sulak PJ, Kuehl TJ. Long-term assessment of symptomatology and satisfaction of an extended oral contraceptive regimen. Contraception. 2007;75(6):444-9.
4. Edelman A, Gallo MF, Nichols MD, Jensen JT, Schulz KF, Grimes DA. Continuous versus cyclic use of combined oral contraceptives for contraception: systematic Cochrane review of randomized controlled trials. Hum Reprod. 2006;21(3):573-8.
5. "Black box" warning added to contraceptive injection. FDA Consum. 2005;39(2):3.
6. Cromer BA, Scholes D, Berenson A, Cundy T, Clark MK, Kaunitz AM, et al. Depot medroxyprogesterone acetate and bone mineral density in adolescents—the Black Box warning: a position paper of the society for adolescent medicine. J Adolesc Health. 2006;39(2):296-301.
7. Vandenbroucke JP, Rosing J, Bloemenkamp KW, Middeldorp S, Helmerhorst FM, Bouma BN, et al. Oral contraceptives and the risk of venous thrombosis. N Engl J Med. 2001;344(20):1527-35.
8. Douketis JD, Ginsberg JS, Holbrook A, Crowther M, Duku EK, Burrows RF. A reevaluation of the risk for venous thromboembolism with the use of oral contraceptives and hormone replacement therapy. Arch Intern Med. 1997;157(14):1522-30.
9. Bloemenkamp KW, Rosendaal FR, Buller HR, Helmerhorst FM, Colly LP, Vandenbroucke JP. Risk of venous thrombosis with use of current low-dose oral contraceptives is not explained by diagnostic suspicion and referral bias. Arch Intern Med. 1999;159(1):65-70.
10. PhVWP Monthly report on safety concerns, guidelines and general matters. European Medicines Agency; 2012.

11. Rosing J, Tans G, Nicolaes GA, Thomassen MC, van Oerle R, van der Ploeg PM, et al. Oral contraceptives and venous thrombosis: different sensitivities to activated protein C in women using second- and third-generation oral contraceptives. Br J Haematol. 1997;97(1):233-8.
12. Rosing J, Middeldorp S, Curvers J, Christella M, Thomassen LG, Nicolaes GA, et al. Low-dose oral contraceptives and acquired resistance to activated protein C: a randomised cross-over study. Lancet. 1999;354(9195):2036-40.
13. Middeldorp S, Meijers JC, van den Ende AE, van Enk A, Bouma BN, Tans G, et al. Effects on coagulation of levonorgestrel- and desogestrel-containing low dose oral contraceptives: a cross-over study. Thromb Haemost. 2000; 84(1):4-8.
14. Kemmeren JM, Algra A, Meijers JC, Bouma BN, Grobbee DE. Effects of second and third generation oral contraceptives and their respective progestagens on the coagulation system in the absence or presence of the factor VLeiden mutation. Thromb Haemost. 2002;87(2):199-205.
15. Kemmeren JM, Algra A, Meijers JC, Tans G, Bouma BN, Curvers J, et al. Effect of second- and third-generation oral contraceptives on the protein C system in the absence or presence of the factor VLeiden mutation: a randomized trial. Blood. 2004;103(3):927-33.
16. Sidney S, Petitti DB, Soff GA, Cundiff DL, Tolan KK, Quesenberry CP Jr. Venous thromboembolic disease in users of low-estrogen combined estrogen-progestin oral contraceptives. Contraception. 2004;70(1):3-10.
17. Pomp ER, le Cessie S, Rosendaal FR, Doggen CJ. Risk of venous thrombosis: obesity and its joint effect with oral contraceptive use and prothrombotic mutations. Br J Haematol. 2007;139(2):289-96.
18. Abdollahi M, Cushman M, Rosendaal FR. Obesity: risk of venous thrombosis and the interaction with coagulation factor levels and oral contraceptive use. Thromb Haemost. 2003;89(3):493-8.
19. Nightingale AL, Lawrenson RA, Simpson EL, Williams TJ, MacRae KD, Farmer RD. The effects of age, body mass index, smoking and general health on the risk of venous thromboembolism in users of combined oral contraceptives. Eur J Contracept Reprod Health Care. 2000;5(4):265-74.
20. Louv WC, Austin H, Perlman J, Alexander WJ. Oral contraceptive use and the risk of chlamydial and gonococcal infections. Am J Obstet Gynecol. 1989;160(2):396-402.
21. Rubin GL, Ory HW, Layde PM. Oral contraceptives and pelvic inflammatory disease. Am J Obstet Gynecol. 1982;144(6):630-5.
22. Ness RB, Keder LM, Soper DE, Amortegui AJ, Gluck J, Wiesenfeld H, et al. Oral contraception and the recognition of endometritis. Am J Obstet Gynecol. 1997;176(3):580-5.
23. Wolner-Hanssen P, Svensson L, Mardh PA, Westrom L. Laparoscopic findings and contraceptive use in women with signs and symptoms suggestive of acute salpingitis. Obstet Gynecol. 1985;66(2):233-8.
24. Ness RB, Soper DE, Holley RL, Peipert J, Randall H, Sweet RL, et al. Hormonal and barrier contraception and risk of upper genital tract disease in the PID Evaluation and Clinical Health (PEACH) study. Am J Obstet Gynecol. 2001;185(1): 121-7.
25. Stanwood NL, Garrett JM, Konrad TR. Obstetrician-gynecologists and the intrauterine device: a survey of attitudes and practice. Obstet Gynecol. 2002;99(2):275-80.
26. Committee on Adolescent Health Care Long-Acting Reversible Contraception Working Group, TACoO Gynecologists. Committee opinion no. 539: adolescents and long-acting reversible contraception: implants and intrauterine devices. Obstet Gynecol. 2012;120(4):983-8.
27. American College of Obstetricians and Gynecologists Committee on Gynecologic Practice; Long-Acting Reversible Contraception Working Group. ACOG Committee Opinion no. 450: Increasing use of contraceptive implants and intrauterine devices to reduce unintended pregnancy. Obstet Gynecol. 2009;114(6):1434-8.
28. Teal SB, Romer SE, Goldthwaite LM, Peters MG, Kaplan DW, Sheeder J. Insertion characteristics of intrauterine devices in adolescents and young women: success, ancillary measures, and complications. Am J Obstet Gynecol. 2015;213(4):515. e1-5.
29. WHO. Medical Eligibility Criteria for Contraceptive Use: A WHO Family Planning Cornerstone. 4th edition. Geneva: WHO; 2010.
30. Stanford JB, Mikolajczyk RT. Mechanisms of action of intrauterine devices: update and estimation of postfertilization effects. Am J Obstet Gynecol. 2002;187(6):1699-708.
31. Ott MA, Sucato GS, Committee on Adolescence. Contraception for adolescents. Pediatrics. 2014;134(4):e1257-81.
32. Steiner MJ, Kwok C, Stanback J, Byamugisha JK, Chipato T, Magwali T, et al. Injectable contraception: what should the longest interval be for reinjections? Contraception. 2008;77(6):410-4.
33. Mulders TM, Dieben TO. Use of the novel combined contraceptive vaginal ring NuvaRing for ovulation inhibition. Fertil Steril. 2001;75(5):865-70.
34. Barreiros FA, Guazzelli CA, Barbosa R, de Assis F, de Araujo FF. Extended regimens of the contraceptive vaginal ring: evaluation of clinical aspects. Contraception. 2010;81(3): 223-5.
35. Miller L, Verhoeven CH, Hout J. Extended regimens of the contraceptive vaginal ring: a randomized trial. Obstet Gynecol. 2005;106(3):473-82.
36. Barreiros FA, Guazzelli CA, de Araujo FF, Barbosa R. Bleeding patterns of women using extended regimens of the contraceptive vaginal ring. Contraception. 2007;75(3): 204-8.
37. Guazzelli CA, Barreiros FA, Barbosa R, de Araujo FF, Moron AF. Extended regimens of the vaginal contraceptive ring: cycle control. Contraception. 2009;80(5):430-5.
38. Barreiros FA, Guazzelli CA, Barbosa R, Torloni MR, Barbieri M, Araujo FF. Extended regimens of the combined contraceptive vaginal ring containing etonogestrel and ethinyl estradiol: effects on lipid metabolism. Contraception. 2011;84(2):155-9.

39. Zacur HA, Hedon B, Mansour D, Shangold GA, Fisher AC, Creasy GW. Integrated summary of ortho Evra/Evra contraceptive patch adhesion in varied climates and conditions. Fertil Steril. 2002;77(2 Suppl 2):S32-5.
40. Kapp N, Abitbol JL, Mathe H, Scherrer B, Guillard H, Gainer E, et al. Effect of body weight and BMI on the efficacy of levonorgestrel emergency contraception. Contraception. 2015;91(2):97-104.
41. Levonorgestrel and ulipristal remain suitable emergency contraceptives for all women, regardless of bodyweight. European Medicines Agency; 2014
42. Salcedo J, Rodriguez MI, Curtis KM, Kapp N. When can a woman resume or initiate contraception after taking emergency contraceptive pills? A systematic review. Contraception. 2013;87(5):602-4.
43. Practice Bulletin No. 152: Emergency Contraception. Obstet Gynecol. 2015;126(3):e1-11.
44. Ulipristal acetate. US FDA approved product information. National Library of Medicine.
45. Clinical Effectiveness Unit. Combined hormonal contraception. London (UK): Faculty of Sexual and Reproductive Healthcare; 2011.

CHAPTER

Modern Assessment of Early Pregnancy

28

Tamara Illescas, Asim Kurjak

INTRODUCTION

The use of ultrasound (US) for the evaluation of early pregnancy is very common in the context of assisted reproduction techniques; the need to confirm the success or failure of an assisted reproduction therapy and to follow-up the evolution of the pregnancy in the first days of gestation leads to certain particularities of these early sonographic scans.

Early pregnancy is a period of uncertainty, especially during the first three postconceptional weeks, because the size of the structures will not be within the range for ultrasound evaluation.

The early pregnancy US examination must be performed by adequately trained and accredited professionals since a profound knowledge of embryology and pregnancy development features is mandatory to get to a safe interpretation of the US findings.

The main indications for an early pregnancy ultrasound scan are:[1,2]

- *To evaluate location and viability of the pregnancy:* Therapeutic decisions must be never taken until we are not certain of these two facts, as long as the mother remains clinically stable. This means that sometimes the only option to reach a definitive diagnosis is watchful waiting and follow-up scans in order to distinguish definitive findings from the uncertain ones that will require further evaluation.
- *To ascertain the number of embryos,* the number of placentas (chorionicity) and the number of sacs (amnionicity).
- *Early assessment of symptomatic pregnant women,* presenting with vaginal bleeding and/or abdominal pain, to rule out first trimester complications such as miscarriage, ectopic pregnancy, or trophoblastic disease.

In the early first trimester, the use of transvaginal (TV) ultrasound probes is crucial, since the structures to be studied are tiny and may be beyond the resolution limits of transabdominal (TA) probes. Usually, the combined use of both probes can be helpful to first achieve a good survey of the pelvic anatomy and then to proceed into the detailed study of smaller structures.[3]

- Transabdominal curvilinear transducer (4–7 MHz probe) to obtain a global view of the pelvis and exclude any pelvic pathology (fibroids, ovarian cysts, suspicion of ectopic pregnancy).
- Transvaginal curvilinear high-frequency transducer (9–12 MHz probe): Closer proximity of the transducer to the structures results in a better display of the pelvic anatomy.

Determination of β-hCG maternal serum levels is an important complementary diagnostic tool for the evaluation of early pregnancy and the detection of pathological situations.

EARLY PREGNANCY FEATURES

The *decidual reaction* is the first manifestation of an early pregnancy, resulting of increased hormonal serum levels and at this early stage it will be present regardless of the location of the gestational sac: it consists of a thickened echogenic and homogeneous endometrium of ≈15 mm which sonographically presents with posterior acoustic enhancement.

The *gestational sac* is expected to be visualized by TV ultrasound at 4.5–5 weeks gestation (serum β-hCG level >1,500 mUI/mL), as an anechoic image of 1–2 mm eccentrically placed in one of the endometrial leafs and usually in the upper half of the uterine cavity. It is surrounded by an echogenic rim corresponding to the *trophoblast reaction*. From 25 to 28 postconceptional days a "double-ring" image can be identified: the inner ring corresponds to the decidua capsularis, the chorionic villi and the chorion itself; the outer ring corresponds to the decidua parietalis. There is a narrow anechoic band between the two rings, corresponding to the uterine cavity which is not yet obliterated[4] (Fig. 28.1).

The *yolk sac* is the first structure to be identified within the gestational sac and its visualization confirms

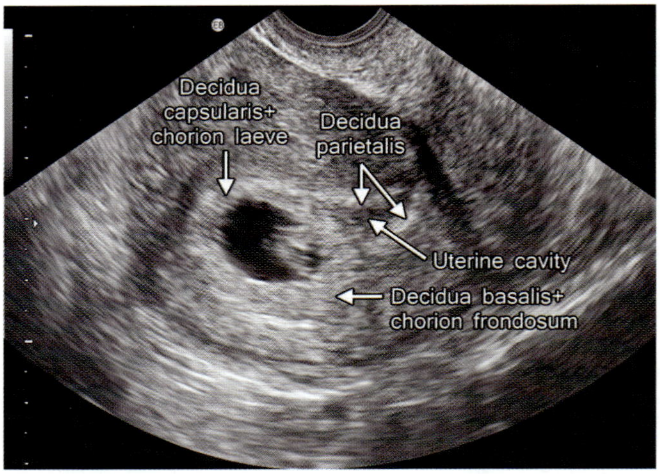

Fig. 28.1: Seven-week-pregnancy image to illustrate the different decidual and chorionic layers: The characteristic double ring is interrupted in the zone where the chorionic villi join the decidua basalis to form the chorion frondosum near the yolk sac. On the opposite side, in the area of the decidua capsularis, the chorionic villi will transform into an avascular shell (chorion laeve). There is a triangular anechoic area corresponding to the uterine cavity which is not yet obliterated. The patient had a former C-section and the uterine scar on the anterior wall of the uterus casts some acoustic shadowing.
Source: Hospital Universitari Vall d'Hebron, Barcelona, Spain.

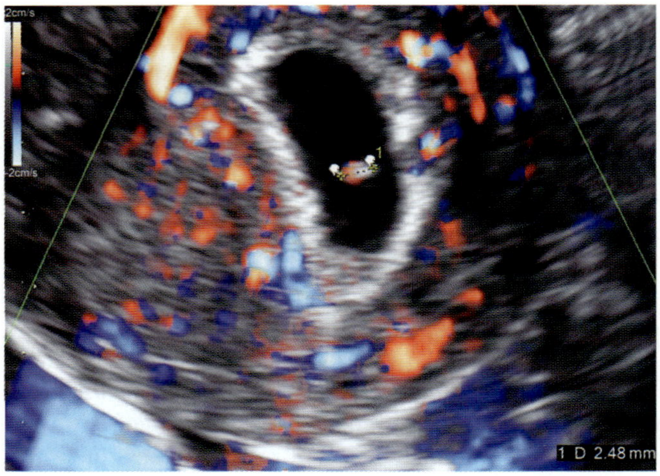

Fig. 28.2: Embryonic heart activity can be demonstrated from the third postovulation week, when the cardiac primordium appears. A significant proportion of the times the heart activity cannot be ascertained before the embryo's size is 3–4 mm; however, in this case, the cardiac activity can be demonstrated with the use of color Doppler.
Source: Delta Ultrasound Diagnostic Center in Obstetrics and Gynecology, Madrid, Spain.

an intrauterine pregnancy and rules out the possibility of an ectopic pregnancy pseudosac. It is visible from the fifth postmenstrual week, as a round structure of hyperechoic rim and sonoluscent content, located outside the amniotic cavity, in the extraembryonic coelom. Its mean diameter is 5 mm and it usually disappears between the 10th and 12th weeks[5] (Fig. 28.2).

The *embryo* heart activity may be demonstrated from the third postovulation week, when the cardiac primordium appears, but in a significant proportion of cases the heart activity cannot be ascertained before the embryo's size gets 7 mm at least (Fig. 28.2).

At 6–8 weeks of gestation the *amnion* is visualized as a thin rounded structure encircling the embryo. Mean amniotic sac diameter is approximately equal to the embryonic crown-to-rump length (CRL) in normal very early pregnancies,[6] therefore, at these stages, it is not unusual that the embryo is identified before the amnion can be visualized.

The amniotic cavity size increases with gestation and the distance between the amnion and the chorion is progressively reduced until they are completely fused by the end of the first trimester.

The number of embryos must be ascertained as soon as possible, especially in pregnancies achieved by assisted reproductive techniques. Early scanning will easily confirm embryo number and the position of each one in the case of a multiple pregnancy. The number and position of placentas should be determined, in particular, by examining the placental-membrane junction for the presence or absence of the *lambda sign* (chorionicity) (Fig. 28.3). In monochorionic twins (Fig. 28.4), the amniotic membranes should be further assessed to determine if the embryos are in separate amniotic sacs (amnionicity). The first trimester is the optimal gestation to investigate all these aspects.[2,3]

UNCERTAIN FINDINGS IN EARLY PREGNANCY: PREGNANCY OF UNKNOWN LOCATION AND PREGNANCY OF UNKNOWN VIABILITY

The following findings are uncertain and need further evaluation on a subsequent scan, thus no therapeutic decisions should be taken until a definite diagnosis has been confirmed.[7]

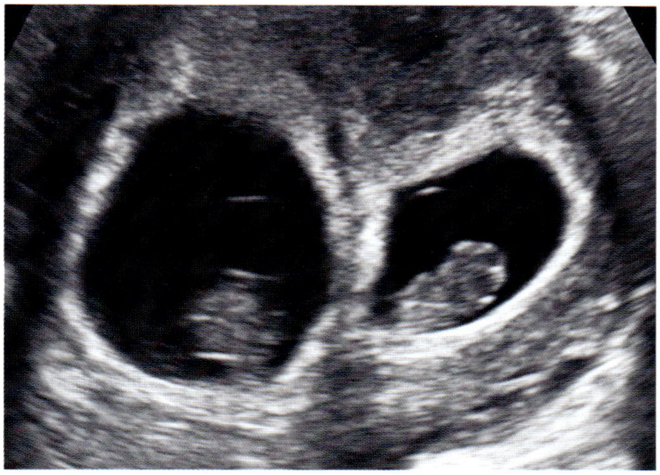

Fig. 28.3: Lambda sign in early twin pregnancy: two embryos can be identified. Their separating wall is thick, indicating that there are both amnion and chorion between the twins. This stands for a dichorionic diamniotic twin pregnancy.
Source: Hospital Universitari Vall d'Hebron, Barcelona, Spain.

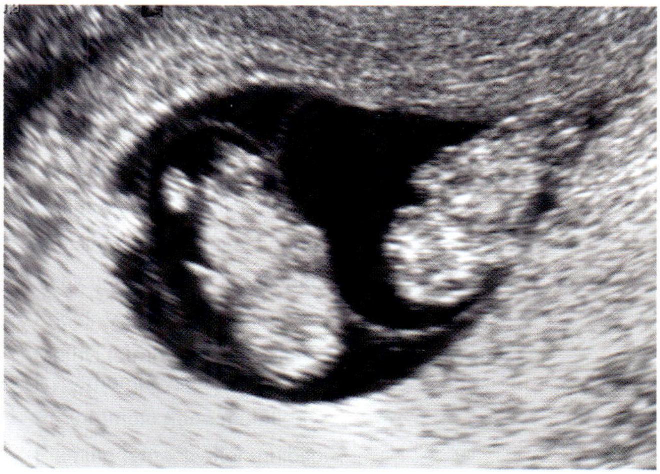

Fig. 28.4: Absent lambda sign in early twin pregnancy: The separating wall between the embryos is thin, indicating that there is only amnion between the two twins. This stands for a monochorionic diamniotic twin pregnancy.
Source: Hospital Universitari Vall d'Hebron, Barcelona, Spain.

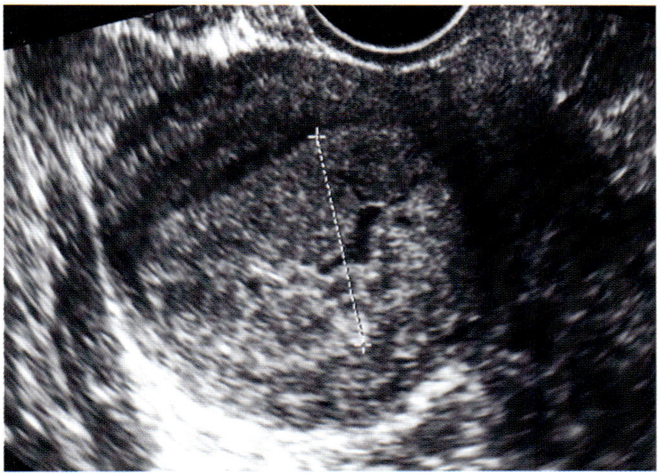

Fig. 28.5: Pregnancy of unknown location, There is a thickened echogenic endometrium, corresponding to the decidual reaction that will manifest, under the hormonal influence, regardless of the location of the gestational sac thus the first days after a positive pregnancy test are uncertain and sonographically correspond to a PUL. The gestational sac is not visible yet, but there is a small amount of fluid between the two layers of thickened endometrium: This is the classical image of a pseudosac that sometimes may be difficult to distinguish from a true gestational sac.
Source: Hospital Universitari Vall d'Hebron, Barcelona, Spain.

Pregnancy of Unknown Location (PUL)

This is a transient state of early pregnancy when no definite image of an intrauterine pregnancy can be identified by TV ultrasound and the adnexa look normal, overall conforming a normal pelvic US scan. During the first days after a positive pregnancy test the only sonographic finding will be the *decidual reaction*[5] (Fig. 28.5). In this situation, the three main diagnostic possibilities include:

- Intrauterine pregnancy
- Ectopic pregnancy
- Pregnancy failure

In this situation, a single determination of β-hCG maternal serum level does not allow reliable differentiation among the three possibilities, thus close surveillance with follow-up US scans and repeated determination of β-hCG maternal serum levels is indicated.

Intrauterine Pregnancy of Unknown Viability

This term can apply to either normal situations before the embryonic cardiac activity is detectable or cases of pregnancy failure. The findings may include[8] the following:

- an empty intrauterine gestational sac less than 25 mm,
- a gestational sac with a yolk sac but no embryo (Fig. 28.6), and
- a gestational sac with a yolk sac and an embryo with a CRL less than 7 mm and no sonographic evidence of cardiac activity (Fig. 28.7).

Monitoring the serum level of β-hCG can be useful as a complement for diagnosis and follow-up of a PUL. Once

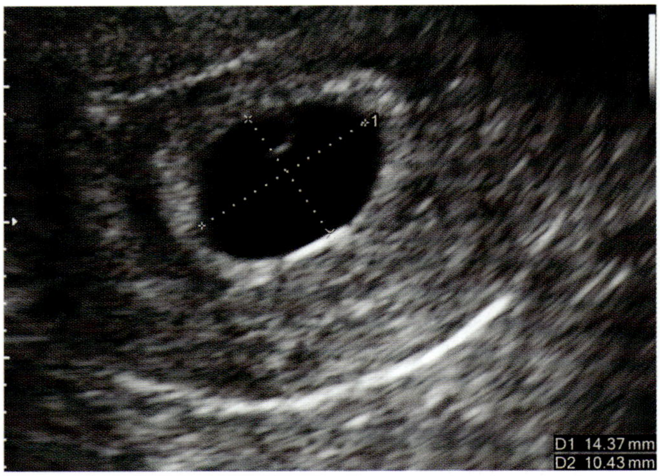

Fig. 28.6: Intrauterine pregnancy of unknown viability. There is a gestational sac with a yolk sac but no embryo can be identified yet. Monitoring and follow-up with a new scan a few days later is necessary to get to a definitive diagnosis.
Source: Hospital Universitari Vall d'Hebron, Barcelona, Spain.

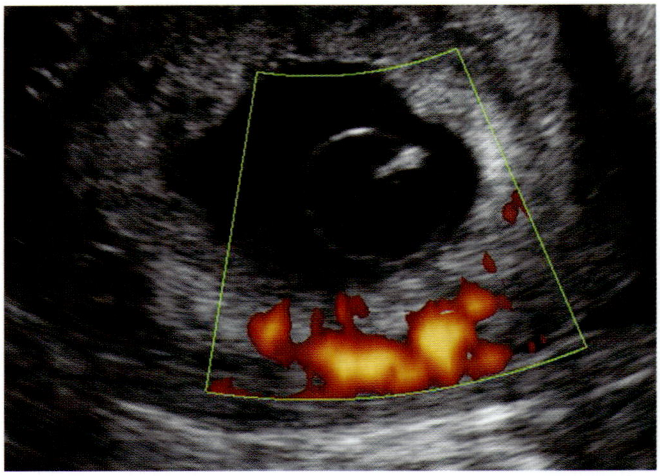

Fig. 28.7: Intrauterine pregnancy of unknown viability. There is a gestational sac with a yolk sac and an embryo with a CRL = 4.5 mm, not displaying cardiac activity. There are certain signs indicating a poor prognosis: the CRL is smaller than expected for the LMP and the gestational sac shape is irregular.
Source: Delta Ultrasound Diagnostic Center in Obstetrics and Gynecology, Madrid, Spain.

the pregnancy has been located by ultrasound, subsequent determination of maternal serum level of β-hCG is no longer necessary.

With serum β-hCG levels below 1,000 mUI/mL, the pregnancy is not supposedly amenable to US visualization; when the levels are over 1,500 mUI/mL, intrauterine pregnancies can be ascertained by TV US in more than 90% of cases. The yolk sac should be observed inside the gestational sac with a β-hCG level of 7,000–10,000 mUI/mL. An embryo with positive heart activity should be seen when the β-hCG level is over 10,800 mUI/mL.[5] These levels must not be considered absolutely discriminatory, thus no definite diagnosis must be made on its basis: even though the likelihood of an ectopic pregnancy is very increased if we have an empty uterus and a β-hCG level higher than 3,000 mUI/mL, there is still a 0.5% likelihood of a viable IUP in this case.[7,8]

ABNORMAL EARLY PREGNANCY

Before 11 weeks of gestation, a routine scan should not usually be offered if the patient remains asymptomatic,[1] the earlier the gestation the higher the likelihood for uncertain findings, which would increase the anxiety of the patient, the risk for iatrogenic interventions and the cost of repeated interventions.

However, in cases of vaginal bleeding or abdominal pain, an US scan must be performed to rule out the most frequent complications of pregnancy in the early first trimester.[1,7]

Ectopic Pregnancy

In cases when the decidual reaction is present but no gestational sac is visualized inside the uterine cavity by TV ultrasound, an ectopic pregnancy must be suspected, especially when the maternal serum β-hCG levels are more than 1,500 mUI/mL and the patient presents with vaginal bleeding and/or abdominal pain.[8]

Sometimes an indeterminate intrauterine fluid collection can be visualized. The image of a pseudosac may be difficult to distinguish from a true gestational sac, although the gestational sac is rounder, it is eccentric with respect to the uterine cavity midline and it shows the trophoblastic echogenic enhancement ("double-ring" sign). The pseudosac usually consists of a small amount of blood trapped between the two layers of thickened endometrium; therefore, it usually takes the shape of a spindle. Color Doppler will show either absent or very low velocity blood flow with moderate resistance index (whereas an IUP shows high velocity and low resistance flow around the gestational sac).[6]

The adnexa must be carefully scanned in search for any suspicious signs of an ectopic pregnancy. If no diagnostic image can be ascertained in the US scan, then monitoring with serial determinations of maternal serum

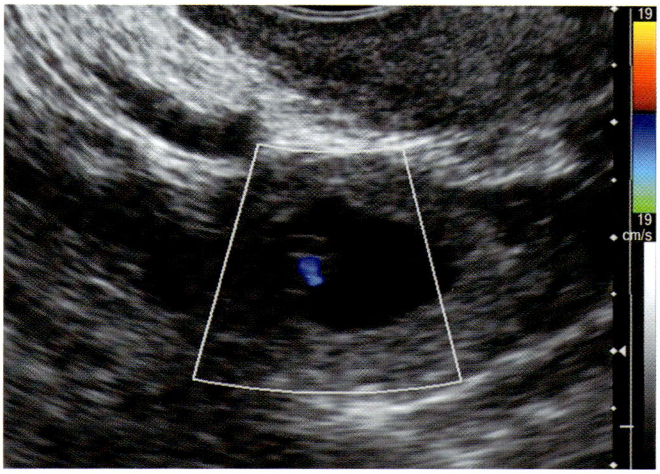

Fig. 28.8: Ectopic pregnancy. There is an extrauterine gestational sac with an embryo inside and the heart activity is visible with color Doppler.
Source: Hospital Universitari Vall d'Hebron, Barcelona, Spain.

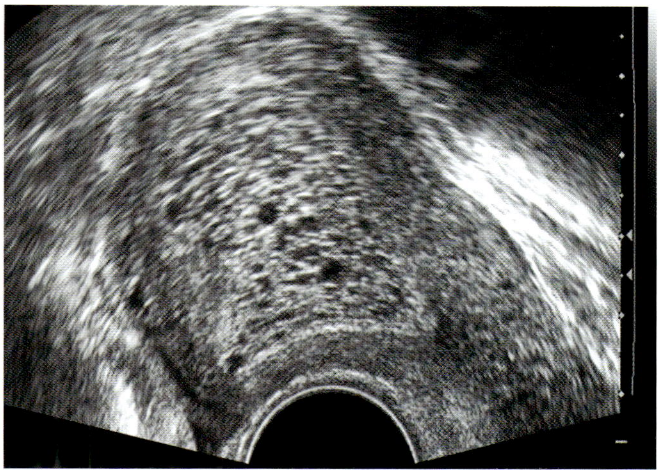

Fig. 28.9: Molar pregnancy. Classical ultrasound "snowstorm" or "honeycomb" pattern.
Source: Hospital Universitari Vall d'Hebron, Barcelona, Spain.

β-hCG levels and US examinations may be of help for the confirmation.

In recent years, the treatment options for ectopic pregnancy have evolved from surgery to medical treatment with methotrexate in selected cases. However, it is of paramount importance to remember that, as long as there is any possibility of an IUP, methotrexate must be never administered to the patient[7] (Fig. 28.8).

Trophoblastic Disease or Molar Pregnancy

In the first weeks of pregnancy, the implantation of the embryo will determine the site of the uterus where the placenta will be located. Usually the placental echo-structure is homogeneous and hypoechoic. In the first trimester of pregnancy, it is possible to notice anechoic cystic areas within the placenta, which would raise the suspicion for a partial or total molar pregnancy. The classical ultrasound features of a total molar pregnancy are the display of vesicles ("snowstorm" or "honey comb" pattern) and the presence of theca-lutein ovarian cysts[9] (Fig. 28.9). The uterus is enlarged and the β-hCG serum levels are very increased and not correlating with gestational age.

EARLY PREGNANCY FAILURE—MISCARRIAGE

Miscarriage, also called spontaneous abortion, is the loss of the products of conception, usually during the first half of the pregnancy. This is a frequent event in human pregnancies. The rate of miscarriage can be up to 30–40% for pregnancies confirmed biochemically but not yet visible by US (preclinical or biochemical miscarriage); once the pregnancy can be ascertained by US the rate of miscarriage decreases to 10–15%; after confirming the presence of a live embryo, the possibility of a miscarriage is only 3–4%.[5]

The main causes for first trimester miscarriage, accounting for at least 80–90% of the cases, are aneuploidies and structural anomalies. After the 10th week of gestation, the predominant factors are maternal or environmental. Miscarriage is considered as a natural selection process that would spontaneously clear 95% of morphological and genetic errors.[7]

There are different clinical situations corresponding to different types of miscarriage.[5]

Vaginal bleeding associated to mild hypogastric pain appears in up to 25% of pregnancies. Some of these episodes would actually correspond to implantation hemorrhage, but these cases should be always regarded and followed up as *threatened miscarriage* episodes. Most of these pregnancies will go on if we can ascertain the embryonic cardiac activity by US. The uterine cervix does not appear dilated to physical examination.

On the contrary, if we find a dilated cervix through which part of the products of conception have been expelled, then we have an *incomplete miscarriage*. The ultrasound scan will show a heterogeneous uterine content

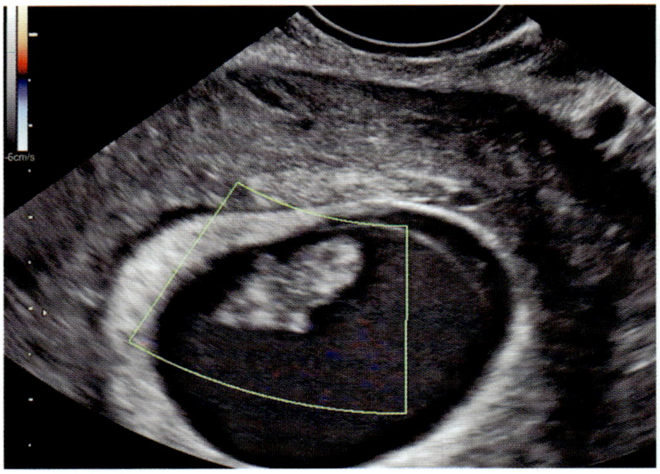

Fig. 28.10: Missed abortion. The CRL is 12 mm, projecting to a gestational age of 7 weeks 3 days; no cardiac activity can be demonstrated with color Doppler.
Source: Delta Ultrasound Diagnostic Center in Obstetrics and Gynecology, Madrid, Spain.

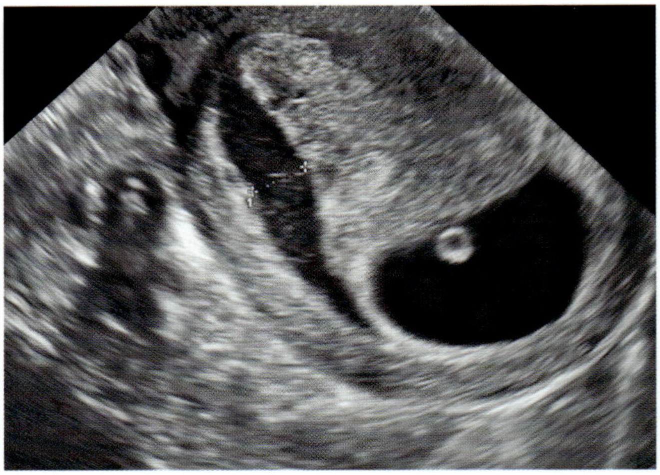

Fig. 28.11: Crescent-shaped hematoma in an early pregnancy.
Source: Delta Ultrasound Diagnostic Center in Obstetrics and Gynecology, Madrid, Spain.

more than 15 mm thick. The *miscarriage* will be *complete* if all the products of conception have been expelled from the body; the cervix is not dilated anymore, the decidua thickness is less than 15 mm and the pain and the bleeding progressively disappear.

Sometimes the pregnancy is no longer developing but there are not any clinical manifestations yet. If there is a gestational sac more than or equal to 25 mm diameter, with no embryo inside, then the diagnosis is a *blighted ovum* (*anembryonic pregnancy*). When the ultrasound shows an embryo without cardiac activity we have a *missed abortion* (Fig. 28.10). In this context, if we see the amnion or the yolk sac inside the gestational sac, even if we can no longer see the embryo, we should rule out the possibility of a blighted ovum because these structures need the presence of an embryo to develop.

PREDICTION AND DIAGNOSIS OF MISCARRIAGE

The anamnesis and the physical examination are mandatory to get to the diagnosis of a miscarriage. Sometimes the findings would be evident enough to ascertain the diagnosis (significant vaginal bleeding, dilated cervix, products of conception expelled through the vagina). Most of the times, though, an US examination is needed for confirmation; furthermore, repeat US examination is often required, especially in very early pregnancies. Before starting the US scan, we should obtain some information from the patient's background, such as age, parity, mode of conception, previous use and type of contraception, any gynecological diseases and other medical conditions.[7] We also need certain information for the right estimation of the gestational age:[5]

- Last menstrual period (LMP): It should be correlated to the sonographically estimated date of delivery (by measuring the CRL if the embryo is visible).
- Duration and regularity of the menstrual periods.
- Date of the first positive pregnancy test.

In cases where the US findings are not definitive and the gestational age cannot be confidently ascertained, it is always preferable to rescan the patient 1 week later to confirm the diagnosis.

Some clinical factors are associated to a poor prognosis for the pregnancy:[5]

- Maternal age more than 35 years.
- β-hCG plasma levels not properly increasing.
- History of recurrent miscarriage.
- Uterine malformations or fibroids, especially if multiple or submucous.
- Intrauterine hematomas: they consist of a collection of blood between the uterine wall and the gestational sac, either asymptomatic or associated to vaginal bleeding. They are a quite common finding during the first trimester scans (Fig. 28.11). The main prognostic factor is location, the retroplacental collections being the

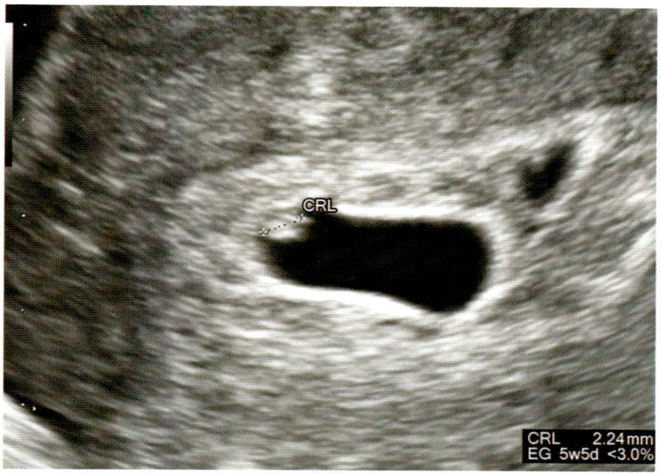

Fig. 28.12: Early pregnancy with signs for poor prognosis. The CRL is smaller than expected and the gestational sac is slightly irregular. To the right of the picture there is a smaller sac image, probably corresponding to a blighted twin.
Source: Delta Ultrasound Diagnostic Center in Obstetrics and Gynecology, Madrid, Spain.

worst due to the risk of placental detachment.[6,10] A close sonographic and clinical (amount of vaginal bleeding) follow-up is needed. Intrauterine hematomas must be differentiated from a nonevolving second gestational sac (blighted twin): the hematomas are usually crescent-shaped whereas a gestational sac tends to be round and appears as an echogenic trophoblast ring (Fig. 28.12).

Diagnostic Confirmation of Early Pregnancy Loss: Ultrasound Criteria

The US findings that allow definitive diagnostic confirmation of a pregnancy loss are described below:[5,11]

1. Absent cardiac activity in an embryo with a CRL more than or equal to 7 mm: The embryonic cardiac activity is present several days before we can actually ascertain it by US. The previous reported cutoff of more than or equal to 5 mm has been proven unsafe thus more recent publications[8,11] recommend to reschedule the patient for a new scan 7 days later in cases with a CRL less than 7 mm and no evidence of cardiac activity, as long as the clinical conditions are stable[7] (Fig. 28.10).
2. Subsequent US scans with no significant changes in the sac's size or embryonic development:[8,11]
   - Persistent absent embryonic cardiac activity on two US scans, 7 days apart.
   - Absence of an embryo with heart activity 10 days after the initial scan showed a gestational sac more than or equal to 12 mm or a gestational sac with a yolk sac inside.
   - Absence of an embryo with heart activity and no significant growth of the gestational sac 14 days after the initial scan showed a gestational sac less than 12 mm or a gestational sac without a yolk sac inside.
3. Anembryonic pregnancy (blighted ovum): There is a gestational sac of more than or equal to 25 mm with no embryo inside.

These cutoffs are general recommendations to apply according to the examination conditions, in case the operator's expertise or the equipment resolution are suboptimal, the patient should be rescheduled for a follow-up scan some days later in order to confirm or rule out the diagnosis.

Predictors for Early Pregnancy Loss: Ultrasound High-risk Indicators

There are some ultrasound findings in the first trimester that, although not diagnostic, are strongly predictive of poor pregnancy outcomes. These findings work as markers for a high risk of miscarriage, but they are not the cause of it (Table 28.1). They usually appear some days before the pregnancy stops evolving, but the definitive confirmation of a missed abortion requires any of the diagnostic criteria listed above.[7]

1. *Trophoblast:* Findings such as a too thin or too thick trophoblast with an abnormal sonographic appearance or multiple small vesicles or a poor vascularization pattern with color Doppler are signs of a bad prognosis.
2. *Gestational sac:*
   - Abnormal size (less than expected for gestational age), growth, shape or implantation site within the uterine cavity are predictors for bad outcomes in early pregnancy.
   - *Empty amnion or "two-bubble" sign:* The combination of the amnion with the yolk sac, identified as two round adjacent structures, with no image corresponding to the embryo, is abnormal and the suspicion of a missed abortion must be raised, especially when the gestational sac diameter is more than 16 mm[12,13] (Fig. 28.13).
3. *Yolk sac:* Abnormalities of the yolk sac have been attributed some predictive value for adverse outcomes in early pregnancy[6,14] (Table 28.1).

Table 28.1: Risk ultrasound indicators for early pregnancy loss. These findings work as markers for a high risk of miscarriage, but they are not the cause of it. The best predictive features are indicated in bold.

Trophoblast	Thickness: Discrepancies >3 mm
	Anomalous sonographic appearance, with multiple small vesicles
	Poor trophoblastic vascularization (scarce signal with color Doppler)
Gestational sac	**Abnormal size (less than expected for gestational age)**
	Early oligohydramnios: Difference between the CRL and the mean sac diameter less than 5 mm
	Sac not growing in subsequent scans
	"Two-bubble" sign or "empty amnion"
	Irregular shape
	Low-set gestational sac
	Absent double-ring sign
	Too thin decidual reaction
Yolk sac	Nonvisible yolk sac
	Too large or too small yolk sac
	Irregular shape
	Calcification of the yolk sac
	Double yolk sac in a singleton pregnancy
Embryo	**CRL smaller than expected for gestational age** (especially if >1 week)
	Slow or absent embryonic movements
	Bradycardia (<80–90 bpm below the 7th week and <100 bpm beyond the 7th week) **or arrhythmia**

4. Embryo:
   - *Crown to rump length smaller than expected for gestational age:* The CRL is measured in a midsagittal section from the top of the head (crown) to the end of the rump of the embryo by TV ultrasound.[3] When the difference between the observed and the expected CRL is more than 1 week there is a threefold increase in the risk for miscarriage,[15] especially in women with regular menstrual periods (Fig. 28.7).
   - *Slow or absent embryonic movements,* especially after the eighth week.
   - *Low embryonic heart rate* (<80–90 bpm below the seventh week and <100 bpm from the seventh week on) or *arrhythmia* are usually ominous signs with a high risk of miscarriage, but only the absence of the heart rate permits to ascertain the diagnosis of a pregnancy failure.[16]

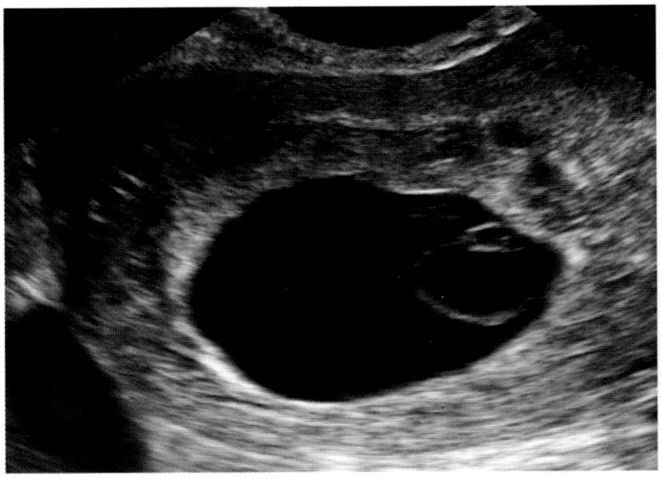

Fig. 28.13: "Two-bubble" sign or "empty amnion". The combination of the amnion with the yolk sac, identified as two round adjacent structures, with no image corresponding to the embryo, is abnormal. The suspicion of a missed abortion must be raised especially when the gestational sac diameter is more than 16 mm. *Source:* Obtained at Delta Ultrasound Diagnostic Center in Obstetrics and Gynecology, Madrid, Spain.

CONCLUSION: PRACTICAL CONSIDERATIONS

Transvaginal ultrasound and determination of maternal serum β-hCG levels are the two main tools for evaluation of early pregnancy.[8] The diagnosis of early pregnancy loss must be based only on diagnostic features since, after this point, irreversible therapeutic decisions are to be made.

If the findings are not definitive the patient must be reevaluated, as long as she is clinically stable, until a definitive diagnosis is reached.

The possible findings in an early pregnancy ultrasound scan are summarized below:[5,8,11]

1. *Abnormal early pregnancy:* The relevant therapeutic actions can be initiated at this point.
   - *Ectopic pregnancy:* The gestational sac is outside the uterus (Fig. 28.8).
   - *Trophoblast disease:* β-hCG serum levels increased high; ultrasound "snowstorm" or "honey comb" pattern and theca-lutein ovarian cysts.[9]
   - *Miscarriage:* Empty gestational sac more than or equal to 25 mm, absent cardiac activity in an embryo more than or equal to 7 mm.
2. *Uncertain findings:* The patient should be rescheduled for surveillance and followed up to get to a definite diagnosis. Sometimes serial determination of

serum β-hCG levels can provide additional useful information.

- *Pregnancy of unknown location:* Only the decidual reaction is present and the gestational sac cannot be ascertained yet.
- *Intrauterine pregnancy of unknown viability:*
  i. An empty intrauterine gestational sac less than 25 mm is visible.
  ii. Only the gestational sac and the yolk sac are visible.
  iii. There is an embryo less than 7 mm without evidence of cardiac activity.

3. *Normal early pregnancy:* There is a gestational sac and the yolk sac is visible; there is an embryo with present cardiac activity. The patient would be scheduled for the routine follow-up according to the local protocols.

REFERENCES

1. Salomon LJ, Alfirevic Z, Bilardo CM, Chalouhi GE, Ghi T, Kagan KO, et al. ISUOG Practice Guidelines: performance of first-trimester fetal ultrasound scan. Ultrasound Obstet Gynecol. 2013;41(1):102-13.
2. Illescas T. Rational use of ultrasound in normal and abnormal early pregnancy. DSJUOG. 2015;9(2):205-10.
3. Illescas T. 11 to 14 weeks' scan. In: Donald School Textbook of Power Point Presentations on Advanced Ultrasound in Obstetrics and Gynecology, 1st edition. New Delhi: Jaypee Brothers Medical Publishers; 2015.
4. Sadler TW. Langman's Medical Embryology, 12th edition. Lippincott Williams and Wilkins. Wolters Kluwer Health; 2012.
5. Illescas Molina T, Martínez Ten P, Bajo Arenas JM. Miscarriage and threatened miscarriage. In: Ecografía Obstétrica. Madrid: SEGO; 2011.
6. Ulrich H, Asim K, Giovanni M. Normal and abnormal early pregnancy. In: Donald School Textbook of Ultrasound in Obstetrics and Gynecology, 3rd edition. New Delhi: Jaypee Brothers Medical Publishers; 2011.
7. Illescas T, Sepulveda W. Normal and abnormal early pregnancy. In: Donald School Textbook of Ultrasound in Obstetrics and Gynecology, 4th edition. New Delhi: Jaypee Brothers Medical Publishers; 2017.
8. Rodgers SK, Chang C, DeBardeleben JT, Horrow MM. Normal and abnormal US findings in early first-trimester pregnancy: review of the society of radiologists in ultrasound 2012 consensus panel recommendations. Radiographics. 2015;35(7):2135-48.
9. Stevens FT, Katzorke N, Tempfer C, Kreimer U, Bizjak GI, Fleisch MC, et al. Gestational trophoblastic disorders: an update in 2015. Geburtshilfe Frauenheilkd. 2015;75(10): 1043-50.
10. Kurjak A, Schulman H, Zudenigo D, Kupesic S, Kos M, Goldenberg M. Subchorionic hematomas in early pregnancy: clinical outcome and blood flow patterns. J Matern Fetal Med. 1996;5:41-4.
11. Preisler J, Kopeika J, Ismail L, Vathanan V, Farren J, Abdallah Y, et al. Defining safe criteria to diagnose miscarriage: prospective observational multicentre study. BMJ. 2015;351:h4579.
12. McKenna KM, Feldstein VA, Goldstein RB, Filly RA. The empty amnion: a sign of early pregnancy failure. J Ultrasound Med. 1995;14:117-21.
13. Yegul NT, Filly RA. Further observations on the empty "amnion sign". J Clin Ultrasound. 2010;38:113-7.
14. Varelas, FK, Prapas, NM, Liang RI, Prapas IM, Makedos GA. Yolk sac size and embryonic heart rate as prognostic factors of first trimester pregnancy outcome. Eur J Obstet Gynecol Reprod Biol. 2008;138:10-3.
15. Koornstra G, Exalto N. Echography in the first pregnancy trimester has prognostic value. Ned Tijdschr Geneeskd. 1991;135:2231-5.
16. Doubilet PM, Benson CB, Chow JS. Long-term prognosis of pregnancies complicated by slow embryonic heart rates in the early first trimester. J Ultrasound Med. 1999;18:537-41.

Index

Page numbers followed by *f* refer to figure, *fc* refer to flowchart, and *t* refer to table.

P

T